CATHETER BASED DEVICES

FOR THE TREATMENT OF NON-CORONARY CARDIOVASCULAR DISEASE IN ADULTS AND CHILDREN

CATHETER BASED DEVICES

FOR THE TREATMENT OF NON-CORONARY CARDIOVASCULAR DISEASE IN ADULTS AND CHILDREN

Editors

P. SYAMASUNDAR RAO, MD

Professor of Pediatrics, Medicine, and Cardiology
Department of Pediatrics
University of Texas-Houston Medical School
Director, Division of Pediatric Cardiology
Memorial Hermann Children's Hospital
Houston, Texas

MORTON J. KERN, MD

Professor of Medicine
Division of Cardiology
Saint Louis University
Director, JG Mudd Cardiac Catheterization Laboratory
Saint Louis University Hospital
Saint Louis, Missouri

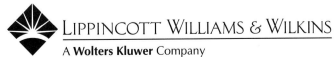

LIPPINCOTT WILLIAMS & WILKINS
A **Wolters Kluwer** Company
Philadelphia • Baltimore • New York • London
Buenos Aires • Hong Kong • Sydney • Tokyo

Acquisitions Editor: Ruth W. Weinberg
Developmental Editor: Erin McMullan
Production Editor: Rakesh Rampertab
Manufacturing Manager: Benjamin Rivera
Cover Designer: David Levy
Compositor: Lippincott Williams & Wilkins Desktop Division
Printer: Maple Press

© 2003 by LIPPINCOTT WILLIAMS & WILKINS
530 Walnut Street
Philadelphia, PA 19106 USA
LWW.com

Printed in the USA

Library of Congress Cataloging-in-Publication Data

Catheter based devices: for the treatment of non-coronary cardiovascular disease in adults and children / editors, P. Syamasundar Rao, Morton J. Kern.
    p.; cm.
  Includes bibliographical references and index.
  ISBN 0-7817-4230-7
    1. Cardiac catheterization. 2. Heart—Surgery. I. Rao, P. Syamasundar, 1941–
II. Kern, Morton J.
    [DNLM: 1. Cardiovascular Diseases—therapy. 2. Catheters, Indwelling. 3. Heart
    Catheterization—methods. WG 141.5.C2 C363 2003]
    RD598.35.C35 C38 2003
    616.1′806—dc21
                                                    2002043086

Care has been taken to confirm the accuracy of the information presented and to describe generally accepted practices. However, the authors, editors, and publisher are not responsible for errors or omissions or for any consequences from application of the information in this book and make no warranty, expressed or implied, with respect to the currency, completeness, or accuracy of the contents of the publication. Application of this information in a particular situation remains the professional responsibility of the practitioner.

The authors, editors, and publisher have exerted every effort to ensure that drug selection and dosage set forth in this text are in accordance with current recommendations and practice at the time of publication. However, in view of ongoing research, changes in government regulations, and the constant flow of information relating to drug therapy and drug reactions, the reader is urged to check the package insert for each drug for any change in indications and dosage and for added warnings and precautions. This is particularly important when the recommended agent is a new or infrequently employed drug.

Some drugs and medical devices presented in this publication have Food and Drug Administration (FDA) clearance for limited use in restricted research settings. It is the responsibility of the health care provider to ascertain the FDA status of each drug or device planned for use in their clinical practice.

10 9 8 7 6 5 4 3 2 1

This book is dedicated to the innumerable patients and parents who graciously served as volunteer research subjects in many of the clinical trials cited in this book, and to their physicians, nurses, and cardiologists who had the courage and wisdom to encourage their patients to participate in the trials. Through their generous efforts, these individuals have helped to create a knowledge base that now forms a foundation of great value to serve generations of patients yet to come.

CONTENTS

CONTRIBUTING AUTHORS

Nadim Al-Mubarak, MD Associate Professor, Case-Western Reserve University, Director, Endovascular Therapeutics, University Hospital System of Cleveland, Cleveland, Ohio

Maja Babic, MD Internal Medicine Resident, Cardiac Clinic Babic, Belgrad, Yugoslavia

Uros U. Babic, MD Babic Cardiology Clinic, Belgrad, Yugoslavia

Anirban Banerjee, MD Associate Professor, Division of Pediatric Cardiology, Tufts University School of Medicine; Director of Pediatric Echocardiography, Division of Pediatric Cardiology, Tufts-New England Medical Center, Boston, Massachusetts

Riyaz Bashir, MD Assistant Professor of Medicine, Internal Medicine, Director of Cardiovascular Diseases, Medical College of Ohio, Toledo, Ohio

Rolf G. Bennhagen, MD Interventional Fellow, Division of Cardiology, The Hospital for Sick Children, Toronto, Ontario, Canada

Lee N. Benson, MD Professor, Department of Pediatrics, Division of Cardiology, University of Toronto School of Medicine; Director, Cardiac Catheterization Laboratories, Division of Cardiology, The Hospital for Sick Children, Toronto, Ontario, Canada

Felix Berger, MD Consultant, Department of Congenital Heart Disease, University of Zürich Children's Hospital, Zürich, Switzerland

Saad R. Bitar, MD Clinical Assistant Professor of Medicine, Department of Internal Medicine, Saint Louis University; Director, Coronary Care Unit, Department of Medicine, Division of Cardiology, Saint Louis University Hospital, Saint Louis, Missouri

Preben Bjerregaard, MD Professor, Department of Medicine, Division of Cardiology; Director, Electrophysiology and Pacemaker Service, Saint Louis University Hospital, Saint Louis, Missouri

Philipp Bonhoeffer, MD Director, Cardiac Catheterization Laboratory, Hospital for Sick Children, Great Ormond Street Hospital, London, United Kingdom

Yones Boudjemline, MD Service de Cardiologic Pédiatrique, Hôspital Necker-Enfants Malades, Paris, France

Qi-Ling Cao, MD Assitant Professor, Department of Pediatric Cardiology, University of Chicago; Director, Pediatric Echocardiography Research Laboratory, University of Chicago Children Hospital, Chicago, Illinois

John P. Cheatham, MD Professor, Department of Pediatrics, Ohio State University Medical Center; Director, Cardiac Catheterization and Interventions, The Heart Center at Columbus Children's Hospital, Columbus, Ohio

John D. Coulson, MD Pediatric Cardiology Clinic, Children's Hospital of Central California, Bakersfield, California

Gladwin S. Das, MD Associate Professor of Medicine and Pediatrics, Cardiovascular Division, University of Minnesota Medical School, Minneapolis, Minnesota

Michael D. Eisenhauer, MD Assistant Professor of Medicine, Department of Medicine, Uniformed Services Health Sciences University, Bethesda, Maryland; Chief, Cardiology Service, Department of Medicine, William Beaumont Army Medical Center, El Paso, Texas

Allen D. Everett, MD Associate Professor, Department of Pediatrics, University of Virginia, Charlottesville, Virginia

Peter Ewert, MD Department of Congenital Heart Disease, German Heart Institute, Deutsches Herzzentram Berlin, Berlin, Germany

Dieter Fassbender, MD Herz-und Diabetes-Zentrum, Badoeynhausen, Germany

Franz Freudenthal, MD Fellow, Department of Radiology, Technical University of Aachen, Pauwelsstr, Germany

T. H. Goh, MD Deputy Director of Cardiology, Royal Children's Hospital, Melbourne, Victoria, Australia

Ralph G. Grabitz, MD Associate Professor, Department of Pediatric Cardiology, University of Kiel, Kiel, Germany

Ronald G. Grifka, MD Associate Professor of Pediatrics, Baylor University School of Medicine; Director, Cardiac Catheterization Laboratory, Texas Children's Hospital, Houston, Texas

Mohamed A. Hamdan, MD Jordan University of Science and Technology, Irbid, Jordan

J. Kevin Harrison, MD Assistant Professor of Medicine, Duke University Medical Center, Durham, North Carolina

Gerd Hausdorf, MD *(Deceased)*

William E. Hellenbrand, MD Professor of Clinical Pediatrics, Department of Pediatrics, Columbia University College of Physicians and Surgeons; Director, Pediatric Cardiac Catheterization Laboratory, Children's Hospital of New York, New York, New York

Ziyad M. Hijazi, MD Professor of Pediatrics and Medicine, Department of Pediatrics, University of Chicago; Director, Pediatric Cardiology, University of Chicago Hospital, Chicago, Illinois

Keiji Igaki, PhD President, Igaki Medical Planning Company, Limited, Yomashina-ku, Kyoto, Japan

Frank F. Ing, MD Clinical Associate Professor, Department of Pediatrics, University of California; Director, Cardiac Catheterization Laboratoy, Department of Pediatric Cardiology, Children's Hospital of San Diego, San Diego, California

Sriram S. Iyer, MD Clinical Associate Professor, Department of Medicine, New York School of Medicine; Associate Chief, Endovascular Services, International Cardiology, Lenox Hill Hospital, New York, New York

K. Anitha Jayakumar, MBBS, MRCP Instructor in Pediatrics, Department of Pediatrics, Columbia University College of Physicians and Surgeons; Pediatric Cardiologist, Department of Pediatric Cardiology, Children's Hospital of New York, New York, New York

Morton J. Kern, MD Professor of Medicine, Division of Cardiology, Saint Louis University; Director, JG Mudd Cardiac Catheterization Laboratory, Saint Louis University Hospital, Saint Louis, Missouri

Terry D. King, MD Director, Pediatric Cardiology, Department of Pediatrics, St. Francis Medical Cebter, Monroe, Louisiana

Michael J. Landzberg, MD Assistant Professor, Department of Medicine, Harvard University; Director, Boston Adult Congenital Heart (BACH) Service, Department of Cardiology, Brigham and Women's Hospital and Children's Hospital, Boston, Massachusetts

Larry A. Latson, MD Chairman of Pediatric Cardiology, Medical Director of Center for Pediatric and Congenital Heart Disease, Cleveland Clinic Foundation, Cleveland, Ohio

Trong-Phi Lê, MD Consultant, Department of Pediatric Cardiology, University of Hamburg, Hamburg, Germany; Chief, Department of Pediatric Cardiology, Central Hospital links der Weser, Bremen, Germany

Andrew F. Lennox MD, FRACS Vascular Fellow, Department of Vascular Surgery, Royal Prince Alfred Hospital, Sydney, New South Wales, Australia

Audrey C. Marshall, MD Instructor in Pediatrics, Department of Pediatrics, Harvard Medical School; Assistant in Cardiology, Department of Cardiology, Children's Hospital, Boston, Massachusetts

James May MD, FACS, FRACS Bosch Professor of Surgery, Department of Vascular Surgery, University of Sydney, Sydney, New South Wales, Australia

Peter McLaughlin, MD The University Health Network, Toronto General Hospital, University of Toronto School of Medicine, Toronto, Ontario, Canada

Colin J. McMahon, MB, BCh Senior Fellow in Pediatric Cardiology, Texas Children's Hospital, Houston, Texas

Bernhard Meier, MD Professor of Cardiology, Department of Cardiology, Swiss Cardiovascular Center of Bern, University Hospital, Bern, Switzerland

John W. Moore, MD, MPH Professor, Department of Pediatrics, The David Geffen School of Medicine at UCLA; Director, Cardiac Catheterization Laboratory, Mattel Children's Hospital at UCLA, Los Angeles, California

Malte B. Neuss, MD German Heart Center Berlin, Augustenburger Platz, Berlin, Germany

Gishel New, MD, PhD Associate Professor, Department of Cardiology, Monash University; Director of Cardiology, Department of Cardiology, Box Hill Hospital, Melbourne, Australia

Michael R. Nihill, MD Professor of Pediatrics, Department of Pediatrics, Baylor College of Medicine; Attending Cardiologist, Department of Cardiology, Texas Children's Hospital, Houston, Texas

Martin P. O'Laughlin, MD Associate Professor of Pediatrics, Duke University Medical Center, Durham, North Carolina

Carl. Y. Owada, MD Director, Cardiac Catheterization Laboratory, Department of Cardiology and Cardiothoracic Surgery, Children's Hospital of Central California, Madera, California

Natesa G. Pandian, MD   Director, Cardiovascular Imaging and Hemodynamics Laboratory, Tufts-New England Medical Center, Boston, Massachusetts

Hitendra T. Patel, MD   Pediatric Cardiologist, Department of Cardiology, Children's Hospital Oakland, Oakland, California

Dušan Pavčnik, MD, PhD   Research Professor, Dotter Institute, Oregon Health and Science University; Joseph Rosch Chair, Dotter Interventional Institute, Portland, Oregon

Stanton B. Perry, MD   Associate Professor, Department of Pediatrics, Stanford School of Medicine, Stanford, California; Director of Pediatric Cardiac, Department of Catherization, Lucile Packard Children's Hospital, Palo Alto, California

Shakeel A. Qureshi, MBCHB, FRCP   Senior Lecturer, Department of Congenital Heart Disease, Guy's, King's and St. Thomas Medical Schools; Consultant Pediatric Cardiologist, Department of Congenital Heart Disease, Guy's Hospital, London, United Kingdom

P. Syamasundar Rao, MD   Professor of Pediatrics, Medicine, and Cardiology, Department of Pediatrics, University of Texas–Houston Medical School; Director, Division of Pediatric Cardiology, Memorial Hermann Children's Hospital, Houston, Texas

Jonathan J. Rome, MD   Associate Professor of Pediatrics, University of Pennsylvania, Director, Cardiac Catheterization Laboratory, Children's Hospital of Philadelphia, Philadelphia, Pennsylvania

Kenneth Rosenfield, MD   Director, Cardiac and Vascular Invasive Services, Cardiology Division, Massachusetts General Hospital, Boston, Masschusetts

Gary S. Roubin, MD, PhD   Clinical Professor of Medicine, New York University School of Medicine, New York University; Chief, Endovascular Services, Interventional Cardiology, Lenox Hill Hospital, New York, New York

Carlos E. Ruiz, MD, PhD   Professor of Pediatrics and Medicine, University of Illinois at Chicago; Chief, Division of Pediatric Cardiology, Division of Pediatric Cardiology, University of Illinois at Chicago Medical Center, Chicago, Illinois

Timothy A. Sanborn, MD   Professor of Medicine, Department of Medicine, Division of Cardiology, The Feinberg School of Medicine Northwestern University; Head, Division of Cardiology, Evanston Northwestern Healthcare, Evanston, Illinois

Satinder K. Sandhu, MD   Associate Professor of Pediatrics, Louisiana State University Health Sciences Center; Director, Pediatric Cardiology, Children's Hospital, New Orleans, Louisiana

Douglas J. Schneider, MD   Assistant Professor of Pediatrics, Drexel University School of Medicine, Philadelphia, Pennsylvania; Director, Cardiac Catheterization Laboratory, St. Christopher Hospital for Children, Philadelphia, Pennsylvania

Martin Schneider, MD   Assistant Professor of Pediatrics and, Division of Pediatric Cardiology, Charite University, Berlin, Germany

Rainer Schräder, MD   Professor, Markus-Krankenhaus-CCB, Frankfurt Am Main, Germany

Venerando S. Seguritan, MD   Director, Interventional Radiology, Department of Radiology, William Beaumont Army Medical Center, El Paso, Texas

Eleftherios B. Sideris, MD   Director, Athenian Institute of Pediatric Cardiology, Athens, Greece

Horst Sievert, MD   Professor of Internal Medicine and Cardiology, Cardiovascular Center Bethanien, Frankfurt, Germany

Gautam K. Singh, MD   Associate Professor, Department of Pediatrics, Saint Louis University; Echo-Laboratory Director, Division of Pediatric Cardiology, Cardinal Glennon Children's Hospital, Saint Louis, Missouri

Narayanswami Sreeram, MD   Director, Division of Cardiology, Wilhelmina Children's Hospital, University Medical Center, Utrecht, Netherlands

S. William Stavropoulos, MD   Assistant Professor, Department of Radiology, University of Pennsylvania School of Medicine, Philadelphia, Pennsylvania

Ruth H. Strasser, MD   Klinik für Kardiologie, Technishe Universität, Dresden, Germany

William B. Strong, MD   Leon Henry Charbonier Professor of Pediatrics, Chief, Section of Pediatric Cardiology, Medical College of Georgia, Augusta, Georgia

Hideo Tamai, MD   Managing Director, Department of Cardiology, Shiga Medical Center for Adults, Shiga, Japan

Takafumi Tsuji, MD   Interventional Cardiologist, Department of Cardiology, Shiga Medical Center for Adults, Moriyama, Shiga, Japan

Peter Vaessen, MD   Fellow, Department of Pediatric Cardiology, University of Achen, Achen, Germany

Peter Vale, MD   Departments of Vascular Medicine, Saint Elizabeth's Medical Center, Tuft's University School of Medicine, Boston, Massachusetts

Jiri J. Vitek, MD, PhD   Interventional Neuroradiologist, Interventional Cardiology, Lenox Hill Hospital, New York, New York

David J. Waight, MD Assistant Professor of Clinical Pediatrics, Department of Pediatrics, University of Chicago; Cardiologist, Department of Pediatrics, University of Chicago Pritzker School of Medicine, Chicago, Illinois

Geoffrey H. White, MD Associate Professor of Surgery, Department of Vascular Surgery, University of Sydney, Sydney, New South Wales, Australia

Neil Wilson, MD Consultant Pediatric Cardiologist, Royal Hospital for Sick Children, Yorkhill, Glasgow, Scotland

Stephan Windecker, MD Department of Cardiology, Swiss Cardiovascular Center of Bern, University Hospital, Bern, Switzerland

Robert N. Wood-Morris, MD Resident, Internal Medicine, Department of Medicine, William Beaumont Army Medical Center, El Paso, Texas

Sing-Chien Yap, MD Division of Cardiology, Wilhelmina Children's Hospital, University Medical Center, Utrecht, Netherlands

Evan M. Zahn, MD Director, Cardiac Catheterization Laboratory, Miami Children's Hospital, Miami, Florida

FOREWORD

In the foreword to Rao's "Transcatheter Therapy in Pediatric Cardiology," contributions of Dr. Rao and the pioneers in this exciting subspecialty were addressed. Over the ensuing decade he has continued to explore, publish and interact with the interventionalist community. He is a tireless worker. This monograph "Catheter Based Devices: for the Treatment of Non-coronary Cardiovascular Disease in Adults and Children" is coedited by Dr. Morton Kern. Drs. Rao and Kern have gathered a comprehensive and extensive international group of interventional cardiologists to address both the results of the earlier intervention techniques and devices as well as the advances over the last decade.

It would seem to the noninterventional cardiologist that each month at least one of the cardiology journals is publishing information about a new device, the application of an old device or a critique of one of the devices that the author of the article does not prefer. As a noninterventional pediatric cardiologist, I am very impressed by the abilities and accomplishments of my colleagues. The imagination required to develop the devices as well as the facileness to deploy them successfully is to be admired. As a senior member of the pediatric cardiology community I marvel at how far we have come since I performed my first Rashkind procedure in 1967. The thirty-five years that have elapsed since Rashkind and Miller published their original results have seen a quantum leap in our technical abilities. The benefits and the risks associated with the atrial septostomy have certainly stood the test of time. The development of registries to evaluate the risks and successes of the newer techniques is essential. Will we be able to say thirty-five years from now that the newer techniques have contributed to the well being of our patients? Hopefully the registries will continue to provide information on which we can base our decisions.

Are we doing what is best for our patients or are we doing some procedures for the sake of doing procedures (and cynically, being able to bill for them). Let us not lose sight of the natural history of these defects. Let us learn the natural/unnatural history of the devices and procedures. Technology and progress are mandatory. Risks must be taken. They must be justifiable.

As a digression, twenty years ago a soft systolic murmur at the upper left sternal border with an otherwise normal examination would have been considered a normal pulmonary flow murmur. Two-dimensional echocardiography with color flow demonstrated some of these individuals had tiny silent patent ductus arteriosus. The test generated more income. These patent ductus arteriosus (PDAs) were hemodynamically insignificant. There was none or virtually no known risk of bacterial endocarditis. Transcatheter closure of the PDA became available and thousands of these silent PDAs were closed because they were there. In at least one instance with which I am familiar, the PDA was so small that it had to be dilated in order to coil it. Cost? Dr. Rao addressed this issue in 1996 (*American Heart Journal* 1996;132:905–9).

Let us not become so consumed by our technical know how to lose sight of what it is we are attempting to accomplish. Let us keep an open mind as we advance our profession and the well being of our patients. Let us do no harm. This thoughtfully put together monograph will help us make the best decisions.

William B. Strong, MD
Augusta, Georgia

PREFACE

Although the seeds of interventional cardiology were planted by Rubio–Alverez and Limon–Lason in the 1950s and by Dotter, Rashkind, Portsman and their associates in the 1960s, it is not until Gruntzig applied the percutaneous transluminal balloon angioplasty technique in the 1970s that the discipline of interventional cardiology developed as a true subspecialty. Transcatheter implantable device technology largely began in the 1970s with continuing works of Portsman and his colleagues in occluding the patent ductus arteriosus, King and Rashkind and their coinvestigators in closing atrial septal defects, and Gianturco and his associates in occluding blood vessels. In the 1980s, Palmaz and coworkers extended Dotter's late 1960s concept by introducing balloon expanding metallic stents to treat stenotic vascular lesions. Further refinements of the technology continue to take place by the diligent studies by these and other investigators. The largest proliferation of device technology occurred in the last decade of twentieth century.

The purpose of this book is to bring together all the available transcatheter implantable device technology and to present the state-of-the-art of this new discipline. Since there are many other books and monographs dealing with coronary artery interventions, this book will address treatment of non-coronary cardiovascular disease in both children and adults.

We have gathered experts from around the world to contribute to this book; in the majority of chapters, we have been able to get either the inventor of the device/method or a major investigator of a particular device or method to write the chapters. The device description, indications for implantation and results of each device will be discussed, along with alternative management strategies, if any. The devices that are generally considered a "pediatric" device will include a section dealing with device application in adult subjects. The book is divided into six sections. The first section discusses transcatheter occlusion of atrial septal defects. The second section deals with closure of patent ductus arteriosus by transcatheter route. The next section describes transcatheter closure of both congenital and post-myocardial infarction ventricular septal defects and paravalvular leaks. The role of intravascular stents in the management of congenital and acquired stenotic vascular obstructive lesions in both children and adults is reviewed in section four. The fifth section deals with a number of diverse topics, including vascular embolization, device management of arrhythmias, vena caval filters to prevent pulmonary embolism, vascular closure devices, transcatheter implantation of prosthetic valves, and other miscellaneous devices. Role of echocardiography is discussed in this and other sections. We conclude in the final section.

This emerging technology will be of great interest to adult and pediatric cardiologists and interventional radiologists. Cardiovascular surgeons will find this book useful in that this technology serves to compliment their work and in some patients, a collaborative treatment plan, since both transcatheter device and surgical methodology may be the best for some patients. Cardiovascular technologists and nurses will also find this a more than suitable reference and introduction to these techniques and outcomes. Finally, this book will serve as a reference to the internist, pediatrician, and family practitioner who care for cardiovascular patients.

It is hoped that this book will answer many questions in interventional cardiology and radiology, stimulate interest in device technology and most importantly promote further research on issues related to the theme of this book, devices delivered via catheters.

P. Syamasundar Rao, MD
Morton J. Kern, MD

ACKNOWLEDGMENTS

Liberal use of case material that we encountered at the University of Wisconsin Hospitals and Clinics, Madison, Wisconsin, Saint Louis University Hospital, St. Louis, Missouri and Cardinal Glennon Children's Hospital, St. Louis, Missouri was made in several chapters of this book. We acknowledge contribution to these data made by past and present colleagues at these institutions, including Drs. Richard R. Bach, Ian C. Balfour, Adam S. Betkowski, Saad R. Bitar, Scott H. Buck, Su-chiung Chen, Paramjeet S. Chopra, David J. Ende, Andrew C. Fiore, Vinod K. Gupta, Cesar Keller, Jay M. Levey, Saadeh B. Jureidini, Gautam K. Singh and Allen D. Wilson. In addition, there were many trainees who also contributed to this clinical material. Our thanks are also due to a number of people in cardiology nursing, catheterization laboratory and echocardiography laboratory for their help in patient/parent preparation, data acquisition and data collection. These dedicated people include Pam Ameis, David Bash, James Dozier, the late Jan Ewenko, Cindy Marino, Donna Marshall, Mary Meyer, Colleen Puers, Christie Short, Pat Smith, Joyce Tackle, and Kathy Tinker.

We appreciate the efforts of each of the contributors in preparing high quality chapters. Our particular thanks go to authors who have been assigned to write on old and no longer used devices, despite their expertise with current technology.

Kay Thompson spent long hours in preparing multiple revisions of the chapters and was of great help throughout the preparation of this book. We appreciate her efforts and thank her for uncompromised cooperation. We also thank Marcellus Duffy, our computer specialist who helped us translate many a different formats that we received into a cohesive format preparatory to publication. Finally, we thank Ms. Erin McMullan, Mr. Rakesh Rampertab, and Ms. Ruth Weinberg of Lippincott Williams and Wilkins for their help, advice, and patience.

P. Syamasundar Rao, MD
Morton J. Kern, MD

CATHETER BASED DEVICES

FOR THE TREATMENT OF NON-CORONARY CARDIOVASCULAR DISEASE IN ADULTS AND CHILDREN

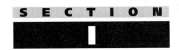

SECTION

I

DEVICE OCCLUSION OF ATRIAL SEPTAL DEFECTS

HISTORY OF ATRIAL SEPTAL OCCLUSION DEVICES

P. SYAMASUNDAR RAO

Following the description of surgical closure of atrial septal defect (ASD) in the early 1950s (1–3), it rapidly became a standard therapy of atrial defects. Surgical closure of ostium secundum ASDs is safe and effective with negligible mortality (4–6), but the morbidity associated with sternotomy/thoracotomy, cardiopulmonary bypass, and potential for postoperative complications cannot be avoided. Other disadvantages of surgical therapy are the expense associated with surgical correction, residual surgical scar, and psychologic trauma to the patients and/or the parents. Presumably because of these reasons, several groups of cardiologists embarked upon developing transcatheter methods of closure of the ASD. The studies of King (7–9), Rashkind (10–12), and their associates paved the way for the future development of transcatheter ASD device occlusion methodology. This chapter reviews the history of development of ASD closure devices.

KING AND MILL'S DEVICE

King and his associates were successful in occluding the ASD via a transcatheter-delivered occluding device. They were the first in doing so and reported their studies in the mid-1970s (7–9). This device is composed of paired, Dacron-covered stainless steel umbrellas collapsed into a capsule at the tip of a catheter (Figure 1.1). A number of sizes of the umbrella were manufactured. Stretched ASD diameter was measured by balloon sizing (13), and a device 10 mm larger than the stretched ASD diameter was selected for deployment. The device delivery catheter was inserted through the saphenous vein at the saphenofemoral venous junction by cut-down. The catheter tip was positioned into the left atrium through the ASD. The distal umbrella was extruded in the body of the left atrium, and the catheter is

withdrawn into the right atrium. Then the distal (left atrial) umbrella was fixed against the left side of the atrial septum and the proximal (right atrial) umbrella was opened in the right atrium. The umbrellas were locked to each other with a special locking mechanism. After the device was in place, the obturator wire was unscrewed and withdrawn, thus releasing the device.

King and Mills (7) initially attempted this technique in experimental animal models. ASDs were created by a punch biopsy technique in adult dogs. Successful device deployment was achieved in five of nine dogs in which the procedure was attempted. Complete closure of the ASD and endothelialization of the implanted umbrellas were observed during the follow-up. Following this experience in the dog model, the technique was extended to human subjects (8,9). Eighteen patients were taken to the catheterization laboratory and ten (56%) of these were considered suitable candidates for device closure. The device was suc-

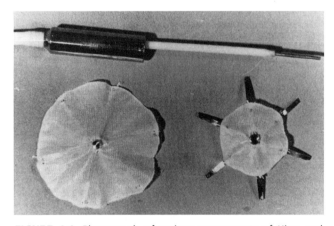

FIGURE 1.1. Photograph of various components of King and Mill's device. Dacron-covered stainless steel left atrial *(lower left)* and right atrial *(lower right)* umbrellas are shown. The device delivery catheter, the capsule into which the device components are folded, and the obturator wire are shown at the top of the figure. (From King TD, Thompson SL, Steiner C, et al. Secundum atrial septal defect: nonoperative closure during cardiac catheterization. *JAMA* 1976;235:2506–2509, with permission.)

P. Syamasundar Rao: Professor of Pediatrics, Medicine, and Cardiology, Department of Pediatrics, University of Texas–Houston Medical School; Director, Division of Pediatric Cardiology, Memorial Hermann Children's Hospital, Houston, Texas

cessfully implanted in five (50%) patients. Their ages were 17 to 75 years, with a median of 24. The stretched ASD diameter was 18 to 26 mm by balloon sizing. Ostium secundum ASDs with left-to-right shunt were present in four patients. The final patient had an atrial defect with presumed paradoxical embolism and a stroke. Symptoms improved and the heart size decreased during observed follow-up. Repeat cardiac catheterization data did not show shunts by oximetry. However, trivial shunts were observed by hydrogen curves.

Although these results are encouraging, King and his associates did not continue their use, nor did any other investigator pursue the technique. This may be related to the need for a large delivery sheath and complicated maneuvering required for implantation of the device.

RASHKIND'S DEVICES

Rashkind developed a slightly different type of ASD closure device. Rashkind's investigations appear to be parallel to those of King and Mills (14). The first Rashkind umbrella consisted of three stainless steel arms covered with medical foam (11). The central ends of the stainless steel arms are attached to miniature springs, which in turn are welded to a small central hub. The outer end of the stainless steel arm ended in a miniature "fishhook." Rashkind modified this umbrella so that there are six stainless steel arms, with the alternate arms carrying the hook (Figure 1.2). He also designed an elaborate centering mechanism, which consisted of five arms bent to produce a gentle outward curve. The umbrella delivery mechanism is built on a 6F catheter with locking tip, which interlocks with the central hub of the device. The entire system (Figure 1.3) is threaded over a

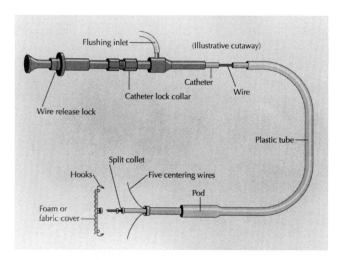

FIGURE 1.3. Detailed sketch of Rashkind's hooked atrial septal defect (ASD) device delivery system. Note the side profile of the hooked device and the pod (PD) marked red. Wire release lock, catheter lock collar, catheter, wire, plastic tube, and five centering wires are shown. (Courtesy of the late William J. Rashkind, MD.)

guide wire. Withdrawal of the guide wire after implantation of the device will unlock the mechanism, thereby disconnecting the umbrella from the delivery system. The umbrella collapsed into a pod, the centering mechanism folded and the delivery system can all be loaded into a 14 or 16F long sheath. The umbrellas were manufactured in three sizes: 25, 30, and 35 mm. An umbrella that is approximately twice the stretched size of the ASD is chosen for implantation. First, the tip of the pod containing the umbrella is advanced into the left atrium through the ASD. Then the umbrella and centering mechanism are delivered into the middle left atrium by retracting the tip of the sheath or pod. The entire system is then slowly withdrawn. The centering mechanism keeps the umbrella centered over the ASD. Further withdrawal results in embedding the hooks of the umbrella onto the left atrial side of the atrial septum (Figure 1.4). After the umbrella is fixed to the atrial septum, the umbrella delivery system is disconnected and removed. Experimental studies in closing surgically created ASDs in dogs and calves have indicated the feasibility of the method with excellent endothelialization of the umbrella components (10).

The author had the privilege of spending a month-long mini-sabbatical with Dr. William Rashkind in mid-1979, when he had the opportunity of performing ASD device closures with the hooked device, both in calf model and in patients under the direction of Dr. Rashkind. Rashkind's enthusiasm and dedication in developing transcatheter closure methodology are laudable, and the diligence with which he pursued the project is admirable. Subsequently, he obtained investigational device exemption from the FDA and began organizing multiinstitutional clinical trials in the United States in the early 1980s. This is probably the first

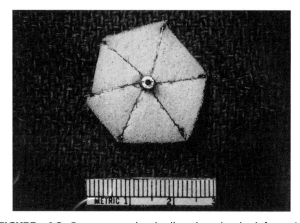

FIGURE 1.2. Foam-covered, six-rib, three-hook left atrial umbrella designed by Rashkind. The helical turns at internal end of each rib (wire) allows recoil of the umbrella from a folded position. The outer end of alternate rib ends in a hook designed to attach to the left atrial aspect of the interatrial septum. Metric ruler (centimeters marked) is shown at the bottom. (Courtesy of the late William J. Rashkind, MD.)

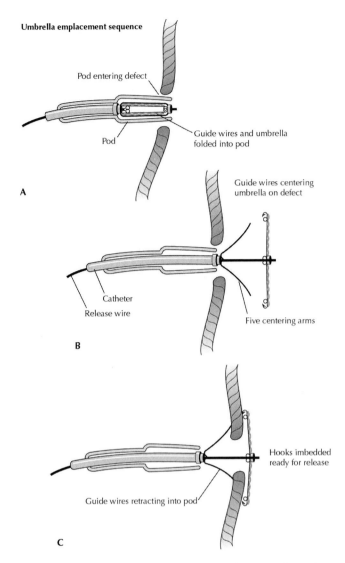

Umbrella emplacement sequence

Pod entering defect

Pod

Guide wires and umbrella folded into pod

A

Guide wires centering umbrella on defect

Catheter

Release wire

Five centering arms

B

Hooks imbedded ready for release

Guide wires retracting into pod

C

FIGURE 1.4. Sequence of hooked prosthesis implantation. (From Rashkind WJ, Tait MA, Gibson RJ, Jr. Interventional cardiac catheterization in congenital heart disease. *Int J Cardiol* 1985;7: 1–11, with permission.)

clinical trial for device implantation in pediatric cardiac practice. Unfortunately, Dr. Rashkind did not live to witness the conclusion of these trials or to see the monumental effect that his work had on the evolution of transcatheter occlusion technology.

Following experimental studies in animal models, Rashkind studied ASD closure in human subjects (11,12,14). Thirty-three patients were recruited for the clinical trial. Device implantation was not attempted in ten patients because the defect was too large ($N = 6$) to safely implant the device or too small ($N = 4$) to warrant the potential risk of device placement. In the remaining 23 patients, 14 (61%) had adequate ASD closure; in nine (39%) the results were considered unsatisfactory. The initial

six device implantations were three-rib umbrellas, and the remaining were six-rib prostheses. Urgent surgical intervention was required in some patients to address the unsatisfactory implantations, and others underwent elective surgery. However, in all subjects the ASD was closed surgically without complications and the device was removed. Clinical application in a limited number of patients by Beekman et al. (15) showed similar results.

Although good results were achieved in more than 50% of patients, a number of problems were identified: requirement of a large sheath for implantation, uncertainty of whether the tissue would bind to the entire rim of the single-disk device, and difficulty in disengaging and repositioning the device if the hooks of the umbrella accidentally engaged onto the left atrial wall or mitral valve. Therefore Rashkind modified this device into a double-disk prosthesis and successfully used it to close an ASD in a cow (12). This device is similar to Rashkind's patent ductus arteriosus occluding device (12,16), which he developed concurrently.

RASHKIND TO CLAMSHELL

Other workers subsequently used the double-umbrella Rashkind device to close ASDs (17–19). Although the results appeared good, the difficulty in delivering umbrellas on either side of the defect, the difficulty in centering the device because of the angle of the delivery catheter (18), and the inability to fold the umbrellas back against each other made it necessary to modify the device by introducing a second spring in the center of the arms (19). This device was named the *Lock clamshell occluder.*The clamshell device was utilized to occlude experimentally created ASDs in lambs. Six of the eight attempted implantations were successful. The remaining two embolized. Complete occlusion of the ASD was noted in four lambs monitored for more than 1 day. Endothelialization of the device components was demonstrated in two lambs observed for 1 and 2 months, respectively, following device implantation.

The clamshell device is composed of two opposing umbrellas made of four steel arms covered with woven Dacron material (Figure 1.5). The steel arms are hinged together in the center of the device, and the springs in the middle of the arm, as alluded to, facilitate folding back of the umbrellas against each other, thereby creating a clamshell configuration. The device is delivered through an 11F sheath, a definitive improvement compared with the sheath size required to implant King's and Rashkind's devices. Several device sizes were manufactured: 17, 23, 28, and 33 mm. Balloon-stretched diameters of the ASD were measured as in the previous device implantations. A device at least 1.6 times larger than the stretched ASD diameter was recommended for device placement. The delivery

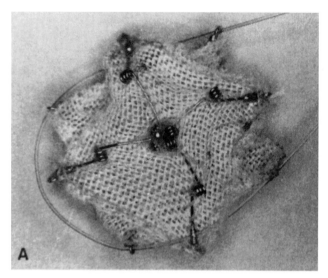
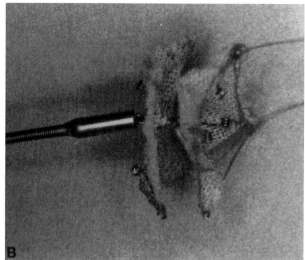

FIGURE 1.5. Photographs of clamshell device are shown on face view **(A)** and side view **(B)**. (From Hellenbrand WE, Fahey JT, McGowan FX, et al. Transesophageal echocardiographic guidance of transcatheter closure of atrial septal defect. *Am J Cardiol* 1990;66:207–213, with permission.)

catheter was advanced into the left atrium across the ASD, and its tip was positioned in the middle left atrium. The distal arms of the device were opened and the device was withdrawn against the atrial septum until the arms were seen to bend. The sheath was pulled back while keeping the device in position, with resultant opening of the proximal arms in the right atrium. After ensuring the stability of the device across the atrial septum by fluoroscopic and echographic imaging, the device was released by activating the pin-to-pin mechanism.

The preliminary clinical experience included 17 clamshell device implantations (17). This report (17) combines the results of implantation of the Rashkind double umbrella, prototype clamshell, and clamshell devices; therefore the exact clamshell results are difficult to discern. Forty patients were taken to the catheterization laboratory with intent to close. Of these, 34 (85%) had implantation of the device. With the exception of one major complication (death secondary to cerebral embolus, presumably related to dislodgment of iliac vein thrombus during placement of device delivery sheath), the procedures were successful. Embolization of the device into the descending aorta at iliac bifurcation occurred in two (6%) patients. The embolized devices were transcatheter retrieved and the patients were sent to elective closure of their ASDs. At short-term follow-up, 12 (63%) of 19 who had adequate echocardiographic study had no residual shunts.

Hellenbrand et al. (20) described their experience with this device. Device implantation was successful in ten of 11 patients. The patients were 13 months to 46 years of age. The single failure was in their youngest patient, who weighed 11 kg. The procedures were performed under gen-

eral anesthesia with endotracheal intubation and transesophageal echo-Doppler monitoring. Residual shunt was present in one (10%) patient. In another study (21), residual shunt was present in 91% immediately following device placement. The residual shunts decreased to 53% at a mean follow-up of 10 months. Actuarial analysis indicated progressive reduction of shunt with time (21). Clinical trials by these and other investigators continued (21–23). However, fractures of the arms of the device were reported in 40% to 84% of implanted devices with occasional embolization (23–25), which were of concern. Therefore further clinical trials with the device were suspended in 1991 by the investigators and the FDA. Subsequently, the device was modified, which will be reviewed later in this chapter.

BUTTONED DEVICE

Sideris et al. (26) described a buttoned device at about the time of the transformation of the Rashkind double-disk device to clamshell device. Atrial septal defects were produced in piglets. The buttoned device was successfully implanted in 17 (85%) of 20 attempts. The failures were in the first three animals and were presume to relate to inexperience of the operator and design imperfections (26). Full occlusion of the ASD and endothelialization of the device were demonstrated in all 17 successful implantations. Following preliminary clinical trials (27–29), the device was modified into second-, third- (30), and fourth-generation (31) devices; centering buttoned device (32); inverted buttoned device (33); and a centering-on-demand device (34). The device has also been successfully used to close atrial defects presumed to be responsible for paradoxical embolism and cerebrovascular accidents (35). A number of single institutional (27–29,36–40) and multiinstitutional (30,31,41–44) clinical trials were undertaken that demonstrated feasibility, safety, and effectiveness of this device. Detailed review of the device description and results will be addressed in a separate chapter.

OTHER ATTEMPTS

Pavčnik et al. (45) designed a monodisk device. The device consists of a stainless steel ring constructed with wire coil covered with two layers of nylon mesh. Three hollow pieces of braided stainless steel wires were sutured onto the right atrial side of the device. Three strands of monofilament nylon pass through, one in each of the hollow wires. The nylon thread also passes through the delivery catheter. The entire system can be loaded and the device delivered through a 9F sheath. Once the device is opened in the left atrium, it is withdrawn against the atrial septum so that the hollow wires are positioned onto the right atrial side of the septum. The nylon filaments are cut, which allows the wires to spring back and detach the device from the delivery catheter. Devices were implanted that occluded five experimentally created ASDs in dogs. The position of the device was good in all dogs and there was no residual shunt. In four dogs, postmortem studies were performed 6 months later that showed the device to be in place with incorporation into the atrial septum and excellent endothelialization. The device was used successfully in two patients with secundum ASD (*personal communication,* D. Pavčnik, December 2000). More recently, the device was modified: The stainless steel ring was replaced with Nitinol wire and Dacron with biomaterial. The new device is retrievable and can be implanted via an 8F sheath. Animal experimentation is planned for the near future (*personal communication,* D. Pavčnik, December 2000).

Redington and Rigby (46) modified the Rashkind patent ductus ateriosus (PDA) umbrella device by bending the arms of the device such that there is better apposition of the umbrellas against each other and the atrial septum. The device was used to occlude four ASDs with left-to-right shunt. In two (50%) patients, the ASD was successfully closed. The remaining two (50%) patients required surgical removal of the device along with closure of the ASD. The device was also used to occlude 11 fenestrated Fontans. In nine patients there was improvement in oxygen saturation. In the remaining two (18%) the procedure failed. To my knowledge, there are no other reports on the use of this modification by this or other workers. In addition, a similar bend placed in the clamshell device has resulted in breakage of the arms, forcing its removal from use. Therefore the advisability of introducing such a bend in the Rashkind PDA device was questioned (47).

NEW DEVICES

The decade of the 1990s witnessed a number of new ASD-closing devices. Babic and his associates (48) described a double-umbrella device implanted via arteriovenous guide wire loop in 1991. They named it the atrial septal defect occluding system (ASDOS). Clinical trials in Europe began in 1995 (49). In 1993, Das and his colleagues (50) designed a self-centering device delivered transvenously via an 11F sheath, named the Das Angel Wing Device. Clinical trials were undertaken in the United States and abroad. The device was modified recently to address some problems discovered during the initial experience, and clinical trials with the modified device, now named Angel Wing II, are likely to start soon (51). In 1997, a new self-expanding Nitinol prosthesis was developed that consists of two self-expandable round disks connected to each other with a 4-mm-wide waist (52) and is commonly referred to as the Amplatzer septal occluder. A number of clinical trials worldwide, including the United States, are under way, as detailed elsewhere (53). As mentioned in the previous section of this paper, following withdrawal of clamshell device because of breakage of arms, the device was redesigned by introducing an additional bend in the arms and was named CardioSeal (54). More recently, the device was further modified by attaching microsprings between the umbrellas and was named StarFlex (55). Clinical trials with these devices are also proceeding worldwide. The final device of the decade was the Helex (56). It consists of a single Nitinol wire with a sleevelike expanded polytetrafluoroethylene membrane attached to it. The wire is preshaped to form two disks that can be delivered transvenously via an 8 or a 9F sheath. Clinical trials with this device are also under way.

The currently utilized ASD occluding devices are double-disk devices with wire components and have some limitations. The major disadvantages are requirement of sufficient septal rims, the need for the device to be 1.5 to 2.0 times the stretched ASD diameter, and complications related to wire components. To circumvent these problems, Sideris and colleagues developed wireless devices and transcatheter-implantable patches to occlude large ASDs (57). Zamora and his associates have reviewed these devices (58). Each of the devices reviewed in this section will be discussed in greater detail in several chapters to follow.

CLOSURE OF ATRIAL DEFECTS TO PREVENT RECURRENCE OF PARADOXIC EMBOLISM

Some cerebrovascular accidents and other systemic arterial emboli, especially in young subjects, are presumed to be due to paradoxic embolism through an atrial defect, most frequently a patent foramen ovale. Closure of such defects is an alternative option to lifelong anticoagulation. Nonsurgical transcatheter occlusion of such a defect was first reported with King's device in 1976 (8). Mills and King effectively occluded an atrial defect with a 25-mm device in a 17-year-old male who had a hemiparetic stroke secondary to paradoxic embolism. Subsequently, clamshell (59) and buttoned (29,35,60) devices have been used to successfully occlude atrial defects presumed to be the site of paradoxical embolism. Most of the devices described in the preceding section have also been used to close patent foramen ovale to prevent recurrence of embolism. Some (61) were modified to address the anatomic features of the foramen ovale.

More recently, a device named PFO-Star was developed and was designed specifically to occlude patent foramen ovale (62). It is composed of two square-shaped Ivalon sails, each made up of four standard Nitinol wires connected to a central pin made of platinum/iridium, covered with polyvinyl alcohol foam (Ivalon). Results of detailed investigation of this device to close patent foramen ovale will be reviewed in a separate chapter. This device has not been used for occluding secundum ASDs with left-to-right shunts.

SUMMARY AND CONCLUSION

This chapter reviews historical aspects of transcatheter atrial septal occluding devices. Since the first description of an ASD closing device by King, a large number of single-disk and double-disk devices have been designed and tested in animal models, followed by clinical trials in human subjects. Feasibility, safety, and effectiveness have been demonstrated with most devices. However, design, redesign, testing, and retesting have been the typical path with most devices. Whereas no device has been approved for general clinical use at the time of this writing, the new millennium may bring a change in that at least a few of the devices may be approved by the regulatory authorities so that they will be available for general clinical use to treat atrial septal defects nonsurgically.

REFERENCES

1. Bigelow WG, Lindsey WE, Greenwood WF. Hypothermia: its possible role in cardiac surgery. *Ann Surg* 1950;132:849–866.
2. Lewis FJ, Tauffic M. Closure of atrial septal defects with the aid of hypothermia: experimental accomplishments and the report of one successful case. *Surgery* 1953;32:52–59.
3. Gibbon JH, Jr. Application of a mechanical heart and lung apparatus to cardiac surgery. In: Gibbon JH, Jr, ed. *Recent advances in cardiovascular physiology and surgery.* Minneapolis: University of Minnesota, 1953:107–113.
4. Murphy JG, Gersh BJ, McGoon MD, et al. Long-term outcome after surgical repair of isolated atrial septal defect. *N Engl J Med* 1990;323:1645–1650.
5. Galal MO, Wobst A, Halees Z, et al. Perioperative complications following surgical closure of atrial septal defect type II in 232 patients: a baseline study. *Eur Heart J* 1994;15:1381–1384.

6. Pastorek JS, Allen HD, Davis JT. Current outcomes of surgical closure of secundum atrial septal defect. *Am J Cardiol* 1994;74:75–79.
7. King TD, Mills NL. Nonoperative closure of atrial septal defects. *Surgery* 1974;75:383–388.
8. Mills NL, King TD. Nonoperative closure of left-to-right shunts. *J Thorac Cardiovasc Surg* 1976;72:371–378.
9. King TD, Thompson SL, Steiner C, et al. Secundum atrial septal defect: nonoperative closure during cardiac catheterization. *JAMA* 1976;235:2506–2509.
10. Rashkind WJ. Experimental transvenous closure of atrial and ventricular septal defects. *Circulation* 1975;52:II-8.
11. Rashkind WJ, Cuaso CE. Transcatheter closure of atrial septal defects in children. *Eur J Cardiol* 1977;8:119–120.
12. Rashkind WJ. Transcatheter treatment of congenital heart disease. *Circulation* 1983;67:711–716.
13. King TD, Thompson SL, Steiner C, et al. Measurement of atrial septal defect during cardiac catheterization: experimental and clinical trials. *Am J Cardiol* 1978;41:537–542.
14. Rashkind WJ, Tait MA, Gibson RJ, Jr. Interventional cardiac catheterization in congenital heart disease. *Int J Cardiol* 1985;7:1–11.
15. Beekman RH, Rocchini AP, Snider AR, et al. Transcatheter atrial septal defect closure: preliminary experience with the Rashkind occluder device. *J Interv Cardiol* 1989;1:35–41.
16. Rashkind WJ, Mullins CE, Hellenbrand WE, et al. Non-surgical closure of patent ductus arteriosus: clinical applications of the Rashkind PDA occluder system. *Circulation* 1987;75:583–592.
17. Rome JJ, Keane JF, Perry SB, et al. Double-umbrella closure of atrial defects: initial clinical applications. *Circulation* 1990;82:751–758.
18. Lock JE, Cockerham JT, Keane JF, et al. Transcatheter umbrella closure of congenital heart defects. *Circulation* 1987;75:593–599.
19. Lock JE, Rome JJ, Davis R, et al. Transcatheter closure of atrial septal defects: experimental studies. *Circulation* 1989;79:1091–1099.
20. Hellenbrand WE, Fahey JT, McGowan FX, et al. Transesophageal echocardiographic guidance of transcatheter closure of atrial septal defect. *Am J Cardiol* 1990;66:207–213.
21. Boutin C, Musewe NN, Smallhorn JF, et al. Echocardiographic follow-up of atrial septal defect after catheter closure by double-umbrella device. *Circulation* 1993;88:621–627.
22. Latson LA. Transcatheter closure of atrial septal defects. In: Rao PS, ed. *Transcatheter therapy in pediatric cardiology.* New York: Wiley-Liss, 1993:335–348.
23. Perry SB, Van der Velde ME, Bridges ND, et al. Transcatheter closure of atrial and ventricular septal defects. *Herz* 1993;18:135–142.
24. Justo RN, Nykanen DG, Boutin C, et al. Clinical impact of transcatheter closure of secundum atrial septal defects with double umbrella device. *Am J Cardiol* 1996;77:889–892.
25. Prieto LR, Foreman CK, Cheatham JP, et al. Intermediate-term outcome of transcatheter secundum atrial septal defect closure using Bard clamshell septal umbrella. *Am J Cardiol* 1996;778:1310–1312.
26. Sideris EB, Sideris SE, Fowlkes JP, et al. Transvenous atrial septal occlusion in piglets using a "buttoned" double-disc device. *Circulation* 1990;81:312–318.
27. Sideris EB, Sideris SE, Thanopoulos BD, et al. Transvenous atrial septal defect occlusion by the "buttoned" device. *Am J Cardiol* 1990;66:1524–1526.
28. Rao PS, Sideris EB, Chopra PS. Catheter closure of atrial septal defect: successful use in a 3.6 kg infant. *Am Heart J* 1991;121:1826–1829.

29. Rao PS, Wilson AD, Levy JM, et al. Role of "buttoned" double-disc device in the management of atrial septal defects. *Am Heart J* 1992;123:191–200.

30. Rao PS, Sideris EB, Hausdorf G, et al. International experience with secundum atrial septal defect occlusion by the buttoned device. *Am Heart J* 1994;128:1022–1035.

31. Rao PS, Berger F, Rey C, et al. Transvenous occlusion of secundum atrial septal defects with 4th generation buttoned device: comparison with 1st, 2nd and 3rd generation devices. *J Am Coll Cardiol* 2000;36:583–592.

32. Sideris EB, Leung M, Yoon JH, et al. Occlusion of large atrial septal defects with a centering device: early clinical experience. *Am Heart J* 1996;131:356–359.

33. Rao PS, Chander JS, Sideris EB. Role of inverted buttoned device in transcatheter occlusion of atrial septal defects or patent foramen ovale with right-to-left shunting associated with previously operated complex congenital cardiac anomalies. *Am J Cardiol* 1997;80:914–921.

34. Sideris EB, Rey C, Schrader R, et al. Occlusion of large atrial septal defects by buttoned devices; comparison of centering and the fourth generation devices [abstract]. *Circulation* 1997;96:I–99.

35. Ende DJ, Chopra PS, Rao PS. Prevention of recurrence of paradoxic embolism: mid-term follow-up after transcatheter closure of atrial defects with buttoned device. *Am J Cardiol* 1996;78:233–236.

36. Rao PS, Wilson AD, Chopra PS. Transcatheter closure of atrial septal defects by "buttoned" devices. *Am J Cardiol* 1992;69:1056–1061.

37. Rao PS, Ende DJ, Wilson AD, et al. Follow-up results of transcatheter occlusion of atrial septal defects with buttoned device. *Can J Cardiol* 1995;11:695–701.

38. Arora R, Trehan VK, Karla GS, et al. Transcatheter closure of atrial septal defect using buttoned device; Indian experience. *Indian Heart J* 1996;48:145–149.

39. Haddad J, Secches A, Finzi L, et al. Atrial septal defect: percutaneous transvenous occlusion with the buttoned device. *Arq Bras Cardiol* 1996;67:17–22.

40. Worms AM, Rey C, Bourlan F, et al. French experience in the closure of atrial septal defects of the ostium secundum type with Sideris buttoned occluder. *Arch Mal Coeur Vaiss* 1996;89:509–515.

41. Lloyd TR, Rao PS, Beekman RH III, et al. Atrial septal defect occlusion with the buttoned device: a multi-institutional U.S. trial. *Am J Cardiol* 1994;73:286–291.

42. Zamora R, Rao PS, Lloyd TR, et al. Intermediate-term results of Phase I FDA trials of buttoned device occlusion of secundum atrial septal defects. *J Am Coll Cardiol* 1998;31:674–678.

43. Rao PS, Sideris EB, Rey C, et al. Echo-Doppler follow-up evaluation after transcatheter occlusion of atrial septal defects with the buttoned device. In Imai I, Momma K, eds. *Proceedings of the Second World Congress of Pediatric Cardiology and Cardiac Surgery.* Armonk, NY: Futura, 1998:197–200.

44. Rao PS, Sideris EB. Buttoned device closure of the atrial septal defect. *J Interv Cardiol* 1998;11:467–484.

45. Pavčnik D, Wright KC, Wallace S. Monodisk: device for percutaneous transcatheter closure of cardiac septal defects. *Cardiovasc Interv Radiol* 1993;16:308–312.

46. Redington AN, Rigby ML. Transcatheter closure of interatrial communication with a modified umbrella device. *Br Heart J* 1994;72:372–377.

47. Rao PS, Sideris EB. Transcatheter occlusion of cardiac defects [letter]. *Br Heart J* 1995;73:585–586.

48. Babic UU, Grujicic S, Popvic Z, et al. Double-umbrella device for transvenous closure of patent ductus arteriosus and atrial septal defect: first clinical experience. *J Interv Cardiol* 1991;4:283–294.

49. Sievert H, Babic UU, Hausdorf G, et al. Transcatheter closure of atrial septal defect and patent foramen ovale with ASDOS device (a multi-institutional European trial). *Am J Cardiol* 1998;82:1405–1413.

50. Das GS, Voss G, Jarvis G, et al. Experimental atrial septal defect closure with a new, transcatheter, self-centering device. *Circulation* 1993;88:1754–1764.

51. Das GS, Harrison JK, O'Laughlin MP. The Angel Wings Das device for atrial septal defect closure. *Curr Interv Cardiol Rep* 2000;2:78–85.

52. Sharafuddin MJA, Gu X, Titus JL, et al. Transvenous closure of secundum atrial septal defects: preliminary results with a new self-expanding Nitinol prosthesis in a swine model. *Circulation* 1997;95:2162–2168.

53. Waight DJ, Koenig PR, Cao Q, et al. Transcatheter closure of secundum atrial septal defects using Amplatzer Septal Occluder; clinical experience and technical considerations. *Curr Interv Cardiol Rep* 2000;2:70–77.

54. Ryan C, Opolski S, Wright J, et al. Structural considerations in the development of the CardioSeal septal occluder. In Imai Y, Momma K, eds. *Proceedings of the Second World Congress of Pediatric Cardiology and Cardiac Surgery.* Armonk, NY: Futura, 1998:191–193.

55. Hausdorf G, Kaulitz R, Paul T. Transcatheter closure of atrial septal defect with a new flexible, self-centering device (the Starflex occluder). *Am Heart J* 1999;84:1113–1116.

56. Latson LA, Zahn EW, Wilson N. Helex septal occluder for closure of atrial septal defects. *Curr Interv Cardiol Rep* 2000;2:268–273.

57. Sideris EB, Sideris SE, Kaneva A, et al. Transcatheter occlusion of experimental atrial septal defects by wireless occluders and patches [abstract]. *Cardiol Young* 1999;9:92.

58. Zamora R, Rao PS, Sideris EB. Buttoned device for atrial septal defect occlusion. *Curr Interv Cardiol Rep* 2000;2:167–176.

59. Bridges ND, Hellenbrand W, Latson L, et al. Transcatheter closure of patent foramen ovale after presumed paradoxical embolism. *Circulation* 1992;16:83–84.

60. Chandar JS, Rao PS, Lloyd TR, et al. Atrial septal defect closure with 4th generation buttoned device: results of US multicenter FDA Phase II clinical trial [abstract]. *Circulation* 1999;100:I–708.

61. Han Y, Gu X, Titus JL, et al. New self-expanding patent foramen ovale occlusion device. *Cathet Cardiovasc Interv* 1999;47:370–376.

62. Keppeier P, Rux S, Dirks J, et al. Transcatheter closure of 100 patent foramina ovalia in patients with unexplained stroke and suspected paradoxic embolism: a comparison of five different devices [abstract]. *Eur Heart J* 1999;20:196.

Catheter Based Devices: For the Treatment of Non-coronary Cardiovascular Diseases in Adults and Children. Edited by P. Syamasundar Rao and Morton J. Kern, Lippincott Williams & Wilkins, Philadelphia © 2003.

2

CLAMSHELL DEVICES

JONATHAN J. ROME

In 1987, Lock and coworkers reported use of the double-umbrella Rashkind PDA device for closure of a variety of intracardiac defects, including atrial septal defects (1). The success of this limited clinical experience prompted development of a double-umbrella device (2) by modifying Rashkind's atrial septal defect closure device (3). This new device, the Clamshell Occluder (C. R. Bard, Inc., Billerica, MA) was designed to allow the two umbrellas to fold back toward the septum and one another by incorporating springs into each of the umbrella arms. Thus the device would fix to the atrial septum via spring tension rather than hooks, as had been the case with the previous Rashkind ASD device (3). The Clamshell was the first device used successfully to close atrial septal defects in a large number of children and adults. More than 800 patients received the original Clamshell umbrella, including more than 300 with atrial septal defects. Because of an unacceptably high incidence of arm fractures on follow-up evaluation, the Clamshell umbrella was never marketed. Rather, the device was modified (Clamshell II, C.R. Bard, Inc.; and CardioSEAL Septal Occluder, Nitinol Medical Technology, Inc., Boston, MA). The modified versions of this initial design will be discussed in a subsequent chapter. Patients who received the Clamshell device constitute a large cohort with intracardiac devices for which long-term follow-up is available.

DEVICE

The Clamshell Occluder has the configuration of a double umbrella designed to cover, rather than plug, an atrial defect (Figure 2.1). The device is symmetric in design. Each side is composed of four 0.007-inch stainless steel arms. Each arm has two hinges: the first where it attaches to the center of the device, and a second midway between device center and perimeter. On the right atrial side of the device,

a locking pin protrudes from the center pole. Square woven Dacron patches suture attached to each set of arms form the two umbrellas of the device. The Clamshell delivery catheter is similar in design to that of the Rashkind PDA Occluder (3). It attaches to the device by means of a central pin and a locking sleeve. The end of the catheter is fitted with a steel pod into which the collapsed device is withdrawn. The Clamshell Occluder was manufactured in five sizes: 17, 23, 28, 33, and 40 mm. Device sizes refer to the diagonal measurement of the occluder umbrella from arm tip to arm tip.

Patient Selection

Before clinical trials with the Clamshell device were initiated, anatomic studies were performed to define the spectrum of secundum atrial septal defects and assess their potential suitability for closure with the device (2). The mean age among the 50 cases examined was 2.8 years (1day to 36 years). Single defects were present in 70%; defects were generally elliptical in shape. The average ratio of shortest to longest diameter was 0.8. The average size of these holes was 8 by 10 mm. Eighty percent of the defects were judged suitable for device closure based on the criteria that a single hole was less than 25 mm and had a circumferential rim of 2 mm or greater. If multiple holes were present, they were judged closeable if a single device could be expected to completely cover both (Figure 2.2).

Selection criteria for Clamshell closure of atrial septal defects evolved somewhat over the years of the use of this device. However, the basic factors considered remained remarkably constant. Patients had to be large enough for their femoral vein to accommodate an 11F delivery sheath. Further criteria were evaluated by transthoracic echocardiography in most instances. These criteria included the following: (a) presence of a single atrial defect (fenestrated defects were acceptable), (b) the ASD was no more than 50% the diameter of the umbrella, (c) the dimension of the atrial septum was large enough to accommodate the device, (d) at least 4 mm separated the defect from atrioventricular valves, venae cavae, and pulmonary veins. Final criteria for

Jonathan J. Rome: Associate Professor of Pediatrics, University of Pennsylvania; Director, Cardiac Catheterization Laboratory, Children's Hospital of Philadelphia, Philadelphia, Pennsylvania

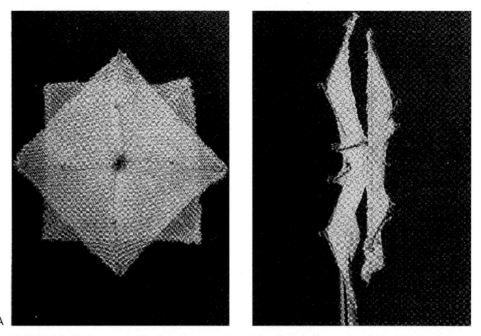

A   B

FIGURE 2.1. En face and side-view photographs of the Clamshell septal occluder. The device configuration is that of a double umbrella. Four stainless steel arms form the frame for each umbrella. Each arm has two hinges, one at the center of the device, and a second midway between device center and perimeter. On the right atrial side of the device, a locking pin protrudes from the center pole. Square woven Dacron patches suture attached to each set of arms to form the two umbrellas of the device. (From Lock JE, Rome JJ, Davis R, et al. Transcatheter closure of atrial septal defects: experimental studies. *Circulation* 1989;79:1091–1099, with permission.)

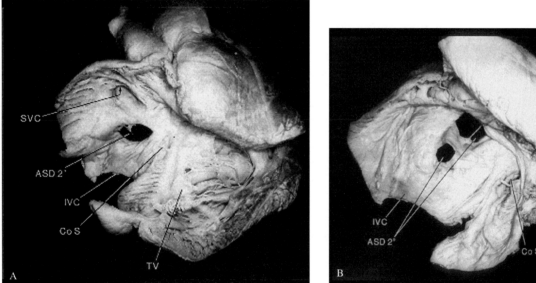

A   B

FIGURE 2.2. Right atrial views of pathologic specimens demonstrating secundum atrial septal defects. **A:** This defect is single with a circumferential septal rim and was therefore considered appropriate for device closure. **B:** Two separate defects are present in this specimen, and this defect was not considered an appropriate candidate for device closure. ASD, atrial septal defect; CoS, coronary sinus; IVC, inferior vena cava; SVC, superior vena cava; TV, tricuspid valve. (From Lock JE, Rome JJ, Davis R, et al. Transcatheter closure of atrial septal defects: experimental studies. *Circulation* 1989;79:1091–1099, with permission.)

device placement were determined at catheterization. Atrial septal defects were measured by balloon sizing. In general, the largest hole that could be closed was 20 mm if the patient's atrium was large enough to accommodate a 40-mm device. Through the years of the Clamshell experience, transesophageal echocardiography became commonly used to aid in device delivery (4). However, transesophageal echocardiograms were rarely used as a method of selecting patients for catheterization (5).

Implantation Technique

In spite of multiple modifications to delivery system and device, the technique originally described for deployment of the Clamshell device has remained largely unchanged with subsequent designs (Clamshell II and CardioSEAL). Femoral venous access is obtained; the right is slightly preferable, and the patient is fully heparinized. After diagnostic right heart catheterization, an angiogram is performed from the right upper pulmonary vein in the hepatoclavicular view. Typically, the defect is well profiled in this projection, allowing optimal angiographic measurement. A second angiogram is then performed left anterior oblique (LAO) 45 degrees without the cranial angulation to demonstrate landmarks in this, the optimal camera angle for device deployment. The other camera is usually positioned right anterior oblique (RAO) for this angiogram. The RAO view is very useful in identifying the location of pulmonary veins and mitral valve. A 0.035-inch exchange guide wire is positioned in the left upper pulmonary vein and the atrial defect is balloon-sized. For the years of the Clamshell experience, the available sizing balloons (Meditech, Inc., Quincy, MA) were "apple-shaped." Sizing was performed by gently pulling the balloon through the hole while deflating it. The ASD created an indentation as the balloon pulled through. Because of a tendency for the shoulder of the balloon to catch the edge of the defect, this maneuver was also performed while pushing the balloon from the right to the left atrium as well. Subsequently, balloons allowing static sizing have been developed (NMT, Boston, MA). When transesophageal echocardiography is being employed, the defect is evaluated before sizing. During balloon occlusion, the atrial septum is interrogated with color Doppler for the presence of other defects. In cases of multiple fenestrations, echocardiography is used to confirm wire position through the primary (largest) defect. The Clamshell device is selected to be twice the balloon-sized defect diameter but less than the dimension of the atrial septum. An 11F Mullins sheath is carefully flushed. A number of strategies were developed to minimize the risk of air embolus from the long sheath. One such strategy involves attaching a large (60-mL) syringe to the Mullins dilator via a Y-adapter. The adapter is tightened and the dilator is flushed. After the skin and fascia are predilated with a 12F dilator, the long sheath and dilator are advanced over the wire. The Y-adapter is kept snug over the wire to prevent

loss of flush out the backstop. The sheath assembly is advanced over the exchange wire into to the left atrium. The exchange wire is withdrawn into the dilator. Then the dilator is continuously flushed while it is withdrawn from the sheath, thus backfilling the sheath completely. The sheath is then flushed.

With the delivery sheath in place, the device is loaded into the delivery catheter. After inspection, the device is submerged in saline. It is then locked to the catheter by pulling the opposing locking pins into the locking sleeve. Once thus attached, the left atrial umbrella of the device is collapsed by applying traction on the loading suture attached to the left atrial umbrella arms. The device is then fully collapsed by pulling it into a plastic loading tube. The collapsed device is withdrawn into the metal pod on the delivery catheter. The delivery catheter is advanced into the Mullins sheath until the metal pod is visible at the floor of the right atrium. Using the control wire, the device is pushed out of the metal pod into the sheath and advanced to the end of the sheath (Figure 2.3A). The sheath position

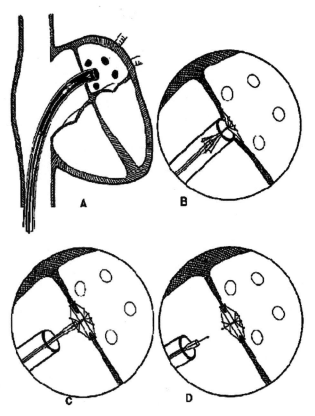

FIGURE 2.3. Diagram demonstrating deployment of Clamshell device in an atrial septal defect. **A:** The device is advanced with the long sheath positioned in the left atrium. **B:** The distal umbrella is deployed on the left atrial side of the defect. **C:** The long sheath is pulled back, allowing the proximal arms to open on the right side of the defect. **D:** The device is released from the delivery catheter. (From Lock JE, Rome JJ, Davis R, et al. Transcatheter closure of atrial septal defects: experimental studies. *Circulation* 1989;79:1091–1099, with permission.)

is verified free in the left atrium away from pulmonary veins or left atrial appendage (by echo, fluoroscopy, or both) and the distal arms of the umbrella are opened (Figure 2.3B). The device and sheath are pulled back as a unit until the atrial septum is engaged. This is determined fluoroscopically by observing flexion of the inferior arms of the device. Vertical plane transesophageal echocardiography demonstrates the inferior device arms engaged against the septum and the superior arms just opposed to it. The device position is held constant while the Mullins sheath is withdrawn, allowing the proximal umbrella to open (Figure 2.3C). In the absence of echocardiographic guidance, correct device positioning is confirmed by observing separation of the right and left atrial arms with very gentle "push/pull" on the delivery wire. Because the septal position is significantly distorted when the device is still attached to the delivery system, this maneuver has the potential of pulling one of the superior arms through the defect. When echo imaging is employed, it is generally sufficient to confirm appropriate positioning, rendering the "push/pull" unnecessary. After correct position is demonstrated, the device is released by pushing forward the locking pin (Figure 2.3D). Final device position is confirmed either echocardiographically or by angiography.

Results

The first report documenting the use of the Clamshell device included 23 patients with secundum atrial septal defects. There was one major complication. This occurred in a 70-year-old patient who sustained an embolic stroke on positioning of the Mullins sheath. One device embolized; this occurred in a patient with right-to-left atrial shunting. Though follow-up in the series was limited to less than 1 year, initial clinical outcomes were quite favorable (6). Subsequent single-center reports have evaluated clinical outcome as well as residual shunting by color Doppler echocardiographic evaluation at intermediate term. Device embolization or malposition requiring surgical removal occurred in two of 76 cases (7,8). These studies have clarified the fact that residual leaks around the device tend to decrease with increasing time after device deployment. In an actuarial analysis, 81% of patients had residual leaks at hospital discharge; this decreased to 36% 4 years after the procedure (8).

Follow-up studies of patients with Clamshell ASD devices demonstrated a prevalence of patients with radiographic evidence of arm fractures. Fractures typically occurred in the middle of the arms near the spring. Though early reports suggested a fracture rate of 10% as more information accrued, it became clear that the fracture rate was substantially greater. Actuarial analysis demonstrated increasing prevalence of fractures with time after device placement, reaching 71% at 4 years (8). The recognition of this phenomenon led to the removal of the Clamshell

device from clinical use and subsequent redesign. Extensive follow-up of this cohort of patients has revealed no discernible sequelae in the great majority of those with documented device arm fracture (see following).

The final IDE progress report for the Clamshell device was submitted to the FDA in January 1998 (C.R. Bard, Inc):. Almost 1,000 devices were implanted in more than 800 patients between December 1988 and June 1995. More than 300 were implanted in atrial septal defects. Fewer than 3% of devices embolized, most very shortly after implantation. It is important to note that device embolization did not lead to hemodynamic instability in any patient. Echocardiographic evaluation at hospital discharge demonstrated complete or virtually complete closure in about two-thirds of cases. Consistent with previous data, the prevalence of residual shunting decreased over time. At the final evaluation, complete closure was noted in two-thirds of the patients; moderate residual leaks were found in 2%. No patients had large (>4-mm) leaks.

Arm fractures were documented in 60% of patients with atrial septal defect devices. Sequellae likely related to arm fracture included atrial masses observed in three cases, and four cases with adherent thrombi. Some of these patients were treated conservatively (anticoagulation for thrombi and observation for masses); some underwent device explant and surgical ASD closure. The abnormalities resolved in all instances. Other important adverse events reported as probably related to device procedures included CVA in two patients (the one noted earlier and one other) and one cardiac perforation.

DISCUSSION

The Clamshell experience demonstrated effective closure of atrial septal defects in more than 94% of cases. The complication rate with this newly designed device was remarkably low. It is not overstating the case to suggest that the development of the Clamshell occluder represents a watershed moment in the evolution of device closure for cardiac defects. After the application of this device, the question was no longer whether or not most atrial septal defects could effectively be closed with devices, but how best to accomplish this achievable end. The Clamshell device is important for its design characteristics, including flexibility and low profile. The added importance of this device's development for the field as a whole can be realized best by considering the spectrum of clinical investigation that occurred as a result of the Clamshell experience. Studies were performed to better delineate atrial defect anatomy relevant for catheter techniques (2,9). Echocardiographers worked to better understand and image atrial anatomy with transesophageal and three-dimensional techniques (4,5,10). Better sizing balloon catheters were developed for device deployment. The shortcomings of the Clamshell device were perhaps even more important in providing the impetus for developments. The arm fracture experience led to a better understanding of the biomechanical forces to which devices were subject, resulting in improved *in vitro* device testing. The occurrence of arm fractures as well as residual leaks led to redesign with new materials and improved arm flexibility (11). Finally, the Clamshell design and experience became a springboard for the development of a host of other closure devices. These alternative designs will be discussed in subsequent chapters.

REFERENCES

1. Lock JE, Cockerham JT, Keane JF, et al. Transcatheter umbrella closure of congenital heart defects. *Circulation* 1987;75:593–599.
2. Lock JE, Rome JJ, Davis R, et al. Transcatheter closure of atrial septal defects: experimental studies. *Circulation* 1989;79:1091–1099.
3. Rashkind WJ. Transcatheter treatment of congenital heart disease. *Circulation* 1983;67:711–716.
4. Hellenbrand WE, Fahey JT, McGowan FX, et al. Transesophageal echocardiographic guidance of transcatheter closure of atrial septal defect. *Am J Cardiol* 1990;66:207–213.
5. Rosenfeld HM, van der Velde ME, Sanders SP, et al. Echocardiographic predictors of candidacy for successful transcatheter atrial septal defect closure. *Cathet Cardiovasc Diagn* 1995;34:29–34.
6. Rome JJ, Keane JF, Perry SB, et al. Double-umbrella closure of atrial defects: initial clinical applications. *Circulation* 1990;82:751–758.
7. Prieto LR, Foreman CK, Cheatham JP, et al. Intermediate-term outcome of transcatheter secundum atrial septal defect closure using the Bard Clamshell Septal Umbrella. *Am J Cardiol* 1996;78:1310–1312.
8. Justo RN, Nykanen DG, Boutin C, et al. Clinical impact of transcatheter closure of secundum atrial septal defects with the double umbrella device. *Am J Cardiol* 1898;77:889–892.
9. Chan KC, Godman MJ. Morphological variations of fossa ovalis atrial septal defects (secundum): feasibility for transcutaneous closure with the clam-shell device. *Br Heart J* 1993;69:52–55.
10. Maeno YV, Benson LN, Boutin C. Impact of dynamic 3D transoesophageal echocardiography in the assessment of atrial septal defects and occlusion by the double-umbrella device (CardioSEAL) [see comments]. *Cardiol Young* 1998;8:368–378.
11. Latson LA. Per-catheter ASD closure. *Pediatr Cardiol* 1998;19:86–93; discussion 94.

3

THE BUTTONED DEVICE

P. SYAMASUNDAR RAO

Since the first description of the atrial septal defect (ASD) occluding transcatheter device by King and Mills (1–3) in the mid-1970s, a number of other devices have been designed and tested in animal models. These tests were followed by trials in human subjects. These, along with the epidemic of device proliferation technology in the last decade of twentieth century, have been reviewed elsewhere (4). The buttoned device, initially described in late 1980s (5), has been used for more than a decade and is the oldest of the ASD occluding devices currently in clinical trials with larger clinical experience than the other devices. This chapter reviews the buttoned device and its modifications along with the results of implantation.

THE DEVICE AND ITS MODIFICATIONS

The Original Device (First Generation)

The device consists of an occluder and a counteroccluder (5). The *occluder* is composed of an x-shaped wire skeleton covered with 0.125-inch polyurethane foam and goes onto the left atrial side of the ASD. The wire skeleton is made up of 0.035-inch Teflon-coated stainless steel guide-wire pieces. The peripheral ends of the wires are devoid of central core wire such that the ends are not injurious to the cardiac tissue. By folding the wire skeleton, the wires become parallel so that the occluder can be introduced through an 8 French (F) sheath, and thus be deliverable to the implantation site via the sheath, where it springs open to assume its original square shape. A 2-mm-long silk string loop is attached to the center of the occluder, which is closed with a 1-mm knot, the *button.* The *counteroccluder* is made up of a rhomboid-shaped 0.125-inch polyurethane foam covering a single-strand Teflon-coated stainless steel wire skeleton. A rubber piece is sewn in the center of the counteroccluder and becomes a *buttonhole.* The wire components of both the occluder and counteroccluder are radiopaque.

P. Syamasundar Rao: Professor of Pediatrics, Medicine, and Cardiology, Department of Pediatrics, University of Texas-Houston Medical School; Director, Division of Pediatric Cardiology, Memorial Hermann Children's Hospital, Houston, Texas

The device delivery and buttoning systems consist of (a) a Teflon-coated 0.035-inch guide wire, the *loading wire*; (b) a folded 0.008-inch nylon thread passing through the loading wire after having its core wire removed (the loop of the folded nylon thread passes through the button loop attached to the center of the occluder [Figure 3.1, left]); (c) a *pusher catheter* used to advance the occluder and counteroccluder within the sheath; and (d) a long 8F (or 9F for larger devices) sheath through which the device implantation is performed.

After the occluder is delivered into the left atrium and positioned on the left atrial aspect of the ASD, the tip of the sheath is withdrawn into the low right atrium and the counteroccluder is delivered into the right atrium. The counteroccluder is gently pushed with tip of the sheath over the loading wire while applying gentle traction on the loading wire, thus advancing the rubber piece (buttonhole) of the counteroccluder over the knot (button) of the loop attached to the occluder. Once the button passes the buttonhole, the rubber piece constricts, which holds the occluder and counteroccluder across the atrial septum, thus justifying the name *buttoned device.*

Second-Generation Device

The experience with the initial clinical trial (6) suggested that introducing a radiopaque component into the button would simplify the procedure because verification that the buttoning had taken place (Figure 3.2) could be undertaken by fluoroscopy. Therefore the button was made radiopaque. At the same time, several other modifications were introduced (7), including (a) the button loop was strengthened by replacing silk with 4-lb proof nylon; (b) the folded double thread in the loading wire was exchanged with a stronger, 4-lb proof nylon; and (c) the 0.125-inch polyurethane foam covering the wire skeleton of the occluder and counteroccluder was replaced with thinner, 0.0625-inch polyurethane foam.

Third-Generation Device

Introduction of radiopacity facilitated visualization of buttoning by fluoroscopy, but the button became eccentric

2nd Generation Device   **3rd Generation Device**   **4th Generation Device**

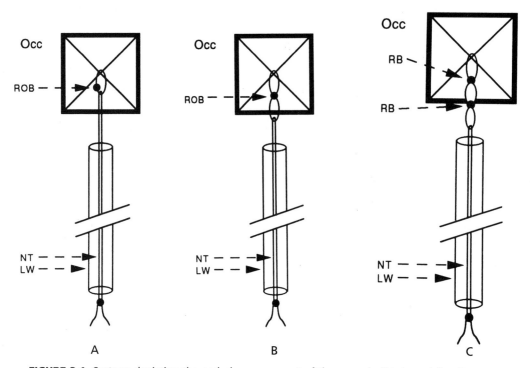

A   B   C

FIGURE 3.1. Cartoon depicting the occluder component of the second-, third-, and fourth-generation buttoned device. The occluder (Occ) in all devices is composed of an x-shaped wire skeleton covered with 1/16-inch polyurethane foam. In the second-generation device (left) a 2-mm string loop is attached to the center of the occluder. The loop is closed with a knot (button) made radiopaque. This radiopaque button (ROB) can easily be visualized by fluoroscopy. In the first-generation device (not shown), the button was *not* radiopaque. A folded 0.008-inch nylon thread (NT) passes through the hollow loading wire (LW) after passing through the loop in the center of the occluder. In the third-generation device (middle) an extra loop is added immediately beneath the radiopaque button. This modification converted the eccentric button of the second-generation device to be aligned straight, thus making it easier to button the Occ and counteroccluder across the atrial septum. In the fourth-generation device (right), the button loop is replaced with two "spring" radiopaque buttons (RB), mounted 4 mm apart. The intent was to reduce unbuttoning seen with earlier-generation devices. (Reproduced from Rao PS, Berger F, Rey C, et al. Results of transvenous occlusion of secundum atrial septal defects with the fourth generation buttoned device: comparison with first, second and third generation devices. *J Am Coll Cardiol* 2000;36;583–592, with permission.)

(Figure 3.1, left), thereby creating difficulty in buttoning. To rectify this problem, an additional loop of nylon thread was added to the button loop (Figure 3.1, center) so that the eccentric button of the second-generation device became aligned straight and was easier to button than was true of earlier versions of the device.

Fourth-Generation Device

In theory, once buttoned, the occluder and counteroccluder should stay together. But separation of both components, termed *unbuttoning*, occurred in 7.2% of the first 180 consecutive device implantations (7). When we examined the unbuttoning rate with successive generations of the device (Figure 3.3), the unbuttoning rate decreased from 11.1% in the first generation to 9.4% in the second and 3.1% in the third generation. But this decrease did not seem to attain statistical significance. To further decrease the unbuttoning rate, the device was modified by incorporating two radiopaque buttons in series [Figures 3.1 (right) and 3.4]. This has substantially reduced the unbuttoning rate (8,9).

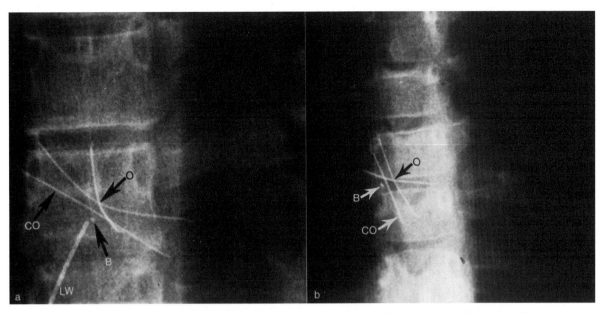

FIGURE 3.2. Selected cineradiographic frames of the device after its implantation across the atrial septum prior to **(a)** and after **(b)** disconnecting the device from the loading wire (LW) showing the occluder (O), counteroccluder (Co), and radiopaque button (B). Note that the radiopaque wire of the Co passed the radiopaque button, thus ensuring that buttoning had taken place. The cine frames were recorded in different projections and magnifications. (From Rao PS, Wilson AD, Levy JM, et al. Role of "buttoned" double-disc device in the management of atrial septal defects. *Am Heart J* 1992;123:191–200, with permission.)

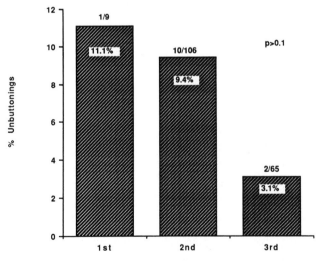

FIGURE 3.3. Bar graph showing prevalence of unbuttoning with each generation of the device during its evolution. There is no significant (*p* = .99) difference between first- and second-generation devices. Although there appears to be a trend toward lower prevalence of unbuttoning with the third-generation devices, this difference did not attain statistical significance (*p* = .135). (From Rao PS, Sideris EB, Hausdorf G, et al. International experience with secundum atrial septal defect occlusion by the buttoned device. *Am Heart J* 1994;128:1022–1035, with permission.)

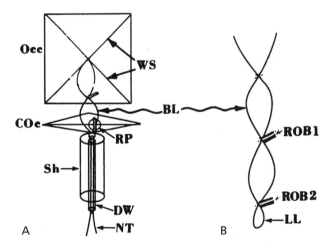

FIGURE 3.4. Cartoon of the fourth-generation buttoned device **(A)** with details of the buttoned loop **(B)**. The buttoned loop (BL) includes two "spring" buttons positioned 4 mm apart. During buttoning the spring button becomes straightened in line with the button loop. After buttoning, the radiopaque spring button becomes perpendicular, preventing unbuttoning. COc, counteroccluder; DW, delivery (loading) wire; LL, lower loop; NT, nylon thread; Occ, occluder; ROB1, radiopaque button 1; ROB2, radiopaque button 2; RP, rubber piece; Sh, sheath. (Reproduced from Sideris EB, Rao PS. Transcatheter closure of atrial septal defects: role of buttoned devices. *J Invasive Cardiol* 1996;8:289–296, with permission.)

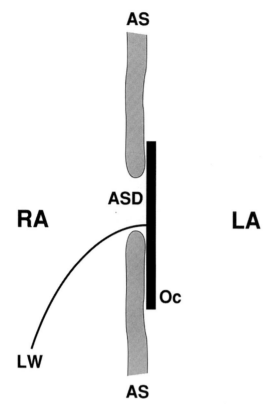

FIGURE 3.5. Artist's diagram of atrial septum (AS) separating left (LA) and right (RA) atria, showing atrial septal defect (ASD). The occluder (Oc) of the device has been delivered into the LA. As the loading wire (LW) is gently pulled, the occluder positions itself with its center at the lower margin of the ASD. If the Oc is less than double the size of the ASD, it is likely to flip back into the RA. If the Oc is larger than two times the size of the ASD, it is likely to be held in position in the LA, as shown in the figure. If a centering mechanism is incorporated into the Oc, the Oc does not have to be two times as large as the ASD. (From Rao PS, Wilson AD, Levy JM, et al. Role of "buttoned" double-disc device in the management of atrial septal defects. *Am Heart J* 1992;123:191–200, with permission.)

Centering-on-Demand Device

Based on theoretical considerations (Figure 3.5), described in detail elsewhere (6), the device size should be slightly larger than two times the stretched diameter of the ASD. Indeed, in practice, the sizes of the devices used were 2.3 to 2.35 times the size of the ASD (9). The button loop in the center of the device does not allow for centering of the device. The requirement for a large device is a definitive disadvantage in patients with relatively small atria, in that the device may impinge upon the mitral valve or pulmonary veins. Therefore the device was modified, incorporating a centering mechanism (Figure 3.6). The centering ring or rings are sutured at the center of the occluder. After the device is delivered into the left atrium, the centering rings are pulled through the ASD, which will result in centering the device over the ASD. Then the centering rings are folded onto the right atrial aspect of the septum. If centering is not required (e.g., fenestrated ASD or patent foramen ovale), the centering ring is folded onto the device in the left atrium before implanting onto the atrial septum, thus the name *centering on demand* (COD). At the time of introduction of the centering mechanism, the device is made circular instead of its prior square shape. The remaining features are similar to the fourth-generation device. In summary, the COD device is a rounded fourth-generation device with a centering mechanism. The recommended device/defect ratio is 1.8. The objectives of these design modifications are to decrease the device/defect ratio so that larger defects in smaller left atria could be occluded and to reduce residual shunts by eliminating the potential for leaving part of the ASD uncovered while at the same time retaining the favorable features of the fourth-generation device.

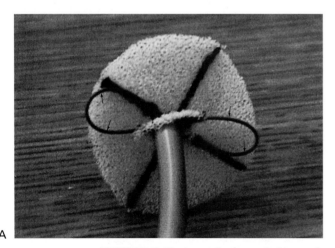

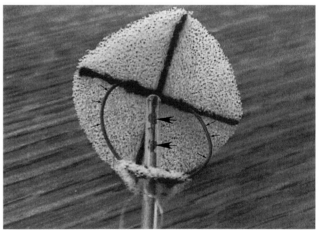

A   B

FIGURE 3.6. Photograph of a centering-on-demand buttoned device. Note the circular appearance of the device. The centering ring *(small arrows)* is attached to two arms of the device wire **(A)**. Radiopaque buttons are similar to a fourth-generation device (Figure 3.1, right) and are barely seen within the pusher catheter *(large arrow)* **(B)**. (Courtesy of E. B. Sideris, MD.)

PROTOCOL

Transcatheter occlusion of ASDs with the buttoned device was performed initially under a custom-made device protocol approved by the local Institution Review Boards (IRBs) in the first nine cases (6,10,11). Subsequent device implantations were undertaken as part of FDA-approved (US Food and Drug Administration) clinical trials with an IDE (Investigational Device Exemption) along with the approval of local IRBs in US institutions and with the approval of local IRBs at the participating institutions outside the United States, as per local regulations (7,9).

SELECTION OF PATIENTS

Ostium secundum ASDs with right ventricular volume overload are selected for closure. When hemodynamic data are known, a Qp:Qs ≥ 1.5:1 is considered a criterion for inclusion. Ostium primum ASDs and sinus venosus ASDs with partial anomalous pulmonary venous return are not candidates for closure. Patients who have developed pulmonary vascular obstructive disease are also excluded.

Precordial echocardiographic screening is generally considered adequate in children, whereas transesophageal echocardiography is generally required in adult subjects. Multiple echocardiographic views are examined to ensure adequacy of septal rims. Generally, a 3- to 4-mm rim is required except for the anterior rim adjacent to the aorta in the transesophageal aortic root short-axis view. Whereas the stretched diameter of the ASD can be estimated with reasonable certainty (12,13), there are occasions when such estimates are different. Therefore we make the final decision to implant the device following balloon sizing of the atrial septal defect (12–14). During the initial phases of the study (7) ASDs with a stretched diameter of more than 25 mm were not included for closure because devices larger than 55 mm are unavailable in the United States. Larger defects have been included from institutions outside the United States because of the availability of 60-mm devices outside the United States. With the advent of the COD device, defects as large as 30 mm are included. Finally, the length of the atrial septum measured by echocardiography and/or by left atrial angiography (left axial oblique view) should be of sufficient size to accommodate the selected size of the device.

In summary, ostium secundum ASDs with right ventricular volume overloading, without associated partial anomalous pulmonary venous return or pulmonary vascular obstructive disease, with adequate septal rims (>4 mm), a Qp:Qs ≥ 1.5:1 when such data are available, stretched diameter ≤ 25 or ≤ 30 mm, depending upon the location and timing, and septal lengths adequate to accommodate the selected device are candidates for buttoned device closure.

CLINICAL TRIALS AND PATIENT COHORTS

As mentioned in the protocol section, the device closures have been performed with the approval of local IRBs and under FDA supervision in US institutions and as per local regulations in non-US institutions. A large number of studies detailing single institutional (6,10,15–18) and multiinstitutional (7,9,19–26) experience with the buttoned device have been published and have demonstrated feasibility, safety, and effectiveness in occluding ostium secundum ASDs. More than 1,500 ASDs have been occluded in the United States and international buttoned-device clinical trials. Three cohorts (Table 3.1) have been selected for presentation in this chapter.

COHORT I

Cohort I is composed of the first 180 buttoned-device implantations performed (7) in the international trial with first-, second-, and third-generation devices, all with a sin-

TABLE 3.1. CHARACTERISTICS OF THE COHORTS

	Cohort I	Cohort II	Cohort III
Type of device	Single button	Double button	Double button plus centering on demand
Generation	First, Second, and Third	Fourth	Rounded fourth with centering mechanism
Time period	1989–1993	1993–1997	1999–2000
Number of implantations	180*	423†	76†

*168 Ostium secundum atrial septal defects (ASDs) and 12 were patent foramen ovale presumed to be the site of paradoxic embolism.
†All are ostium secundum ASDs.

gle button (Table 3.1). This cohort includes all first- and second-generation devices and only a portion of third-generation devices. The cohort includes all patients in Phase I FDA trial in the United States.

Technique

Informed consent was obtained from the patients or parents, as appropriate. Conscious sedation or general anesthesia was used, depending upon whether transthoracic or transesophageal monitoring was selected by the investigator (7,22). Cardiac catheterization, usually via the right femoral vein, was performed to confirm the clinical and echocardiographic diagnosis and to exclude other cardiac anomalies, particularly partial anomalous pulmonary venous return. Left atrial cineangiogram was performed in a left axial oblique view. This is useful to visualize multiple defects (in addition to transesophageal echocardiography), to measure the atrial septal length and to serve as a landmark for the left atrium during device implantation. The stretched diameter of the ASD was measured by balloon sizing (12–14) under both fluoroscopic and echocardiographic monitoring.

An 8 or 9F long sheath (Cordis Corporation, Miami, FL; or Cook, Inc., Bloomington, IN) was inserted and its tip positioned in the left atrium, while taking usual precautions to prevent vacuum creation and air entry. The sheath was clamped and cut, saving the valved portion of the sheath. The occluder was folded and introduced into the cut end of the sheath. The pusher catheter was introduced over the loading wire. The cut end of the saved valved component was reintroduced, and the system was flushed to eliminate any air. Then the clamp was released. The occluder was advanced with the pusher catheter and delivered into the left atrium. The occluder was then positioned over the atrial septum occluding the defect under fluoroscopic and echocardiographic monitoring. The pusher catheter was removed and the sheath was clamped. The valved sheath piece was detached. The counteroccluder was loaded over the loading wire and advanced into the sheath. The valved sheath was reinserted, the system was flushed, and the clamp was removed. The counteroccluder was advanced over the wire with the pusher catheter and delivered into the right atrium while still on the loading wire. After ensuring that the occluder is in place, buttoning was performed by advancing the counteroccluder over the wire with the tip of the sheath, while applying gentle traction on the occluder with the delivery wire. Once the buttonhole of the counteroccluder passes over the button of the occluder loop, buttoning has taken place and can be verified by fluoroscopy (Figure 3.2). The radiopaque component of the counteroccluder is past the radiopaque button. The position of the device was verified by echocardiography and the device was disconnected by initially cutting the loading wire and withdrawing it, fol-

lowed by the removal of the folded nylon thread. During the latter two maneuvers, the tip of the sheath was held against the device to prevent applying excessive force on the device. The sheath tip was then withdrawn into the abdominal inferior vena cava. A final echocardiogram was performed to document the position of the device and residual shunts, if any. Repeat oxygen saturation data and pulmonary arteriogram to visualize the levoangiographic phase were performed in the first 80 patients in this series. During the subsequent cases, these data were not recorded because of concern of the potential for device dislodgment; echocardiographic data were used instead to assess residual shunts.

Heparin was administered before introducing the long sheath. Additional doses were given, depending on activated clotting time (ACT) levels and maintain them above 200s. The femoral arterial line was placed for monitoring blood pressure during the procedure. Ancef 25 mg/kg (or 1 g in adults) was given in the catheterization laboratory and two additional doses were given 6 and 12 hours later. Oral aspirin (5 to 10 mg/kg/day as a single dose or 325 mg in adults) was given for 6 to 12 weeks. Most, if not all, patients were discharged on the morning following the procedure after a chest x-ray and echocardiogram were repeated.

Study Subjects

Between September 1989 and February 1993, 180 patients underwent closure of their ASDs with first-, second-, and third-generation buttoned devices (single button). These device implantations were from among 200 patients taken to the catheterization laboratory with intent to occlude at 16 institutions around the world (7). Twenty patients did not undergo closure for various reasons. The patients were 0.6 to 76 years of age, with a median of 7 years. Their weights varied between 3.6 and 105 kg (median, 22 kg).

ASDs

Ostium secundum ASD with left-to-right shunt was the reason for closure in 168 children and adults. Patent foramen ovale or ASD presumed to be the site of paradoxic embolism was the reason for closure in the remaining 12 adults. The echocardiographic diameter of the ASD was 10.6 ± 3.8 mm (range, 5 to 25 mm). Pulmonary-to-systemic flow ratio (Qp:Qs) varied from 1.5 to 3.8 (2.1 ± 0.6). Balloon-stretched diameter was 15.8 ± 4.6 mm, with a range of 5 to 25 mm.

Devices

Implanted device size varied between 25 and 50 mm. The most commonly used devices were 40 (N = 52) and 35 mm (N = 50). Nine first-generation, 106 second-generation, and 65 third-generation devices were used. The devices were delivered to implantation site via 8F sheath in 148 patients and via 9F sheath in the remaining 32 patients.

Immediate Results

The device was successfully implanted in 166 (92%) of 180 patients. The unsuccessful implantations will be detailed in the "Complications" section to follow. The Qp:Qs decreased (2.1 ± 0.6 versus 1.05 ± 0.1; $p < .01$) in the 80 patients in whom such data were recorded. Auscultatory finding of ASD disappeared. Right ventricular volume over-loading improved on postdevice echocardiograms. The device is seen well positioned across the defect (Figure 3.7). Effective occlusion, defined as trivial ($N = 62$) or no ($N = 92$) residual shunt (Table 3.2) was found in 154 (92%) patients.

Complications

Separation of the occluder and counteroccluder from each other, termed *unbuttoning,* occurred in 13 (7.2%) patients. The entire device was seen embolizing into the main pulmonary artery in one (0.6%) child. Device dislodgments occurred while the patients were in the catheterization laboratory in ten patients. In the remaining four patients,

device dislodgments were observed 4 hours to 4 weeks after the procedure. In ten patients urgent surgery was performed to retrieve the device and the ASD was closed at the same time. In the remaining four patients, transcatheter retrieval of the device was performed in the catheterization laboratory and the ASDs were closed surgically later. No other major complications occurred.

The causes of unbuttoning were investigated in terms of cardiologist's experience and device type. Unbuttoning occurred in 12 instances in the hands of an inexperienced operator, defined as having performed fewer than ten cases. Whereas this was higher (Figure 3.8) than that seen with experienced investigators, this difference did not attain statistical significance ($p = .06$). There was decreasing unbuttoning rate (Figure 3.3) with successive generations of the device, but again, this was not statistically different ($p > .1$).

Follow-up

Clinical, chest x-ray and echocardiographic evaluation were performed 1, 6, and 12 months after device closure and yearly thereafter. Follow-up data were available for review in all patients. The duration of follow-up was 1 to 7 years, with a median of 4 years (46 ± 20 months) (22,24). Fourteen (8%) patients underwent surgical ($N = 13$) or transcatheter ($N = 1$) intervention to treat residual shunts ($N = 12$) or core-wire migration ($N = 2$). Actuarial event-free

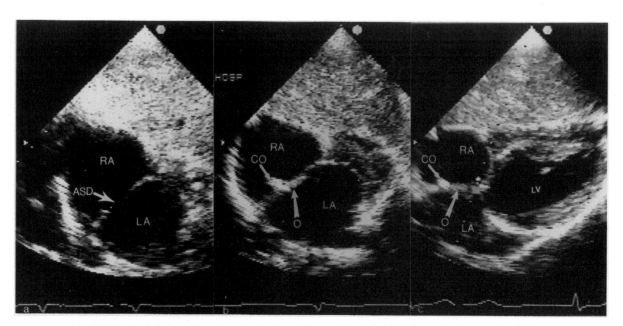

FIGURE 3.7. Subcostal four-chamber echocardiographic views of the interatrial septum showing an atrial septal defect (ASD) prior to closure (a) and the device in place in the afternoon (b) and 3 months (c) after implantation of the device. Large arrows in b and c point to the occluder (O) on the left atrial (LA) side of the atrial septum and smaller arrows show counteroccluder (Co) on end in the right atrium (RA). LV, left ventricle. (From Rao PS, Wilson AD, Levy JM, et al. Role of "buttoned" double-disc device in the management of atrial septal defects. *Am Heart J* 1992;123: 191–200, with permission.)

TABLE 3.2. GRADING OF THE ATRIAL SHUNT BY ECHO-DOPPLER STUDIES

Grade	Criteria
None	No defect by two-dimensional echocardiogram
	No color Doppler disturbance on the right atrial side of the device
	No RV volume overload*
Trivial	No defect by two-dimensional echocardiogram
	Minimal color disturbance on the right atrial side of the device (<1 mm width at the origin of the color Doppler jet)
	No RV volume overload*
Small	No defect by two-dimensional echocardiogram
	1 to 2 mm width of color Doppler jet, either in the center or on the periphery of the device
	No RV volume overload*
Moderate	Defect visualized on two-dimensional echocardiogram
	>2 mm width of color jet
	RV volume overload* may be present
Large	Defect visualized on two-dimensional echocardiogram
	Large and/or multiple color Doppler jets
	RV volume overload* present

RV, right ventricle.
*RV volume overload is defined as enlarged RV (>95th percentile for patient's body surface area) and flat to paradoxical septal motion.
From Rao PS, Sideris EB, Hausdorf G, et al. International experience with secundum atrial septal defect occlusion by the buttoned device. *Am Heart J* 1994;128:1022–1035, with permission.

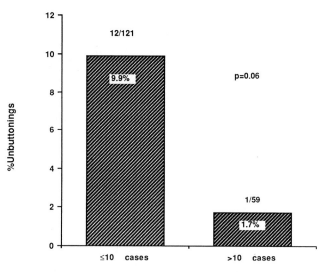

FIGURE 3.8. Bar graph demonstrating the effect of learning curve on the incidence of unbuttoning. Although there is a trend, the decrease in the unbuttoning rate with experience does not attain statistical significance (*p* = .06). (From Rao PS, Sideris EB. Buttoned device closure of the atrial septal defect. *J Interv Cardiol* 1998;11:467–484, with permission.)

rates are shown in Figure 3.9. Event-free rates were 85% at 5 and 7 years, respectively.

Core-wire migration occurred in two patients. The devices implanted were from a single batch of defectively manufactured devices that have since been withdrawn and for which the defect has been corrected. No other wire-related problems occurred.

The devices remained in place with incorporation into the atrial septum (Figures 3.7 and 3.10). There was gradual reduction in residual shunt rate (Figure 3.11). No evidence for thrombus formation or vegetations was observed during the echocardiographic evaluation.

COHORT II

Cohort II consists of 423 fourth-generation buttoned-device implantations (9), all with two radiopaque buttons, in the international trial (Table 3.1). The cohort does not include all fourth-generation devices but does include all patients in Phase II FDA-supervised trials up to September 1997.

Technique

The technique of implantation of the fourth-generation devices is similar to that described in the section on Cohort

I. However, two modifications of the technique were introduced during the double-button device trial: valve bypass and over-the-wire technique.

Valve Bypass

In the valve bypass technique, cutting of the valve component of the long sheath to introduce the device into the sheath is avoided. Instead, the occluder was loaded into a short sheath piece (similar to the French size of the long sheath) and the entire system was introduced through the

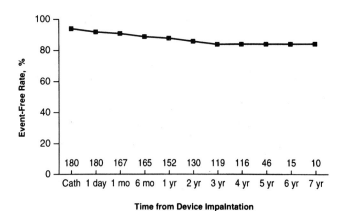

FIGURE 3.9. Graph showing actuarial event-free rates after transcatheter buttoned-device occlusion of atrial septal defects. Note high (85%) event-free rates at 6 years following device implantation. (From Rao PS, Sideris EB. Buttoned device closure of the atrial septal defect. *J Interv Cardiol* 1998;11:467–484, with permission.)

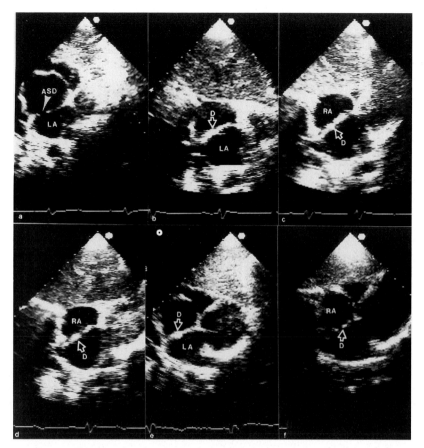

FIGURE 3.10. Selected frames from video recordings of two-dimensional echocardiographic studies in subcostal four-chamber view of the atrial septum. Before **(a)**, immediately after **(b)**, and 1 **(c)**, 6 **(d)**, 12 **(e)**, and 24 months **(f)** following buttoned-device implantation across the atrial septum to occlude ostium secundum atrial septal defect (ASD) (*arrowhead*). Note the stable position of the device (D) (*arrows*) on the atrial septum, which appears to be incorporated into the atrial septum **(f)**. There was no evidence for shunt across the device/atrial septum on pulsed or color Doppler study (not shown). LA, left atrium, RA, right atrium. (From Rao PS, Ende DJ, Wilson AD, et al. Follow-up results of transcatheter occlusion of atrial septal defects with buttoned device. *Can J Cardiol* 1995;11:695–701, with permission.)

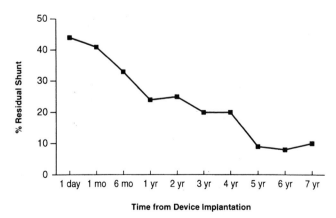

FIGURE 3.11. Resolution of residual shunts for patients who had shunts one day following device placement. (Reproduced from Rao PS, Sideris EB. Buttoned device closure of the atrial septal defect. *J Interv Cardiol* 1998;11:467–484, with permission.)

valve of the long sheath. The device was extruded into the sheath and the short sheath piece was removed. The system was then flushed and the clamp was removed. The same procedure was repeated during the introduction of the counteroccluder as well. This modification preserves the integrity of the sheath and decreases/eliminates the potential for any accidental air entry into the system. Now the short sheath piece is supplied with the device by the manufacturer.

Over-the-Wire Technique

The over-the-wire procedure is similar to the direct-delivery technique with the following exceptions: (a) a 0.025-inch Amplatz extra-stiff guide wire was used to introduce the long sheath (the dilator was removed but the wire was left in place) and (b) the foam part of the occluder (close to the middle of x) was pierced with the end of the 0.025 Amplatz wire and was retained throughout the procedure. At the end of the procedure, the guide wire was removed.

Transesophageal echographic and fluoroscopic appearances obtained during the over-the-wire technique of implantation are shown in Figures 3.12 and 3.13. This modification requires a sheath 1F size larger than the size required for direct device delivery. The advantages of this technique are (a) if the occluder slips through the ASD it can be readvanced/repositioned into the left atrium without much difficulty, (b) the occluder is easily positioned over the left atrial side of the defect and is less operator dependent, and (c) injury to the atrial walls and mitral valve is avoided (8,27).

Study Subjects

Between October 1993 and September 1997, 475 patients were taken to the catheterization laboratory with intent to occlude the ASD. Fourth-generation devices were implanted in 423 (89%) patients at 40 institutions around the world (9). The patients' age varied between 1.5 and 80 years, with a median of 16 years. The weights varied between 7 and 125 kg, with a median of 35 kg.

ASDs

The Qp:Qs was 2.1 ± 1.4, with a range of 1.5 to 3.7. The stretched diameter varied between 5 and 30 mm, with a median of 17 mm.

Devices

The size of devices used varied between 25 and 60-mm; the most commonly used devices were 35 mm ($N = 71$), 40 mm ($N = 109$), and 45 mm ($N = 73$).

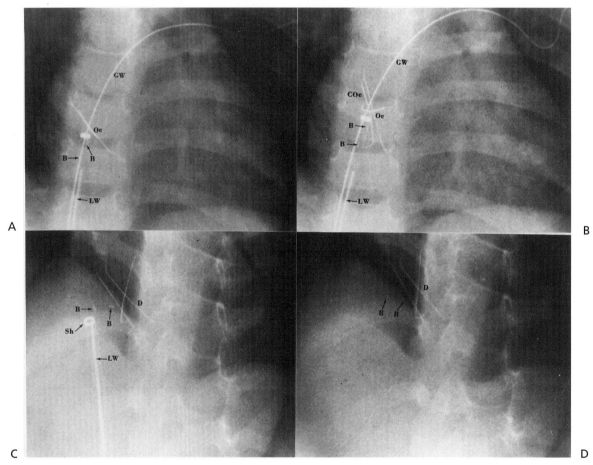

FIGURE 3.12. Selected cineradiographs demonstrating the over-the-wire device implantation. Posteroanterior views of the heart showing the position of the guide wire (GW) in the left upper pulmonary vein **(A** and **B)** with the occluder (Occ) in the left atrium **(A)** and the counteroccluder (COc) in the right atrium **(B)**. The sheath with the radiopaque tip (Sh) is in the right atrium. Radiopaque buttons (B), the loading wire (LW), and the GW are seen lodged within the sheath. Left axial oblique (30-degree LAO and 30-degree cranial) views following buttoning **(C** and **D)** demonstrate the radiopaque wire of COc is past both buttons. After removal of GW **(C)**, the device and buttons are well visualized and the sheath and LW are seen. After disconnecting the device from the LW and removal of the sheath, the device components including the buttons are well positioned **(D)** across the atrial septum (by echo). (From Rao PS, Sideris EB. Buttoned device closure of the atrial septal defect. *J Interv Cardiol* 1998;11:467–484, with permission.)

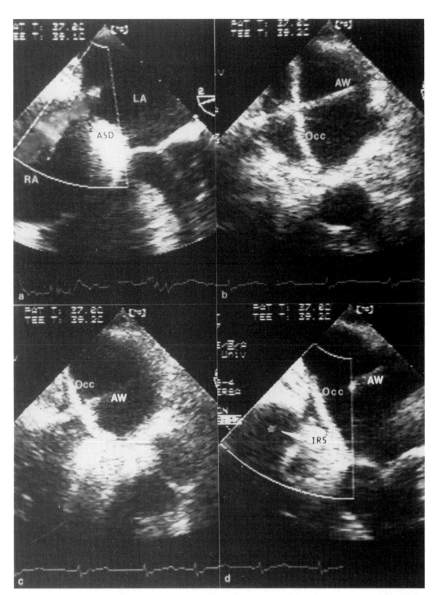

FIGURE 3.13. Selected video frames from transesophageal echocardiographic studies performed during an over-the-wire implantation of a fourth-generation buttoned device. **a:** Atrial septal defect (ASD) is shown *(arrow)*. **b, c:** The occluder (Occ) component of the device in various positions in the left atrium (LA) and the Amplatz wire (AW) passing the ASD and Occ are shown. **d:** The Occ on the left atrial side, well opposed to the ASD, is seen with tiny residual shunt (TRS).

Immediate Results

The device was successfully implanted in 422 (99.8%) of 423 patients in whom the device was released. Unbuttoning ($N = 4$) or whole-device embolization ($N = 1$) occurred in five (1.2%), and these will be described in the complications section. Effective occlusion, defined as trivial ($N = 34$) or no ($N = 343$) residual shunt (Table 3.2) on echo-Doppler study performed within 24 hours after the procedure was found in 377 (90%) of the remaining 417 patients. Detailed statistical analysis did not identify any factors predictive of residual shunts.

Complications

Major complications were encountered in six (1.4%) patients. Unbuttoning occurred in 4 (0.9%) of 423 patients. When the experience of cardiologists performing the procedure was compared [two (0.94%) in 214 versus two (0.96%) in 209; $p > .1$], there was no difference in unbuttoning rates between cardiologist with (more than ten cases performed) and without [less than ten cases performed (7)] experience. Whole-device embolization occurred in one patient. All these complications were discovered either in the catheterization laboratory ($N = 2$) or within 24 hours of the procedure (*N* = 3). In four of these patients, the device was catheter-retrieved and the patients underwent successful surgical closure of the ASD later. In the remaining patient, urgent surgical retrieval of the device along with surgical closure of the ASD were undertaken at the discretion of the primary cardiologist. In the final patient, the device was straddling the ASD on the day after the procedure. There was also a small pericardial effusion. The device was removed surgically and ASD was closed. A small perforation in the right atrium was found, which was repaired at the same time. All six patients made uneventful recovery following surgery. No other complications were observed.

Follow-up

Follow-up clinical and echo-Doppler data were available in 333 (80%) of 417 eligible patients; the median was 24 months, with a range of 1 to 60 months (9). Reintervention to treat residual shunts (*N* = 20) or mitral insufficiency (*N* = 1) was required in 21 (5%) patients. Actuarial reintervention-free rates are shown in Figure 3.14; the reintervention-free rates were 91% and 89% at 2 and 5 years, respectively. The residual shunts were treated either by surgical closure (*N* = 11) or with a second device (*N* = 9) 3 to 30 months (median 13) after device placement. The second device used to close the residual shunt was either an Amplatzer (*N* = 2) or a second buttoned device (*N* = 7) as per the preference of the primary cardiologist. In the remaining patients there was gradual decrease in the residual shunt (Figure 3.15) (9).

As seen with Cohort I, there was no evidence for vegetations or thrombus formation. No wire fractures were observed during the period of observation.

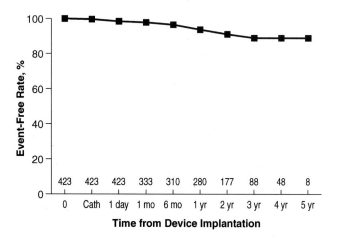

FIGURE 3.14. Graph showing actuarial event-free rates after implantation of fourth-generation buttoned device to occlude the ASD. (From Rao PS, Berger F, Rey C, et al. Results of transvenous occlusion of secundum atrial septal defects with the fourth generation buttoned device: comparison with first, second and third generation devices. *J Am Coll Cardiol* 2000;36;583–592, with permission.)

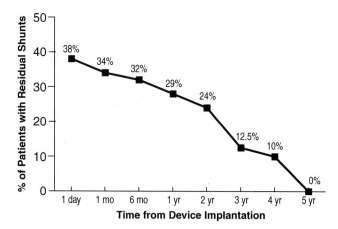

FIGURE 3.15. Time course of percent residual atrial shunts following fourth-generation buttoned-device implantation. (From Rao PS, Berger F, Rey C, et al. Results of transvenous occlusion of secundum atrial septal defects with the fourth generation buttoned device: comparison with first, second and third generation devices. *J Am Coll Cardiol* 2000;36;583–592, with permission.)

COHORT III

Cohort III consists of 76 COD buttoned-device implantations from January 1999 through December 2000 in the international trial including patients in the FDA-supervised COD buttoned-device trials in the United States. This cohort includes 65 patients whose results were described elsewhere (28).

Technique

The device implantation technique is similar to the implantation of previous buttoned devices with some exceptions. Use of the valve bypass technique by loading the device into a loading sheath has become a standard part of the procedure. Ten to 12F long sheaths are required to deliver the device. Following the delivery of the entire device into the left atrium, the pusher catheter was advanced so that it is against the center of the device and the knots (buttons) are drawn into it. While keeping the device in the left atrium, the delivery sheath is withdrawn into the right atrium. The centering ring was then pulled with the nylon threads attached to it so that the centering rings come through the ASD (Figure 3.16), thus centering the device within the atrial defect. The nylon thread connected to the centering ring(s) is cut and removed. The loading wire is held stable while pushing the centering ring with the tip of the sheath, thus folding the centering wire onto the right atrial side of the atrial septum. The centering ring then assumes a figure-8 configuration (Figure 3.16c). The entire procedure is performed under both fluoroscopic (Figure 3.16) and transesophageal echocardiographic (Figure 3.17) monitoring. Delivering the counteroccluder, buttoning, and disconnecting the device are similar to what was described for Cohorts I and II. If centering is not needed, the centering wires can be folded onto the device in

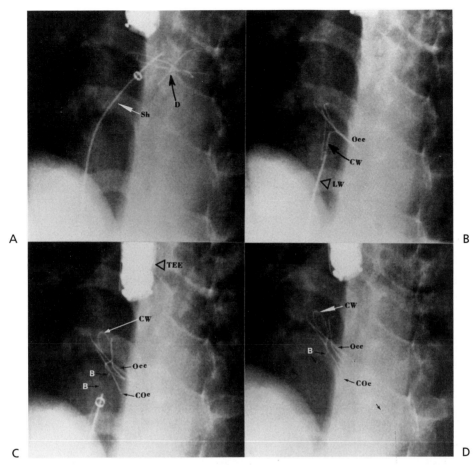

FIGURE 3.16. Selected cineradiographic frames in a left axial oblique view showing various steps in the delivery and implantation of the centering-on-demand device. **A:** Device (D) delivered into the left atrium. **B:** Occluder (Occ) is positioned against the atrial septum, and the centering wire (CW) is drawn through the atrial defect. **C:** Centering ring is folded and the counteroccluder (COc) is delivered and buttoned (B). **D:** Device after detachment from the loading wire (LW). Sh, sheath; TEE, transesophageal echo probe.

the left atrium and then the procedure can be performed in a manner similar to that of fourth-generation device implantation. In the presence of an atrial septal aneurysm (Figure 3.18), a square-shaped counteroccluder of the inverted buttoned device (29) may be positioned on the right atrial side of the aneurysm and the aneurysm can be sandwiched (Figure 3.18c,d) between the occluder and the square-shaped counteroccluder (hybrid device).

Study Subjects

During an 18-month period ending in December 2000, 80 patients with ostium secundum ASD were taken to the catheterization laboratory with intent to occlude the ASD. Of these, 76 (95%) underwent device implantation. Their ages were 1.5 to 70 years, with a median of 9 years. Their weights varied between 9.2 and 100 kg, with a median of 28 kg.

ASDs

On echocardiography, the ASDs measured 5 to 18 mm (10.5 ± 3.5 mm). Their Qp:Qs was 2.1 ± 0.7. Balloon-stretched diameter was 17.1 ± 5.8 mm; range, 9 to 30 mm.

Devices

Twenty-five- to 60-mm devices were implanted. The most commonly used device sizes were 30 mm ($N = 17$) and 35 mm ($N = 19$).

Immediate Results

The device was successfully implanted in 76 (95%) of 80 patients taken to catheterization laboratory with intent to occlude. In four patients the device was not implanted, either because rims were deficient ($N = 2$) or because the device was unstable ($N = 2$). Successful elective surgical clo-

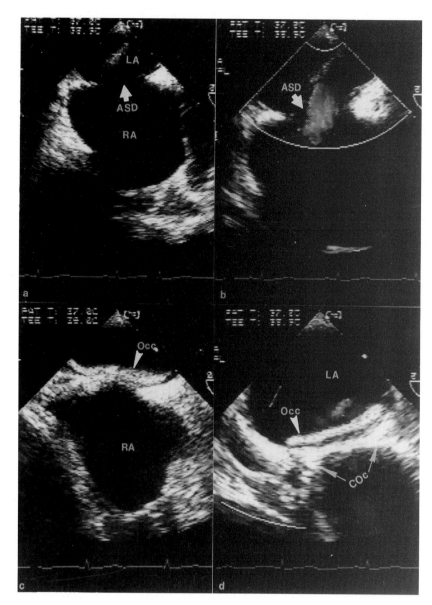

FIGURE 3.17. Selected video images from trans-esophageal echocardiographic study demonstrating the device position during centering-on-demand buttoned device implantation. Atrial septal defect (ASD) (*arrow*) is shown in **(a)** with left to right shunt (*arrow*) in **(b)**. The occluder (Occ) in **(c)** and **(d)** (*arrowheads*) and the counter–occluder (*arrows*) in **(d)** are seen across the ASD, occluding it. LA, left atrium; RA, right atrium.

sure was undertaken in all four patients. Effective occlusion, again defined as no (*N* = 51; 68%) or trivial (7) (*N* = 20; 27%) residual shunt, was observed in 71 (95%) of 76 implantations. The residual shunt was small (Table 3.2) in the remaining three patients.

Complications

A small echo-density was seen on the occluder by trans-esophageal echocardiography in one patient at the conclusion of the procedure; this was presumed to be a thrombus. Thrombolysis with tPA was opted by the primary cardiologist because of high risk for surgery in that patient (chronic lung disease and tracheostomy). The thrombus completely resorbed and the patient was discharged home 4 days after device deployment. No embolic complications were seen in

the child. No other complications were seen in the other patients in this cohort.

Follow-up

Follow-up data were available for 1 to 12 months. No reinterventions were necessary during this short period of observation.

Comparison of Cohorts

Table 3.3 compares the patient, ASD, and device characteristics of all three cohorts. As seen in the table, although there are differences in ages and weights of the cohorts, the sizes of the ASD as assessed by Qp:Qs and stretched diameter are similar in cohorts II and III. The device/defect

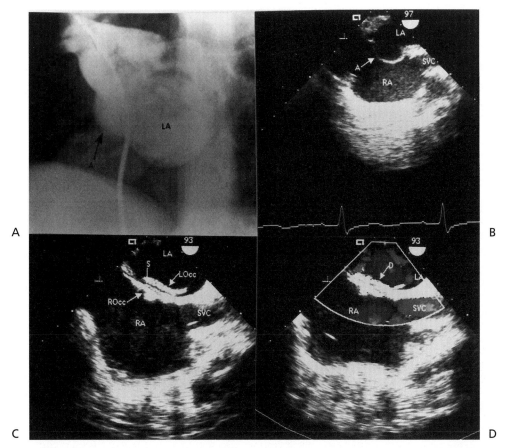

FIGURE 3.18. Selected cineangiographic and transesophageal echocardiographic frames demonstrating an atrial septal aneurysm **(A, B)** and its appearance following device implantation, sandwiching between the components of a hybrid device **(C,D)**.

TABLE 3.3. COMPARISON OF PATIENT, DEFECT AND DEVICE CHARACTERISTICS

	First-, Second-, and Third-Generation Buttoned Device	P Value	Fourth-Generation Buttoned Device	P Value	COD Buttoned Device
Total number of patients (intent to close)	200	—	475	—	80
Number (%) of patients in whom the device was implanted	180 (90%)	>0.1	423 (89%)	>0.1	76 (96%)
Age, years	14.6 ± 16.8 (range, 0.6 to 76; median, 7)	<0.001	20.8 ± 19.4 (range, 1.5 to 80; median, 16)	<0.01	15.0 ± 16.0 (range, 1.5 to 70; median, 11)
Weight, kg	31.6 ± 21.4 (range, 3.6 to 105; median, 22)	<0.001	39.6 ± 22.7 (range, 7 to 125; median, 35)	<0.05	33.8 ± 22.0 (range, 9.2 to 100; median, 28)
Size of ASD Qp:Qs	2.1 ± 0.6 (range, 1.5 to 3.8)	>0.1	2.1 ± 1.4 (range, 1.5 to 3.7)	>0.1	2.1 ± 0.7 (range, 1.5 to 4.2)
Stretched diameter, mm	15.8 ± 3.8 (range, 5 to 24)	<0.001	17.3 ± 5.3 (range, 5 to 30)	>0.1	17.1 ± 5.8 (range, 9 to 30)
Devices used	25 to 50 mm	—	25 to 60 mm	—	25 to 60 mm
Device/defect ratio	2.3 ± 0.3	>0.1	2.35 ± 0.8	<0.01	2.1 ± 0.2

ASD, atrial septal defect; COD, centering on demand.

TABLE 3.4. COMPARISON OF IMMEDIATE AND FOLLOW-UP RESULTS

	First-, Second-, and Third-Generation Buttoned Devices	P Value	Fourth-Generation Buttoned Devices	P Value	COD Buttoned Devices
Ratio of device implants to number of subjects taken to catheterization lab	180/200 (90%)	>0.1	423/475 (89%)	<0.01	76/80 (95%)
Ratio of successful implants/ number implanted	166/180 (92.2%)	<0.001	417/423 (98.6%)	>0.1	76/76 (100%)
Total major complications	14/180 (7.8%)	<0.001	6/423 (1.4%)	>0.1	1/76 (1.3%)
Unbuttoning rates	13/180 (7.2%)	<0.001	4/423 (0.9%)	>0.1	0/76 (0)
Effective occlusion rates	154/168 (92%)	>0.1	377/417 (90%)	>0.1	72/76 (95%)
Duration of follow-up	46 ± 20 (1 mo to 7 yr)	<0.001	23 ± 15 (1 mo to 5 yr)	<0.001	6 ± 6 (1 to 12 mo)
Reintervention rates	14/166 (8%)	<0.02	21/417 (5%)	<0.02	0/76 (0)
Actuarial reintervention-free rates at 1, 2, and 5 years, respectively, after successful implantation	93.5%, 92.1%, and 89.8%	>0.1	95.3%, 92.6%, and 90.5%	>0.1	100%

COD, centering-on-demand.

diameter ratio was similar ($p > .1$) between cohorts I and II but was smaller ($p < .01$) in Cohort III.

Table 3.4 summarizes the immediate and follow-up results in all three cohorts. With the COD device there was improvement in the device implantation rates. The unbuttoning rates decreased with successive cohorts. The effective occlusion rates improved with the COD device. The reintervention-free rates improved with each successive cohort, although the duration of follow-up was too short with COD devices to make any valid conclusions.

OTHER APPLICATIONS OF THE BUTTONED DEVICE

The buttoned device has also been effectively used in occluding the following:

1. ASDs/patent foramen ovale (PFO) associated with cerebrovascular accidents and transient ischemic attacks presumed to be related paradoxical embolism (7,26,30).
2. ASDs/PFOs causing right-to-left shunt and systemic arterial hypoxemia in association with postoperative complex cardiac defects, including fenestrated Fontan (29).
3. ASDs/PFOs that are sites of right-to-left shunt in platypnea/orthodeoxia syndrome of the elderly (31,32).

The device is also useful in occluding patent ductus arteriosus (33–35), ventricular septal defect (36), and aortopulmonary window (37). Some of these are discussed in greater detail in other chapters in this book.

APPLICABILITY IN ADULT SUBJECTS

In the preceding three cohorts, adult subjects have been included and were 32 (18%) in Cohort I, 183 (43%) in

Cohort II, and 22 (29%) in Cohort III. Generally, the results in adults paralleled those observed in the pediatric patients. A careful comparison (38,39) of adult subjects in Cohorts I and II (Table 3.5) revealed reduction of unbuttoning rates (12% versus 1.6%; $p < .01$) while maintaining similar effective occlusion rates (96% versus 85%; $p > .1$). the reintervention rates during follow-up also appear to have decreased (11% versus 3.5%; $p < .05$). In adult subjects of Cohort III, there was continued improvement in feasibility and effectiveness. The results of buttoned-device occlusion in adult subjects are similar to those seen in children, and there was progressive improvement of device performance with successive modifications of the device.

DISCUSSION

The COD buttoned-device results are good and are better than earlier generations of the device. The unbuttoning rate decreased after introduction of double button, but after the introduction of the COD device, the unbuttoning is eliminated. The effective occlusion rates are similar in cohorts I and II (92% and 90%), and remain excellent (95%) in the COD cohort. There was progressive improvement of the reintervention-free rates with the successive cohorts. The minor disadvantages of the COD devices are the requirement of a slightly larger (10F) sheath and a slightly more complex device implantation procedure than with the fourth-generation device.

All the devices in clinical trials, including the COD buttoned device, are double-disk devices with wire components. Therefore the requirement of sufficient septal rims to hold the device and complications associated with wire components are disadvantages with the use of these devices. Balloon-based

TABLE 3.5. BUTTONED DEVICE CLOSURE OF ASD IN ADULTS: IMMEDIATE AND FOLLOW-UP RESULTS

	Number Implanted	Unbuttoning Rate	Effective Occlusion	Follow-up Period	Reintervention Rate
Second and Third generation	32	12%	95%	44 ± 18 mo	11%
P value	—	<0.01	>0.1	<0.01	<0.05
Fourth generation	183	1.6%	85%	18 ± 12 mo	3.5%
P value	—	<0.05	>0.1	<0.05	<0.05
COD device	22	0	95%	6 ± 6 mo	0

ASD, atrial septal defect; COD, centering on demand.

and transcatheter patch closure techniques, described elsewhere (25) and in a chapter in this book, may be useful in closing defects not amenable to double-disk devices.

CURRENT STATUS

The device is under FDA-approved clinical trials in the United States. It is, however, available outside the United States for general clinical use with the approval of local IRBs.

CONCLUSION

A number of modifications have been undertaken since the initial descriptions of the buttoned device in late 1980s. The latest modification is the COD device, which is a rounded fourth-generation double-button device with a centering mechanism. The ratio of successful device implantations to the number of subjects taken to the catheterization laboratory with intent to treat has increased with this new device. Defects larger than what could be occluded with earlier-generation devices can be effectively closed with the COD device. Because of the centering mechanism, smaller devices than needed in earlier-generation devices are adequate. Unbuttoning of the device components has been abolished, and effective occlusion rates remained good. However, longer-term follow-up data than are currently available are needed to further substantiate the utility of the COD buttoned device.

ACKNOWLEDGMENT

The author acknowledges the contributions of E. B. Sideris, MD, for his innovative efforts in the development of the buttoned device discussed in this chapter. The author also thanks the investigators listed in authorship and acknowledgement sections of references 7 and 9 for their contributions to the clinical material related to the buttoned device.

REFERENCES

1. King TD, Mills NL. Nonoperative closure of atrial septal defects. *Surgery* 1974;75:383–388.
2. Mills NL, King TD. Nonoperative closure of left-to-right shunts. *J Thorac Cardiovasc Surg* 1976;72:371–378.
3. King TD, Thompson SL, Steiner C, et al. Secundum atrial septal defect; nonoperative closure during cardiac catheterization. *JAMA* 1976;235:2506–2509.
4. Chopra PS, Rao PS. History of the development of atrial septal defect occlusion devices. *Curr Interv Cardiol Rep* 2000;2:63–69.
5. Sideris EB, Sideris SE, Fowlkes JP, et al. Transvenous atrial septal occlusion in piglets using a "buttoned" double-disc device. *Circulation* 1990;81:312–318.
6. Rao PS, Wilson AD, Levy JM, et al. Role of "buttoned" double-disc device in the management of atrial septal defects. *Am Heart J* 1992;123:191–200.
7. Rao PS, Sideris EB, Hausdorf G, et al. International experience with secundum atrial septal defect occlusion by the buttoned device. *Am Heart J* 1994;128:1022–1035.
8. Sideris EB, Rao PS. Transcatheter closure of atrial septal defects: role of buttoned devices. *J Invasive Cardiol* 1996;8:289–296.
9. Rao PS, Berger F, Rey C, et al. Results of transvenous occlusion of secundum atrial septal defects with the fourth generation buttoned device: comparison with first, second and third generation devices. *J Am Coll Cardiol* 2000;36:583–592.
10. Sideris EB, Sideris SE, Thanopoulos BD, et al. Transvenous atrial septal defect occlusion by the "buttoned" device. *Am J Cardiol* 1990;66:1524–1526.
11. Rao PS, Sideris EB, Chopra PS. Catheter closure of atrial septal defect: successful use in a 3.6 kg infant. *Am Heart J* 1991;121:1826–1829.
12. Rao PS, Langhough R. Relationship to echographic, shunt flow, and angiographic size to the stretched diameter of the atrial septal defect. *Am Heart J* 1991;122:505–508.
13. Rao PS, Langhough R, Beekman RH, et al. Echocardiographic estimation of balloon-stretched diameter of secundum atrial septal defects for transcatheter occlusion. *Am Heart J* 1992;124:172–175.
14. King TD, Thompson SL, Steiner C, et al. Measurement of atrial septal defect during cardiac catheterization: experimental and clinical trials. *Am J Cardiol* 1978;41:537–542.
15. Rao PS, Wilson AD, Chopra PS. Transcatheter closure of atrial septal defects by "buttoned" devices. *Am J Cardiol* 1992;69:1056–1061.
16. Arora R, Trehan VK, Karla GS, et al. Transcatheter closure of atrial septal defect using buttoned device: Indian experience. *Indian Heart J* 1996;48:145–149.
17. Haddad J, Secches A, Finzi L, et al. Atrial septal defect: percutaneous transvenous occlusion with the buttoned device. *Arq Bras Cardiol* 1996;67:17–22.
18. Rao PS, Ende DJ, Wilson AD, et al. Follow-up results of transcatheter occlusion of atrial septal defects with buttoned device. *Can J Cardiol* 1995;11:695–701.
19. Lloyd TR, Rao PS, Beekman RH III, et al. Atrial septal defect

occlusion with the buttoned device: a multi-institutional U.S. trial. *Am J Cardiol* 1994;73:286–291.

20. Worms AM, Bourlon F, Hausdorf G, et al. European clinical trials of atrial septal defect closure with buttoned device: early and mid-term results in 125 patients. *Cardiol Young* 1994(Suppl).

21. Worms AM, Rey C, Bourlan F, et al. French experience in the closure of atrial septal defects of the ostium secundum type with Sideris buttoned occluder. *Arch Mal Coeur Vaiss* 1996;89:509–515.

22. Rao PS, Sideris EB. Buttoned device closure of the atrial septal defect. *J Interv Cardiol* 1998;11:467–484.

23. Zamora R, Rao PS, Lloyd TR, et al. Intermediate-term results of Phase I FDA trial of buttoned device occlusion of secundum atrial septal defects. *J Am Coll Cardiol* 1998;31:674–678.

24. Rao PS, Sideris EB, Rey C, et al. Echo-Doppler follow-up evaluation after transcatheter occlusion of atrial septal defects with the buttoned device. In: Imai Y, Momma K, eds. *Proceedings of the Second World Congress of Pediatric Cardiology and Cardiac Surgery.* Armonk, NY: Futura, 1998:197–200.

25. Zamora R, Rao PS, Sideris EB. Buttoned device for atrial septal defect occlusion. *Curr Interv Cardiol Rep* 2000;2:167–176.

26. Chandar JS, Rao PS, Lloyd TR, et al. Atrial septal defect closure with 4th generation buttoned device; results of US multicenter FDA Phase II clinical trial (abstract). *Circulation* 1999;100:I–708.

27. Onorato E, Berger F, Rey C, et al. Atrial septal defect repair by the buttoned device placed over a wire; early follow-up results, comparison to direct placement (Abstract). *Cardiol Young* 1996;(Suppl)6:5.

28. Rao PS, Sideris EB. Centering-on-demand buttoned device: its role in transcatheter occlusion of atrial septal defects. *J Interv Cardiol* 2001;14:

29. Rao PS, Chandar JS, Sideris EB. Role of inverted buttoned device in transcatheter occlusion of atrial septal defects or patent foramen ovale with right-to-left shunting associated with previously operated complex congenital cardiac anomalies. *Am J Cardiol* 1997;80:914–921.

30. Ende DJ, Chopra PS, Rao PS. Prevention of recurrence of paradoxic embolism: mid-term follow-up after transcatheter closure of atrial defects with buttoned device. *Am J Cardiol* 1996;78:233–236.

31. Godort F, Porte HL, Rey C, et al. Post-pneumonectomy interatrial right-to-left shunting successful percutaneous treatment. *Ann Thorac Surg* 1997;64:834–836.

32. Rao PS, Palacios IF, Bach RG, et al. Platypnea-orthodeoxia: management by transcatheter buttoned device implantation (Abstract). *J Am Coll Cardiol* 2000;35:199A.

33. Rao PS, Sideris EB, Haddad J, et al. Transcatheter occlusion of patent ductus arteriosus with adjustable buttoned device: initial clinical applications. *Circulation* 1993;88:1119–1126.

34. Rao PS, Kim SH, Rey C, et al. Results of transvenous buttoned device occlusion of patent ductus arteriosus in adults. *Am J Cardiol* 1998;8:827–829.

35. Rao PS, Kim SH, Choi J, et al. Follow-up results of transvenous occlusion of patent ductus arteriosus with the buttoned device. *J Am Coll Cardiol* 1999;33:820–826.

36. Sideris EB, Walsh KP, Haddad J, et al. Occlusion of congenital ventricular septal defects by the buttoned device. *Heart* 1997;77:276–279.

37. Jureidini SB, Spadaro JJ, Rao PS. Aortopulmonary window: successful transcatheter closure with buttoned device in an adult. *Am J Cardiol* 1998;81:371–372.

38. Rao PS, Sideris EB, Bourlon F, et al. Transcatheter buttoned device closure of secundum atrial septal defects in adults. follow-up results (Abstract). *Circulation* 1997;96(Suppl) I–217.

39. Rao PS, Berger F, Schrader R, et al. Transvenous occlusion of atrial septal defects in adults with fourth generation buttoned device (Abstract). *Circulation* 1998;98(Suppl) I–716.

4

ASDOS—ATRIAL SEPTAL DEFECT OCCLUDER SYSTEM

UROS U. BABIC
HORST SIEVERT
MARTIN SCHNEIDER
MAJA BABIC

Porstmann pioneered the catheter-based closure of cardiovascular defects in 1967 (1). King and, later on, Rashkind extended these adventurous attempts to intracardiac communications (2,3).

In the late 1980s no device for transcatheter closure of atrial septal defects (ASD) was commercially available in Europe. Between 1985 and 1990, a large number of patients with mitral valve stenosis underwent balloon dilatation of the mitral valve throughout the world. In addition to the congenital interatrial defects, a new large patient population with iatrogenic ASD created during the balloon dilatation of mitral valve emerged. The need for an ASD occlusion system (ASDOS) was obvious. The ASDOS was conceived to overcome this shortage.

THE ASDOS PROTOTYPE

The device consisted of two self-opening umbrellas made of stainless steel. A patch of homologous pericardium was sewn on the left atrial umbrella. This patch was obtained and preserved by the method used for the aortic valve homograft (4). To ensure device centering, compressed Ivalon (polyvinyl alcohol, which swells on contact with blood) was placed between the two umbrellas. The implantation technique was different from that used with previous devices in that it required the creation of a venoarterial long wire track using the technique originally reported by Babic et al. (5,6). This wire track was covered with the 6F catheter from the arterial side and with the 14F introducing sheath from the venous side. The left atrial umbrella, then the Ivalon, and the right

Uros U. Babic: Internal Medicine Resident, Babic Cardiology Clinic, Belgrade, Yugoslavia

Horst Sievert: Professor of Internal Medicine and Cardiology, Cardiovascular Center Bethanien, Frankfurt, Germany

Martin Schneider: Assistant Professor of Pediatrics, Division of Pediatric Cardiology, Charite University, Berlin, Germany

Maja Babic: Babic Cardiology Clinic, Belgrade, Yugoslavia

atrial umbrella were introduced transvenously, one after the other over the wire track. The hypothetical advantages of the loop technique were the following:

1. Ability to introduce the components of the occluder separately and to manipulate them on both septal sides.
2. Versatility of the system to achieve an optimal positioning before definite device anchoring.
3. No risk of loosening the device during implantation.
4. Possibility of performing simultaneous selective left atriography to check the amount of residual shunting during positioning maneuver.

Mounted on the tracking wire (which had a conus barrier at its middle to prevent distal movement of the device toward the mitral valve), the screw of the left atrial umbrella pointed toward the right umbrella, which had the fitting thread for the screw. The guide wire went through the center of both umbrellas and the center of Ivalon. The umbrellas were joined and interlocked at the level of the ASD, compressing the Ivalon between them and thus enabling a good centering (Figure 4.1). The positioning of the system was controlled by selective left atriography. Once interlocked, the umbrellas could not be separated (which was a big disadvantage of this ASDOS prototype). In case the position of the interlocked system was not satisfactory, it had to be retrieved surgically. The initial experience with this prototype on a small number of patients was promising (7,8). In 1994, Osypka Company GmbH of Germany licensed the ASDOS system for further refinement and commercialization.

THE CERTIFIED ASDOS DEVICE

The ASDOS (Atrial Septal Defect Occluder System; Osypka GmbH, Germany) consists of two major components: delivery system (Figure 4.2) and prosthesis consisting of two self-opening umbrellas made of a Nitinol wire frame and a thin membrane of polyurethane. Each umbrella has

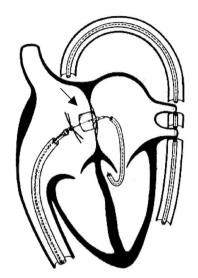

FIGURE 4.1. The ASDOS prototype had an Ivalon plug *(arrow)* between the umbrellas which provided an easier centering.

five arms that assume a round shape in the open position. When joined together, the umbrellas assume a discoid shape in profile and a "flower" shape in the frontal view.

TECHNIQUE

General anesthesia was used in children and those adults who could not tolerate a transesophageal echocardiographic (TEE) probe well. The right femoral venous and left femoral arterial access was accomplished and heparin was given to achieve an activated clotting time of more than 300 seconds. Fluid was administered intravenously to increase the right atrial pressure to more than zero. The 11F long introducer sheath with the

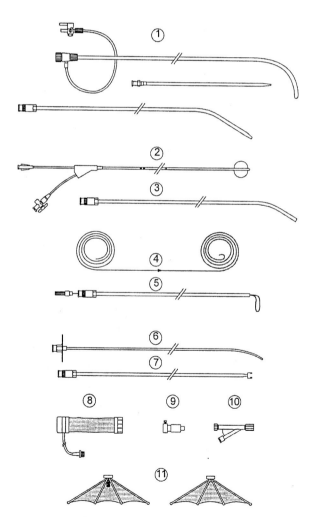

FIGURE 4.2. ASDOS system scheme: *1,* 11F long introducing sheath; *2,* 7F end-open floating balloon catheter; *3,* 6F arterial (i.e., left atrial catheter); *4,* 0.014-inch, 450 cm long, ASDOS Nitinol J guide wire with a conus; *5,* snare catheter; *6,* 20-gauge metal cannula; *7,* torquer catheter; *8,* air embolism protector "air back"; *9,* contact keeper; *10,* Y connector; *11,* umbrellas.

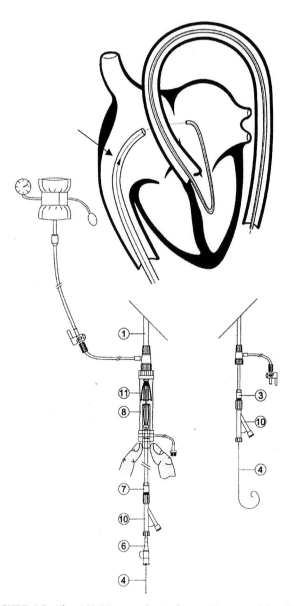

FIGURE 4.3. The ASDOS procedure scheme. Venoarterial guide wire track is arranged. The conus on the long wire within the long sheath *(arrow).* The umbrellas are folded and introduced into the plastic bag "air back," where the air bubbles are removed. Numbering is as in Figure 4.2.

fluid-filled plastic bag ("air bag") attached to its proximal end was placed transvenously into the left atrium. A pressurized infusion line was connected to the side arm of the long sheath. The venoarterial wire track was created with the 0.014- inch, 450-cm-long ASDOS J-wire. Over this wire, a 6F left coronary guiding catheter was advanced transarterially to the left atrium. The assembled occluder system was introduced over the long wire into the fluid-filled plastic bag, where the air bubbles were removed (Figure 4.3). The unit was advanced until the left atrial umbrella was at the tip of the introducer sheath situated within the left atrium. Extrusion of the left umbrella was achieved by retracting the introducer sheath. The metal conus on the long wire prevented any distal movement of the umbrella. When the long wire was pulled from the venous side, the left atrial umbrella was secured to the tip

of the transseptal cannula from the right side and to the metal conus from the left side. When the torquer catheter was pushed over the metal cannula, the right atrial umbrella was advanced to the right atrium, where it was opened by retracting the sheath (Figure 4.4A). The appropriate anchoring place was found by individual manipulation with the metal cannula and torquer catheter. The umbrellas were then interlocked by the screw mechanism (Figure 4.4B). The torquer catheter and the metal cannula were released from the umbrellas and retracted into the lower right atrium, leaving the interlocked umbrellas anchored but still on the long guide wire (Figure 4.4C). The positioning was guided by the TEE and selective simultaneous left atriography. If the position was not satisfactory, the metal cannula and the torquer catheter were readvanced, and the umbrellas were separated from each other and

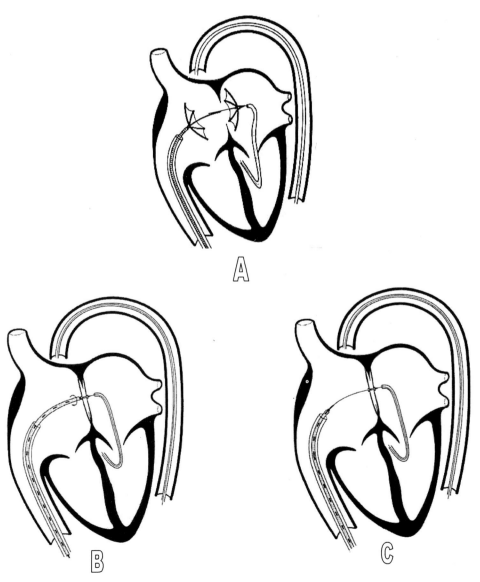

FIGURE 4.4. The scheme of the ASDOS procedure. **A:** The system is being held on the continuous wire, the umbrellas open within the atria. **B:** The umbrellas are centered with the transseptal cannula and screwed together with the torquer. **C:** The device is anchored but still held on the wire, which (if the occluder position is good) is withdrawn via the left atrial catheter.

repositioned. This maneuver could be repeated several times until a good position was found. If the position and stability of the placed umbrellas appeared good, the tracking wire was removed via the left atrial catheter out the femoral artery. Systemic anticoagulation with warfarin (for adults) or antiaggregation with aspirin (for children) was administered for 6 months. Endocarditis prophylaxis was recommended for 12 months. If the umbrellas could not be anchored satisfactorily, they were retrieved through the same 11F introducing sheath. The umbrellas were separated from each other. The right umbrella was taken with the torquer catheter and withdrawn together with the metal cannula. The cannula was readvanced to affix the left atrial umbrella. The snare catheter was advanced over the metal cannula and over the left atrial umbrella through the same sheath. Its snare was opened and advanced over the left umbrella to catch the middle of the long wire leftward from the umbrella. The middle of the long wire was then exteriorized through the sheath, turning round the left atrial umbrella toward the sheath. This enabled the pulling of the left umbrella into the sheath and its removal (9).

ANIMAL EXPERIMENTAL STUDY

The experiments were performed in the laboratory of The Institute of Experimental Clinical Research at Skejby Sygehus, Aarhus University Hospital, Denmark (10,11). The ASDOS implantation technique was utilized on 20 mixed-breed pigs, Danish Landrace and Yorkshire, of both genders, weighing around 30 kg. The interatrial communication was created with a dilatation balloon and subsequently closed with the ASDOS. After 3, 4, and 6 months, respectively, the animals were taken to the laboratory to be reexamined and euthanized. All devices were completely covered with smooth, scarlike tissue after 3 months. No leg fractures occurred. No sign of thrombotic material or excrescences were seen. Signs of chronic inflammation around the device were detected in all cases. The inflammatory response declined with increasing distance from the device, and a pseudomembrane delimited the device from the surrounding tissue. Thus a foreign-body reaction of variable degree was found. This reaction declined with increased interval from the time of implantation. In one case there was evidence of pericardial adhesions indicating a possible inflammatory etiology. No injury of the mitral valve and nearby cardiac structures was observed. No evidence for hemolysis or systemic immunologic reaction was observed.

EXPERIENCE WITH CLINICAL USE OF ASDOS

The refined ASDOS version was first utilized for closure of large ASDs in Frankfurt by Sievert et al. (12,13). The defects of 26 to 35 mm were closed with ASDOS umbrellas 45 to 60 mm in diameter in five adult patients who opted for catheter closure before undergoing surgery, which was recommended. The procedure was guided by selective

left atriography without TEE. The prosthesis was implanted in all patients (one required a second session). Dislodgment of 60-mm umbrellas and left atrial perforation with a 55-mm prosthesis required surgery in two patients 8 hours and 2 weeks after the procedure, respectively. A single umbrella-arm fracture was noticed in one patient 4 months after the implantation. Hausdorf and Schneider initiated the use of the ASDOS for closure of ASDs in pediatric patients (14). Ten children with a secundum ASD 10 to 20 mm in diameter underwent the catheter closure with ASDOS prostheses 25 to 40 mm in diameter. The closure was successful in nine out of ten patients. Except for a transitory atrioventricular (AV) block in one case, no complications were observed. The procedure was guided by the echocardiography. A trace of residual shunt could be detected in one patient months after implantation. Between 1995 and 1997, a multiinstitutional clinical trial was conducted in 20 European institutions to assess the feasibility, safety, and efficacy of the ASDOS for catheter-based closure of secundum ASD (154 patients) and patent foramen ovale (PFO) after episodes of cerebral embolism (46 patients). There were 62 children and 138 adults. Patients were included in this study if they had a secundum ASD of less than 20 mm, as determined by echocardiography, or less than 25 mm, as measured by balloon sizing; a septal rim of more than 5 mm; or a PFO and repeated neurologic events. The procedure was guided by selective atriography and by the TEE (15). The procedure failed in 26 patients (13%). Procedure-related complications necessitating surgical removal of the device included device embolization in two, device entrapment within the Chiari network in one, frame fracture in one, and perforation of atrial wall in two patients. An additional 11 patients (11%) underwent surgical removal of the device during follow-up. There were 163 patients (81%) with an implanted ASDOS at follow-up of from 6 to 36 months. Dislodgment, thrombus formation, perforation, and infection were identified as implant-related complications (16). The overall use of the ASDOS was centrally registered (Sulzer-Osypka ASDOS registry) from 1995 to 1998. The data of 350 patients were available (17). There were 261 patients with a secundum ASD and 89 patients with a PFO. Table 4.1 lists the overall success and failure

TABLE 4.1. RESULTS OF ASD (261) AND PFO (89) CLOSURE WITH ASDOS

	n	%
Closure attempted	350	100
Failure	32	9
Device retrieved per catheter	26	7
Retrieved per surgery	6	2
Successfully implanted	318	91
Extracted surgically during the follow-up	11	3
Occluder in place at the present follow-up	307	87

ASDOS, atrial septal defect occluder system; PFO, patent foramen ovale.

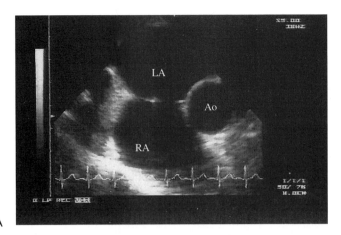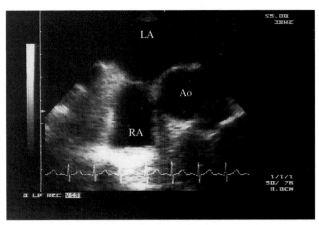

A

B

FIGURE 4.5. Transesophageal echocardiography in a patient with a hyperdynamic defect. **A:** During atrial diastole. **B:** During atrial systole. Note the significant reduction of the distance between the posterior aorta and interatrial groove during the atrial systole. Ao, aorta; LA, left atrium; RA, right atrium.

rates. Out of more than 800 preselected patients with a secundum ASD only 261 were accepted for a closure attempt with ASDOS. The most common reason for nonsuitability was the inadequacy of the residual septum posterior to the aorta. In some patients with hyperdynamic atrial excursions the diameter of the ASD during atrial diastole was larger than the diameter of the whole atrial septum during the atrial systole (Figure 4.5A, B). Implantation of a

device big enough to cover the defect and to provide a stable attachment onto the residual tissue may lead to mechanical injury of the free atrial wall in such patients. Little attention was paid to defining the texture of the residual septal tissue. In one patient a frail atrial septum could not hold the occluder and disrupted over time, leading to reappearance of the shunt, but the implant remained stable (Figure 4.6). The versatility of the ASDOS system proved

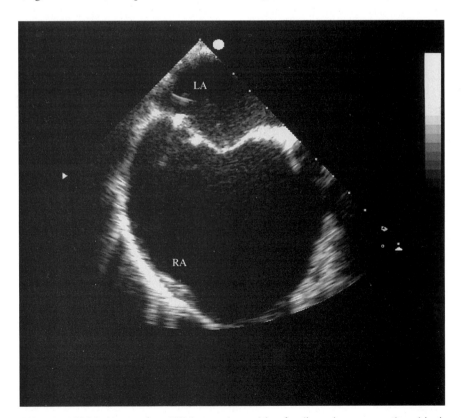

FIGURE 4.6. ASDOS closure of an ASD in a patient with a fragile and aneurysmatic residual septum. The device was too small to cover the solid portions of the residual septum and thus did not immobilize the aneurysm. In addition, there was shunt reappearance after 3 years, most probably caused by the disruption of the posterior septal portion. LA, left atrium; RA, right atrium.

to be useful for closure of secundum defects situated at the higher or at the lower portion of the atrial septum. Since the ASDOS implant was firmly attached, compressing the residual tissue between the two umbrellas, it did not move after deployment. It was possible to anchor the prosthesis at any septal level the operator regarded as appropriate. In most patients several positioning and repositioning maneuvers (up to 17 repositions in one patient) were needed to center the prosthesis properly before deployment (i.e., before removal of the tracking wire). In patients with a vertical septal orientation, pulling the device toward the inferior caval vein led to prolapse of the device (Figure 4.7B). In such cases the right atrial umbrella was first aligned to the septum by advancing it over the curved metal cannula (Figure 4.7C). The left atrial umbrella was then approached to the left septal side and the parallel alignment was achieved, enabling an optimal closure (Figure 4.7A). In patients with an oblique-horizontal topography of the septum the closure procedure was much easier.

Patients with multiperforated defects could be treated with ASDOS by placing one device that covered the whole septum through the central defect. In patients with aneurysmatic residual septum, only a large device that could be anchored onto the stable portion of the residual septum resulted in an immobilization of the septal aneurysm. The eccentrically situated defects were not regarded as suitable for closure with ASDOS. Only in cases where the eccentric defect was small and the residual tissue large, the residual septum was punctured at its center under TEE control. Subsequently, the ASDOS device was placed centrally through the puncture site covering the whole septum, including the defect situated at the periphery.

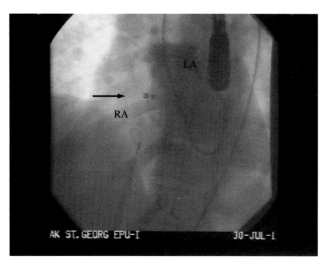

A

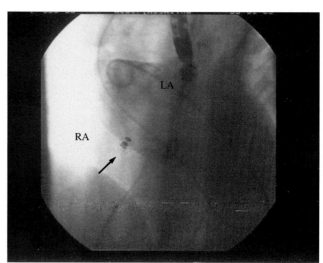

D

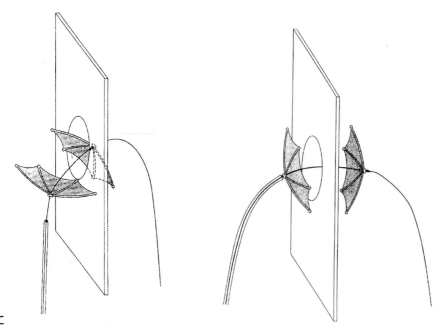

B,C

FIGURE 4.7. ASD closure in a patient with a vertical atrial septum. **A:** Selective left atriography showing a closed ASD in a patient with vertical atrial septum (*arrow*). **B:** Scheme of device prolapse by pulling it toward the inferior caval vein. **C:** Individual alignment of the both umbrellas parallel to the septum by advancing the right atrial umbrella first over the curved metal cannula. **D:** The closure is much easier in a patient with an oblique-horizontal septum (*arrow*).

Immediately after procedure, a small residual shunt remained in 28% of patients. In a very small number of these patients the shunt disappeared with time. A medium/large residual shunt was present in 8% of patients, all of whom underwent uneventful surgical closure subsequently.

COMPLICATIONS

Procedure-Related Complications

Procedure-related complications included groin hematoma (0.8%); intimal injury of the left iliac artery, which required surgical treatment in one (0.3%) patient; air embolism of the right coronary artery in two (0.6%) (terminated spontaneously); transient AV block in two (0.6%); and transient dysrhythmia in three (0.9%) patients.

Implantation-Related Complications

Frame fracture was detected in 20% of patients who had been examined by cineradiography. In two cases a fragmentation and clinically silent embolization of the fragmented arms to the right ventricle and pulmonary artery, respectively, were observed (Sievert, Hausdorf- discussion on international symposium, Frankfurt, 2000).

Thrombus formation was found in most adult patients who underwent TEE control examination during the first postocclusion week. This echo formation was limited to a 3- to 4-mm echo-layer around the device. In about 25% of these patients the TEE revealed "hamburger-like" thrombi. The thrombi reduced in size and disappeared spontaneously over time (18).

Thromboembolism occurred in three adult patients. One of these patients had a deficiency of coagulation factor XII. He suffered cerebral thromboembolism with a significant neurologic deficit and a delayed recovery (19). In a young patient who had had diagnostic catheterization via the right groin years before, venography showed a closed right iliac vein. Although the study protocol did not allow acceptance of patients with chronic venous thrombosis, the closure procedure was successfully performed from the left groin. One week after closure he developed a thromboembolism of the aortic bifurcation. The TEE revealed a thrombus on the left side of the occluder. He underwent surgery with an uneventful course. The third thromboembolism occurred in a patient after PFO closure. The thrombus embolized to the leg and had to be removed surgically. The TEE revealed a small transitory left-to-right shunt, which disappeared over the following days.

Infection occurred in two adult patients who were assumed to have a prosthetic endocarditis and underwent surgery. No hemodynamic compromise was present in either of these two patients before surgery. The described intraoperative gross findings were not convincingly suggestive of the inflammatory process. There was no access to the results of the microscopic analysis of the explanted specimens. Both of these two surgical interventions had a fatal outcome.

Dislodgment of the device occurred in five patients (two adults and three pediatric) during the first postclosure day. In one, the connected umbrellas dislodged to the right ventricle and had to be retrieved surgically. In the other four patients the joined umbrellas separated ("unbuttoning") from each other and embolized to the abdominal aorta and pulmonary artery, respectively. In one of these patients the umbrellas were removed percutaneously. The other three patients underwent surgical removal of the embolized umbrellas and ASD closure with uneventful course. There was no late device dislodgment.

Perforation of the free atrial wall with tamponade (in three) and hemopericardium (in two) occurred in five adult patients, 1 day to 8 months after implantation (20,21). All underwent surgery with an uneventful postoperative course. The perforation site could be identified only intraoperatively in two of these patients.

DISCUSSION AND CONCLUSION

The ASDOS system has existed for more than 10 years. Initially, the system had an Ivalon plug between the two umbrellas, which provided good centering and allowed closure of defects with much smaller devices. However, the incorporated device with Ivalon appeared too bulky in surgeons' eyes some months after implantation. The plug is no longer used. Instead a sophisticated delivery system provides the umbrellas with versatility. The venoarterial long tracking wire technique made the procedure much safer. The umbrellas could easily be retrieved through the same 11F sheath, and another pair of umbrellas of different size could be attempted over the same tracking wire. Since it was firmly affixed onto the septum, the implanted ASDOS prosthesis did not move after deployment. Consequently, no mechanical injury of the mitral valve occurred after ASDOS. Requiring an 11F venous and a 6F arterial access, the procedure proved applicable to both children and adults. All patients with a medium/large residual shunt after ASDOS implantation underwent surgery. Although the residual defects in some of these patients appeared amenable to closure with an additional occluder, no attempts were made to implant a second ASDOS device. After ASDOS implantation, if needed later on in the patient's life, the interatrial septum remains amenable to transseptal left heart catheterization, whether it is diagnostic or therapeutic. This might be at least of some hypothetical value. The procedure was complex and required a long learning curve. It was good for closure of a centrally situated ASD and for PFO. The PFO closure with ASDOS did not necessitate TEE guidance (nor did it require general anesthesia), since the selective left atriography provided good topographic orientation during the procedure. The results of PFO closure in reducing the number and frequency of neurologic events were encouraging. The utilization of oversized umbrellas was the biggest mistake. Very often the diameter of the implanted occluder exceeded or was equal to the septal length, and it was significantly larger than the distance between the aorta and the posterior interatrial groove. This resulted in perforation of the free atrial wall in some patients. Patients with a fragile texture of the residual septum and those with hyperdynamic defects are not good candidates for ASDOS. The experience with separation ("unbuttoning") of the implanted umbrellas in four patients indicates the need for improvement of the safety of the interlocking mechanism. The two cases of suggestive prosthetic endocarditis emphasized the need for endocarditis prophylaxis and for sterile conditions under which a permanent intracardiac prosthesis is implanted. Unfortunately, there will be no protection against possible thromboembolic complication after ASD closure with an occluder. The systemic anticoagulation appeared in our experience of no help. Therefore it seems wise to renounce it. To minimize the possibility of mechanical injury of the free atrial wall, much smaller devices should be used. In addition, the wire frame should be made softer. The improved ASDOS version is aimed at fulfilling these expectations. This latest version contains a wire stent between the umbrellas that provide optimal centering (Figure 4.8). The stent is compressed between the umbrellas, which not only avoids its protrusion into the atrial cavity but stabilizes the anchoring of the prosthesis onto the septum. In this way, a much smaller device will be sufficient to close even eccentrically situated defects. Unfortunately, this version is presently not available for clinical use.

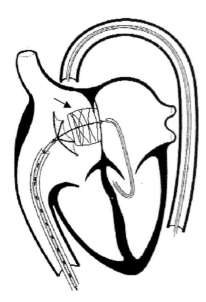

FIGURE 4.8. Latest ASDOS version contains a nitinol wire sent (*arrow*) between two umbrellas which provides a self-centering and allows the use of much smaller umbrella diameters.

CURRENT STATUS

The ASDOS system (Osypka GmbH, Rheinfelden, Germany) obtained the European Certification (CE) 3 years ago. No FDA approval is planned. Only one registered multiinstitutional European study has been conducted. The centralized registry of ASDOS use existed until the end of 1998. An improved version has been conceptualized but is unavailable for clinical use. The certified version is used occasionally in some European centers.

REFERENCES

1. Porstmann W, Wierny L, Warnke H. Der Verschluss des Ductus arteriosus persistens ohne Thoracotomie. 1. Mitteilung. *Thoraxchirurgie* 1967;15:199–203.
2. King TD, Mills NL. Secundum atrial septal defect: Nonoperative closure during cardiac Catheterization. *JAMA* 1976;235:2506–2509.
3. Rashkind WJ. Transcatheter treatment of congenital heart disease. *Circulation* 1983;67:711–716.
4. Collins LJ, Clarke DB, Smith AR. *D'Abreu's practice of cardiothoracic surgery.* London: Edward Arnold, 1976:457–460.
5. Babic UU, Pejcic P, Djurisic Z, et al. Percutaneous transarterial balloon valvuloplasty for mitral valve stenosis. *Am J Cardiol* 1986;57:1101–1104.
6. Babic UU, Dorros G, Pejcic P, et al. Percutaneous mitral valvuloplasty: retrograde, transarterial double-balloon technique utilizing the transseptal approach. *Cathet Cardiovasc Diagn* 1988;14:229–237.
7. Babic UU, Grujicic S, Djurisic Z, et al. Transcatheter closure of atrial septal defect (letter). *Lancet* 1990;336:566–567.
8. Babic UU, Grujicic S, Popovic Z, et al. Double-umbrella device for transvenous closure of patent ductus arteriosus and atrial septal defect: first experience. *J Interv Cardiol* 1991;4:283–294.
9. Babic UU. The ASDOS device: technique and guidelines for clinical use. *J Interv Cardiol* 1998;11:485–494.
10. Schneider M, Babic U, Thomsen BA, et al. Das ASDOS-Implantat: Tierexperimentelle Erprobung. *Z.Kardiologie* 1995(Suppl);84:9.
11. Thomsen-Bloch A. Closure of atrial septal defects with catheter technique: an animal experimental study. Doctoral diploma thesis. Aarhus University Hospital, Aarhus, Denmark, 1995.
12. Sievert H, Babic UU, Ensslen R, et al. Transcatheter closure of large atrial septal defects with the Babic system. *Cathet Cardiovasc Diagn* 1995;36:232–240.
13. Sievert H, Babic UU, Ensslen R, et al. Verschluss des Vorhofseptumdefektes mit einem neuem Okklusionssystem. *Z Kardiol* 1996;85:97–103.
14. Hausdorf G, Schneider M, Franzbach B, et al. Transcatheter closure of secundum atrial septal defects with the atrial septal defect occlusion system (ASDOS): initial experience in children. *Heart* 1996;75:83–88.
15. Fehske W, Pfeiffer D, Babic UU, et al. Multiplane transoesophageal imaging during transcatheter closure of an atrial septal defect. *Circulation* 1997;96:1702–1703.
16. Sievert H, Babic UU, Hausdorf G, et al. Transcatheter closure of atrial septal defect and patent foramen ovale with the ASDOS device (a multi-institutional European trial). *Am J Cardiol* 1998;82:1405–1413.
17. Babic UU. Experience with ASDOS for transcatheter closure of atrial septal defect and patent foramen ovale. *Curr Interv Cardiol Rep* 2000;2:177–183.

18. La Rosee K, Deutsch JH, Schnabel P, et al. Thrombus formation after transcatheter closure of atrial septal defect. *Am J Cardiol* 1999;84:356–359.

19. Gastmann O, Werner GS, Babic UU, et al. Thrombus formation on transcatheter ASD occluder device in a patient with coagulation factor XII deficiency. *Cathet Cardiovasc Diagn* 1998;43:81–83.

20. Bohm j, Bittigau K, Koehler F, et al. Surgical removal of atrial septal defect occlusion system devices. *Eur J Cardiol Thorac Surg* 1997;12:869–872.

21. Pfeiffer D, Omran H, Otto J, et al. Transvasal closure of interatrial defects using the Babic double-umbrella occluder system. *Thorac Cardiovasc Surg* 1998;46:134–140.

Catheter Based Devices: For the Treatment of Non-coronary Cardiovascular Diseases in Adults and Children. Edited by P. Syamasundar Rao and Morton J. Kern, Lippincott Williams & Wilkins, Philadelphia © 2003.

5

THE ANGEL WINGS DAS DEVICE

GLADWIN S. DAS
J. KEVIN HARRISON
MARTIN P. O'LAUGHLIN

In 1993 we reported (1) on the successful closure of atrial septal defects in dogs using a Nitinol–polyester atrial septal defect (ASD) closure device with a true self-centering mechanism. We postulated that self-centering of ASD occluders would be critical for complete closure of defects. Our initial experience with the Angel Wings Das device (Microvena Corporation, White Bear Lake, Minnesota) validated the critical role of self-centering the occluder for obtaining complete occlusions and laid the foundation for the development of the Angel Wings II , now renamed, Guardian Angel device.

THE ANGEL WINGS PROSTHESIS AND DELIVERY SYSTEM

The Angel Wings device consists of two square frames made of "superelastic" Nitinol wire (0.012-inch diameter) with radiopaque markers of platinum at each corner. Each square frame has a flexible eyelet at each corner and at the midpoint of each side of the square. These flexible eyelets function as torsion springs that permit the device to be collapsed and loaded into the delivery catheter. Polyester fabric that is sewn onto the wire frames after being stretched taut covers the wire frames. A circular hole of a diameter equal to half the length of the side of the square disk is punched out from the right atrial disk, and the margin of this orifice is sewn onto the fabric of the left-sided patch to form a conjoint suture ring. The device is available in a range of sizes from 12 to 40 mm, although most of the devices implanted were 18-, 22-, 25-, and 30-mm squares. The size of the device refers to the length of each side of the square.

Gladwin S. Das: Associate Professor of Medicine and Pediatrics, Cardiovascular Division, University of Minnesota Medical School, Minneapolis, Minnesota

J. Kevin Harrison: Assistant Professor of Medicine, Duke University Medical Center, Durham, North Carolina

Martin P. O' Laughlin: Associate Professor of Pediatrics, Duke University Medical Center, Durham, North Carolina

The device has a delivery system that consists of a control handle connected to an 11, 12, or 13F size delivery catheter (11F for the 12-mm device; 12F for the 18-, 22-, and 25-mm devices; and 13F for the 30-, 35-, and 40-mm devices). The control handle has a Y connector that permits the delivery catheter to be flushed with heparinized saline. A coaxial pusher rod within the delivery catheter permits the device to be advanced from the catheter and thereby deployed in a gradual manner by rotation of the blue actuator ring on the control handle clockwise. The device is preloaded, in the manufacturing facility, by inserting one of the eyelets of the right atrial disk into the attach–release fixture at the end of the pusher rod (1).

The Angel Wings device is locked in place by a wire running through the hollow pusher rod and placed through the attachment eyelet of the right atrial disk. The attach–release fixture is a slot in a short tube, at the tip of the pusher rod with a length of Nitinol wire that runs throughout the length of the hollow coaxial pusher rod and delivery catheter (1). This attach–release wire is fixed to the red release knob on the end of the control handle. The red release knob is first unscrewed and then withdrawn to detach and release the device from the delivery catheter.

PATIENT SELECTION

Patients with secundum atrial septal defects that were less than 20 mm in diameter, with a distance of at least 4 mm from the atrioventricular valves, coronary sinus, and pulmonary veins were considered for percutaneous closure. On echocardiography the atrial septal defect had to be central in location. The presence of a deficient anterior rim was not considered to be an exclusion, because the aortic root behaves as the anterior rim in those patients. Patients with atrial septal defects also required evidence of right ventricular volume overload on echocardiography for inclusion.

In addition, patients who have a patent foramen ovale with a presumed paradoxical embolism, patients with significant residual shunts following previous surgical or device closure, and patients with a fenestrated Fontan or baffle leaks were considered for closure worldwide between February 1995 and 1998. All patients gave informed consent. This narrative highlights the experience only with atrial septal defect closures in the trials approved by the FDA in the United States. The study protocol was approved by the Investigational Review Boards or ethics committees of the individual centers involved, and was approved for clinical investigation by the FDA in the United States.

CATHETERIZATION AND DEFECT CLOSURE PROTOCOL

All procedures were performed in the cardiac catheterization laboratory under general anesthesia. Transesophageal echocardiography (TEE) was used to help guide the device deployment. Access was gained percutaneously from both the femoral veins and the left femoral artery. After a right heart catheterization the atrial septal defect was crossed with an NIH angiographic catheter (USCI, Bard, Inc., Tewkesbury, MA). Left atrial angiograms were performed in the 30-degree left anterior oblique (LAO) projection with 30-degree cranial angulation and in the straight posteroanterior (PA) projection. These views were obtained primarily to provide "road maps" to guide deployment of the device.

The atrial septal defect was then recrossed with an endhole catheter and a 0.038-inch, 260-cm-length Amplatz Superstiff exchange wire (Meditech, Watertown, MA) was placed across the defect. A 27- or 33-mm balloon occlusion catheter (Meditech, Watertown, MA) was calibrated outside the body by inflating it with measured volumes of diluted radiographic contrast. The diameter of the balloon for every 1-mL increase in volume was measured. The balloon catheter was then passed over the Amplatz wire into the left atrium. The balloon was inflated to a size larger than the defect and was withdrawn into the ASD using gentle traction. The volume of the balloon was gradually decreased, and the minimum diameter of the balloon that could not be pulled across the atrial septum through the defect was determined. This diameter was referred to as the balloon occlusive diameter (BOD). In patients with patent foramen ovale (PFO) the sizing was done in both directions, and the larger diameter was selected if there was a difference. The ratio of device (D) size to balloon occlusive diameter (D:BOD) was variable. A ratio of 1.5 was recommended. The appropriate-sized (11, 12, or 13F) Mullins transseptal sheath (Cook, Inc., Bloomington, IN) was passed via the femoral vein, over the exchange wire, with the tip positioned in the left atrium. To prevent air entry into the Mullins sheath, the sheath was continuously flushed with saline while the dilator and the guide wire were removed. The sheath was filled with contrast in order to detect subsequent air entry into the sheath. The appropri-

ate-sized device in its delivery catheter was then inserted into the Mullins sheath. The delivery catheter was inserted into the sheath with the hub of the sheath immersed in saline, again to prevent air entry into the sheath. The delivery catheter was advanced until the tip of the delivery catheter exited the tip of the sheath in the left atrium.

After it was ascertained by TEE that the tip of the delivery catheter was in the middle portion of the left atrium, away from the atrial appendage and mitral valve, the blue actuator ring was torqued clockwise to deploy the LA disk. The Mullins sheath and the delivery catheter were then held as a unit and withdrawn until the LA disk was seated flush against the left side of the atrial septum. In some cases, torquing of the sheath and delivery catheter, and readvancing and withdrawing the delivery system were required to position the left atrial disk properly. Gentle traction on the delivery system was employed to maintain proper position of the left atrial disk, while further clockwise rotation of the blue actuator ring gradually pushed the right atrial disk from the delivery catheter, allowing it to open against the right side of atrial septum. Fluoroscopy, right atrial cineangiography, and transesophageal echocardiography were used to evaluate the position of the Angel Wings device after deployment while the device was still attached to the delivery catheter via a right atrial corner eyelet. If these images demonstrated proper position of both disks the red release knob was unscrewed and withdrawn, and the Angel Wings device was released from its delivery catheter. Following release of the device, right atrial angiography and transesophageal echocardiography were repeated to evaluate the final position of the Angel Wings device and to evaluate residual shunting. During the procedure the patients were heparinized to obtain an activated clotting time (ACT) of more than 300 seconds. At the completion of the procedure, protamine sulfate reversed the effects of heparin. Patients received intravenous cefazolin as prophylaxis for 24 hours following the procedure. The patients were allowed to recover from anesthesia, were observed overnight, and were discharged from the hospital the following morning.

FOLLOW-UP

Patients were clinically evaluated 24 hours after the procedure. This evaluation included an electrocardiogram, a chest radiograph, and a transthoracic echocardiogram. All adult patients were given aspirin 325 mg daily (children 10 mg/kg/day) for a period of 6 months and were prescribed subacute bacterial endocarditis prophylaxis for dental work. Echocardiographic residual shunting was graded according to the classification proposed by Boutin (2). Patients underwent repeat transthoracic echocardiography within 6 months of the procedure. In the US trials and a few international sites transesophageal echocardiography was performed as well. Patients underwent yearly reevaluation, including a chest radiograph, electrocardiogram, and clinical examination, and transthoracic echocardiogram.

EXPERIENCE IN THE UNITED STATES

The device was evaluated in a FDA-approved clinical trial from 1995 through 1998. The Phase I trial established the feasibility and safety of this device, which was then evaluated in a Phase II trial. The Phase II trial was terminated prematurely to redesign the device (Guardian Angel). A total of 90 patients underwent 91 closures in the Phase I study. Table 5.1 summarizes the clinical characteristics of these patients. A total of 50 patients had a diagnosis of secundum atrial septal defect, and 34 of these had no coexisting diseases. The rest of the ASD patients either were at high risk for surgery because of coexistent medical illnesses or had paradoxical embolization or right-to-left shunting. The ASD defect diameter was 10.5 mm ± 4.6 mm, with a median diameter of 11 mm measured on transesophageal echocardiography (range, 2 to 20 mm). The balloon occlusive diameter was 15.6 ± 3.9 mm, with a median of 16 (range, 8 to 23 mm).

The device size used was 24.7 ± 4.1 mm, with a median of 25 and a range of 18 to 35 mm. The device-to-balloon occlusive diameter was variable in the clinical trials. In the initial phase in an attempt to understand the optimal device size to be used, ratios as small as 1.1 were used. Subsequently, a ratio of 1.5 was utilized. The device-to-balloon occlusive diameter ratio was 1.57:1. Forty-six of these 50 patients had successful deployment of the device, giving an implantation success rate of 92%. Four closures were unsuccessful. In two

of these the right atrial (RA) disk was accidentally deployed into the left atrium (LA). In one patient the device was deployed with the RA disk straddling the atrial septum, and in a fourth patient the LA disk was pulled into the RA. These patients underwent surgical retrieval of the device and defect closure with no complications. Thirty-four patients with secundum ASDs had transesophageal echocardiograms within 3 to 6 months of closures. Of these, 31 had no shunt, or less than a 2-mm shunt; three patients had a shunt more than 3 mm in diameter. Residual shunts greater than 3 mm were usually related to prolapse of a corner of the LA disk across the atrial septal defect or to the use of a device with a small device-to-balloon occlusive diameter ratio.

Significant procedural or device-related complications included the following: transient 2:1 atrioventricular block and ST segment elevations due to possible air embolism in one patient; paroxysmal atrial fibrillation in one; and transient ischemic attack in one.

PHASE II CLINICAL TRIALS

After completion of the Phase I trials the FDA approved a Phase II trial. In the Phase II trial a total of 47 patients with secundum ADS underwent closure. The ASD diameter on transesophageal echo was 9.7 ± 4.1 mm, with a median of 10, range of 2 to 18 mm, and device size of 25.2 ± 4.1. The balloon occlusive diameter was 15.9 ± 3.2, with a range of 9 to 23 mm. The device-to-balloon occlusive diameter ratio used was 1.59:1. The device was successfully deployed in 44 of 47 attempted closures (success rate, 94%). There were three unsuccessful closures. In two the failure was related to the left atrial disk being pulled into the RA. In another the

TABLE 5.1. CLINICAL CHARACTERISTICS, PHASE I US TRIALS

Characteristic	Value
Age (years)	36 ± 22
Range	3.63 to 86
Median	32.9
Sex	
Male	56
Female	34
Weight (kg)	63.5 ± 23.46
Range	13.7 to 115.8
Median	65.45
DIAGNOSIS	
1. Atrial septal defect (ASD)	34
2. Patent foramen ovale (PFO) with unexplained stroke/TIA	16
3. ASD—postsurgical residual shunt	6
4. ASD—postdevice closure residual shunt	1*
5. Fenestrated fontan/baffle leaks	7
6. PFOs R → L shunts, orthodeoxia platypnea, etc.	17
7. ASD, High surgical risk patients	10
Total	91

*, a second closure.
R → L, right to left; TIA, transient ischemic attacks.

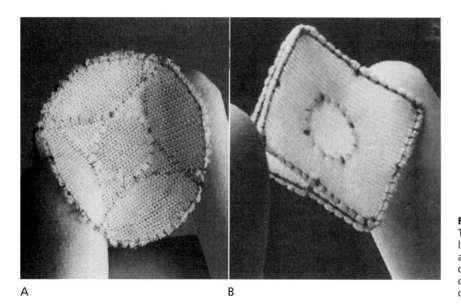

A   B

FIGURE 5.1. The Angel Wings devices. **A:** This illustration highlights the circular outline of the disks, the central conjoint ring, and the low profile of the Guardian Angel device. **B:** In contrast, the Angel Wings I device is square shaped, but similar in all other respects.

right atrial disk was deployed straddling the atrial septum. In one of the patients the device was retrieved percutaneously. In the other two, surgical retrieval and closure were without complication. Residual shunts at 24 hours in 44 patients revealed that 29 had no residual shunts, nine had less than a 1-mm shunt, and six had 1- to 2-mm residual shunts. There were no patients with 3-mm shunts or more in the Phase II trials. Significant procedural and device-related complications included the following: paroxysmal atrial fibrillation in two patients; pulmonary embolism in one; small clot on the LA disk requiring warfarin in one; and a stroke in one. There were no procedural or device-related deaths, embolization after device deployment, or infective endocarditis.

After the initiation of the Phase II trials in the United States and the clinical use of the device in Europe, a decision was made to prematurely stop the clinical trials for the device to be redesigned with three design features: (a) circular LA and RA disks, (b) the ability to be retrievable and repositionable, (c) retention of the central feature of self-centering of the device. The device has been so modified and is to reenter clinical use under the new name of Guardian Angel device (Figure 5.1).

DISCUSSION

The device reported in this study was designed to achieve complete occlusion of defects due to its unique ability to self-center. To make the deployment process user-friendly, a customized delivery system was developed. The success rate in the present study is excellent, especially considering that this was the initial use of this device. The rate of complete closure assessed by echocardiography is high. Significant residual shunts were usually procedure related, due to a cor-

ner of the left atrial disk prolapsing across the atrial septal defect or devices that were small in relation to the occlusive diameter of the ASD. This initial experience also represents the learning curve of several investigators.

One concern with this device is that percutaneous retrieval of suboptimally deployed devices has been difficult and retrievability into the delivery catheter impossible once either the LA disk or both are deployed. Even though we have demonstrated that devices are retrievable using snares in an animal model, we have been apprehensive in making vigorous attempts to retrieve this device with a snare for fear of perforation of one of the cardiac chambers or the inferior vena cava. Hence we adopted a deliberate policy of surgical conversion if percutaneous device retrieval was not easily attainable. This also provided the impetus to enhance the performance of the device by modifying it to be retrievable and repositionable.

This experience supports our earlier hypothesis (1) that a truly self-centering device would afford almost complete occlusion of atrial septal defects. These results are comparable with those of open-heart surgery (3–7). Following the demonstration in clinical trials of the effective occlusion of defects with the self-centering mechanism of the Angel Wings device, there has been widespread acceptance of this concept, demonstrated by the development of other self-centering devices, including the Amplatzer device (8) and self-centering variants of the "Buttoned" device and the "CardioSEAL" device with the "STARFlex centering system."

THE GUARDIAN ANGEL DEVICE

The clinical experience with the Angel Wings device has validated the efficacy of the self-centering mechanism in occluding atrial septal defects. The device is made primarily of polyester fabric, with the metallic framework occupying an insignificant proportion of the whole device. The device splays well around the aorta, and it has a very low profile. In addition, because of its unique design, the device has not embolized after successful deployment and release. However, larger devices have a considerable learning curve for manipulating the square disks in small atria, and the lack of retrievability has proven to be a challenge in retrieving suboptimally deployed devices. To permit a more user-friendly device than Angel Wings I and obviate the need for surgical retrieval of the device, the Guardian Angel device has been developed. This has two disks that have a circular outline with a central conjoint ring. The device has a novel delivery system that permits one or both disks that are deployed to be retrieved into the delivery catheter. Guardian Angel should obviate the need for surgical retrieval. In addition, the delivery system permits the deployed device to "hang loose" without any traction by the delivery catheter. If the deployment is optimal, the device can be released. If it is suboptimal it can be retrieved into the delivery catheter.

CONCLUSION

The initial clinical experience with the Angel Wings device has firmly established high rates of nearly complete occlusion of defects due to the self-centering feature of the device. This provides results easily comparable with surgery. A low profile of the device, nonembolization of the device after successful deployment, and absence of infective endocarditis are strengths of the device. Difficulties in deployment and retrieval due to the square-shaped device have led to the development of Guardian Angel. This has two circular disks, self-centers, has a low profile, and can be retrieved into the delivery catheter or repositioned. This obviates the need for surgical retrieval and enhances the performance of this device. Guardian Angel is to enter clinical trials in the near future.

ACKNOWLEDGMENT

We would like to acknowledge all the investigators of the Angel Wings device in the United States who provided data about their patients. We would also like to acknowledge the assistance of Carole Gallagher, RN, Cardiovascular Division, University of Minnesota, in collating the data and the excellent secretarial assistance of Ms. Teresa Nesbit, of the Cardiovascular Division of the University of Minnesota.

REFERENCES

1. Das GS, Voss G, Jarvis G, et al. Experimental atrial septal defect closure with a new, transcatheter, self-centering device. *Circulation* 1993;88:1754–1764.
2. Boutin C, Musewe NN, Smallhorn JF, et al. Echocardiographic follow-up of atrial septal defect after catheter closure by double-umbrella device. *Circulation* 1993; 88:621–627.
3. Meijboom F, Hess J, Szatmari A, et al. Long-term follow-up (9 to 20 years) after surgical closure of atrial septal defect at a young age. *Am J Cardiol* 1993;72:1431–1434.
4. Pastorek JS, Allen HD, Davis JT. Current outcomes of surgical closure of secundum atrial septal defect. *Am J Cardiol* 1994;74: 75–77.
5. Nasrallah AT, Hall RJ, Garcia E, et al. Surgical repair of atrial septal defect in patients over 60 years of age: long term results. *Circulation* 1976;53:329–331.
6. Konstantinides S, Geibel A, Olschewski M, et al. A comparison of surgical and medical therapy for atrial septal defect in adults. *N Engl J Med* 1995;333:469–473.
7. Horvath KA, Burke RP, Collins JJ, Jr, et al. Surgical treatment of adult atrial septal defect: early and long-term results. *J Am Coll Cardiol* 1992;20:1156–1159.
8. Sharafudin MJ, Gu X, Titus JL, et al. Secundum-ASD closure with a new self-expanding prosthesis in swine. *Circulation* 1996; 94:I–57.

6

AMPLATZER SEPTAL OCCLUDER

MOHAMED A. HAMDAN
QI-LING CAO
ZIYAD M. HIJAZI

The Amplatzer Septal Occluder (ASO) is a unique device that combines the advantages of being a double-disk device with a self-centering mechanism. Although relatively new, it has proved to be an important device to consider for catheter closure of various defects, including secundum atrial septal defect (ASD), patent foramen ovale (PFO), and Fontan fenestration. Its remarkable ease of implantation, small delivery sheaths, simple mechanics, high complete-closure rates achieved immediately after closure, and excellent short- and mid-term results resulted in this device being the one most widely used for catheter closure of such defects.

DEVICE

The ASO device (AGA Medical Corp., Golden Valley, MN) is constructed from a 0.004- to 0.0075-inch Nitinol (55% nickel, 45% titanium) wire mesh that is tightly woven into two flat disks (Figure 6.1). There is a 4-mm connecting waist between the two disks that corresponds to the thickness of the atrial septum (1). Nitinol has superelastic properties with shape memory. This allows the device to be stretched into an almost linear configuration and placed inside a small sheath for delivery and then to reform to its original configuration within the heart when not constrained by the sheath. Nitinol also has been proven to have excellent biocompatibility. The device size is determined by the diameter of its waist and is constructed in various sizes, ranging from 4 to 40 mm (1-mm increment up to 20 mm; 2-mm increments up to the largest device currently available at 40 mm) (2). The two

flat disks extend radially beyond the central waist to provide secure anchorage. Patients with ASD usually have left-to-right shunt. Therefore the left atrial disk is larger than the right atrial disk. For devices 4 to 10 mm, the left atrial disk is 12 mm and the right atrial disk is 8 mm larger than the waist. However, for devices larger than 11 mm, the left atrial disk is 14 mm and the right atrial disk is 10 mm larger than the connecting waist (3). Both disks are angled slightly toward each other to ensure firm contact of the disks to the atrial septum. Three Dacron polyester patches are sewn securely with polyester thread into each disk and the connecting waist to increase the thrombogenicity of the device. A stainless steel sleeve with a female thread is laser-welded to the right atrial disk. This sleeve is used to screw the delivery cable to the device. For device deployment we recommend a 6F delivery system for devices smaller than 10 mm in diameter. We suggest a 7F delivery system for devices 10 to 15 mm, an 8F sheath for devices 16 to 22 mm, a 9F sheath for devices 24 to 28 mm, a 10F sheath for devices 30 to 34 mm, a 12F sheath for the 36- and 38-mm device, and we use a 14F sheath for the 40-mm device.

PATIENT SELECTION

In theory, ASO devices can be used in any patient with an ostium secundum ASD if there is an adequate rim of tissue of more than 5 mm from the margins of the defect to the adjacent mitral and tricuspid valves, superior vena cava, right upper pulmonary vein, and coronary sinus (1,4,5). The presence of an anterior rim (toward the aorta) is not essential for the Amplatzer. As a matter of fact, many of our patients lack such a rim. Defects up to 33-mm anatomic diameter by two-dimensional transesophageal echocardiography (TEE) (40- to 42-mm balloon stretched) were closed successfully using the ASO (6,7). However, the experience with defects larger than 34 mm unstretched is still limited.

Mohamed A. Hamdan: Pediatric Cardiology, Jordan University of Science and Technology, Irbid, Jordan

Qi-Ling Cao: Assistant Professor, Department of Pediatric Cardiology, University of Chicago; Director, Pediatric Echocardiography Research, University of Chicago Children's Laboratory Hospital, Chicago, Illinois

Ziyad M. Hijazi: Professor of Pediatrics and Medicine, Department of Pediatrics, University of Chicago; Director, Pediatric Cardiology, University of Chicago Hospital, Chicago, Illinois

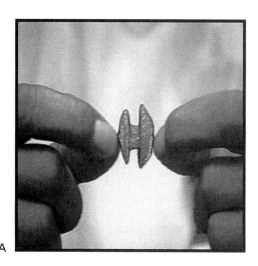

A

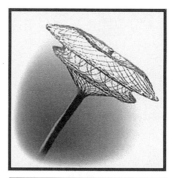

B

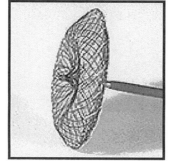

C

FIGURE 6.1. The Amplatzer septal occluder device. **A:** The device consists of three components: a left atrial disk, a connecting waist, and a right atrial disk. **B:** The sheath and delivery cable are attached to the device. **C:** The device is retracted slightly into the sheath.

DEVICE IMPLANTATION TECHNIQUE

The procedure is usually done under general endotracheal anesthesia, especially if TEE is planned. Successful implantation with conscious sedation under TEE guidance only has been accomplished (8) where patients had similar procedure time and overall success rate relative to control. Most recently, we have been performing the closure of ASD and PFO under continuous intracardiac echocardiographic (ICE) guidance using the new 10F (3.2-mm), 5.5- to 10-MHz ultrasound tipped catheter (Acuson Corporation, Mountain View, CA) without anesthesia and without TEE. The catheter tip contains a 64-element vector phased array transducer that scans in the longitudinal plane, providing a 90-degree-sector image with tissue penetration of 12 cm.

The protocol for closure under TEE or ICE guidance consists of obtaining vascular access in the femoral vein and artery. The artery is used only for monitoring the arterial pressure and blood gases during the procedure. Heparin is given at 100 IU/kg to keep the activated clotting time (ACT) above 200 seconds. Complete right and left heart hemodynamic evaluation is performed prior to angiography. Single-plane fluoroscopy is usually sufficient. An angiogram in the right upper pulmonary vein is performed in the four-chamber view (35 degrees cranial/35 degrees left anterior oblique) to profile the atrial septum. The presence of partial anomalous pulmonary venous drainage should be excluded using the TEE or ICE. An end-hole catheter (multipurpose) is manipulated through the ASD into the left upper pulmonary vein. Using an exchange length Amplatz extra- or suprastiff

guide wire, a sizing balloon catheter is exchanged for the catheter. Balloon sizing of the ASD is a very important step (9). The static method is less time-consuming and relatively easier than the pulling technique (10). We use either the AGA sizing balloon (AGA Medical, Golden Valley, MN) catheter or the NuMED sizing balloon catheter (NuMED, Inc., Hopkinton, NY) (2,10). These balloon catheters have 1-cm markers inside for calibration. The balloon is positioned in the middle of the septum across the defect. The balloon is inflated under fluoroscopic and echocardiographic (TEE or ICE) guidance until waisting and disappearance of the shunt occur. The stretched diameter of the defect is then measured by both echocardiography and a spot cine after correction for magnification. Figures 6.2 to 6.4 demonstrate the steps of closure by cine fluoroscopy, TEE, and ICE, respectively. Once the stretched diameter of the ASD is determined, the balloon is removed, keeping the guide wire in the left upper pulmonary vein. The device size chosen is usually the same ± 2 mm of the stretched diameter, depending on the size of the patient's left atrium. The proper size of delivery sheath is advanced over the guide wire to the left upper pulmonary vein. Both dilator and wire are removed, keeping the tip of the sheath inside the left upper pulmonary vein. Extreme care must be exercised not to allow passage of air inside the delivery sheath. The device is then screwed to the tip of the delivery cable, immersed in normal saline, and drawn into the loader underwater seal to expel air bubbles out of the system. A Y-connector is applied to the proximal end of the loader to allow flushing with saline. The loader containing the device is attached to the proxi-

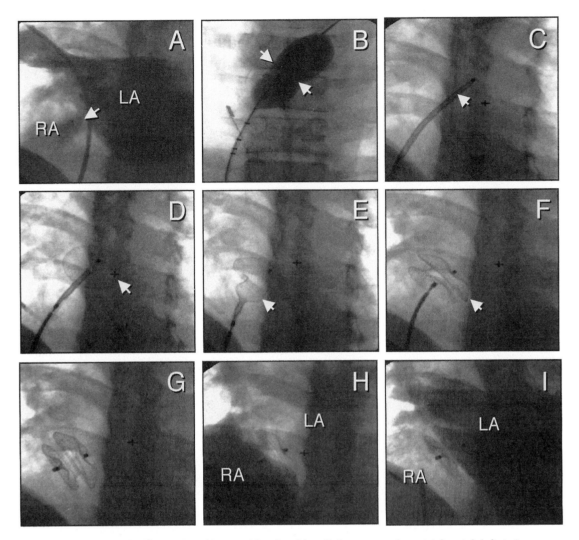

FIGURE 6.2. Cine frames in a 22-year-old male with a 12.9-mm secundum atrial septal defect. **A:** Angiogram in the right upper pulmonary vein in the four-chamber view demonstrating left to right shunt at the atrial level *(arrow)*. **B:** Balloon sizing of the defect demonstrating waisting (stretched diameter of 16 mm) in the middle of the balloon *(arrows)*. **C:** Delivery sheath with device inside in the middle of left atrium *(arrow)*. **D:** Deployment of the left atrial disk *(arrow)* of an 18-mm Amplatzer septal occluder. **E:** Deployment of the connecting waist *(arrow)* in the defect. **F:** The device *(arrow)* is deployed (both disks) but not released yet. **G:** Device released across the defect. **H:** Angiogram in the right atrium demonstrating the atrial septum and the right atrial disk. Note that the left atrial disk has no contrast, which indicates good device position. **I:** Pulmonary levophase of the previous angiogram, revealing good device position with no residual shunt. LA, left atrium; RA, right atrium.

mal hub of the delivery sheath. The cable with the ASO device is advanced to the distal tip of the sheath, taking care not to rotate the cable while advancing it in the long sheath to prevent premature unscrewing of the device. Both cable and delivery sheath are pulled back as one unit to the middle of the left atrium. Position of the sheath can be verified using TEE or ICE.

The left atrial disk is deployed first under fluoroscopic and/or echocardiographic guidance. Caution should be taken not to interfere with the left atrial appendage. Part

of the connecting waist should be deployed in the left atrium, very close (a few millimeters) to the atrial septum (the mechanism of ASD closure using the ASO is stenting of the defect). While applying constant pulling of the entire assembly and withdrawing the delivery sheath off the cable, the connecting waist and the right atrial disk are deployed in the ASD itself and in the right atrium, respectively. Proper device position can be verified using fluoroscopy or TEE/ICE. Before device release, the cable is pushed forward and backward (the "Minnesota Wiggle")

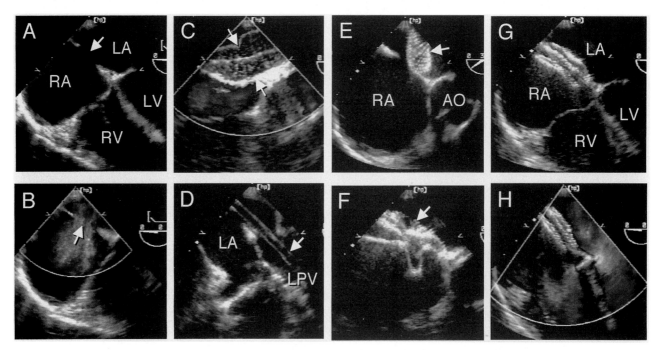

FIGURE 6.3 Transesophageal echocardiographic (TEE) images in the four-chamber view in a 17-year-old female with moderate ASD *(arrow)* measuring 14 mm without (**A**) and with (**B**) color flow, demonstrating left-to-right shunt. **C:** Balloon sizing of the defect for measuring the stretched diameter (20 mm) of the defect *(arrow)*. **D:** The delivery sheath *(arrow)* is positioned in the left pulmonary vein (LPV). **E:** Deployment of the left atrial disk *(arrow)* in the left atrium. **F:** The device *(arrow)* is deployed across the defect but still attached to cable. TEE images immediately after deployment of a 20-mm device without (**G**) and with (**H**) color flow, demonstrating good device position and no residual shunt. AO, aortic valve; LA, left atrium; LV, left ventricle; RA, right atrium; RV, right ventricle.

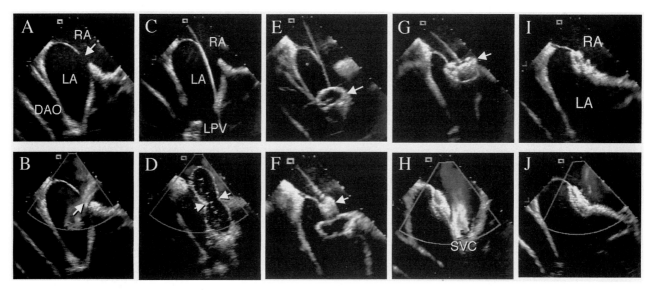

FIGURE 6.4. A–J: Intracardiac echocardiographic (ICE) images in a 28-year-old female with a 10-mm secundum atrial septal defect demonstrating the protocol of device deployment as obtained by ICE. Two-chamber (right and left atrium) view without (**A**) and with (**B**) color Doppler, demonstrating the defect *(arrow)* and the atria as well as the descending aorta. **C:** the guide wire is through the defect into the left upper pulmonary vein (LPV). **D:** measurement of the balloon-stretched (11 mm) diameter *(arrows)*. **E:** Deployment of the left atrial disk of a 14-mm Amplazter septal occluder far in the left atrium *(arrow)*. **F:** Deployment of the connecting waist *(arrow)* partly in the left atrium and defect. ICE images after the device has been deployed *(arrow)* across the defect but not released without (**G**) and with (**H**) color, demonstrating good device position. ICE images after the device has been released without (**I**) and with (**J**) color, demonstrating good device position and no residual shunt. Note the unobstructed SVC flow. DAO, descending aorta; LA, left atrium; RA, right atrium; SVC, superior vena cava.

(3,9). Adequate device position manifests by the lack of movement of the device in either direction. Another method of verifying device position can be achieved by contrast injection in the right atrium using the side arm of the delivery sheath with pulmonary levophase. If device position is not certain or questionable, the device can be recaptured entirely or partly and repositioned following similar steps. Once the device position is verified, the device is released by counterclockwise rotation of the delivery cable using a pin vise. There is often a notable change in the angle of the device as it is released from the slight tension of the delivery cable and it self-centers within the ASD and aligns with the interatrial septum. To assess result of closure, repeat TEE/ICE and angiography in the right atrium with pulmonary levophase are performed. The patients receive a dose of an appropriate antibiotic (commonly cefazolin at 20 mg/kg) during the catheterization procedure and two further doses at 8-hour intervals. Patients are also asked to take endocarditis prophylaxis when necessary for 6 months after the procedure, as well as aspirin 5 mg/kg orally once daily for 6 months. Full activity, including competitive sports, is usually allowed after 4 weeks of implantation (9). Magnetic resonance imaging (if required) can be done any time after implantation (9,11).

RESULTS

Since the introduction of the ASO device in 1996, there have been numerous studies to evaluate its immediate and short-term results in different parts of the world. In the first paper describing the device, Sharafuddin et al. (1) implanted 15 devices in 15 minipigs with surgically created ASDs. Using devices up to 16 mm in diameter, acute complete closure was achieved in eight of 12 animals (66.7%), with only trace or small residual shunt noted in the rest of the animals, resulting in an overall success rate of 100%. At 1-month follow-up, complete closure increased to 87.5%. Device displacement resulting in significant shunt occurred in one of eight animals at 1-month follow-up. Histopathologic examination of the device in the sacrificed animals after 1 week of implantation showed complete investment of the wire mesh in a layer of organized fibrinous thrombus. By 3 months there was complete layering with neo-endothelium covering both atrial disks, which was in close continuity with the endocardium of the surrounding atrial septal rim.

Immediate Results

Results of Phase II trials in the United States submitted to the FDA were presented at the 49th Scientific Sessions of the American Heart Association (November 1999) (6).

Two hundred and twenty-nine devices were implanted in 219 patients with median weight of 27 kg and median age of 8.3 years, using devices up to 34 mm in diameter. The success rate (defined as complete closure and/or trace or small residual shunt ≤ 2 mm in jet width) was achieved in 98.1% immediately and at 6 months after implantation. Significant residual shunting (moderate or large shunt with jet width of more than 2 mm) occurred only in 1.9% of patients, both immediately after implantation and at their 6-month follow-up. Complications were rare and occurred in ten of 210 patients (4.6%). They included embolization of the device in five; atrial tachycardia in two; complete AV block in one; esophageal tear due to TEE in one; and embolization of the marker band in one. Only three of ten patients required surgical intervention.

Other studies have reported similar results and are included in Table 6.1. Complete closure in the catheterization laboratory ranged from 36.7% to 85% (3,4,6,7,12), with slightly better acute results for devices of less than 28 mm than for the larger devices (more than 34 mm). This could be explained partly by the fact that larger devices were not available initially, so larger defects may have been closed than with undersized devices. Trace or small residual shunts occurred in 15% to 61.4% of patients (3,4,6,7,12). However, as early as 24 hours after implantation, complete closure increased to 80% to 87.5% of patients (4,7,10,13), indicating a high rate of thrombogenicity of the device. Significant residual shunting was more common when the ASD diameter was ≥ 2 mm larger than the diameter of the chosen device (9).

Our experience using the Amplatzer consists of 140 patients (101 female, 39 male). These patients had secundum ASD in 121, PFO associated with either a stroke or a transient ischemic attack (TIA) in 13, and Fontan fenestration in six patients. Closure was performed at a median age of 24.8 years (range, 5.5 months to 87.5 years) and median weight of 57.8 kg (range, 4 to 130 kg). The median Qp:Qs ratio was 1.9 (range, 0.7 to 10.0). The median size of the defect as measured by TEE was 12.5 mm (2 to 33 mm), the median stretched diameter of the defect was 18 mm (range, 7 to 40 mm), and the median size of the device used was 18.5 mm (range, 5 to 38 mm). There was complete immediate closure in 110 of 140 patients (78.6%), six patients had trivial residual shunt (4.3%), and 21 had small residual shunt (15%). In one patient each, the procedure failed or there was moderate or large residual shunt. At 24-hour follow-up the complete closure rate increased to 90.6% (126 out of 139 patients). Five patients had trivial residual shunt and six had small residual shunt. The median fluoroscopy time was 8.8 minutes (range, 3.3 to 38.3 minutes) and the median total procedure time (sheath in and sheath out) was 63 minutes (range, 21 to 181 minutes).

TABLE 6.1. IMMEDIATE AND SHORT-TERM RESULTS OF ATRIAL SEPTAL DEFECT CLOSURE USING THE AMPLATZER SEPTAL OCCLUDER AS REPORTED BY DIFFERENT OPERATORS

Author	#	Age	Wt	Size (TEE) (mm)	SD (mm)	Qp:Qs	FT	PT (minutes)	Immed C	Immed TS/SS	Immed MS/LS	>3–6 mo C	>3–6 mo TS/SS	>3–6 mo MS/LS	6–12 mo C	6–12 mo Ts/SS	6–12 mo Ms/LS	CX
Masura	30	6.1	22	12.5	14	2.3	15	92.5	80%	13.3%	6.7%		N/A			N/A		None
Thanopoulos	16	9.0	35	14	17	2.0	20	67.5	81.3%	18.8%	0.0	91.5%	N/A			N/A		6.3%
Hijazi (1999)	219	8.3	27	12	16.3	1.9	17	N/A	36.7%	61.4%	1.9%		6.6%	1.9%		N/A		4.6%
Dhillon	20	44.2	18	N/A	20	2.5	15.2	61	90%	10%	0.0	95%	5%	0.0	95%	5%	0.0%	None
Walsh	104	6.8	22	11	11	2.0	12.6	N/A	68%	N/A	N/A		N/A		90%	N/A	N/A	3.8%
Berger	200	29.8	51.5	12	N/A	1.6	10.2	109	95.5%	4.5%	0.0		N/A		98.5%	1.5%	0.0	1.0%
Wilkinson	27	8.1	21	11.8	16.1	N/A	N/A	N/A	61.5%	38.5%	0.0		N/A			N/A		11.5%
Chan	100	13.2	32.5	N/A	N/A	N/A	16	92.4	84.8%	N/A	N/A		N/A			N/A		5.0%
Hijazi (2000)	40	47.9	63.8	14	18.5	1.9	9.3	65	87.5%	10%	2.5%	92%	4%	4%		N/A		2.5%
Vogel	12	1.4	N/A	12	N/A	2.1	12.8	162		N/A	N/A		N/A		83%	N/A	N/A	25%

#, number of patients in series; age, years; wt, weight in kg; TEE, transesophageal echocardiography; mm, millimeter; SD, stretched diameter of defect; FT, fluoroscopy time; PT, procedure time; Immed, immediate; C, complete closure; TS, trivial residual shunt (color jet width <1 mm); SS, small residual shunt (color jet width 1–2 mm); MS, moderate residual shunt; (color jet width 2–4 mm); LS, large residual shunt (color jet width >4 mm); mo, months; CX, complications.

Complications

Reported complications were rare and could be managed in the catheterization laboratory. Most of the complications occur in the immediate period after implantation. There is a wide range in the complication rate because of the learning curve of the operators, widely varying patients' ages and sizes, and the complexity of their anatomy (Table 6.2). The complication rate ranges from 0 to 11.5% (2–7,9,12–15). Complications tend to be relatively more frequent with larger devices and with younger patients. Vogel et al. (16) reported a complication rate of 25% (three of 12) in children less than 2 years of age with symptomatic ASD. This is in comparison to the 4.6% rate reported by Hijazi et al. (6) in older children and adults, and 2.5% in adults with ASD/PFO (7). The most common complication is device displacement and/or embolization, which occurs in 1% to 7.4% (2,4–7, 9,13,15) of patients after ASO implantation. Most of these incidents result in transcatheter retrieval of the device, with the occasional need for surgery. Device displacement can be minimized by appropriate sizing of the ASD and choosing devices that are at least the same size as the defect in small to medium-sized defects, and 1 to 2 mm above the diameter of the ASD in larger defects. Arrhythmias were reported as late as 10 days after implantation in 0.9% to 2.9% of patients after ASO implantation (6,13). Despite being quite rare, complications were observed beyond the immediate period. Wilkinson et al. (15) reported a case of bacterial endocarditis in a 10-month-old infant who had complete closure of an 11-mm ASD. The patient developed staphylococcus septicemia 6 weeks after implantation related to multiple noncardiac invasive procedures. Vegetations were found on the implanted device, requiring elective surgical removal and ASD closure thereafter. The authors concluded that the multiple invasive procedures and the suboptimal antibiotic therapy during septicemia could have contributed to this complication during the first 1 to 3 months of implantation before full endothelialization of the device. Atrial arrhythmias were reported in 0.9% to 2.9% of patients as late as 10 days after ASO implantation (6,9). Walsh et al. (9) reported three patients in their series who developed supraventricular arrhythmias 6 hours to 10 days after ASO implantation. Two patients were easily controlled on antiarrhythmia medications, and the third (who developed atrial flutter) converted spontaneously to sinus rhythm without treatment.

In our series of 140 patients, seven patients developed complications, which included device embolization in two patients (one immediate and another 24 hours later) (2). Both devices were retrieved in the catheterization laboratory and both patients underwent a second attempt a few months later with complete closure of the defects. Another patient developed complete heart block that required placement of a dual-chamber pacemaker after 6 months (2,17). Three patients developed atrial arrhythmias (flutter/fibrillation), which required cardioversion in two patients. One patient developed a large thrombus on the left and right atrial disks of the device. This 62-year-old patient with a history of hypoplastic right ventricle, bidirectional Glenn anastomosis,

TABLE 6.2. COMPLICATIONS ENCOUNTERED DURING CATHETER CLOSURE OF ATRIAL COMMUNICATIONS USING THE AMPLATZER SEPTAL OCCLUDER DEVICE

Author	#	Age	SD (mm)	Device (mm)	# CX (%)	Type of CX	Action Taken
Thanopoulos	16	9.0	17	16.6	1 (6.3%)	Displacement of device	Catheter retrieval
Hijazi (1999)	219	8.3	16.3	17	10 (4.6%)	5: device displacement	3: catheter retrieval; 2: surgery
						2: SVT	Spontaneous resolution
						1: complete heart block	Transvenous pacemaker
						1: marker band embolization	No intervention required
						1: esophageal tear	No intervention needed
Walsh	104	6.8	11	7–34	7 (6.7%)	2: device displacement	Surgical removal
						2: deep venous thrombosis	Anticoagulation
						3: atrial arrhythmias	2: antiarrhythmia meds; 1: spontan
Berger	200	29.8	12	12	2 (1%)	2: device displacement	Catheter retrieval
Wilkinson	27	8.1	16.1	16.3	3 (11.1%)	2: device displacement	Catheter retrieval
						1: bacterial endocarditis	Surgical removal + antibiotics
Chan	100	13.2	N/A	N/A	5 (5%)	1: device displacement	Surgical removal
						1: transient ST elevation	No intervention
						1: transient AV block	No intervention
						1: transient ischemic attack	Anticoagulation/full recovery
						1: deep venous thrombosis	Anticoagulation/full recovery
Hijazi (2000)	40	47.9	18.5	20	1 (2.5%)	Displacement of device	Catheter retrieval second device
Vogel	12	1.4	12	N/A	3 (25%)	2: device displacement	Surgical removal
						1: stroke	Anticoagulation/full recovery

#, number of patients in series; SD, stretched diameter; CX, complications; SVT, supraventricular tachycardia; meds, medications; spontan, spontaneous.

and frequent clot formation requiring vena cava filter placement underwent placement of a 22-mm ASO. During the recovery, Coumadin and aspirin therapy was discontinued inadvertently. Transthoracic echocardiography a few days later revealed the presence of large clots on both sides of the device. Heparin therapy resulted in full resolution of these clots. However, this patient succumbed to her disease 6 weeks later due to low cardiac output and septicemia.

Follow-up

Only short-term follow-up results are available for ASO. A complete closure rate occurred in up to 97% of patients at 1 and 3 months after implantation (4,13,18) and in 92% to 95% of patients at 6 months (7,8,12). At 1-year follow-up, both Walsh et al. (14) and Dhillon et al. (12) reported complete closure in 93% to 95% of the patients using devices 8 to 28 mm in diameter. In our series of 140 patients, two patients died. (In addition to the previously mentioned patient, a 5.5-month-old baby with trisomy-21 and severe pulmonary artery hypertension and right ventricle failure died 6 weeks after closure of the ASD.) Autopsy revealed the device to be in good position, with histopathologic findings in the lungs consistent with severe pulmonary vascular disease. Ninety-three patients reached the 6-month follow-up and underwent TEE evaluation. Out of 93 patients, 86 (92.5%) had complete closure and four patients (4.3%) had small residual shunt. Therefore the success rate of the procedure was 96.8%. Two patients had moderate shunt and one patient had large shunt. The patient with the large shunt underwent a second procedure with complete closure of the defect. The other two patients are being followed medically.

APPLICABILITY IN ADULT SUBJECTS

Results in adult patients are no different from those in the pediatric patient population (Table 6.1). Dhillon et al. (12) reported complete complication-free closure rates for patients 16 to 60 years old of 90%, 95%, and 95% at 1 day, 6 months, and 1 year, respectively, after implantation of devices up to 28 mm in diameter. The same results hold true for larger devices. Using devices up to 35 mm, Hijazi et al. (7) had an acute success rate of 97.5% in 40 adult patients, 33 of whom had ASD. One patient, however, developed large shunt due to device displacement shortly after implantation. This patient underwent a second procedure with placement of a second device, resulting in complete closure. In the 26 patients who completed their 6-month follow-up, 24 had complete closure, one had trace shunt, and one had large shunt. In the study by Berger et al. (5) 200 patients with a mean age of 30 years underwent ASO implantation. Of these, 127 adults had ASD, 68 had PFO, and 21 had fenestrated Fontan. Complete closure occurred in 95.5% to 98.5% of the patients acutely and up to 3 months after implantation. Complications occurred in only 1% of the patients.

In our cohort of 140 patients, 74 were adults more than 18 years of age. Fifty-eight of the 74 patients had secundum ASD, 12 had PFO associated with TIA, and four had Fontan fenestration. The median weight was 67.5 kg (range, 48 to 130 kg) and the median Qp:Qs ratio was 1.8 (range, 0.7 to 7.5). The median size of defect as measured by TEE was 14 mm (range, 2 to 33 mm) and the median balloon-stretched diameter was 19 mm (range, 10 to 40 mm). Patients with PFO did not undergo balloon sizing of their defects. The median size of device implanted was 21 mm (range, 10 to 38 mm). Immediate complete closure was documented by color Doppler TEE in 55 of 74 patients (74.3%), four patients had trivial shunt (5.4%), 14 of 74 had small shunt (18.9%), and one had moderate residual shunt. Therefore the success rate of the procedure was 98.6%. The median fluoroscopy time was 9.6 minutes (range, 3.6 to 32 minutes) and the median total procedure time was 61.5 minutes (range, 21 to 138 minutes). Forty-two patients reached the 6-month follow-up. TEE revealed complete closure in 38 (90.5%) patients, three patients had small residual shunt (7%), and one patient developed large residual shunt requiring a second procedure with complete closure.

DISCUSSION

Although surgical closure of ostium secundum ASD can be performed with low mortality (<1%), considerable morbidity is associated with general anesthesia, sternotomy, cardiopulmonary bypass, and postoperative recovery for several days in the hospital. Added to that, there are psychologic aspects related to the disfigurement associated with the operative scar. Berger et al. (19) recently compared the results of surgical and transcatheter treatment of ASD using ASO. Although both groups had a similar high incidence of complete closure (98%), and complication rate, duration of the hospital stay was significantly shorter in the ASO treatment group. ASO clearly has several advantages over both the surgical treatment of ASD and other currently available devices. ASO is delivered through relatively smaller sheaths (6 to 14F), which facilitates its application in smaller patients. It is a user-friendly device with simple mechanics. The operator can easily reposition or recapture the device should misplacement occur. Such advantages resulted in higher closure rates with shorter fluoroscopy and procedure time (1–4). The ability to recapture and reposition the device enabled operators to close multiple and complex atrial septal defects (20,21).

The bulkiness "profile" of the device has caused some concern. On follow-up, the profile of the device decreases significantly from the implantation profile. This is clearly due to the shape memory property of the Nitinol metal. The risks of developing atrial arrhythmias due to the profile of the device were analyzed in a study performed on patients receiving the device. Ambulatory EKG monitoring was performed before and immediately after device implantation (17). There was no added risk in patients who had the ASO. However, one patient who had slow junctional rhythm before device implantation developed heart block that required pacemaker implantation after device closure (2,17).

Long-term results on safety and efficacy, as well as results involving larger defects, are being collected.

CURRENT STATUS

The device was initially used under IDE protocol. However, the data of more than 450 patients who enrolled in Phase I and Phase II trials have been submitted to the US Food and Drug Administration for premarket approval of the device.

CONCLUSION

The ASO device has a unique design that combines such features as high complete closure rates; ease of implantation; ability to retrieve, reposition, or recapture the device before release; and small delivery system. Acute and short-term results are encouraging, with high success rate and low risk of complications, both in pediatric patients and adults. Long-term evaluation is under way.

ACKNOWLEDGMENT

We wish to thank Ms. Mary Heitschmidt, RN, for data collection, and the nursing, technical, and echocardiography staff at the Section of Pediatric Cardiology at the University of Chicago Children's hospital for their hard work during the clinical trials of the Amplatzer septal occluder.

REFERENCES

1. Sharafuddin MJA, Gu X, Titus JL, et al. Transvenous closure of secundum atrial septal defects: preliminary results with a new self-expanding Nitinol prosthesis in a swine model. *Circulation* 1997;95:2162–2168.
2. Hijazi ZM, Cao QL, Patel HT, et al. Transesophageal echocardiographic results of catheter closure of atrial septal defect in children and adults using the Amplatzer device. *Am J Cardiol* 2000;85:1387–1390.
3. Masura J, Gavora P, Formanek A, et al. Transcatheter closure of secundum atrial septal defects using the new self-centering Amplatzer septal occluder: initial human experience. *Cathet Cardiovasc Diagn* 1997;42:388–393.
4. Thanopoulos BD, Laskari CV, Tsaousis GS, et al. Closure of atrial septal defects with the Amplatzer occlusion device: preliminary results. *J Am Coll Cardiol* 1998;31:1110–1116..
5. Berger F, Ewert P, Bjornsted PG, et al. Transcatheter closure as standard treatment for most interatrial defects: experience in 200 patients treated with the Amplatzer septal occluder. *Cardiol Young* 1999;9:468–473..
6. Hijazi ZM, Radtke W, Ebeid MR, et al. Transcatheter closure of secundum atrial septal defects using the Amplatzer septal occluder: results of Phase II US multicenter clinical trial. *Circulation* 1999;100(Suppl I):804.
7. Hijazi ZM, Cao QL, Patel HT, et al. Transcatheter closure of atrial communications (ASD/PFO) in adult patients >18 years of age using the Amplatzer septal occluder: immediate and mid-term results. *J Am Coll Cardiol* 2000;35(Suppl A):522A.
8. Ewert P, Berger F, Daehnert I, et al. Transcatheter closure of atrial septal defects without fluoroscopy: feasibility of a new method. *Circulation* 2000;101:847–849.
9. Walsh KP, Maadi IM. The Amplatzer septal occluder. *Cardiol Young* 2000;10:493–501.
10. Gu X, Han YM, Berry J, et al. A new technique for sizing of atrial septal defects. *Cathet Cardiovasc Interv* 1999;46:51–57.
11. El-Helw T, Bhadelia RA, Hanlon K, et al. Radiological appearances of Amplatzer septal occluder after transcatheter closure of atrial communications. *Radiology* 1999;213:554.
12. Dhillon R, Thanopoulos B, Tsaousis G, et al. Transcatheter closure of atrial septal defects in adults with the Amplatzer septal occluder. *Heart* 1999;82:559–562.
13. Chan KC, Godman MJ, Walsh K, et al. Transcatheter closure of atrial septal defect and interatrial communications with a new self-expanding Nitinol double disc device (Amplatzer septal occluder): multicenter UK experience. *Heart* 1999;82:300–306..
14. Walsh KP, Tofeig M, Kitchiner DJ, et al. Comparison of the Sideris and Amplatzer septal occlusion devices. *Am J Cardiol* 1999;83:933–936.
15. Wilkinson JL, Goh TH. Early clinical experience with the use of the "Amplatzer septal occluder" device for atrial septal defect. *Cardiol Young* 1998;8:295–302.
16. Vogel M, Berger F, Dahnert I, et al. Treatment of atrial septal defects in symptomatic children aged less than 2 years of age using the Amplatzer septal occluder. *Cardiol Young* 2000;10:534–537.
17. Hill SL, Berul CI, Patel HT, et al. Early ECG abnormalities associated with transcatheter closure of atrial septal defects using the Amplatzer septal occluder. *J Interv Cardiol Electrophysiol* 2000;4:469–474.
18. Fischer G, Kramer HH, Stieh J, et al. Transcatheter closure of secundum atrial septal defects with the new self-centering Amplatzer septal occluder. *Eur Heart J* 1999;20:541–549.
19. Berger F, Vogel M, Alexi-Mekishvili V, et al. Comparison of results and complications of surgical and Amplatzer device closure of atrial septal defects. *J Thorac Cardiovasc Surg* 1999;118:674–678.
20. Suarez DJ, Medina A, Pan M, et al. Transcatheter occlusion of complex atrial septal defects. *Catheter Cardiovasc Interv* 2000;51:33–41.
21. Cao Q, Radtke W, Berger F, et al. Transcatheter closure of multiple atrial septal defects. Initial results and value of two- and three-dimensional transesophageal echocardiography. *Eur Heart J* 2000;21:941–947.

Catheter Based Devices: For the Treatment of Non-coronary Cardiovascular Diseases in Adults and Children. Edited by P. Syamasundar Rao and Morton J. Kern, Lippincott Williams & Wilkins, Philadelphia © 2003.

7

CARDIOSEAL AND STARFLEX DEVICES

ROLF G. BENNHAGEN
PETER MCLAUGHLIN
LEE N. BENSON

Atrial septal defects are common cardiac lesions, varying in frequency between 5% and 15% of all congenital heart lesions (1–4). Surgical correction, requiring cardiopulmonary bypass and cardioplegia, is generally successful in achieving complete defect closure in most patients. Surgery carries nearly zero risk of mortality, and low morbidity, which includes pericardial or pleural effusions, arrhythmias, postoperative bleeding, atelectasis, pneumonia, and septicemia with or without renal failure (5,6). Sternotomy is associated with pain, the risk of a wound infection, postoperative immobilization, and a permanent surgical scar. As interventional procedures evolved, it was a natural evolution that an interest in the development of a nonsurgical technique for defect closure would be developed (7–10). Two such cardiac implants, under investigational use, are the CardioSEAL (CardioSEAL Septal Occlusion System) and the STARFlex (CardioSEAL Septal Occluder implant with STARFlex Centering System) septal occluders manufactured by Nitinol Medical Technologies, Inc., in Boston, Massachusetts.

THE DEVICES

The CardioSEAL

The earlier version of this double-disk occluder was the earlier Bard Clamshell Septal Umbrella (C.R. Bard, Inc, Billerica, MA) produced in 1989. This implant was tested in more than 700 patients, before the current, sec-

ond-generation CardioSEAL emerged. The original design was withdrawn from clinical trials due to stress fractures in the supporting arms. The present device consists of two self-expanding square umbrella-like disks that, after implantation, fix by spring tension to either side of the atrial septum. Four metal arms, made of the metal alloy MP35N, radiate via hinges from each of the two disk centers to each corner of the disk (Figure 7.1). A knitted polyester fabric (Dacron) covers the disks, including the supporting arms. This framework design facilitates conformability of the implant to variations in the septal topography, as well as giving the device a low profile along the septum after deployment. Two coil joints or hinges in each arm (added in the redesign) displace stress during atrial contraction and contribute to improved fracture resistance (11). The spring-back characteristics allow the disk/umbrella frames to assume their original shape after reexpansion upon device delivery. The metal arms of the device are considered to be more resistant to fatigue fracture and than the original stainless steel formulation in Clamshell implant (11). The alloy is nonferromagnetic, making MRI an investigative option in patients having this implant. The CardioSEAL device is front-loaded into the distal pod of the delivery catheter with the aid of a plastic loader and attached to the delivery catheter through a pin-to-pin attachment mechanism. An 11F sheath is required for the implantation. CardioSEAL is available in five sizes (17, 23, 28, 33, 40 mm), corresponding to the diagonal length of each umbrella. Device diameter is selected to be one and one-half to two times the size of the balloon-stretched diameter (see later). In the United States, CardioSEAL has FDA approval under humanitarian device exemption (HDE) for closure of patent foramen ovale (PFO), ventricular septal defects, and fenestrated Fontan communications in selected patients. General use in patients with an isolated atrial septal defect awaits results of ongoing clinical trial. In 1997, the CardioSEAL was awarded the CE mark in Europe.

Rolf G. Bennhagen: Interventional Fellow, Division of Cardiology, The Hospital for Sick Children, Toronto, Ontario, Canada

Peter McLaughlin: The University Health Network, Toronto General Hospital, University of Toronto School of Medicine, Toronto, Ontario, Canada

Lee N. Benson: Professor, Department of Pediatrics, Division of Cardiology, University of Toronto School of Medicine; Director, Cardiac Catheterization Laboratories, Division of Cardiology, The Hospital for Sick Children, Toronto, Ontario, Canada

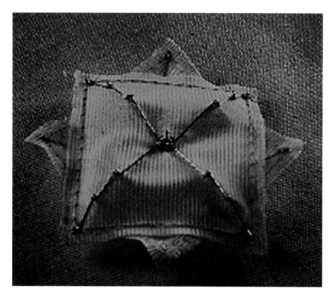

FIGURE 7.1. The CardioSEAL implant. Note the two elbows within each supporting arm.

The STARFlex

The STARFlex implant is a modification of the CardioSEAL implant. The unique difference consists of a flexible, autoadjusting, and self-centering spring mechanism. Soft, flexible metallic microsprings made from Nitinol are attached using polyester sutures along the circumference of the two disk frames alternating between the two umbrellas (12). These microsprings allow the left atrial disk to pivot against the left atrial aspect of the septum during deployment and facilitate the centering of the device within the defect. STARFlex is currently available in four sizes: 23, 28, 33, and 40 mm. It uses a smaller 10F transseptal delivery sheath than the CardioSEAL. The attachment of the device to the delivery catheter uses a pin-to-pin mechanism, similar to that of the CardioSEAL. The length of the pin-to-pin attachment, however, allows the device to rotate through its attachment, reducing tension between device and intraatrial septum. Additionally, the attachment wire is made of a smaller-diameter metal than in the CardioSEAL system, allowing greater flexibility after the right atrial disk is opened. Both, these design changes allow the device to attain the anatomic atrial position before final release (11). The loading system and implantation are similar to those of CardioSEAL, although a new rapid-loading mechanism has recently been made available that reduces handling before implantation and allows air to be easily removed from the catheter before placement into the vascular system. Because of the implant's self-centering properties, larger defects, up to 25 mm (balloon-stretched) in diameter, can be addressed. As such, the ratio of defect size (stretched-diameter) to device diameter can be selected so that the

ratio diameters are in the 1.5:1 to 1.6:1 range (12). High-risk defect clinical trials under FDA guidelines are under way in North America, and the CE mark award was obtained in Europe in 1998.

PATIENT SELECTION

Indications for transcatheter closure of atrial septal defects are similar to those for surgical closure, which include a defect in the septum secundum resulting in right heart volume and a pulmonary-to-systemic flow ratio of greater than 1.5:1 (5). Unfavorable defects for catheter closure are the superior sinus venosus defect, unroofed or partially unroofed coronary sinus defects, primum atrial defects, and inferior sinus venosus defect. In addition, those defects whose rims include the orifice of the inferior caval vein are not suitable for closure. Indications for closure are less clear in early childhood and in elderly patients. If the defect is diagnosed in infancy or early childhood, the size of the defect on two-dimensional transthoracic echocardiogram (TTE) or color-coded Doppler flow mapping (CCD) in end-systole can predict its natural history (13). Defects of less than 3 mm will almost uniformly close spontaneously. Defects ≥3 but ≤ 5 mm in diameter will close in up to 90% of cases, >5 but <8 mm in 80%, and in those ≥8 mm rarely. In the absence of symptoms, closure (surgical or catheter based) is generally postponed until 4 to 6 years of age. In the adult patient, surgical defect closure has improved symptoms of exercise intolerance and possibly mortality over the short term. Table 7.1 lists criteria for transcatheter closure with CardioSEAL and STARFlex implants. After initial screening with TTE, chest radiograph, and electrocardiogram, selected pediatric patients are further evaluated by transesophageal echocardiography (TEE) under general anesthesia, although in adults, TEE is normally performed under sedation alone. TEE reassesses size and defect location, the surrounding rims, length of the atrial septum, and proximity to the pulmonary veins. A clearer understanding of interatrial septal anatomy has become apparent with recent three-dimensional transesophageal echocardiographic reconstructions (14–18) and, coupled with improvements in catheter technique, have broadened the selection criteria (Figure 7.2). Patients with partial deficiency of septal rims, a multiperforated septal wall, septal aneurysms in the oval fossa combined with an atrial septal defect or up to two perforations (19), multiple or irregularly shaped atrial defects or unusually located oval defects are also occludable (20). Finally, patients who have had a fenestrated Fontan procedure and individuals suffering from cerebrovascular accidents with an ascertained PFO comprise two recent groups for transcatheter closure of the communication (20–24).

TABLE 7.1. CRITERIA FOR TRANSCATHETER CLOSURE OF SECUNDUM ATRIAL SEPTAL DEFECTS USING CARDIOSEAL OR STARFLEX IMPLANTS

Presence of a secundum atrial septal defect
Documented left-to-right shunting across the defect
Recommended maximal defect diameter of 20 mm. Relative indication if defect ≤24 mm
Dilated right ventricle with evidence of volume overload
A substantial rim, usually 4–5 mm, between the margins of the defect and nearby intracardiac structures (atrioventricular valves, superior and inferior caval vein, pulmonary veins, and coronary sinus)
Adequate rim of tissue around at least 75% of the defect circumference
Atrial volume large enough to accommodate the device, usually an individual >2 years of age or >10 kg. Peripheral venous vasculature should be able to accommodate a 10 or 11 French sheath.

DEVICE IMPLANTATION TECHNIQUE

Preparation

General anesthesia and TEE guidance are prerequisites for optimal device positioning and maximum patient safety (25). Important anatomic landmarks on TEE before closure are the anterosuperior rim (distance to the aorta), the anteroinferior rim (distance to the tricuspid valve annulus), the posterosuperior rim (distance to the superior caval vein) and the posteroinferior rim (distance to the inferior caval vein). After percutaneous entry of the femoral vein, a complete hemodynamic evaluation is generally performed. A contrast injection in the right upper pulmonary vein to outline the atrial wall and defect (30 degrees LAO, 30 degrees CRAN) has largely been replaced by TEE to determine atrial anatomy. After heparinization, an end-hole catheter is passed through the defect into the left upper pulmonary vein. A hand injection of contrast is undertaken to outline the catheter for later use in quantification for magnification correction, although marker catheters and external references have been useful as well. An exchange-length, 260-cm, guide wire (Cook, Bloomington, IN) is then introduced into the catheter and the catheter is removed.

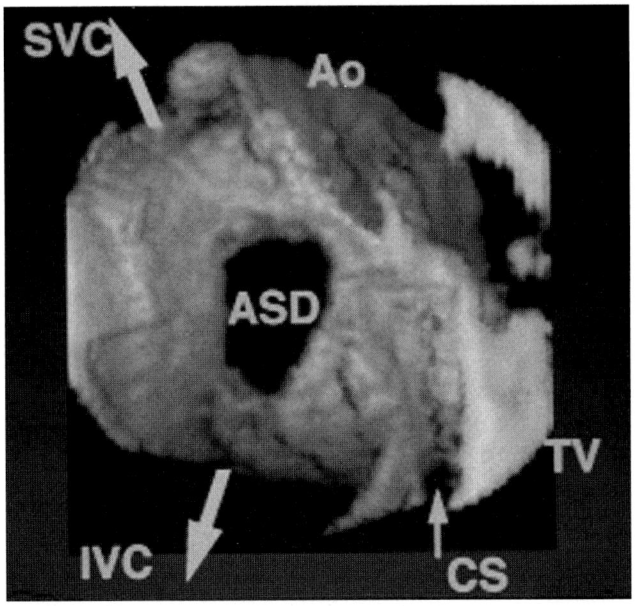

Sizing the Defect

There are several ways to size the defect. Although two- and three-dimensional imaging can define the defect margins, the muscular margins are the effective anchors for the closure. To determine the muscular margins both static and dynamic methods have been employed. Over the guide wire, placed into the pulmonary vein, a round occlusion balloon (Meditech, Watertown, MA) can be advanced through the defect and into the left atrium. The balloon is inflated with a mixture of contrast and saline, and under fluoroscopic and TEE guidance, pulled gently toward the atrial septum. This procedure is repeated, with varying degrees of balloon inflation, until an indentation or deformation is seen on the balloon (Figure 7.3). A cineangiogram is obtained of the deformed balloon. The width of the deformation is measured, and this length is designated as the balloon-stretched diameter. After confirmation of complete balloon occlusion of the defect, TEE interrogates the presence of any additional atrial septal defect(s). If found, their size(s), location(s), and distance(s) from the central defect are defined. The static method of defect diameter determination uses balloons (NuMed, Inc., Nicholville, NY, and AGA Medical, Golden Valley, MN) made from highly compliant materials and oblong in shape. They deform easily when inflated across the defect without the need to pull the balloon against the septum. Inflation is stopped when an indentation is first seen along the balloon length (Figure 7.3). The two methods of defect sizing are not comparable. The first

FIGURE 7.2. Three-dimensional echocardiogram of a typical secundum atrial septal defect. Ao, aorta; ASD, atrial septal defect; CS, coronary sinus; IVC, inferior vena cava; SVC, superior vena cava; TV, tricuspid valve.

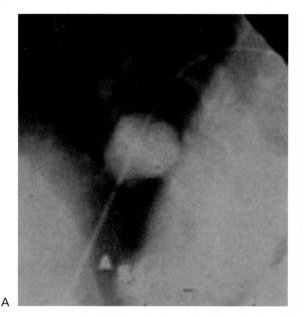

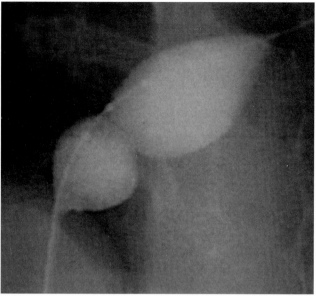

A

B

FIGURE 7.3. A: Dynamic sizing of the atrial septal defect using a pull-back technique. **B:** Static measurement of the defect diameter, using a compliant oblong balloon.

method is truly a stretch defect measurement, as the margins are in contact with the balloon, whereas the second is more filling of the defect. Whether the defect is oblong, circular, or irregular, the former method places tension on the lower margins of the defect (septum primum) but may not stretch the entire lesion circumference. The effect of either sizing technique on oblong, noncircular lesions is not fully understood, regarding the choice of device and device size, although three-dimensional transesophageal echocardiographic reconstructions could be insightful (14–18). Not surprisingly, there is a poor correlation ($r = .41$) between the defect size measured by three-dimensional TEE and the balloon-stretched diameter (16). Moreover, it varies with the shape of the defect, $r = .35$ for complex and $r = .68$ for circular defects (18). Recently, intracardiac echocardiography (AcuNav, Acuson Corporation, Mountain View, CA) has allowed visualization of the atrial septum in real time during the procedure, possibly making TEE unnecessary (26). This latter technology may be very important in the adult, where general anesthesia may be unnecessary.

To avoid implantation of an oversized device, particularly in small patients with large defects, the length of the atrial septum should be measured and compared with the size of the selected device. Depending on the texture and thickness of the interatrial septum, distension and overestimation of the defect size may occur (20). Measurement of a defect considerably smaller than expected suggests passage of the balloon catheter through an unappreciated smaller second defect. When multiple defects are present, a single device can be implanted if it is estimated that the

device would cover all the defects. In this regard, it may be necessary to pass the sheath through the larger or more central defect and TEE may be useful in the catheter location. Two defects distant from each other can also be closed with two devices through two separate sheaths (20). Such devices may overlap slightly after implantation.

Loading of the Device

The selected device is soaked in saline to remove air and then connected to the delivery or core wire (0.014 inch for CardioSEAL, 0.013 inch for STARFlex) by activating the pin-to-pin mechanism. If the retaining sutures attached to the arms of the distal umbrella are pulled, the arms will collapse, allowing the proximal umbrella to be pulled through a loading cylinder. Thereafter the entire device can be loaded into the cylinder. With the delivery wire, the collapsed device is pulled out of the loading cylinder and into a plastic pod at the end of the delivery catheter.

Device Delivery

A 10F long sheath (when using a STARFlex system) with dilator is advanced over the guide wire into the pulmonary vein. To avoid air entry into the system, a continuous infusion of heparinized saline can be maintained through a side arm attached to the dilator of the long sheath. Flushing starts before the system is introduced through the skin. The sheath and dilator are passed to the level of the hepatic portion of the inferior vena cava. While holding the dilator, the sheath is advanced over the guide wire into the left atrium toward the left upper pulmonary vein. During this maneuver, fluid under pressure is continuously passed through the dilator. No attempt to withdraw blood from the sheath is made once it is in position. In the adult, a continuous flushing solution may be unnecessary and the sheath may be aspirated once in the pulmonary vein. After crossing the defect with the sheath, the dilator and the guide wire are carefully removed. It is important to keep the end of the dilator below the level of the heart, or using a water lock, upon withdrawal. The next step is to advance the loaded device with attached delivery wire into the long sheath until the distal arms are fully unfolded into the center of the left atrial cavity. Care is taken to avoid entrapment of the device within the left atrial appendage, pulmonary veins, or mitral valve apparatus. Under TEE guidance, the entire system is pulled back gently toward the left atrial wall, the center of the device is positioned just within the left atrium for the CardioSEAL implant and just until the left atrial umbrella slightly contacts the left side of the atrial septum with the STARFlex. In most cases, this is in the region of the anterosuperior portion of the septum. Attempts should be made to bring the device into a parallel alignment with the atrial septum by rotation of the system (sheath and delivery catheter). The device can be recaptured (i.e., refolded) by retracting the delivery wire with the attached device into the sheath. Preshaping the long sheath, forming a slight curve with a posterior direction at its end, may direct the device more posteriorly in the left atrium. Positioning the sheath into the right upper pulmonary vein is an alternative option. Rotation and/or repositioning the system may also be necessary to achieve optimal contact between device and septum to close multiple or unusually located defects (20). When a satisfactory position toward the atrial septum is obtained, the long sheath is further retracted over the delivery wire (which is kept immobile), thereby unfolding the proximal umbrella in the right atrium, affixing itself against the atrial septum. To avoid distortion of the septum, the sheath is fully retracted to the inferior caval vein. While still connected to the delivery wire, the positioning of the device is confirmed by TEE.

Release of the Device

If the device is in a stable location, not impinging on surrounding structures and with only minor residual shunting through the Dacron disks, the release mechanism is activated by advancement of the delivery wire to disengage the two parts of the pin-to-pin mechanism, resulting in device deployment. Usually, this maneuver will slightly alter the device spatial orientation within the atria.

After Release

TEE is again employed to confirm the final position of the device; evaluate the presence, location, and size of residual shunting; rule out systemic or pulmonary venous obstruction; or compromise atrioventricular valve function. An optional right atrial or inferior caval vein angiogram with follow-through can be done for additional confirmation. Cephalosporins and heparin sulfate are administered before device implantation. A low dose of aspirin (3 to 5 mg/kg daily; maximum, 325 mg) is prescribed for 6 months and endocarditis prophylaxis is recommended for the first 6 months after the procedure.

Retrievability

After release, the devices cannot be refolded, but it can be retrieved with a snare and other snarelike devices.

Practical Considerations

A common pitfall is to unfold the distal (left atrial) umbrella too close to the atrial septum and the defect, which may lead to one of the left disk arms prolapsing through the defect. Another difficulty that might emerge occurs when the curvature of the three-dimensional topology of the atrial septum makes it difficult to adjust the distal umbrella so that it is parallel to the defect. If the distal umbrella can be rotated then toward the right upper pulmonary vein and gently retracted down alongside the septum, it might be possible to keep it parallel with the defect.

STARFlex is implanted in a similar way, as described earlier. The delivery process follows the same steps until the distal arms are unfolded in the left atrium. At this point, to activate the self-centering mechanism, the long sheath is pulled back to a point where the centering microsprings between the umbrellas are uncovered but with the tips of the proximal arms still within the sheath (12). The device can still be recaptured, if not in a favorable position. Although the microsprings are not visible on fluoroscopy, they can be seen on TEE, appearing as a parachute (Figure 7.4). The entire system is pulled back until the distal umbrella slightly touches the left side of atrial septum. Then the proximal umbrella is unfolded by fully retracting the sheath over the delivery wire (which is kept immobile) into the inferior caval vein. If the position is satisfactory on TEE, the device can be released, and the final result can be evaluated. Because of the flexible push wire and the extended pin-to-pin attachment mechanism, there is less device motion (repositioning) of the STARFlex than with other cardiac implants in relation to the atrial septum after release.

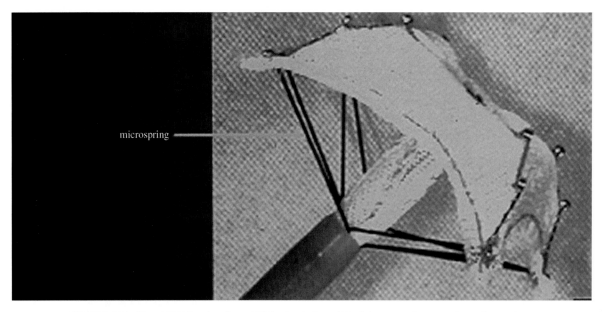

FIGURE 7.4. The STARFlex implant. With the left atrial disk opened, note the microsprings attached to the umbrella disk

RESULTS

Immediate Results

After release of the device, it is unusual to observe changes in position immediately after the procedure, although slight positional alterations have been noted in follow-up (27). In the European multicenter experience (28) with both occluders between 1996 and 1999, the implantation was attempted in 334 patients (mean age, 12 years; mean weight, 44 kg). An isolated defect was found in 73%. Twenty-one patients (6%) had multiple defects; 15 (5%), a defect with a septal aneurysm; 44 (13%), a PFO; and nine (3%), a fenestrated Fontan circulation. The mean defect size was 11.5 mm by TTE, 12 mm by TEE, and 15 mm by balloon-stretched diameter. Mean device-to-balloon-stretched diameter ratio was 2.16 (range, 1.4 to 7). Implantation was accomplished in 325 patients (97.3%) with a mean fluoroscopy time of 18 minutes. A residual leak was detected in 41% immediately after the procedure, decreasing to 31% at time of discharge. Device embolization (minutes to a few hours after implantation) was observed in 13 patients (4%). The devices embolized to the pulmonary artery in 12 cases and once to the left ventricle. Ten of these 13 patients underwent uncomplicated surgical repair, whereas in three cases the devices were retrieved and a second device was successfully reimplanted. The device-to-defect ratio for the embolized devices was 1.8 (range, 1.5 to 2.2). One patient suffered hemiplegia 4 hours after implantation.

At the Hospital for Sick Children, Toronto, 50 patients (median age 9.7 years) underwent percutaneous occlusion of ASD with the CardioSEAL implant between 1996 and 1998 (29). The mean defect diameter, estimated by TEE was 11.9 ± 2.9 mm (range, 7 to 18 mm; median, 12 mm) and by balloon-stretched diameter 13.7 ± 3.2 mm (range, 7.5 to 20 mm; median, 14 mm). Two defects were found in ten patients (20%), and a multiperforated atrial septum was found in one patient (2%). Partial deficiency of septal rims (<4 mm) was present in 19 patients (38%). Before closure Qp:Qs was 1.9 ± 0.7 (range, 1 to 4:1). Fluoroscopy time during the procedure ranged from 7 to 32 minutes (mean, 15.5 ± 5.4 minutes). Device-to-balloon-stretched diameter ratio was 2.5 ± 0.4 (range, 1.9 to 3.6). All patients had successful implantations, although in four (8%) a second device was implanted after removal of a malpositioned initial implant. There were no significant immediate complications. All patients except one were discharged within 24 hours; 40% had a complete closure. Mean follow-up was 9.9 ± 3.2 months (range, 6 to 12 months), and at the latest follow-up, residual shunting was identified in 23 patients (46%). The shunt measured less than 2 mm in 13 patients (26%), 2 to 4 mm in four patients (8%), and more than 4 mm in six patients (12%). Of the six patients with residual shunts of more than 4 mm by CCD, four had normal right ventricular size and septal wall motion. In a univariate analysis, defects with little or no rim, particularly in the anterosuperior portion of the septum, were associated with a higher incidence of residual leaking due to prolapse of one arm through the defect (Figure 7.5). However, in a multivariate analysis, no risk factor was predictive of residual shunting. The right ventricular end-diastolic dimension, corrected for age, decreased from 137 ± 29 to 105 ± 17%, and septal motion abnormalities normalized in all but one

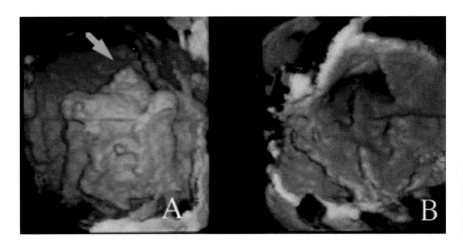

FIGURE 7.5. A three-dimensional echocardiogram after placement of a CardioSEAL implant. The superoanterior rim (*arrow*) was deficient in this patient, and one arm is protruding from left atrium to right atrium. **A:** Right atrial view. **B:** Left atrial view.

patient. Device fractures were detected in seven patients (14%). Prolapse of one arm of the device through the defect was noted in 16 patients (32%). No complications occurred due to device fracture or arm prolapse. Five patients (10%) experienced transient headaches. There were no episodes of device embolization, endocarditis, stroke, or cardiac-related hospital admissions (29).

Healing Process

With the device *in situ* a normal healing process is initiated. In long-term animal studies (30) neointima covered the device surface area to at least 50% by 1 month and completely by 3 months. After 2 years, the encapsulated device becomes more densely organized with fibrous tissue and neovascularized, with a persistent foreign-body reaction between the device and surrounding tissue.

Complications

Device fracture, dislocation, and embolization are possible complications to device implantation, becoming more infrequent with improved device engineering, improved techniques, and experience. One isolated case of left atrial wall erosion has been described (29). Thromboembolic events can occur, despite antiplatelet therapy during and after the intervention, partly depending on the patient's preinterventional condition. Alteration in atrioventricular valve function can be avoided with TEE. With a meticulous implantation technique, air embolism can be eliminated. Finally, the cause of postprocedural headache days after the implantation is not yet fully understood, but generally is well treated with acetaminophen.

Follow-up

Various follow-up protocols are in use; however, there is no standardization. Some authors advocate routine follow-up TEE (20). Right ventricular end-diastolic dimensions have

been measured serially and noted to normalize over time as compared with predicted values for age (31). In the European Multicenter study (28), residual shunting decreased to 24% at 1 month, 21% at 6, months and 20.5% by 12 months after implantation. Two patients underwent elective surgical repair at 6 months. The indication in one patient was device malposition and in another, late device embolization. Device arm fractures were seen in 19 of 309 patients (6.1%). All remain asymptomatic. Such fractures were most common with the larger devices (23 mm: *N* = 1; 28 mm: *N* = 1; 33 mm: *N* = 7; 40 mm: *N* = 10). There were no arrhythmias, endocarditis, valvular distortion, thromboembolic events, or other complications. At 1-year follow-up, clinical success, defined as complete closure of the defect or presence of only a trivial leak, was observed in 99 of 107 patients (92.5%). A study with longer median follow-up (32) (31 months; range, 7 to 56) with the Clamshell device (USCI Angiographics) experienced a higher occurrence of device arm fractures of 42% and a 36% incidence of residual, hemodynamically nonsignificant shunting after 4 years, although progressive spontaneous shunt resolution continued years after implantation.

APPLICABILITY TO ADULT SUBJECTS

Previously undiagnosed secundum atrial septal defects are often detected in adults. A recent study discussed the reversibility of symptoms and effects on the right heart circulation after device closure (33). Forty adults underwent secundum ASD device closure (32 CardioSEAL, eight Amplatzer Septal Occluder). Mean ASD size was 13 mm and device sizes varied from 12 to 40 mm. One month after the procedure, heart size (50% versus 46%), QRS-duration (125 versus 119 ms), right atrial (39 versus 34 mm), and ventricular dimensions (43 versus 41 mm) had decreased significantly. Six months after the procedure, pulmonary arterial pressures began to decline (37 versus 32 mm Hg) and the paradoxical septal motion had completely normalized. Individuals with grown-up congenital heart disease (GUCH) who enter adult life with an atrial communication (i.e., fenestrated Fontan) (34) as well as adults with a PFO experiencing presumed paradoxical embolism (24) or orthodeoxia-platypnea syndrome (35,36) are all possible candidates for transcatheter closure with these devices.

DISCUSSION

The CardioSEAL or STARFlex implants correct the hemodynamic disturbances secondary to the right ventricular volume overload and pulmonary hyperperfusion. Ventricular septal motion, right atrial, and ventricular dimensions normalize. Small residual leaks that can be detected in a few at follow-up appear to be of little clinical importance. Although little data are available, results suggest that the rate of residual leaks is lower with the STARFlex design (28). The low profile of the CardioSEAL and STARFlex designs facilitates endothelialization and minimizes the risk of thrombus formation in the atria. Device fractures have not been completely eliminated with CardioSEAL, although the incidence is clearly lower than that with the Clamshell implant (32,37). The presence of fractures is not associated with an increased rate of residual shunting, device embolization, or other clinical complications. The relatively high incidence of headaches detected after device closure is an interesting observation of unknown etiology. Possible explanations in the genesis of these symptoms include the release of vasoactive mediators from platelets during the early process of endothelialization or the release of vasoactive hormones that increase left atrial or decrease right atrial pressure and volume after defect closure. In comparison, the more flexible microspring centering mechanism in the STARFlex design does not distort the atrial septum during implantation to the same extent as with CardioSEAL (12). The spring coil design allows for positioning of each arm and reduces the stress forces between the device and the atrial septum (12). Because of the STARFlex self-centering mechanism, relatively smaller devices can be used to close similar-sized defects. Correspondingly, larger defects, up to 25-mm balloon-stretched diameter, can be closed with this implant. The issue of the surrounding rim appears to be less critical for implantation with the later design (12).

REFERENCES

1. Feldt RH, Avasthey P, Yosimasu F, et al. Incidence of congenital heart disease in children born to residents of Olmstead County, Minnesota, 1950–1969. *Mayo Clin Proc* 1971;46:794–799.
2. Keith JD. Atrial septal defect: ostium secundum, ostium primum and atrioventricularis communis (common AV canal). In: Keith JD, Rowe RD, Vlad P, eds. *Heart disease in infancy and childhood,* 3rd ed. New York: Macmillan, 1978:380–404.
3. Nakamura FF, Hauck AJ, Nadas AS. Atrial septal defects in infants. *Pediatrics* 1964; 34:101–106.
4. Porter Coburn J, Feldt RH, Edwards WD, et al. Atrial septal defects. In: Emmanouilides GC, Riemen-schneider TA, Allen HD, et al. *Disease in infants, children, and adolescents. Including the fetus and young adults,* 5th ed. Baltimore: William & Wilkins 1995:687–703.
5. Latson LA. Per-catheter ASD closure. *Pediatr Cardiol* 1998;19: 86–93.
6. Galal M, Wobst A, Halees Z, et al. Perioperative complications following surgical closure of atrial septal defect type II in 232 patients: a baseline study. *Eur Heart J* 1994;15:1381–1384.
7. King TD, Thompson SL, Steiner C, et al. Secundum atrial septal defect: nonoperative closure during cardiac catheterization. *JAMA* 1976;235:2506–2509.
8. Lock JE, Rome JJ, Davis R, et al. Transcatheter closure of atrial septal defects: experimental studies. *Circulation* 1989;79: 1091–1099.
9. Rome JJ, Keane JF, Perry SB, et al. Double-umbrella closure of atrial septal defects: initial clinical applications. *Circulation* 1990; 82:751–758.
10. Bjornstad PG. The role of devices in the closure of atrial septal defects in the oval fossa. *Cardiol Young* 1998;8:285–286.
11. Latson LA. The CardioSEAL device: history, techniques, results. *J Interv Cardiol* 1998;11:501–505.
12. Hausdorf G, Kaulitz R, Paul T, Carminati M, et al. Transcatheter closure of atrial septal defect with a new, flexible, self-centering device (the STARFlex occluder). *Am Heart J* 1999;84: 1113–1116.
13. Radzik D, Davignon A, Van Doesburg N, et al. Predictive factors for spontaneous closure of atrial septal defects diagnosed in the first 3 months of life. *J Am Coll Cardiol* 1993;22:851–853.
14. Acar P, Piechaud JF, Bonhoeffer P, et al. Anatomic evaluation of ostium secundum atrial defects by three-dimensional echocardiography. *Arch Mal Coeur Vaiss* 1998;91:543–550.
15. Acar P, Saliba Z, Bonhoeffer P, et al. Influence of atrial septal defect anatomy in patient selection and assessment of closure with the CardioSEAL device: a three-dimensional transoesophageal echocardiographic reconstruction. *Eur Heart J* 2000; 21:573–581.
16. Acar P, Bonhoeffer P, Saliba Z, et al. Three-dimensional reconstruction by transesophageal echocardiography of Amplatzer and CardioSEAL prosthetic devices after percutaneous closure and atrial septal defects. *Arch Mal Coeur Vaiss* 2000;93:539–545.
17. Maeno YV, Benson LN, Boutin C. Impact of dynamic 3D transesophageal echocardiography in the assessment of atrial septal defects and occlusion by the double-umbrella device (CardioSEAL). *Cardiol Young* 1998;8:368–378.
18. Acar P. Three-dimensional echocardiography in transcatheter closure of atrial septal defects. *Cardiol Young* 2000;10:484–492.
19. Ewert P, Berger F, Vogel M, et al. Morphology of perforated atrial septal aneurysm suitable for closure by transcatheter device placement. *Heart* 2000;84:327–331.
20. Kaulitz R, Paul T, Hausdorf G. Extending the limits of transcatheter closure of atrial septal defects with the double umbrella device (CardioSEAL). *Heart* 1998;80:54–59.
21. Chambers J. Should percutaneous devices be used to close a patent foramen ovale after cerebral infarction or TIA? *Heart* 1999;82:537–538.
22. Van Camp G, Schulze D, Cosyns B, et al. Relation between patent foramen ovale and unexplained stroke. *Am J Cardiol* 1993; 71:596–598.
23. Bridges ND, Hellenbrand W, Latson L, et al. Transcatheter closure of presumed paradoxical embolism. *Circulation* 1992;86: 1902–1908.
24. Hung J, Landzberg MJ, Jenkins KJ, et al. Closure of patent fora-

men ovale for paradoxical emboli: intermediate-term risk of recurrent neurological events following transcatheter device placement. *J Am Coll Cardiol* 2000;35:1311–1316.

25. Hellenbrand WE, Fahey JT, McGowan FX, et al. Transoesophageal echocardiographic guidance of transcatheter closure of atrial septal defect. *Am J Cardiol* 1990;66:207–213.

26. Bruce CJ, Packer DL, Belohlavek, M, et al. Intracardiac echocardiography: newest technology. *J Am Loc Echocard* 2000;13:780–795.

27. Boutin C, Musewe NN, Smallhorn JF, et al. Echocardiographic follow-up of atrial septal defect after catheter closure by double umbrella device. *Circulation* 1993;88:621–627.

28. Carminati M, Giusti S, Hausdorf G, et al. A European multicentre experience using the CardioSEAL and STARFlex double umbrella devices to close interatrial communications holes within the oval fossa. *Cardiol Young* 2000;10:519–526.

29. Pedra CAC, Pihkala J, Lee K-J, et al. Transcatheter closure of the atrial septal defects using the CardioSEAL implant. *Heart* 2000;84:320–326.

30. Kuhn MA, Latson LA, Cheatham JP, et al. Biological response to Bard Clamshell Septal Occluders in the canine heart. *Circulation* 1996;93:1459–1463.

31. Meyer RA. *Pediatric echocardiography.* Philadelphia: Lea & Febiger, 1977:291–294.

32. Justo RN, Nykanen DG, Boutin C, et al. Clinical impact of transcatheter closure of secundum atrial septal defects with the double umbrella device. *Am J Cardiol* 1996;77:889–892.

33. Veldtman GR, Razak V, Benson LN, et al. Right ventricular form and function after percutaneous ASD device closure. *J Am Coll Cardiol* 2001;37:2108–2113.

34. Ruiz CE, Austin EH 3rd, Cheatham JP, et al. First Food and Drug Administration approval under humanitarian device exemption of a septal occluder for fenestrated Fontan and muscular ventricular septal defects. *Circulation* 2000;101:E9042.

35. Landzberg MJ, Sloss LJ, Faherty CE, et al. Orthodeoxia-platypnea due to intracardiac shunting: relief with transcatheter double umbrella closure. *Cathet Cardiovasc Diagn* 1995;36:247–250.

36. Waight DJ, Cao Q-L, Hijazi ZM. Closure of patent foramen ovale in patients with orthodeoxia-platypnea using the Amplatzer devices. *Cathet Cardiovasc Interv* 2000;50:195–198.

37. Prieto LR, Foreman CK, Cheatham JP, et al. Intermediate-term outcome of transcatheter secundum atrial septal defect closure using the Bard Clamshell septal umbrella. *Am J Cardiol* 1996;78:1310–1312.

Catheter Based Devices: For the Treatment of Non-coronary Cardiovascular Diseases in Adults and Children. Edited by P. Syamasundar Rao and Morton J. Kern, Lippincott Williams & Wilkins, Philadelphia © 2003.

8

HELEX SEPTAL OCCLUDER

LARRY A. LATSON
NEIL WILSON
EVAN M. ZAHN

The HELEX Septal Occluder is a new double-disk transcatheter occlusion device with some unique features. In the conceptualization and building of this device, the design team sought to create an occluder that emphasized certain characteristics. A round shape using relatively flexible materials was utilized to produce a device that is as atraumatic as possible. The ability to deploy the device and yet maintain the option of easily repositioning or removing it if necessary was considered essential. Materials for the device—Nitinol covered almost entirely by ultrathin ePTFE—were chosen to provide excellent biocompatibility. The final HELEX design has characteristics that may make it an appealing choice for transcatheter treatment of many patients with atrial septal defects (ASDs) (1).

DEVICE

The HELEX Septal Occluder is designed to be nearly linear when elongated for delivery through a catheter and yet form an elegant rounded and relatively flat septal occluder with deployment (Figure 8.1). The frame of the device is constructed from a single strand of Nitinol wire. The superelastic wire can be largely straightened for withdrawal into the delivery catheter. As the Nitinol frame is deployed, it forms into two interconnected circular, disklike structures designed to be deployed on either side of the atrial septum. The Nitinol frame is draped with a sheet of ultrathin ePTFE that is bonded to the wire. When the frame is in its final configuration, the ePTFE forms an occluding membrane to block flow through the ASD. To secure the free edge of the ePTFE membrane at the central portion of the device, the membrane is threaded onto a mandrel around which the Nitinol frame configures itself during deployment (Figure 8.2). The terminal portion of the wire frame forms a locking loop to restrict separation of the three "eyelets" in the frame when the device is fully released.

The HELEX Septal Occluder is delivered through a 9F delivery catheter. Because the frame is formed from a single elongated piece of thin Nitinol wire, the delivery catheter remains relatively flexible even with the device loaded inside. The catheter can therefore be maneuvered directly across the atrial septal defect without first placing a separate long sheath. The HELEX Septal Occluder was designed to maximize safety during deployment. All or a portion of the device can be withdrawn back into the delivery catheter even after complete formation of both occluding disks. This feature allows the operator to change the position of the device if it is initially in an undesirable orientation with respect to the defect. Until the device is released from the mandrel, it can be fully or partially withdrawn back into the delivery catheter and redeployed in a new position. Even after the mandrel has been removed, the device remains attached to the delivery catheter by a loop of ePTFE thread that is anchored at the tip of the control catheter, then threaded through the right atrial eyelet, and back out the end of the control catheter itself (Figure 8.2). The free end of the suture is held in place at the end of the control catheter by a safety cap. This safety cord attachment to the device allows the device to be released from all the formed portions of the delivery system and to achieve its true final resting position. If the device should embolize upon release of the mandrel or if the final resting position without any tension on the device was considered suboptimal, then the device could be withdrawn by pulling it back into the delivery catheter using the safety cord. Withdrawal of the device using the safety cord unlocks the Gore-Tex membrane from the central portion of the frame and renders the device unusable at that point. However, the additional safety feature does allow an extra level of protection of the patient

Larry A. Latson: Chairman of Pediatric Cardiology, Medical Director of Center for Pediatric and Congenital Heart Diseases, Cleveland Clinic Foundation, Department of Pediatric Cardiology, Cleveland, Ohio

Neil Wilson: Consultant Pediatric Cardiologist, Royal Hospital for Sick Children, Yorkhill, Glasgow, Scotland

Evan M. Zahn: Director, Catheterization Laboratory, Miami Children's Hospital, Miami, Florida

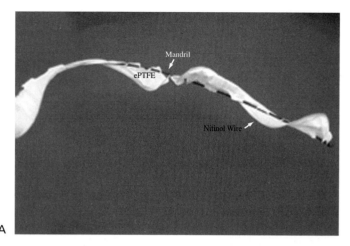

A

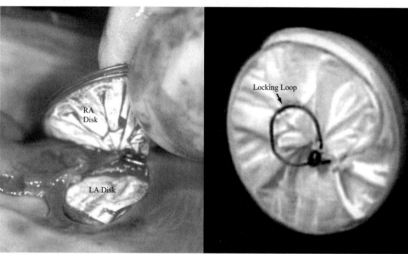

B

FIGURE 8.1. A: Photograph of HELEX device in its nearly completely elongated configuration. The ePTFE membrane has a Nitinol wire frame embedded in the free edge. The device is threaded onto a mandrel that is used during deployment and then removed as one of the final steps of device release. **B:** Photographs of the HELEX Septal Occluder in its final shape. On the left, the device has been placed in an animal with a surgically created ASD. The RA disk is being pulled back to demonstrate the defect, and the LA disk can be seen through the defect in the septum. The disks are quite flexible and there is little distortion of the septal tissue as the right atrial disk is folded back in this photograph. The en fosse view of the right atrial side of the device in the right-hand photograph illustrates the shape of the device. The terminal portion of the Nitinol wire frame of the device forms a locking loop that helps to hold the left and right atrial disks together. LA, left atrium; RA, right atrium.

from error in device placement or very early device embolization.

PATIENT SELECTION

The HELEX Septal Occluder was designed for transcatheter closure of interatrial communications. The available device diameters range from 15 to 35 mm in 5-mm increments. The delivery catheter is advanced through a standard 9F sheath in the femoral vein. Patients as small as 8 kg have been found to easily accommodate this size of sheath in the early clinical trials. Devices such as the HELEX with a narrow central connection between the occluding disks work well for small defects such as patent foramen ovale (PFO) or baffle fenestrations and for patients with multiple defects. In patients with multiple defects, the delivery catheter is placed through one of the more central defects and a device large enough to cover the most distant defect is deployed in this central position. This feature avoids the need for multiple smaller occluders. The currently approved upper size limit for a secundum atrial sep-

tal defect is a stretched diameter of 22 mm. This device is not recommended for primum atrial septal defects or sinus venous atrial septal defects.

Refinements in guidelines for device sizing are still undergoing evaluation. In many patients, one of several sizes could be readily utilized. When small patient size is a concern, device-to-defect-diameter ratios of 1.5 or slightly less have proven to be effective. In medium-sized to large defects, some degree of self-centering appears to be conferred by the spiraling middle portion of the frame and slightly increased bulk of the ePTFE material near the central portion of the device. In small patients, the round and soft frame of the device allows the use of a device that is large enough to be somewhat constrained in its position by the walls of the atrium itself. In larger patients who can readily accommodate large-diameter devices, a device-to-defect ratio exceeding 2 can be utilized to geometrically ensure complete coverage of the defect. The two occluding disks of the device are similar in size and strength so that the device can be used for left-to-right or right-to-left shunts without modification. Placement of more than one device in separate, widely spaced holes is technically feasible. An

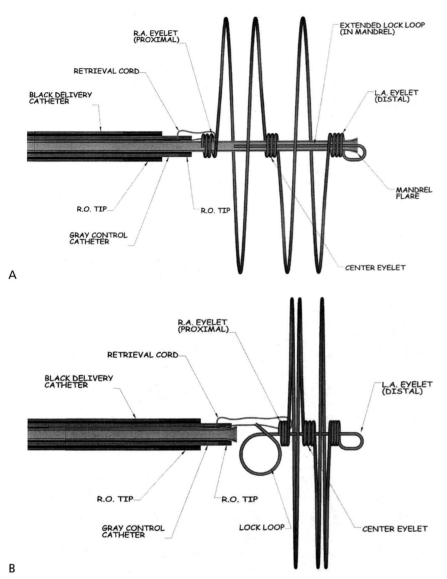

A

B

FIGURE 8.2. Diagrams of HELEX Septal Occluder components. **A:** This diagram illustrates the device and delivery system after both left atrial and right atrial disks have been configured but before release of the device from the mandrel. Note that the frame of the device is composed from a single length of Nitinol wire. One end of the retrieval or safety cord is attached to the tip of the gray control catheter and the cord is then threaded through the right atrial eyelet and back through the lumen of the gray control catheter, where it is secured by a red safety cap (not shown). Thus the gray control catheter controls the proximal portion of the wire frame. The distal portion of the frame is threaded into the mandrel and is held in place by friction and the flare at the end of the mandrel. Pushing the mandrel while holding the gray control catheter in position elongates the frame so that it is straightened and can be withdrawn into the black delivery catheter. **B:** Diagrammatic view of the device after the locking loop has been released. Withdrawal of the mandrel has allowed the distal-most portion of the frame to form into a loop that prevents the eyelets of the device from separating. Note that some slack has been created in the retrieval cord (as described in the text) but that the retrieval cord is still looped through the right atrial eyelet. Thus a flexible attachment to the device is maintained after release from the formed elements of the delivery system as a safety feature in case the device should embolize at the time of release or in case the operator feels that the device position or function is less than optimal and removal of the device is desired. L.A., left atrium; R.A., right atrium; R.O., radiopaque.

experimental study looking at the *in vitro* effects of such deployments is currently under way.

DEVICE IMPLANTATION TECHNIQUE

Most of the steps recommended for implantation of the HELEX Septal Occluder device are similar to those for other devices. Transesophageal echocardiography is recommended to aid in accurate device placement. Therefore most operators prefer to use general anesthesia, especially in younger patients. A right heart catheterization is performed to assess hemodynamics. A pulmonary arteriogram or pulmonary vein angiogram is done to ensure that there are no abnormalities of pulmonary venous return and to produce a road map of the location of the atrial septum radiographically. Some prefer to leave a separate pulmonary artery

catheter in place throughout the delivery of any type of ASD occluder so that repeat hemodynamics and angiography can be performed with minimal catheter manipulation around a freshly deployed device. A right femoral venous catheter is advanced to the left atrium or left pulmonary vein and a guide wire is positioned through this catheter. A sizing balloon with a nominal diameter that is preferably at least 1.5 times the echocardiographic diameter of the ASD is advanced over the guide wire. The sizing balloon is inflated by hand under very low pressure only until the distinct indentation in the balloon caused by the ASD is readily identified (Figure 8.3). The balloon is usually not even fully inflated, to avoid the possibility of inadvertently enlarging the ASD. The diameter of the indentation of the balloon is measured angiographically and by transesophageal echocardiography. Transesophageal echocardiography is also used to be certain that no other sites of left-

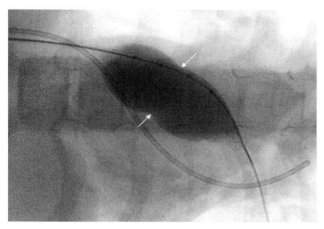

FIGURE 8.3. Determining the stretch diameter of the ASD. A guide wire can be seen extending through the atrial septal defect and into the left upper pulmonary vein. The sizing balloon has been advanced to the level of the atrial septum and has been partially inflated. Indentations from the edges of the defect can be readily visualized *(arrows)*. The diameter of this waist in the balloon is the stretch diameter of the ASD. Note that a second catheter has been placed in the main pulmonary artery to perform pulmonary arteriograms and obtain repeat hemodynamics as desired throughout the procedure.

to-right shunting are identifiable when the sizing balloon is occluding the ASD. A pulmonary arteriogram can be performed with a second catheter to assess any residual shunting angiographically if desired.

An appropriately sized HELEX Septal Occluder device is selected. A side-arm adapter positioned on the delivery catheter is used to flush the catheter and eliminate any trapped air bubbles. During the loading process, the HELEX Septal Occluder is placed in a basin filled with normal saline. The device is loaded by incrementally advancing the mandrel to straighten the frame and withdrawing the gray control catheter to withdraw the frame into the delivery catheter. This entire process is performed with the device held under water to avoid trapping any small air bubbles. The catheter is then flushed thoroughly through the side-arm adapter until no bubbles are visible exiting from the end of the catheter.

The sizing balloon and guide wire are removed and the HELEX Septal Occluder delivery catheter is inserted through the femoral sheath and advanced directly across the ASD to the middle left atrium. The left atrial disk of the device is deployed by incrementally advancing the gray control catheter and withdrawing the mandrel. The left atrial disk can be seen to form around the mandrel. The middle eyelet of the device is readily identifiable fluoroscopically and marks the division between the left atrial and right atrial disks (Figure 8.4). When the left atrial disk is fully formed, the entire system is gently withdrawn toward the atrial septum. The position is checked fluoroscopically and by transesophageal echocardiography. In most cases, mild

tension can be applied to the left atrial disk since no arms or portions of the device are at risk for prolapsing through the defect. If the left atrial disk size and position seem appropriate, the delivery catheter is withdrawn to the inferior vena cava–right atrial junction while the left atrial disk is held in place by maintaining the position of the gray control catheter and mandrel (Figure 8.4B). The right atrial disk is then formed by advancing the gray control catheter over the mandrel. The gray control catheter and the black delivery catheter are then advanced against the device to bring all the central eyelets close together. The position of the device and the presence of any residual leaks are assessed by transesophageal echocardiography. The freshly deployed device is relatively echo-dense and the position of the right atrial disk is best assessed from a transgastric view so that shadowing from the left atrial disk is minimized.

If the device position appears to be suboptimal, the device can be withdrawn back into the delivery catheter by incrementally advancing the mandrel and withdrawing the gray control catheter, as was done during the initial loading process. All or a portion of the device can be withdrawn as needed. The catheter can then be readvanced to the left atrium and the device redeployed in a new orientation.

If the device position is deemed optimal, then the locking loop can be deployed. Before deploying the locking loop, it is advisable to allow approximately 2 cm of slack in the safety cord. This is done by removing the red safety cap at the end of the catheter and then withdrawing the gray control catheter approximately 2 cm while the black delivery catheter remains buttressed against the center portion of the device. The gray control catheter is then readvanced to the device and the black delivery catheter is withdrawn at least 2 cm. To release the terminal portion of the device that forms the locking loop, the mandrel is withdrawn until no further tension is felt. The mandrel is then left in position and the gray control catheter is withdrawn to allow the loop of the locking mechanism to form in the right atrium.

At this point, all the formed portions of the delivery system have been released and the device position can be assessed with no tension on the device (Figure 8.4C). The only attachment to the delivery system is the safety cord, which is looped through the right atrial eyelet. If the device were to embolize through the ASD at this point or if the device position were suboptimal enough that it was felt that device removal was indicated, then replacing the red safety cap would lock the safety cord in position at the end of the catheter. The gray control catheter could then be withdrawn to pull the device back into the delivery catheter. The device is elongated back into its relatively linear configuration of ePTFE-draped Nitinol wire. Removal by this method unzips (or unlocks) the free edge of the ePTFE from the device, and an unzipped device cannot be redeployed. However, another device can be selected and deployed if it is felt that a different size or position would be successful.

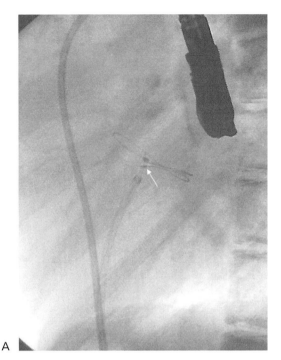

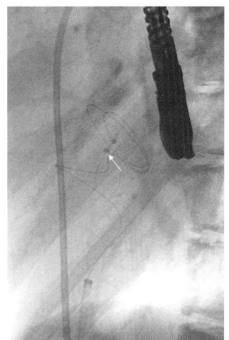

A

B

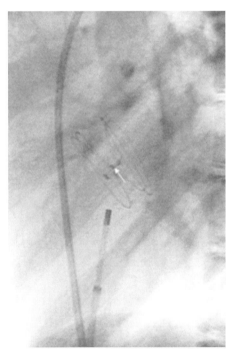

C

FIGURE 8.4. Fluoroscopic views of deployment of HELEX Septal Occluder. **A:** The left atrial disk has been deployed in the left atrium and pulled against the atrial septum. The middle eyelet *(white arrow)* clearly demarcates the division between the left atrial disk and the right atrial disk. **B:** The delivery catheter has been withdrawn to the right atrium–inferior vena cava junction. The gray control catheter (not shown) is being advanced to allow formation of the right atrial disk. Note that the left atrial disk remains in position against the left side of the atrial septum, and the middle eyelet is in the plane of the ASD. **C:** Both the left and right atrial disks have been formed, and the mandrel has been withdrawn to complete delivery of the formed elements of the device. The catheter with the dark tip is the gray control catheter, and a safety cord still is threaded from the tip of this catheter through the right atrial eyelet and then back through the lumen of the catheter (not visible fluoroscopically). A full assessment of the device in its final configuration and orientation can be made. If necessary, the device could still be pulled back into the delivery catheter, even at this point.

If the device position is optimal, then the black delivery catheter can be gently advanced over the safety cord until it is abutting the central portion of the device. The mandrel is then fully withdrawn from the gray control catheter and the gray control catheter is slowly withdrawn to pull the safety cord completely through the right atrial eyelet and totally release the device. Final hemodynamics and a pulmonary arteriogram provide assessment of device positioning and evidence of any residual left-to-right shunting.

RESULTS

The HELEX device is among the newest of the ASD occlusion devices described in this book. The first human implantations of this device were performed in Glasgow, Scotland, by Dr. Neil Wilson in the summer of 1999. The initial US implantations occurred at Miami Children's Hospital and the Cleveland Clinic Children's Hospital, July 2000. The device had undergone extensive engineering and animal trials before the first human implantations (2,3).

At the time of writing of this chapter, the HELEX Septal Occluder had been used to close a hemodynamically significant atrial septal defect in approximately 70 patients, and the available data on follow-up evaluations were limited. Data on the first 46 patients were published in abstract form and presented at the American Heart Association meeting in October 2000 (4). This published experience plus additional preliminary data have shown that the device has an excellent safety record. The device has been used in patients as young as 13 months without difficulty. Defects as large as 22 mm have been closed utilizing the 35-mm-diameter device. The HELEX has proven effective in closing multiple defects with a single device by delivering a device large enough to cover adjacent openings through one of the more central defects. A long sheath has been used in some patients to selectively guide the delivery catheter through a specific central ASD. Small leaks visible at implantation appear to get smaller, and most disappear within 6 months. More long-term follow-up is needed to accurately assess the complete closure rate, but preliminary data are encouraging.

No major complications have been reported in patients undergoing ASD closure with the HELEX Septal Occluder.

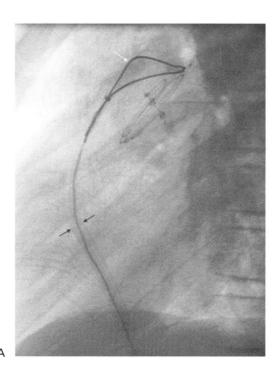
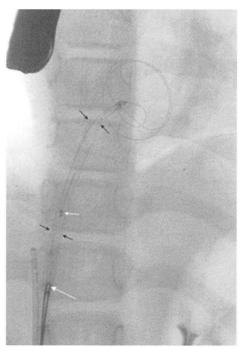

A   B

FIGURE 8.5. Snare retrieval of embolized HELEX Septal Occluder. **A:** Lateral radiograph of HELEX Septal Occluder embolized to the distal main pulmonary artery. An 11F long sheath has been advanced to the right atrium *(black arrows)* and the snare catheter has been advanced to the main pulmonary artery. The gooseneck snare *(white arrow)* was manipulated between the layers of the HELEX Septal Occluder to capture a portion of the frame of the device. **B:** A-P radiograph demonstrating withdrawal of the embolized HELEX Septal Occluder into the 11F long sheath *(black arrows)*. The snare *(large white arrow)* was used to capture a portion of the frame, and the device was withdrawn to the right ventricle. The right atrial eyelet *(small arrow)* is seen in the long sheath. Continued traction on the snare results in the device elongating into its linear form so that it can be completely removed through the long sheath.

One minor procedural complication has been transient ST changes secondary to presumed embolization of small air bubbles during delivery in two patients. These events were transient and did not require specific therapy. They occurred early in the experience with the device and such events should be preventable with proper technique. Early in the experience, several devices were removed because the locking loop did not correctly catch the right atrial eyelet during deployment. The utility of providing additional slack to the safety cord just before deployment was subsequently recognized, and the incidence of missed right atrial eyelet decreased significantly. Determination of optimal device sizing evolved throughout the early experience. Device-to-stretched-diameter ratios as low as 1.3 have been successful. The use of large devices in small patients may result in poor configuration of the device. In one patient, transient complete atrioventricular (AV) block developed as the right atrial disk of an overly large device was configured. In all instances, the devices were easily removed and smaller devices were successfully deployed with device-to-defect ratios of less than 2 to 1.

The effectiveness of the safety features of the device is undeniable. Devices have been removed using the safety cord because of unacceptably large leaks or suboptimal device position after initial deployment. Three undersized devices have embolized after release of the safety cord. Two of these embolizations occurred in the catheterization laboratory and one occurred within the first 12 hours. All devices embolized to the right atrium or right ventricle. There was no hemodynamic instability with the embolizations. All devices were removed uneventfully utilizing a goose-neck snare (Figure 8.5). A larger device was successfully redeployed and remained in place in two patients. The stretch diameter of the third patient was 26 mm, and no additional attempts were made to close the defect with the HELEX Septal Occluder.

APPLICABILITY IN ADULT SUBJECTS

The HELEX Septal Occluder has been used in a number of adult patients with atrial septal defects. There do not appear to be any inherent characteristics that make the HELEX Septal Occluder performance different in adult patients from what it is in pediatric patients. The only limitation is the size of the ASD, which may exceed the maximal allowable stretch diameter of 22 mm in a larger proportion of adult ASD patients than pediatric ASD patients. Although this chapter does not present data on PFO patients following a stroke, the device has been used in this population with excellent early results. The device works well for patients with fenestrated atrial septal defects, since a large device can be used to cover a significant portion of the atrial septum with a single device. Several patients with atrial septum aneurysms have had HELEX Septal Occluders successfully implanted. Use of a relatively large device allows the aneurysm tissue to be sandwiched between the two disks.

DISCUSSION

The HELEX Septal Occluder is a new device for transcatheter ASD closure. A number of advantageous features of the device have been demonstrated in the *in vitro* studies, animal studies, and limited early human clinical studies. Computer modeling of the Nitinol frames and *in vitro* testing of intact devices have shown an extremely low likelihood of frame fracture (2). The ultrathin ePTFE membrane utilized to cover all of the device except for small portions of the central latching mechanism is considered by many to be the best available vascular patch material. Animal studies have demonstrated that the ePTFE membrane allows for cellular adhesion and relatively rapid formation of a fibrointimal layer (2,3). Transesophageal evaluations in living animals and histologic studies of major organs from animals with devices implanted for up to 1 year have demonstrated no evidence of peripheral emboli (3).

Relatively limited clinical studies to date have shown that the device can be deployed safely. More steps are involved in deployment than with some other devices. However, the unique delivery system and safety features of the device have performed as intended. The device is delivered directly by the delivery catheter without the necessity of first placing a long transseptal sheath. No difficulties relating to this delivery method have been discovered. The ability to deploy and then reposition the device has proven to be a significant comfort to the operator and allows for removal or repositioning of the device if the initial deployment seems less than optimal. The safety cord retains a flexible attachment to the device even after release from the major parts of the delivery system. This allows the operator to remove the device easily after assessing its function in the final anatomic position. The rounded shape and flexibility of this device add to the safety of the device if embolizations occur. Numerous purposeful embolizations in animals and three embolizations in humans have demonstrated that the device is very unlikely to cause problems as it travels through the heart. Because the device is relatively easily captured and can be pulled into a long sheath in its linear form, retrieval from distal vascular sites is significantly easier than retrieval of bulky devices that cannot be fully collapsed and must be withdrawn through the heart with portions of the device protruding. Our preliminary experience with this device has convinced us that, although slightly more manual dexterity is required to deploy this device than with some other transcatheter ASD closure devices, the movements can be readily mastered by anyone familiar with catheter interventions. The other advantageous features appear to outweigh the small amount of time required to become familiar with the deployment movements.

CURRENT STATUS

The HELEX Septal Occluder device is currently approved for use in the European market. Company policies require device training before use in each institution. Phase I feasibility trials are under way in the United States. A multicenter pivotal trial of the device began in 2001. Minor modifications of materials used in the delivery system are planned before the pivotal trials. No changes in the design of the device itself are anticipated.

CONCLUSION

The HELEX Septal Occluder for transcatheter ASD closure is still in its infancy in terms of clinical use. Thorough preclinical testing and early limited human trials are very encouraging. Particular strengths of the device include the shape of the device, the materials utilized, ease of deployment of the device without a long sheath, and design features to allow for easy repositioning or withdrawal. Safety features enhance confidence should difficulties be encountered with positioning of the device before or after the device is released from the delivery system. Expanded use of the device commercially in Europe and in a multicenter trial in the United States began in 2001.

REFERENCES

1. Latson LA, Zahn EM, Wilson N. HELEX Septal Occluder for closure of atrial septal defects. *Curr Interv Cardiol Rep* 2000;2: 268–273.
2. Latson, LA, Wilson N. A new transcatheter ASD closure device. Abstract presented at the 48th Annual Scientific Session, March 7–10, 1999. *J Am Coll Cardiol* 1999;33(Suppl):520A.
3. Zahn EM, Latson LA, Wilson N. Acute and long-term follow-up results with the HELEX Septal Occluder in an animal model. Presented at the 49th Annual Scientific Session, March 12–15, 2000. *J Am Coll Cardiol* 2000;35(Suppl):498A.
4. Wilson N, Sievert H, Zahn EM, et al. Total world clinical experience with the HELEX atrial septal defect occlusion device. *Circulation* 2000;102:588.

9

WIRELESS DEVICES

ELEFTHERIOS B. SIDERIS

Surgery has been the traditional method for atrial septal defect repair. It is effective for all defects but is associated with low mortality and significant morbidity (1). Patch material is frequently used, although suture patch placement requires thoracotomy and cardiotomy, which occasionally cause problems (2). A nonsurgical patch placement should offer obvious advantages.

Disk device atrial septal defect occlusion has emerged as an alternative to surgery (3–5); it is only effective in some atrial septal defects (small to moderate secundum ASDs). Imperfect centering and need for a significant rim are the obvious limitations of all disk devices. Device-related problems are mostly related to their skeleton wires. They include wire fractures and component part embolization, atrial perforation, and valve leaflet perforation (6–8). The long-term problems of such wires or alloys are unknown. However, potential hazards related to the nickel content of these alloys include carcinogenicity, coronary spasm, tissue necrosis, and allergy (9).

Wireless devices obviously eliminate wire-related problems. Furthermore, since defect occlusion with these devices is balloon dependent, they have excellent centering and minimal rim requirements. It is reasonable to assume that the wireless devices could have wider application than the disk devices.

THE DEVICES

Two wireless devices will be described: the detachable balloon device and the transcatheter patch.

Detachable Balloon Device

The detachable balloon device (DBD) (Figure 9.1) has the following components: the detachable balloon occluder, the floppy disk, the loading wire, the needle catheter, and the

Eleftherios B. Sideris: Athenian Institute of Pediatric Cardiology, Athens, Greece; Pediatric Cardiology, Amarillo, Texas

counteroccluder. Detachable balloons are made from latex in different sizes; they are attached to a needle catheter. The 0.025-inch needle of the needle catheter is inserted in a protective 10-mm-long 5F catheter piece with several side holes. The needle and the tail of the balloon are tied with a latex tie. The latex tie will seal the balloon after needle/catheter extraction. The floppy disk is made of polyurethane and Nitinol hyperelastic wire and can have different diameters. A regular counteroccluder (similar to the one used with the buttoned device) can be delivered over the loading wire to further support the stability of the device. A double-balloon DBD has been also used (totally wireless device).

Method of Implantation

The procedure includes the following steps:

1. The device is delivered to the left atrium, through a long sheath; the balloon occluder exits at the tip of the sheath first.
2. Inflation of the balloon with a predetermined volume of dilute contrast.
3. The whole complex, including the inflated balloon, is pulled to the septum occluding the defect. Minor adjustments of the balloon volume can be made at this stage to optimize the result.
4. The tip of the long sheath is pulled to the right atrium, liberating the floppy disk.
5. The balloon is detached by pulling and extracting the needle catheter through the long sheath.
6. A counteroccluder is inserted over the loading wire and buttoned with the balloon occluder.
7. The device is released in a similar manner to the buttoned device.

The Transcatheter Patch

The transcatheter patch device (Figure 9.2) consists of the following components: the sleeve patch, the double-balloon support catheter, and the double nylon thread. The transcatheter patch is tailored from polyurethane foam and is

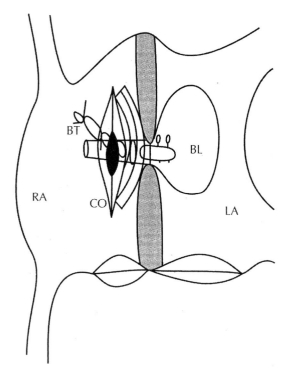

FIGURE 9.1. A drawing of detachable balloon device correction of atrial septal defect. Bl, balloon; Bt, button; COC, counteroccluder; FD, folding disk; LA, left atrium; RA, right atrium.

made in the form of a sleeve covering the distal balloon of the support catheter. A nylon loop 2 mm in diameter is sutured at the apical internal surface of the patch; it is connected to a double nylon thread for retrieval/retraction. A radiopaque thread is sutured on the patch. The supporting double balloon is made up of two latex balloons mounted on a triple-lumen catheter. Each balloon can be filled independently with dilute contrast through its own lumen,

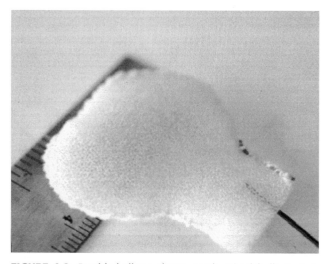

FIGURE 9.2. Double-balloon sleeve patch. Distal balloon supporting the patch, proximal balloon, double nylon thread.

while the central lumen can be used for the over a wire insertion of the device.

Method of Implantation

The procedure of introduction and release (Figure 9.3) is performed under fluoroscopy and echocardiography and includes the following steps:

1. Introduction of the balloon/patch through a short sheath over a wire in the left atrium. Alternatively, the balloon patch can be introduced directly in the left atrium through a long (Mullins-type) sheath.
2. The occluding balloon/patch (distal balloon) is inflated at volumes predetermined by test balloon inflation. A balloon/patch diameter 2 mm larger than the test-occluding diameter is selected.
3. The balloon/patch is pulled to the septum, occluding the defect.
4. The right atrial (proximal) balloon is inflated. Heparin is used during the procedure at 100 U/kg. Aspirin is started within 24 hours and is continued for a month. Antibiotics (cephalosporins) are started in the catheterization laboratory and are continued for 72 hours.
5. The introducing sheath and the outside part of the balloon catheter along with the double nylon thread of the patch are immobilized by suture and adhesive tape on the groin.
6. The patient is taken to intensive care or his room under monitoring and is confined to bed without restraint. A chest x-ray is obtained in bed in 12 hours, and fluoroscopy along with transthoracic echocardiography is done within 24 hours.
7. The patch is released in 48 hours from the placement under fluoroscopy and echocardiography as follows:
   a. The distal balloon is first deflated.
   b. The proximal balloon is deflated next.
   c. Providing that there is a good result and the patch is well attached to the septum, the double nylon thread attached to the patch is removed as a single strand. The balloon catheter and/or the long sheath remain against the patch to counteract tension during pulling.
   d. Extraction of the double-balloon catheter through the sheath; extraction of the sheath.

EXPERIMENTAL STUDIES

DBDs were applied in the occlusion of experimental ASDs in 20 piglets in which the ASDs were created by balloon dilatation of the foramen ovale (10). In 17 experiments the occluder balloon was supported by a floppy disk and a counteroccluder from the right side. In three experiments a double detachable balloon was applied. Full occlusion occurred in all cases.

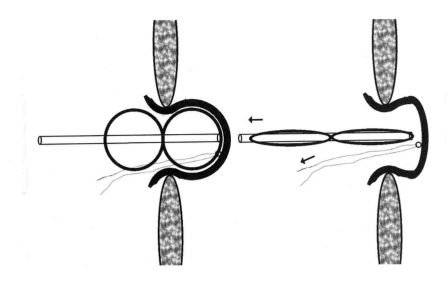

FIGURE 9.3. Method of application of the double-balloon sleeve patch. The distal balloon is supporting the patch from the left atrium with the proximal balloon immobilizing it from the right atrium. In 48 hours the balloons are deflated and the patch is released.

One device was embolized into the descending aorta. In this case only a floppy disk without a counteroccluder was used. The balloon was ruptured using the sharp end of a wire and was retrieved by transcatheter approach.

All animals were followed by echocardiography and fluoroscopy for up to 2 months. The device was covered by tissue within 3 or 4 weeks. The detachable balloon lost its content and became flat in approximately 2 months. All piglets recovered from the procedure in good health and were back in full activity in a few hours.

The transcatheter patch was studied in the piglet model of atrial septal defect (11). Twenty experimental ASDs were created by balloon dilatation of the foramen ovale. They were corrected by custom-tailored polyurethane patches applied and supported temporarily by specially made balloon catheters. Two types of patches were used; a flat patch in ten animals and a sleeve patch in ten. The patches were visualized by echocardiography as well as by fluoroscopy because of their radiopaque threads. They could be retrieved and retracted in the introducing sheath (10F), if necessary. The patches were supported by specially made balloon catheters for periods varying from 1 to 6 days. After this period the supporting catheter was withdrawn. Fluoroscopy and echocardiography were used during implantation and follow-up. All animals were sacrificed up to 14 hours after implantation. Pathologic and histologic studies were performed. There was immediate full occlusion of the experimental ASDs in all animals. Full occlusion was maintained if the supportive catheter was withdrawn 48 hours or more after implantation. In autopsy the patch was safely embedded in the atrial wall at 48 hours or more after implantation. Histologic examination revealed that fibrin and inflammatory cells were responsible for the attachment. The sleeve patch was bulkier but better centered than the flat patch. The conclusion of this experimental study was that the transcatheter patch was effective and safe in the

occlusion of experimental ASDs; it has minimal septal rim requirements and excellent safety characteristics. The only disadvantage of the transcatheter patch is the need for 48-hour balloon support.

PATIENT SELECTION

Both the DBD and the transcatheter patch ASD occlusion are balloon occlusive methods, in principle. A balloon is a three-dimensional structure with certain advantages compared to the two-dimensional disk devices. It is always centered when it is pulled to the atrial septal defect and requires a minimal rim of 1 or 2 mm to sit on the defect, in comparison to a more than 5-mm rim for the disk devices. We should expect therefore a much wider application of the balloon-based occlusive methods than for the disk devices. Using the wireless methods described, the application range of transcatheter ASD occlusion could extend to more secundum ASDs with insufficient rim and to some ostium primum ASDs without mitral insufficiency or sinus venosus ASDs without anomalous pulmonary veins. The limitations of the balloon-based wireless methods for ASD occlusion are related either to the anatomy or to the particular device. A single defect is more appropriate for a balloon-based method than defects with multiple fenestrations; however, a larger balloon might cover more than one fenestration. A large balloon seems inappropriate for a small child with a small left atrium. The exact balloon/septal length ratio has not been established; however, the balloon test occlusion of the defect before the application of the device seems of paramount importance. If the balloon test occlusion achieves full occlusion without impairment of the mitral flow or the pulmonary venous flow, the wireless balloon-based method will most likely be successful.

DBD limitations include size of the introducing sheath (8 to 11F, depending on the balloon size) and slight risk of embolization or balloon leakage. The operator should be able to respond to an unanticipated embolization by breaking the balloon and extracting it percutaneously. No detachable balloon occluders larger than the aortic valve annulus should be used with the current DBD, since the balloon could obstruct the aorta.

Large transcatheter patch devices are bulkier than DBD, requiring currently a 12F introduction. Their use is currently restricted to patients weighing more than 15 kg. However, transcatheter patch devices are much safer with regard to embolization, since they are doubly immobilized inside and outside the heart. In case of any unanticipated problems they can be easily retracted and retrieved through the introducing sheath. A single large balloon/patch device can occlude defects from 20 to 35 mm, in comparison with disk devices, where multiple sizes are required for the same result. As was mentioned before, balloon test occlusion of the defect before the transcatheter patch device application is the most important predictor of the success (full occlusion of the defect, no impairment of mitral flow or pulmonary venous return).

RESULTS

Detachable Balloon Device

A feasibility study was performed in four centers (12). A total of 14 heart defects inappropriate for disk device repair were occluded, including secundum ASD, membranous VSD, and large patent ductus arteriosus (PDA). Six secundum ASDs unsuitable for disk device repair were selected. Reasons for rejection for disk device repair included insufficient rim or insufficient septal length for a disk device. The diameter of the defects varied between 18 and 27 mm (median, 23) and the patient age varied from 6 to 40 years (median, 20). The lowest patient weight was 14 kg.

The detachable balloons were inflated 1 to 2 mm more than the occluding diameter of the defect. A floppy disk approximately twice as long supported them from the right septal side along with a regular counteroccluder(s). There was immediate full occlusion of all defects, and in one case a small residual shunt occurred. Full occlusion was maintained in all cases with successful implantation on the long term, although the latex balloons became flat after approximately 2 months. In the cases with the residual shunt, though, the shunt not only did not improve but increased over the long term. There was one complication. A 26-mm DBD in a 19-year-old was embolized 40 hours after implantation. It was embolized into the descending aorta, causing numbness of the lower extremities. The balloon was ruptured with the sharp end of a wire and the device was retrieved percutaneously uneventfully. All the symptoms disappeared.

Transcatheter Patch

A feasibility trial started in December 1999 (11). The median diameter of the secundum ASDs was 27 mm (range, 13 to 34 mm). The youngest patient was 1.5 years old (range, 1.5 to 58; median, 35). The lowest weight was 11 kg. Most transcatheter patches were supported by double balloons and three by a single balloon with an incorporated floppy disk. Smaller balloon patches up to 15 mm were delivered through 10F sheaths. Larger patches required a 12F introduction.

All patches were successfully implanted; only 2 implantations were unsuccessful in 48 hours and were retrieved. All patients with successful implantations are alive and well. There were 2 cases with significant residual shunt. One of them received a second device six months later with full occlusion.

DISCUSSION

We have shown that wireless ASD occlusion is feasible both with detachable balloons (wireless occluder only) and with the transcatheter patch (total wireless occlusion). The two methods have differences in the need for hospitalization. The detachable balloon method can be done as an outpatient procedure; in contrast, transcatheter patch placement requires at least 48 hours of hospitalization. The results of the detachable balloon device ASD occlusion demonstrated the effectiveness of the method in the occlusion of defects inappropriate for disk device repair (12). Spherical, well-centered, detachable balloons occluded the defects immediately. They were released right after implantation and became flat 2 months later with full occlusion maintained. The minimal rim requirement is an attraction of the method; however, the lack of significant overlapping could result in residual shunts without improvement overtime, as was shown in one case.

There are concerns related to the safety of the detachable balloon device used. The stability of the device was the main concern, since embolization into the descending aorta occurred in one case. The occluder totally obstructed the descending aorta, with temporary symptoms; it was broken by the sharp end of a wire and was retrieved uneventfully. Total obstruction of the ascending aorta can be lethal. Therefore the current DBD device cannot be routinely used, before better stability is ensured. The operator should be ready to rupture and remove the detachable balloon in case of embolization. No defects larger than the aortic root diameter should be occluded. The other concern is the emerging risk of latex allergy (13). Careful history as well as latex antibodies should be obtained, and if there is latex allergy, alternative materials should be used.

The transcatheter patch is balloon delivered; therefore it maintains the advantages of the detachable balloon occlusion, like the minimal rim requirement and excellent centering. In addition, the stability of the device is very good because it is doubly secured inside and outside the heart. The attachment of the patch to the atrial wall is fast (48 hours) and its endothelialization is probably faster than with the disk devices (Figure 9.4A). Histologic examination revealed that the attachment of the patch to the septum is due to fibrin and inflammatory cells (Figure 9.4B). We should be very careful therefore with the duration of heparin treatment, since the patch attachment depends on fibrin. In our experimental study no additional heparin was used, and all patches were securely attached on the septum after 48 hours. The balloon/patch needs to be immobile for fast embedding in the septum. The 24-hour fluoroscopy and echocardiography are very important to verify the position and stability of the patch. Further adjustment is possible at this stage to ensure a good result at 48 hours. Small technical problems like those of premature deflation of the supporting balloons need to be resolved before generalized use of the device is recommended. Deflation of the supporting balloon in less than 24 hours can result in a significant residual shunt.

A

B

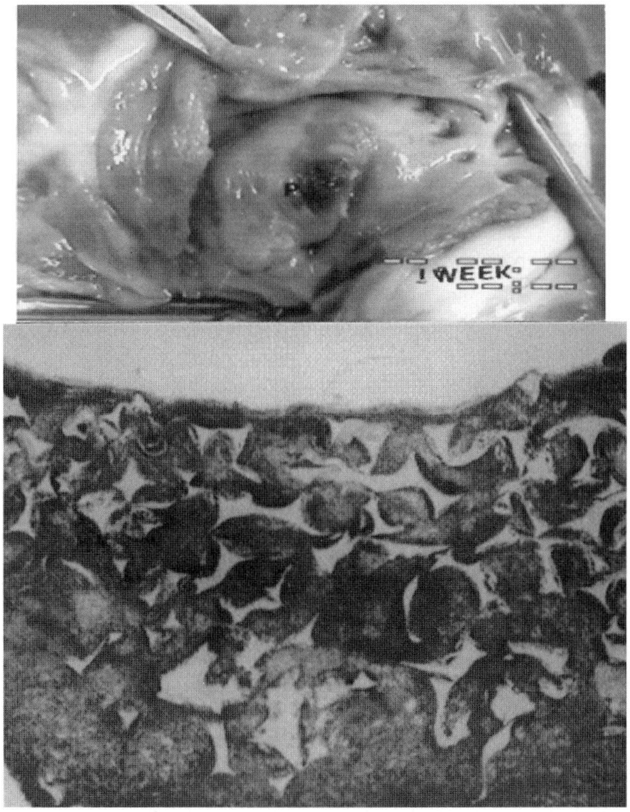

FIGURE 9.4. A: Patch pathology 10 days after implantation. The patch is fully covered by endothelium. **B:** Histology of transcatheter patch 48 hours after implantation. The patch is covered by fibrin and is attached to the endocardium. (See Color Figure 9.4.)

Therefore it is better to be retrieved and replaced by a new one. Retrieval and retraction of the balloon into the introducing sheath is possible the first 24 hours. The patch is not only echogenic but radiopaque, since radiopaque thread is sutured.

Double-balloon supporting catheters were used in most cases so far; they are safer than single-balloon/floppy-disk combinations for large defects. They are currently made with three lumens. The central lumen is used for the over-the-wire introduction of the balloon/patch through a short sheath, thus eliminating the use of the more dangerous long sheath (Mullins type).

The sleeve patch is designed to be used for single defects. An oversized balloon/patch has been used successfully, though, for a case with multiple fenestrations. The transcatheter patch may be useful in the occlusion of lesions other than secundum ASDs like sinus venosus and ostium primum defects because of the minimal rim requirement. The single most useful predictor of a successful patch occlusion is the test occlusion of the defect during sizing. A full occlusion without impairment of the mitral valve or the pulmonary vein flow is a good predictor of success. The disadvantage of the transcatheter patch occlusion is the need for an additional day in the hospital; however, no bed restraint is necessary.

CURRENT STATUS

The use of wireless devices is experimental and is used only under appropriate protocols, approved in each center. The use of transcatheter patches should not require the strict regulations of implantable devices, since custom modification of existing materials (balloon catheters and patch) is only required. However, carefully conceived clinical trials are planned to evaluate its effectiveness and safety. An investigational device exception application has been filed for the performance of FDA-approved clinical trials with the transcatheter patch in the United States.

CONCLUSION

Wireless ASD occlusion is feasible and effective by both detachable balloon devices and transcatheter patches. The transcatheter patch appears safer and should be the preferred wireless method for defects inappropriate for disk device repair. Larger clinical trials are necessary.

REFERENCES

1. Fyler DC. Atrial septal defect secundum. In: Fyler DC, ed. *Nadas' pediatric cardiology.* Philadelphia: Hanley and Belfus, 1992:513–534.

2. Robins RC. Atrial septal defects: surgical procedure. In: Nichols DG, Cameron DE, Greeley WJ, eds. *Critical heart disease in infants and children.* St. Louis: Mosby-Year Book, 1995:584–586.

3. King TD, Mills NL. Nonoperative closure of atrial septal defects. *Surgery* 1974;75:383–388.

4. Rashkind WJ, Cuaso CC. Transcatheter treatment of congenital heart disease. *Circulation* 1983;67:711–716.

5. Sideris EB, Sideris SE, Thanopoulos BD, et al. Transvenous atrial septal defect occlusion by the "buttoned" device. *Am J Cardiol* 1990;123:191–200.

6. Prieto LR, Foreman CK, Cheatham JP, et al. Intermediate-term outcome of transcatheter secundum atrial septal defect closure using the Bard Clamshell septal occluder. *Am J Cardiol* 1996; 78: 1310–1312.

7. Agarwal SK, Ghosh PK, Mittal PK. Failure of devices used for closure of atrial septal defects, mechanisms and management. *J Thorac Cardiovasc Surg* 1996;112:226–230.

8. Rao PS, Sideris EB, Hausdorf G, et al. International experience with secundum atrial septal defect occlusion by the buttoned device. *Am Heart J* 1994;128:1022–1035.

9. Sunderman FW. A review of the metabolism and toxicology of nickel. *Ann Clin Lab Sci* 1977;81:377–398.

10. Sideris E, Kaneva A, Sideris S, et al. Transcatheter atrial septal defect occlusion in piglets by balloon detachable devices. *Catheter Cardiovasc Interv* 2000;51:529–534.

11. Sideris E, Toumanides S, Alekyan B, et al. Transcatheter patch correction of atrial septal defects: Experimental validation and early clinical experience. *Circulation* 2000;102(Suppl. II):588.

12. Sideris EB, Chiang CW, Zhang JC, et al. Transcatheter correction of heart defects by detachable balloon buttoned devices: a feasibility study. *J Am Coll Cardiol* 1999;528A.

13. Tomajic VJ, Withrow TJ, Fisher BR, et al. Short analytical review: latex-associated allergies and anaphylactic reactions. *Clin Immunol Immunopath* 1992;64:89–97.

10

TRANSCATHETER ATRIAL SEPTAL DEFECT CLOSURE WITHOUT FLUOROSCOPY

PETER EWERT
FELIX BERGER

The diagnostic accuracy of two-dimensional and color Doppler ultrasound has led to surgical closure of atrial septal defects (ASDs) without routinely performed preoperative catheterization (1,2). However, with the introduction of new interventional devices for defect closure, catheterization of ASDs has experienced a renaissance. Ease of handling of some devices in routine use has diminished procedure and fluoroscopy times for successful interventions (3,4). On the other hand, the widespread availability of multiplane transesophageal transducers has increased the role of echocardiography in the procedure. Transcatheter ASD closure under echocardiography as the only imaging tool can now be performed without fluoroscopy at all (5).

METHODS

Patient Selection

Patients with an ASD in the fossa ovales or a persistent foramen ovale (PFO) who are suitable for transcatheter closure without fluoroscopy are assessed by an outpatient transthoracic echocardiographic study. No special selection criteria are necessary, in comparison to the conventional procedure.

To become comfortable with the technique, small or medium-sized defects located centrally in the oval fossa with sufficient margins to the atrioventricular valves and the pulmonary and caval veins are advantageous in the initial experience with this procedure.

Diagnostic Catheterization

Before the defect closure, a diagnostic catheterization under echocardiography guidance, including pressure measure-

ments and oximetry for shunt quantification, may be performed. However, meticulous balloon sizing is always necessary but may be abandoned only if an ordinary persistent foramen ovale is present.

After a premedication with intravenous midazolam (0.1 mg/kg, 5 mg maximum) and insertion of a sheath in the right femoral vein under local anesthesia, a 5 or 7F Berman angiographic catheter is advanced into the pulmonary trunk. The pressure curve is used for positioning the catheter. A transthoracic subxyphoidal sagittal echocardiographic view along the inferior caval vein may visualize the advancement of the balloon catheter into the right atrium and through the tricuspid valve. A parasternal short axis view showing both tricuspid and pulmonary valves is helpful to maneuver the catheter through the pulmonary valve and avoid entering the right ventricular apex. After a blood oximetry has been done, the catheter can be pulled back into the right atrium for pressure measurements in the right heart chambers. The distance from the catheter tip in the right atrium to the entrance into the sheath is measured using the scale printed on the catheter. A guide wire with J-formed tip is then advanced that distance, then carefully pushed forward into the superior caval vein and exchanged for a multipurpose or an angulated pigtail catheter. The tip of the pigtail catheter can be recognized in the ultrasound view because the circle is cut through twice, generating two reflections in the view plane. To facilitate a controlled movement with a 7F multipurpose catheter, a 3F Fogarty catheter can be inserted through it, so that the saline-filled balloon marks the tip (Figures 10.1). The wings of the catheter's proximal connectors facilitate an orientation of the angulated distal end. From a subxyphoidal sagittal view the advancement of the wire and the correct position of the catheter can be monitored (Figure 10.2). Oximetry is repeated. Now the catheter can be pulled back into the right atrium; it should be oriented posteriorly and to the left, and then moved through the defect. The subxyphoidal sagittal echocardiographic view (Figure 10.2) can again monitor

Peter Ewert: Department of Congenital Heart Diseases, German Heart Institute, Berlin, Germany
Felix Berger: Consultant, Department of Congenital Heart Disease, University of Zürich, Zürich, Switzerland

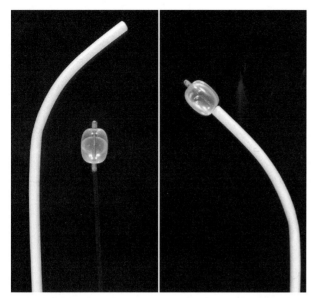

FIGURE 10.1. To visualize the catheter tip under echocardiography, a 3F Fogarty catheter and a 7F multipurpose catheter with an inner diameter of 0.06 inch *(left)* can be used. The Fogarty catheter is inserted into the multipurpose so that the small balloon marks the end *(right)*.

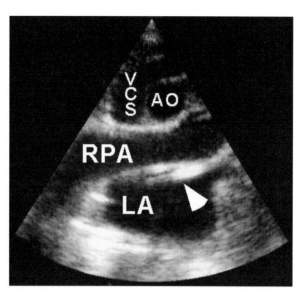

FIGURE 10.3. Suprasternal frontal view. A catheter *(arrowhead)* has been advanced into the left upper pulmonary vein. AO, aorta; LA, left atrium; RPA, right pulmonary artery; VCS, superior caval vein.

these steps. After pressure and oximetry measurements, the catheter can be advanced under slight clockwise rotation into the left upper pulmonary vein, again monitored from a suprasternal frontal view plane (Figure 10.3).

In general, transthoracic view planes are excellent in small children and slim patients. However, whenever the quality of transthoracic views is unsatisfactory, there should be no hesitation to switch to transesophageal echocardiography.

If the procedure is not performed under mechanical ventilation, deep sedation with continuous propofol infusion is preferred. However, the individual patient tolerance of the echo probe varies considerably. Some adults may only need mild sedation (e.g., midazolam) and a good pharyngeal anesthesia.

Crossing the atrial septum can best be performed with the catheter tip slowly pulled down from the superior caval vein into the right atrium. The esophageal probe in a transversal view just above the orifice of the superior caval vein will visualize the catheter tip. As soon as the tip is visible, the probe follows the catheter movement down to the level of the defect. Then a careful clockwise rotation and a slight advancement in case of a PFO lets the tip of the catheter enter the left atrium (Figure 10.4).

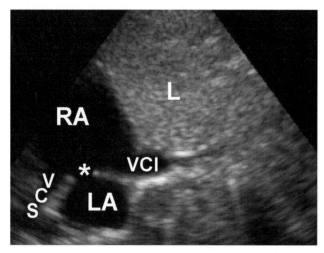

FIGURE 10.2. The subxyphoidal sagittal view is very helpful to determine the inferior and superior posterior rims of the defect and to monitor the catheter movements into the superior caval veins (VCS) or across the defect *(asterisk)*. VCI, inferior caval vein L, liver.

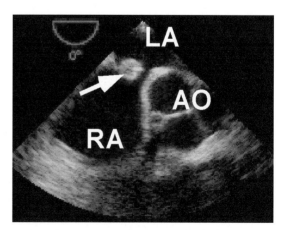

FIGURE 10.4. A transesophageal, transversal (horizontal) echocardiographic viewplane. A multipupose catheter with a 3F Fogarty catheter (Figure 10.1) has been rotated clockwise at the level of the atrial septal defect. The balloon of the Fogarty catheter *(arrow)* is just crossing the defect. AO, aorta; LA, left atrium; RA, right atrium.

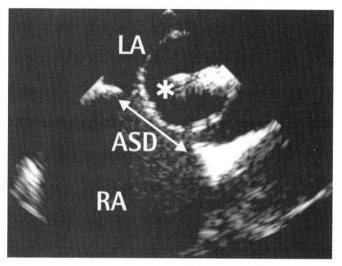 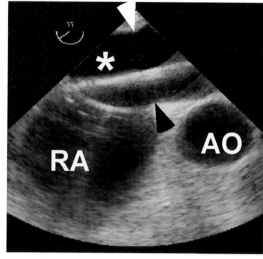

FIGURE 10.5. Sizing under echocardiographic guidance. **A:** A balloon catheter *(asterisk)* is pulled over the wire from the left atrium (LA) against the defect (ASD) to the right atrium (RA). **B:** A large eleastic balloon is positioned in the defect and inflated. In a long-axis cross section through the balloon *(asterisk)* the indentations *(arrowheads)* mark the edges of the defect.

Balloon Sizing

The balloon sizing is performed over the wire and with transesophageal echocardiography. If not already in place, the tip of the catheter can be maneuvered safely under transesophageal echocardiography from the left atrium into the left upper pulmonary vein and exchanged over a stiff guide wire.

Accurate sizing under echocardiography is possible with both the classic "pull-through" and the "notch" techniques (Figure 10.5). Both methods have specific advantages and disadvantages, which are beyond the scope of this chapter.

The sizing balloons are filled with pure saline; no radiopaque contrast medium is needed. A small amount of liquid should already be in the balloon after insertion through the sheath in the inguinal or inferior caval vein, so that the balloon can easily be recognized as soon as it has reached the atrial septum. A 35- to 60-degree angulated view plane best visualizes the balloon catheter.

As with conventional sizing, the balloon is pulled from the left to the right atrium with different filling volumes until moderate resistance is encountered, or until the sizing balloon in the defect produces indentation of the septum that can be measured in a view plane of a longitudinal cut through the balloon (Figure 10.5B). During occlusion of the septal defect with a balloon of appropriate size, color flow mapping is performed to exclude additional defects or residual shunts. The distances to the right pulmonary veins, the mitral valve, and the coronary sinus can be determined. The catheter is removed and the balloon is filled outside the patient with the corresponding volume during the sizing maneuver. The diameter is again estimated with a sizing tablet.

Interventional Closure

A long sheath is advanced over the guide wire placed in the upper left pulmonary vein. Use of a stiff guide wire

and an approximately 45-degree angulated echocardiographic view of the wire across the septum is helpful to safely advance the sheath into the pulmonary vein and avoid having the sheath flip the wire out of the left atrium. The correct position of the sheath in the pulmonary vein can be clearly visualized in a transverse view. An appropriate Amplatzer Septal Occluder (AGA Medical Corporation, Golden Valley, MN) is then introduced and advanced until the device is visible inside the sheath just in front of the orifice of the pulmonary vein (Figure 10.6). With the occluder held in place over the delivery system, careful retraction of the sheath unfolds the distal umbrella under the roof of the left atrium (Figure 10.7). Under

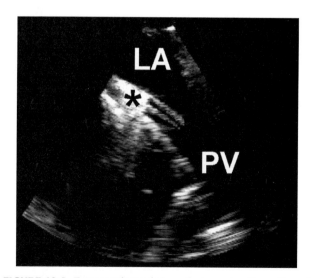

FIGURE 10.6. Transesophageal view of a long sheath positioned in the left upper pulmonary vein (PV). An Amplatzer occluder *(asterisk)* is pushed through the sheath into the left atrium (LA) just in front of the orifice of the pulmonary vein.

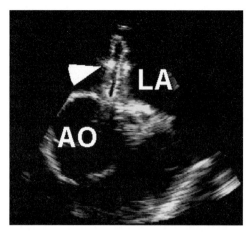

FIGURE 10.7. The left atrial disk of the occluder *(arrowhead)* is configured under the roof of the left atrium (LA) behind the aortic root (AO).

echocardiographic guidance, the occluder is retracted against the rim of the septal defect, the proximal umbrella is unfolded, and the correct position of the occluder is verified by performing the so-called wiggle movement (Figure 10.8). An echocardiographic view in an angulation of approximately 45 to 65 degrees is recommended for the stepwise implantation of the occluder. After exclusion of residual shunts by color flow mapping, the device can be released. The correct position of the released occluder should then be documented from different echocardiographic views.

RESULTS

Immediate Results

From July 1998 to October 2000, successful transcatheter closures of ASD or PFO with Amplatzer devices were possible without fluoroscopy in 39 patients (Table 10.1). In 12 additional patients, the diagnostic and the sizing procedures were performed without fluoroscopy but revealed defects unsuitable for interventional closure. One device was explanted electively, despite complete closure of the septal defect, but because of a mismatch between occluder size and septum length, which had produced a serious complication in a similar case treated conventionally.

Complicatons

During the learning period in six cases, fluoroscopy was used because the operator felt uncomfortable with the procedure, because of the implantation of a new device, or as a means of verifying the correct position of the occluders after successful intervention. However, there was no occasion in any of the procedures in which fluoroscopy was needed to overcome a critical or potential hazardous situation. In one patient atrial flutter occurred during the diagnostic catheterization. Sinus rhythm was established by cardioversion prior to the release of the occluder.

Follow-up

During a follow-up of 18 months (5 to 29 months) echocardiograms and chest x-rays showed no displacement of the occluders. Otherwise no specific occurrences in com-

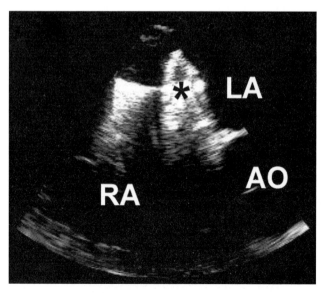 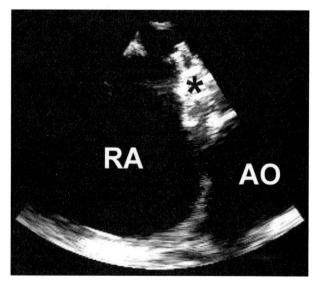

FIGURE 10.8. Transesophageal views of the so-called wiggle maneuver: by pulling (left) and pushing (right) the correct and safe position of the occluder *(asterisk)* is confirmed. AO, aorta; LA, left atrium; RA, right atrium.

TABLE 10.1. DEMOGRAPHIC DATA OF 39 PATIENTS (23 WITH ASD AND 16 WITH PFO) TREATED WITH AMPLATZER OCCLUDER WITHOUT FLUOROSCOPY

| | Age (years) | Weight (kg) | ASD Size* (mm) | Qp:Qs* | Procedure Time (min) | | | | Follow-up (months) |
					Diagnostic	Sizing	Intervention	Total	
Median	21	60	14	1.6	25	25	25	75	18
Mean	28	55	16	1.8	28	26	26	79	18
Minimum	2	13	7	1.2	10	15	10	35	5
Maximum	76	160	28	2.6	80	50	80	130	29

ASD, atrial septal defect; PFO, patent foramen ovale.
*PFO excluded.

parison to the follow-up of conventionally treated patients with fluoroscopy were noted.

APPLICABILITY TO ADULT SUBJECTS

The previously described method is applicable to adults. Only minor modifications are necessary in special situations. For example, in moving the catheter into the pulmonary artery in adult patients with enlarged right ventricular chambers, the catheter is more easily steered under echocardiographic guidance with a stiff guide wire. In patients with a persistent foramen ovale, the left atrium is best entered with a balloon-tipped multipurpose catheter. In case of an ordinary PFO, suitable for an Amplatzer PFO occluder, the sizing procedure can be omitted.

DISCUSSION

With the extensive use of echocardiography for patient selection and intervention, and the development of new occluder systems, the transcatheter closure of ASDs has become a standard technique (3). With increasing operator experience and the development of easy-to-handle devices, x-ray exposure is minimized to several minutes or is even unnecessary (3,6).

The benefits of avoiding fluoroscopy and radiopaque contrast media are obvious. Whether invasive diagnostic hemodynamic measurements like pressure recordings and oximetric shunt estimation prior to a transcatheter closure of uncomplicated ASDs are still necessary may be questioned. However, to avoid the use of fluoroscopy completely, both the technique of device placement and device sizing of the defect itself must be as safe as possible under echocardiographic guidance (7). Echocardiography plays a decisive role in the sizing procedure, delivering information about residual shunts and spatial relationships to adjacent anatomic structures. The saline-filled balloon is clearly visible with ultrasound, and the balloon is safely moved over the wire. Furthermore, comparative measurements of the inflated Amplatzer sizing balloon showed excellent correlations

between angiography and echocardiography. Thus the sizing procedure under echocardiographic guidance is reliable and differs only partially from the conventional sizing maneuver.

For a successful intervention under echocardiographic guidance the self-centering capabilities of an ASD device without arms or edges are fundamental. The Amplatzer devices have excellent occlusion rates (3), are easily retrievable, and have the decisive advantage of remaining rotationally symmetric during the stepwise deployment. Therefore the exact position can be reliably monitored by cross-sectional echocardiographic view planes.

The median procedure time is comparable to that needed for the conventional procedure and is mainly dependent on synchronization between echocardiographer and interventionist.

Because of the longer time for which the transesophageal echo probe must be inserted in comparison to the conventional procedure, higher doses of propofol had to be administered. However, if the procedure is performed under general anesthesia, as some centers do, this issue becomes a minor factor. With increasing experience, successful intervention with more complex defects, such as atrial septal aneurysms or a multiperforated defect, which needed two devices for complete closure, may be possible. In a pregnant patient with recurrent thromboembolic events, a large PFO could be successfully closed without fluoroscopy and with only minimal sedation.

CONCLUSION

We conclude that transcatheter closure of ASD or PFO with Amplatzer devices is possible in most patients under echocardiographic guidance alone with results similar to those of the conventional procedure.

REFERENCES

1. Shub C, Tajik AJ, Seward JB, et al. Surgical repair of uncomplicated atrial septal defect without "routine" preoperative cardiac catheterization. *J Am Coll Cardiol* 1985;6:49–54.
2. Marek J, Skovranek J, Hucin B, et al. Seven-year experience of

noninvasive preoperative diagnostics in children with congenital heart defects: comprehensive analysis of 2,788 consecutive patients. *Cardiology* 1995;86:488–495.

3. Berger F, Ewert P, Björnstad P, et al. Transcatheter closure as standard therapy of most interatrial defects. *Cardiol Young* 1999;9: 468–473.

4. Walsh KP, Tofeig M, Kitchener DJ, et al. Comparison of the Sideris and Amplatzer septal occlusion devices. *Am J Cardiol* 1999; 83:933–936.

5. Ewert P, Daehnert I, Berger F, et al. Closure of an atrial septal defect without surgery and without x-ray [German]. *Z Herz Thorax Gefässchirurgie* 1998;12:221–225.

6. Ewert P, Berger F, Daehnert I, et al. Transcatheter closure of atrial septal defects without fluoroscopy: feasibility of a new method. *Circulation* 2000;101:847–849.

7. Ewert P, Berger F, Daehnert I, et al. Diagnostic catheterization and balloon sizing of atrial septal defects by echocardiographic guidance without fluoroscopy. *Echocardiography* 2000;17:159–163.

Catheter Based Devices: For the Treatment of Non-coronary Cardiovascular Diseases in Adults and Children. Edited by P. Syamasundar Rao and Morton J. Kern, Lippincott Williams & Wilkins, Philadelphia © 2003.

11

COMPARATIVE SUMMARY OF ATRIAL SEPTAL DEFECT OCCLUSION DEVICES

P. SYAMASUNDAR RAO

Following the description by King et al. (1–3), a number of atrial septal defect (ASD) occluding devices have been designed and investigated, reviewed elsewhere (Chapter 1) (4). Most devices were tested initially in animal models; these tests were followed by clinical trials in human subjects. At least seven devices are in various phases of clinical trials at this time. The interventional cardiologist, therefore, has a lot to choose from. However, the selection of one device over the other is difficult in the absence of prospective, randomized clinical trials (5,6). In some studies (7–10), results of ASD occlusions with consecutive use of two to six devices, as the newer devices become available, have been investigated. Unfortunately, most studies examined the results of small cohorts of patients, but more important, these investigations are neither prospective nor randomized in their design; therefore accurate comparison of the devices could not be made. A prospective, randomized clinical trial using all eligible devices is necessary to provide accurate information on usefulness of the devices. The existing technical, medical, ethical, regulatory, and economic considerations are unlikely to be conducive to organize such a study (5,6). Consequently, the choice of the device may have to be based on the results of clinical trials on large patient cohorts with the respective devices, conducted independently, sponsored by the device manufacturer. Apart from the safety and effectiveness data derived from clinical trials, issues such as availability, ease with which device implantation technique may be mastered, size of the device delivery sheath, and cost of the device may have to be considered in the selection of the device for transcatheter occlusion of ASD (5,6). This chapter compares and contrasts the reported experience with ASD closure devices.

P. Syamasundar Rao: Professor of Pediatrics, Medicine, and Cardiology, Department of Pediatrics, University of Texas-Houston Medical School; Director, Division of Pediatric Cardiology, Memorial Hermann Children's Hospital, Houston, Texas

FEASIBILITY, SAFETY, AND EFFECTIVENESS

Feasibility of device implantation to occlude the ASD in human subjects has been demonstrated for most, if not all, devices. Whereas embolization of the device or device components, or device dislodgment have occurred with most of the devices, such events have not resulted in fatality, but required transcatheter or surgical retrieval of the devices. Effectiveness of the device in occluding the ASD has been studied mostly by echocardiography and Doppler examination. These issues will be reviewed by examining acute (<6 months), mid-term (6 to 23 months), and when available, long-term (≥24 months) results.

IMMEDIATE OR ACUTE RESULTS

Feasibility

Feasibility of device implantation may be assessed by examining the ratio of the number of implantations versus the number of subjects taken to the cardiac catheterization laboratory with intent to occlude. This index is expected to indicate the ease with which a given device can be used to occlude the ASD. While there is some disparity in criteria for selection of subjects for intention to treat, the feasibility of implantation for most of the devices is similar, varying from 66% to 97%, as shown in Table 11.1 (Chapters 6, 8, and 9) (2,11–49).

Safety

Embolization of the device or device components, or device dislodgment or misplacement has been observed with most devices. Most investigators undertook surgical retrieval of the devices with concurrent operative closure of the atrial defect during their early experience. With increasing experience, transcatheter retrieval of the device coupled with

TABLE 11.1. IMMEDIATE RESULTS OF DEVICE CLOSURE OF ASD

Device/Authors (Reference)	No. of Subjects Taken to Cath Lab with Intent to Close	No. of Subjects (%) in Whom the Device was Implanted	No. of Subjects (%) in Whom Device Dislodgment/Embolization/ Misplacement Occurred	No. of Subjects (%) with Effective Occlusion*
King's device				
Mills and King (2)	10	5 (50%)	0	4 (80%)
Hooked device				
Rashkind (11)	33	23 (70%)	4 (17%)	14 (61%)
Beekman (12)	3	2 (66%)	1 (50%)	1 (50%)
Clamshell				
Rome et al. (13)	40	34 (85%)	2 (6%)	12 (63%)†
Hellenbrand et al. (14)	11	10 (91%)	0	9 (90%)
Buttoned (first, second, and third)				
Rao et al. (15)	200	180 (90%)	12 (7%)	154 (92%)
Arora et al. (16)	‡	27	3 (11.1%)	17 (71%)
Buttoned (second, third, and fourth)				
Haddad et al. (17)	‡	32	3 (9.4%)	26 (90%)
Worms et al. (18)	140	121 (86%)	5 (4.1%)	102 (88%)
Das angel wing				
Weil et al. (19)	89	56 (63%)	3 (6%)	37 (66%)
Mendelsohn et al. (20)	75	65 (87%)	7 (11%)	‡
Rickers et al. (21)	105	75 (71%)	3 (4%)	52 (72%)
Banerjee et al. (22)	‡	70	5 (7%)	61 (94%)
Das et al. (Phase I) (23)	‡	50	4 (8%)	31 of 34 (91%)
Das et al. (Phase II) (23)	‡	47	3 (6%)	36 (92%)
Das et al. (International) (23)	‡	126	8 (6%)	81 of 96 (94%)
ASDOS				
Sievert et al. (24)	13	12 (92%)	2 (17%)	9 (75%)
Hausdorf et al. (25)	10	9 (90%)	1 (11%)	8 (89%)
Sievert et al. (26)	‡	200	26 (13%)	79/126 (63%)
Babic (27)	‡	350§	32 (9%)	(70–75%)
Amplatzer				
Massura et al. (28)	30	30 (100%)	0	27 (90%)
Thanopoulos et al. (29)	18	16 (89%)	1 (6%)	13 (81%)
Wilkins & Goh (30)	34	26 (76%)	2 (8%)	22 (92%)
Hijazi et al. (31)	19	18 (95%)	1 (5%)	16 (89%)
Chan et al. (32)	‡	100	7 (7%)	79 (85%)
Berger et al. (33)	108	61 (56%)	1 (1.6%)	59 (98%)
Fisher et al. (34)	52	46 (88%)	3 (6.5%)	42 (97%)
Waight et al. (35)	‡	77	2 (2.6%)	74 (99%)
Dhillon et al. (36)	21	20 (95%)	0	18 (90%)
Hijazi et al. (37)	‡	219	6 (2.7%)	210 (98%)
Hijazi et al. (38)	‡	40	1 (2.5%)	38 (98%)
Walsh & Maadi (39)	‡	104	2 (1.9%)	69 (68%)
Vogel et al. (40)	‡	12	2 (16.7%)	‡
Hamdan et al. (Chapter 6)	‡	140	2 (1.4%)	126 (91%)
CardioSeal/StarFlex				
Zahn et al. (41)	33	29 (89%)	0	17 (59%)
Latson (42)	72	56 (78%)	5 (9%)	‡
Moore et al. (43)	157	132 (84%)	2 (1.5%)	84 (63%)
Carminati (44)	334	325 (97%)	13 (4%)	215 (69%)
Pedra et al. (45)	‡	50	4 (8%)	20 (40%)
Buttoned; (fourth generation)				
Rao et al. (46)	475	423 (89%)	6 (1.4%)	377 (90%)

(continued)

TABLE 11.1. *(continued)*

Device/Authors (Reference)	No. of Subjects Taken to Cath Lab with Intent to Close	No. of Subjects (%) in Whom the Device was Implanted	No. of Subjects (%) in Whom Device Dislodgment/Embolization/ Misplacement Occurred	No. of Subjects (%) with Effective Occlusion*
Helex septal occluder Latson et al. (Chapter 8) (47)	‡	703 (4.3%)	‡	‡
COD buttoned device Rao and Sideris (48)	68	65 (96%)	0 (0)	62 (95%)
Transcatheter patch Sideris (Chapter 9)	14	14 (100%)	2 (14%)	10 (83%)

From Rao PS. Summary and comparison of atrial septal defect closure devices. *Curr Interv Cardiol Rep* 2000;2:367–376, with permission.
*Effective occlusion defined as no or trivial residual shunt (15).
†19 of 32 had adequate imaging studies; 12 (63%) of these had no residual shunt.
‡No data.
§Includes Sievert's 200 patients.
ASD, atrial septal defect; ASDOS, atrial septal defect occluding system; cath lab, cardiac catheterization laboratory; COD, centering-on-demand; No., number.

elective surgical closure of the ASD was undertaken by most investigators. Device dislodgment rates are similar with all devices, as shown in Table 11.1.

Death secondary to cerebrovascular accidents (13,50) has been reported. This seems to be related to dislodgment of thrombus from femoral/iliac veins while inserting the device delivery sheath. This was seen in high-risk patients with right-to-left shunts (13,50). Ultrasound/Doppler imaging of iliac/femoral veins in such high-risk patients to exclude intramural thrombi, especially if they had recent cardiac catheterization, as previously suggested (13) is advisable. Cerebrovascular accidents are extremely rare while occluding left-to-right shunt secundum ASDs; the single case cited (Chapter 4) may be related to factor XII deficiency.

Formation of thrombus on the device with or without systemic embolization has been observed (Chapters 4 and 6) (51–55). Whereas some of the thromboses may be related to associated coagulation factor deficiency (Chapter 4) (52), others (Chapter 6) (51,53–55) did not have evidence for coagulation abnormality. Thrombotic complications have been reported more frequently with ASD occlusion system (ASDOS) (Chapter 4) (53,54). However, it is not clear whether this is related to true thrombogenicity of this particular device. Also, endocarditis with vegetation formation following Amplatzer device implantation (30,56) has been reported, thus emphasizing the need for bacterial endocarditis prophylaxis until the device components are endothelialized. Despite implantation of a large number of devices, reports of thrombus/vegetation formation are infrequent. Therefore it is difficult to conclude that a given device is more thrombogenic or infection-prone than another device. Systematic studies to examine these issues are warranted.

Effectiveness

Detailed cardiac catheterization and angiography have been used in the early studies to assess effectiveness. Because of the potential for device dislodgment (13,57) and of the availability of reliable noninvasive technology, two-dimensional echocardiography and Doppler studies are preferred methods of evaluation at this time. Most investigators use effective occlusion, defined as trivial or no shunt (15), as a measure of effectiveness of device closure. Such a definition is appropriate because (a) the reason for closing ASDs is to decrease right ventricular volume overloading and pulmonary blood flow, and (b) the residual shunts decrease and disappear with time (15,26,32,46,58). Effective occlusion rates following device implantation are also shown in Table 11.1, and they reveal similar effective occlusion rates for all devices.

MID-TERM FOLLOW-UP RESULTS

Mid-term (defined as 6 to 23 months) follow-up results have been examined for some of the devices and are tabulated (Table 11.2) (Chapters 4 and 6) (15,26,35,36,38,39, 43–45,48,58–61). The prevalence of residual shunts is variable. It is lowest with Amplatzer (35,36,39) and highest with clamshell device (58). Gradual decrease and disappearance of residual shunt has been observed with most of the devices (15,26,32,58). Data on reintervention rates are sketchy. Wire fractures were observed with clamshell, ASDOS, and CardioSEAL devices; the highest rate of fractures is seen with the clamshell device (60). Migration of the core wire occurred in a single batch of defectively manufactured third-generation buttoned devices. The manufacturing deficiency has since

TABLE 11.2. MID-TERM (6–23 MONTHS) RESULTS OF ASD DEVICE CLOSURES

Device/Authors (Reference)	No. of Subjects with Follow-up Data	Duration of Follow-up Mean/Median (Range)	Percent of Subjects with Residual Shunt	Reintervention Rate	Wire-Related Problems
Clamshell					
Boutin et al. (58)	49	10 mo (1 day–21 mo)	53%	*	*
Latson (59)	100	12 mo	16%	*	*
Perry et al. (60)	150	*	15%	*	40% (WF)
Buttoned (first, second, & third)					
Rao et al. (15)	166	12 mo (1–48 mo)	26%	3.6%	1.2% (WM)
Lloyd et al. (61)	46	11 mo (1–20 mo)	12%	0	None
ASDOS					
Sievert (26)	174	17 mo (6–36 mo)	28%	6%	14% (WF)
Babic et al. (Chapter 4)	318	*	*	3.5%	20% (WF)
Amplatzer					
Waight et al. (35)	52	6 mo (*)	6%	6%	None
Dhillon et al. (36)	20	8 mo (1–12 mo)	5%	*	*
Hijazi et al. (38)	26	12 mo (*)	5%	*	*
Walsh & Maadi (39)	102	6 mo (*)	7.5%	1.1%	*
Hamdan et al. (Chapter 6)	93	6 mo (*)	7.7%	7.7%	*
CardioSeal					
Moore et al. (43)	†	1 year	20.5%	†	6.1% (WF)
Carminati (44)	107	12 mo (*)	20.5%	2%	6.1% (WF)
Pedra et al. (45)	50	10 mo (6 to 12 mo)	46%	0	14% (WF)
COD buttoned					
Rao and Sideris (48)	65	6 mo (1 to 12 mo)	4%	0	None

From Rao PS. Summary and comparison of atrial septal closure devices. *Curr Interv Cardiol Rep* 2000;2:367–376, with permission.
†Two were said to have required surgery during follow-up.
*No data.
mo, months; WF, wire fractures; WM, wire migration.

been rectified. Core wire migration has not been observed with the remaining third-generation, (62) fourth-generation (46), or centering-on-demand (COD) (48) buttoned devices.

LONG-TERM FOLLOW-UP RESULTS

Long-term (defined as mean or median ≥ 24 months) follow-up results are reported for clamshell and buttoned devices and are shown in Table 11.3 (46,62–67).

The clamshell device implantation data in 884 patients have been compiled but not published (68). However, the results of single institutional, small cohorts from this large cohort have been reported (63,64). The data indicate 44% to 45% residual shunts and 42% to 84% wire fractures. This device has been withdrawn from further clinical trials and has since been redesigned into CardioSEAL and STARFlex devices. Long-term follow-up of the latter devices is not yet available.

Follow-up with buttoned device (46,62,65–67) revealed residual shunt rates of 10% to 27% and reintervention rates of 4% to 8% during a follow-up of up to 7 years.

As and when long-term follow-up results for the other devices become available, they should be compared with the existing data on clamshell and buttoned devices.

TABLE 11.3. LONG-TERM (≥24 MONTHS) RESULTS OF ASD DEVICE CLOSURES

Device/Authors (Reference)	No. of Subjects with Follow-up Data	Duration of Follow-up Mean/Median (Range)	Percent of Subjects with Residual Shunt	Reintervention Rate	Wire-Related Problems
Clamshell					
Justo et al. (63)	43	31 mo (7–56 mo)	44%	*	42% (WF)
Prieto et al. (64)	31	41 mo (12–65 mo)	45%	3.2%	84% (WF)
Buttoned (first, second, and third)					
Rao et al. (65)	20	29 mo (16–52 mo)	20%	5%	None
Zamora et al. (66)	46	62 mo (51–68 mo)	27%	4%	None
Rao et al. (62,67)	166	46 mo (12–84 mo)	10%	8%	1.2% (WM)
Buttoned (fourth generation)					
Rao et al. (46)	333	24 mo (1–60 mo)	14%	5%	None

From Rao PS. Summary and comparison of atrial septal closure devices. *Curr Interv Cardiol Rep* 2000;2:367–376, with permission.
*No data.
ASD, atrial septal defect; mo, months; WF, wire fractures; WM, wire migration.

OTHER ISSUES

Discussion of issues other than feasibility, safety, and effectiveness will be limited to the devices that are currently in clinical trials.

PATIENT SELECTION

Patients for transcatheter device occlusion are generally selected from findings of precordial or transesophageal echocardiographic studies. The size of the atrial septal defect and adequacy of septal margins to support the device are the major considerations. The assessment of these parameters is arbitrary and at the discretion of the cardiologist performing the procedure. However, these are dealt with very similarly in the clinical trials of all devices. More recently, the role of three-dimensional echocardiographic reconstruction in the patient selection (Chapter 16) (69) is being explored.

The study protocol for transcatheter device occlusion of the ASD for all devices is approved by the respective institutional review boards (IRBs) as per the local regulations and with investigational device exemption (IDE) from the Food and Drug Administration (FDA) in US cases. Informed consent from the parents or patients, as the case may be, is routine in all device protocols.

Most, if not all, cardiologists perform cardiac catheterization to confirm clinical impression and to exclude other defects, particularly partial anomalous pulmonary venous return.

Balloon-stretched diameter of the atrial septal defect (70–72) is routinely measured with septostomy catheters or venous occlusion catheters. More recently, balloon occlusion diameter, the segment of the balloon that eliminates flow across the ASD, is being considered for selection of device size. The occlusion diameter appears to have a good correlation with three-dimensional echocardiographic diameter of the ASD (73). However, most cardiologists seem to be switching to balloon sizing with compliant PTA-OS balloon catheters (NuMed, Inc, Hopkinton, NY) (74).

DEVICE DELIVERY AND IMPLANTATION

Delivery Sheath

The size of device delivery catheters/sheaths required for implantation of currently used devices has gradually diminished compared with initial King's interlocking umbrellas and Rashkind's hooked devices, which required a 23F and 16F sheath, respectively. The sizes of delivery sheaths required to implant the devices currently in clinical trial are shown in Table 11.4. Amplatzer appears to require a smaller delivery sheath than other devices (Table 11.4). When the device is used in a young/small child, the small delivery sheath is helpful. But in the older child and adult, the size of the delivery sheath, 9 to 12F, required to deliver most of the other devices (Table 11.4) is of no major concern.

Device/Defect Ratio

The size of the device used to close the ASD is larger than the stretched diameter of the device, varying from 1.3 to 2.4 times the size of the defect. To a great degree this is determined by the mechanism by which the device is deemed to be anchored across the defect. In most small to moderate-sized defects, the size of the device is not a major issue. In large defects, however, the size of the device required to occlude the defect may be too large for the atrial septum or may impinge upon the conduction system,

TABLE 11.4. SIZE OF THE DEVICE AND DEVICE DELIVERY CATHETER USED TO OCCLUDE ATRIAL SEPTAL DEFECTS

Device	French Size of Delivery Sheath	Device/Defect* Ratio
Buttoned device (fourth generation)	8F to 11F	2:1
Das angel wing device	11F to 13F	1.6:1
ASDOS	11F	2:1
Amplatzer	6F to 12F	Defect + 14 mm
CardioSEAL/STARFlex	11F	1.6:1
COD buttoned device	10F to 12F	1.8:1
Helex device	9F	1.6:1
Transcatheter patch	10F	2 mm larger than stretched diameter

From Rao PS. Summary and comparison of atrial septal closure devices. *Curr Interv Cardiol Rep* 2000;2:367–376, with permission.
*Stretched diameter of the atrial septal defect.
ASDOS, atrial septal defect occluding system; COD, centering-on-demand; F, French size.

mitral valve, or pulmonary veins. Therefore the devices requiring smaller device/defect ratios (Table 11.4) may have an advantage, especially in occluding large defects.

The Device and Its Implantation

Currently used devices are double-disk devices with or without a self-centering mechanism. Table 11.5 lists the device characteristics. The method of device delivery and implantation is unique for each device. The cardiologists should master the technique prior to embarking upon device implantation independently. The degree of complexity in device delivery, placement, and release varies with each device. Implantation of ASDOS appears most complex, whereas placement of Amplatzer device seems to be the simplest. However, most interventional cardiologists with some instruction and training can master the techniques, which is required prior to embarking on implantation of any device.

COST AND AVAILABILITY

Outside the United States, most devices are available for implantation, although local regulations have to be followed. In the United States, however, only Amplatzer devices are available for general clinical use. Other devices may be used only at institutions participating in the device manufacturer-sponsored, FDA-approved clinical trials under IDE and with the approval of local IRBs. For each device, only a limited number of institutions (usually five to ten) are allowed to participate in clinical trials. More recently, Humanitarian Device Exemption (HDE) for use of CardioSEAL device for closure of fenestrations in Fontan patients has been obtained. While the HDE protocol makes it slightly easier to acquire devices than IDE protocol, restrictions remain, including approval by IRBs and

detailed consent forms. Table 11.6 lists the clinical trial status of devices.

The cost of the device is variable and is listed in Table 11.6. Since the devices are used under FDA supervision, the regulatory authority may also oversee the costs. After approval for general clinical use, the cost will be different; it may increase secondary to regulatory release or due to use of limited number of devices. Alternatively, it may decrease as a consequence of competition or the use of more devices than now.

DISCUSSION

Some observations with regard to the potential utility of the devices, along with their relative advantages and disadvantages, will be made in this section.

Buttoned Device

The buttoned device is the oldest of all the devices currently in clinical trials and has the largest clinical experience. The technique of implantation of the fourth-generation device is simple, but the COD device implantation is more complex, although it can easily be learned. The device delivery catheter is small (10F) for most devices, although larger devices (≥50 mm) require 11 or 12F sheaths. There have been claims of high prevalence of residual shunts and high rates of unbuttoning. A careful review of Table 11.1 suggests that the incidence of residual shunts following buttoned-device implantation is not significantly different from that of the other devices. Nor is the unbuttoning rate different from device dislodgment/misplacement rates of other devices. Furthermore, introduction of the fourth-generation device with two radiopaque buttons has decreased the unbuttoning rate to

TABLE 11.5. DEVICE CHARACTERISTICS

	Buttoned Device 4th Generation	ASDOS	Das Angel-Wing Device	Amplatzer	CardioSEAL Device*	Helex Device	COD Buttoned Device
Device components	Square-shaped occluder on the left atrial side and rhomboid shaped counteroccluder on the right atrial side	Two pentagonal umbrellas, one on either side of the ASD	Two square frames joined together with a conjoint ring	Two unequal sized round disks connected together with a 4mm-wide connecting waist	Two square-shaped umbrellas connected together in the center	Round double-disk device built on a single wire	Rounded fourth generation with centering mechanism
Wire skeleton	Teflon-coated 0.018-inch stainless steel wire	Preshaped Nitinol wire	Superelastic 0.01-inch Nitinol wire	0.005-inch Nitinol wire mesh	Mp35n nonferro magnetic alloy	Nitinol wire	Teflon-coated 0.018-inch stainless steel wire
Fabric covering wire foam skeleton	0.0625-inch polyurethane foam	Thin polyurethane membrane	Dacron fabric with an element of elastic stretch	Filled with Dacron fabric	Woven Dacron cloth	Expanded polytetrafluoroethylene	0.0625-inch polyurethane
Device delivery	Occluder into the left atrium and counter-occluder into the right atrium separately	Separate delivery of left and then right atrial umbrellas over a guidewire loop	Device delivered as one unit	Device delivered as one unit	Device delivered as one unit	Device delivered as one unit	Separate delivery of the left and right atrial components
Device fixation	Knots (buttons) attached to the occluder are pulled through the button hole of the counteroccluder (buttoning)	Bolt of the right atrial umbrella is screwed on to the thread of the left atrial umbrella using a screwdriver catheter	Conjoint ring keeps the disks together	Connecting waist keeps the disks together	Central hub connecting both umbrellas	A single-length wire preshaped into two "umbrellas"	Folded centering wires and buttoning
Device release	Withdrawing the nylon thread passing through the delivery wire and button loop of the occluder	Removal of the arteriovenous guidewire loop via the left atrium and femoral artery	Release of Nitinol wire passing through the notch and one of the corner eyelets of the right atrial disk	Unscrewing by counterclockwise rotation of the delivery cable	Removal of central core wire	Detachment of retrieval cord	Withdrawal of nylon thread
Device retrieval prior to release	Pulling the loading wire into the sheath. Snare to prevent inadvertent disconnection from loading wire	Device withdrawn into the sheath	Device withdrawn into the sheath	Withdrawn into the sheath	Withdrawn into the sheath	Withdrawn into the sheath	Loading wire into the sheath plus snaring device

*Further modification of the device by attaching microsprings between the umbrellas, Starflex centering system, was made to provide centering capability and has features similar to CardioSEAL device.

ASDOS, atrial septal defect occluding system; COD, centering-on-demand.

From Rao PS. Summary and comparison of atrial septal closure devices. *Curr Interv Cardiol Rep* 2000;2:367–376, with permission.

TABLE 11.6. COST* AND CLINICAL TRIAL STATUS OF THE ASD DEVICES

Device	Cost*	Clinical Trial Status
Buttoned device (fourth generation)	$1,300	Phase II trials in the U.S., completed
Das Angel-Wing Device	$4,250†	Phase II trials, discontinued
ASDOS	DM 9,000	Clinical trials outside the U.S.
Amplatzer	$2,700‡	Phase II trials, device approved by FDA, completed
CardioSEAL/STARflex	$2,750	Phase II trials in the U.S.
COD buttoned device	$2,300	Phase II trials in the U.S.
Helex device	§	Phase I trials in the U.S.
Transcatheter patch	$2,300	Clinical trials outside the U.S. U.S. trials to begin soon

ASDOS, atrial septal defect occluding system; COD, centering-on-demand; U.S.A., United States of America; FDA, Food and Drug Administration.
*The amount that the institution participating in clinical trial pays per each device
†The cost of modified device, when available for clinical trials has not been established at the time of this writing.
‡Cost in Europe is approximately $4,500.
§Unable to obtain information at the time of this writing.
From Rao PS. Summary and comparison of atrial septal closure devices. *Curr Interv Cardiol Rep* 2000;2:367–376, with permission.

less than 1% (46). The disadvantage of this device is lack of centering mechanism. Therefore a device at least two times the size of the stretched ASD diameter (75) is required (Table 11.4). Consequently, closure of large defects may become difficult because the required device size may be too large for the atrial septum to accommodate or may impinge upon critical structures. Therefore the device has been modified into a COD device and has been tested in animal models (76). The COD buttoned device has recently been approved by the FDA for clinical trials in the United States and the clinical trials have begun. The clinical experience thus far (48) is encouraging.

Angel Wing Das Device

The Angel Wing Das device has excellent self-centering characteristics, and the incidence of residual shunt is low. However, delivery of the device is complex. It is also difficult to adjust the position of the device, and retrieval of the device, even before detachment, is problematic. Aortic perforation, presumably related to sharp eyelet at the corners of the device, was found during Phase II clinical trials. Because of this the device was withdrawn from further clinical trials. The device has been redesigned to make the disks circular and turn the eyelets inward to prevent aortic perforation (23). It is also planned to introduce transcatheter retrievability feature, while maintaining self-centering characteristics (23). Once the redesigned device receives FDA approval, further clinical trial may resume.

ASDOS

The concept and design of the ASDOS device are attractive; however, the device implantation process is complex. A high incidence of thrombosis is of concern. Fractures of wire frame have been detected by cineradiography in 20% of patients. FDA approval for clinical trials has not been sought and therefore has not been used in the United States. It also appears that there are limited on-going clinical trials outside the United States.

Amplatz Septal Occluder

The Amplatz Septal Occluder is a relatively new double-disk, self-centering device with rapid accumulation of implantation data. Short-term and mid-term follow-up data have been published. Implantation of the device is relatively easy and requires a small delivery sheath. The device can be retrieved with ease into the sheath prior to release. It can also be repositioned. The prevalence of residual shunts is low. Phase II clinical trials have been completed in the United States, and the device recently received approval from the FDA. The device may soon be available for general clinical use. The disadvantages are a thick profile of the device and concern related to a large amount of Nitinol (a nickel-titanium compound) in the device and consequent potential for nickel toxicity.

CardioSEAL/STARFlex Devices

CardioSEAL is a modified/redesigned version of the clamshell device and requires a large delivery sheath, which is difficult to retrieve. The CardioSEAL is not a self-centering device, but the further modified version by STARFlex system made it more self-centering than CardioSEAL. Arm fractures seen with clamshell device have also been reported with this device, thus raising concern about long-term safety.

Helex Device

The Helex device is the newest of the devices. It is a double-disk device built on single-strand Nitinol wire draped with ultrathin ePTEE. It may be delivered via a 9F delivery catheter without a sheath. The implantation of the device is complex, but the device can be withdrawn into the catheter before detachment and redeployed as desired. However, the human experience with this device is limited. FDA-approved clinical trials with an IDE have recently begun.

Transcatheter Patch

The currently used devices are double-disk devices and have similar limitations in that they require septal rims to hold the device. In addition, wire-related problems such as atrial perforation, aortic perforation, mitral valve injury, wire fractures, and embolization may exist in all devices. In response to resolving these problems, wireless devices have been conceived by Sideris (Chapter 9) (76), and detachable-balloon and transcatheter-deliverable patches have been developed. Polyurethane patches, supported by modified balloon catheters are implanted across atrial septal defects, left *in situ* for 48 hours, and are withdrawn by balloon, leaving the patch in place. Following the feasibility and safety studies in piglets (Chapter 9) (77), human trials began outside the United States (Chapter 9). FDA approval for IDE and human trials in United States was recently received and clinical trials will begin soon.

SUMMARY AND CONCLUSION

Following pioneering works of King, Rashkind, and their associates in the mid-1970s of transcatheter device closure of ASD, a number of devices have been designed and tested in animal models. This is followed by subsequent clinical trials. For various reasons, some of the devices have been discontinued and others have been modified or redesigned. At the present time, seven devices are in various phases of clinical trials. The FDA, at this time, has approved only one device for general clinical use. Most are available in US hospitals participating in clinical trials sponsored by device manufacturers with investigational device exemption from the FDA. Most are available in countries outside the United States, with less stringent requirements. Based on independently conducted clinical trials, the feasibility, safety, and effectiveness of all devices appear similar. Considerations pertaining to the size of the device delivery sheath, ease of implantation, cost, and availability are different with each of the devices; some devices have advantages with some aspects and others, with another. Complexity of device implantation (ASDOS and Angel Wing Das device), thrombus formation (ASDOS), removal from clinical trials pending device redesign (Angel Wing Das), and arm fractures (ASDOS and CardioSEAL) make these devices problematic. Currently, the Amplatzer,

COD buttoned device, and Helex device are still in the running. Approval for general clinical use by the FDA and/or other regulatory authorities and good results in large patient cohorts with long-term follow-up are needed to identify devices that are likely to be suitable for routine clinical use for transcatheter closure of ASDs.

REFERENCES

1. King TD, Mills NL. Nonoperative closure of atrial septal defects. *Surgery* 1974;75:383–388.
2. Mills NL, King TD. Nonoperative closure of left-to-right shunts. *J Thorac Cardiovasc Surg* 1976;72:371–378.
3. King TD, Thompson SL, Steiner C, et al. Secundum atrial septal defect: nonoperative closure during cardiac catheterization. *JAMA* 1976;235:2506–2509.
4. Chopra PS, Rao PS. History of development of atrial septal occlusion devices. *Curr Interv Cardiol Rep* 2000;2:63–69.
5. Rao PS. Closure devices for atrial septal defect: which one to chose? [editorial]. *Indian Heart J* 1998;50:379–383.
6. Rao PS. Transcatheter closure of atrial septal defects: Are we there yet? [editorial]. *J Am Coll Cardiol* 1998;31:1117–1119.
7. Walsh KP, Tofeig M, Kitchiner DJ, et al. Comparison of the Sideris and Amplatzer septal occlusion devices. *Am J Cardiol* 1999;83:933–936.
8. Formigari R, Santoro G, Rosetti L, et al. Comparison of three different atrial septal defect occluding devices. *Am J Cardiol* 1998;82:690–692.
9. Sievert H, Koppeler P, Rux S, et al. Percutaneous closure of 176 interatrial defects in adults with different occlusion devices: 6 years experience [abstract]. *J Am Coll Cardiol* 1999;33:519A.
10. Keppeir P, Rux S, Dirko J, et al. Transcatheter closure of 100 patent foramina ovalia in patients with unexplained stroke and suspected paradoxic embolism: a comparison of five different devices [abstract]. *Eur Heart J* 1999;20:196.
11. Rashkind WJ, Tait MA, Gibson RJ, Jr. Interventional cardiac catheterization in congenital heart disease. *Int J Cardiol* 1985;7:1–11.
12. Beekman RH, Rocchini AP, Snider AR, et al. Transcatheter atrial septal defect closure: preliminary experience with the Rashkind occluder device. *J Interv Cardiol* 1989;1:35–41.
13. Rome JJ, Keane JF, Perry SB, et al. Double-umbrella closure of atrial defects: initial clinical applications. *Circulation* 1990;82:751–758.
14. Hellenbrand WE, Fahey JT, McGowan FX, et al. Transesophageal echocardiographic guidance of transcatheter closure of atrial septal defect. *Am J Cardiol* 1990;66:207–213.
15. Rao PS, Sideris EB, Hausdorf G, et al. International experience with secundum atrial septal defect occlusion by the buttoned device. *Am Heart J* 1994;128:1022–1035.
16. Arora R, Trehan VK, Karla GS, et al. Transcatheter closure of atrial septal defect using buttoned device: Indian experience. *Indian Heart J* 1996;48:145–149.
17. Haddad J, Secches A, Finzi L, et al. Atrial septal defect: percutaneous transvenous occlusion with the buttoned device. *Arq Bras Cardiol* 1996;67:17–22.
18. Worms AM, Rey C, Bourlan F, et al. French experience in the closure of atrial septal defects of the ostium secundum type with Sideris buttoned occluder. *Arch Mal Coeur Vaiss* 1996;89:509–515.
19. Weil J, Rickers C, Stern H, et al. Percutaneous closure of secundum atrial septal defect with a new self-centering device ("Angel Wings"): preliminary experience in Germany. In: Imai Y, Momma K, eds. *Proceedings of the Second World Congress of Pedi-*

atric Cardiology and Cardiac Surgery Armonk, NY: Futura, 1998:200–203.

20. Mendelsohn AM, Banerjee A, Schwartz DC, et al. Transcatheter atrial septal defect closure with Das Angel Wings transcatheter ASD occlusion device: the Cincinnati-Rochester experience. *J Interv Cardiol* 1998;11:495–500.

21. Rickers C, Hamm C, Stern H, et al. Percutaneous closure of secundum atrial septal defect with a new self-centering device ("Angel Wings"). *Heart* 1998;80:517–521.

22. Banerjee A, Bengur AR, Li JS, et al. Echocardiographic characteristics of successful deployment of the Das Angel Wings atrial septal defect closure device: initial multicenter experience in the United States. *Am J Cardiol* 1999;83:1236–1241.

23. Das GS, Harrison JK, O'Laughlin MP. The Angel Wing Das devices for atrial septal defect closure. *Curr Interv Cardiol Rep* 2000;2:78–85.

24. Sievert H, Babic UU, Ensslen R, et al. Occlusion of atrial septal defects with a new device. *Z Cardiol* 1996;85:97–103.

25. Hausdorf G, Schneider M, Franzback B, et al. Transcatheter closure of secundum atrial septal defect occluder system (ASDOS): initial experience in children. *Heart* 1996;75:83–88.

26. Sievert H, Babic UU, Hausdorf G, et al. Transcatheter closure of atrial septal defect and patent foramen ovale with the ASDOS device (a multi-institutional European trial). *Am J Cardiol* 1998;82:1405–1413.

27. Babic UU. Experience with ASDOS for transcatheter closure of atrial septal defect and patent foramen ovale. *Curr Interv Cardiol Rep* 2000;2:177–183.

28. Masura J, Gavora P, Formanek A, et al. Transcatheter closure of secundum atrial septal defects using the new self-centering Amplatzer septal occluder: initial human experience. *Cathet Cardiovasc Diagn* 1997;42:388–393.

29. Thanopoulos BD, Laskari CV, Tsaousis GC, et al. Closure of atrial septal defects with the Amplatzer occlusion device: preliminary results. *J Am Coll Cardiol* 1998;31:1110–1116.

30. Wilkins JL, Goh TH. Early clinical experience with the use of the "Amplatzer Septal Occluder" device for atrial septal defect closure. *Cardiol Young* 1998;8:295–302.

31. Hijazi Z, Cao Q, Patel H, et al. Transcatheter closure of atrial communications using the Amplatzer septal occluder. *J Interv Cardiol* 1999;12:51–58.

32. Chan KC, Goodman MJ, Walsh K, et al. Transcatheter closure of atrial septal defect and interatrial communications with a new self-expanding Nitinol double disc device (Amplatzer septal occluder): multicentre UK experience. *Heart* 1999;82:300–306.

33. Berger F, Vogel M, Alexi-Meskishvili V, et al. Comparison of results and complications of surgical and Amplatzer device closure of atrial septal defects. *J Thorac Cardiovasc Surg* 1999;118:674–680.

34. Fisher G, Kramer HH, Stieh J, et al. Transcatheter closure of secundum atrial septal defects with the new self-expanding Amplatzer septal occluder. *Eur Heart J* 1999;20:541–549.

35. Waight DJ, Koenig PR, Cao Q, et al. Transcatheter closure of secundum atrial septal defects using the Amplatzer Septal Occluder: clinical experience and technical considerations. *Curr Interv Cardiol Rep* 2000;2:70–77.

36. Dhillon R, Thanopoulos B, Tsaousis G, et al. Transcatheter closure of atrial septal defects in adults with the Amplatzer septal occluder. *Heart* 1999;82:559–562.

37. Hijazi ZM, Radtke W, Ebeid MR, et al. Transcatheter closure of secundum atrial septal defect using the Amplatzer septal occluder: results of phase II US multicenter clinical trial [Abstract]. *Circulation* 1999;100(Suppl I):I-804.

38. Hajazi ZM, Cao QL, Patel HT, et al. Transcatheter closure of atrial communications (ASD/PFO) in adult patients > 18 yr. of age using Amplatzer septal occluder: immediate and mid-term results [Abstract]. *J Am Coll Cardiol* 2000;35:522A.

39. Walsh KP, Maadi IM. The Amplatzer septal occluder. *Cardiol Young* 2000;10:493–501.

40. Vogel M, Berger F, Dahnert I, et al. Treatment of atrial septal defects in symptomatic children ages less than 2 years of age using Amplatzer septal occluder. *Cardiol Young* 2000;10:534–537.

41. Zahn EM, Benson LN, Hellenbrand WE, et al. Transcatheter closure of secundum ASDs with CardioSEAL septal occluding system: early results of the North American Trial [abstract]. *Circulation* 1997;96:I-568.

42. Latson LA. The CardioSEAL device: history, techniques, results. *J Interv Cardiol* 1998;11:501–505.

43. Moore P, Benson LN, Berman W, Jr. CardioSEAL device closure of secundum ASDs: how effective is it? [abstract]. *Circulation* 1998;8:I-754.

44. Carminati M, Guisti S, Hausdorf G, et al. A European multicenter experience using CardioSEAL and STARFlex double umbrella devices to close interatrial communications/holes within the oval fossa. *Cardiol Young* 2000;10:519–526.

45. Pedra CAC, Pihkala J, Lee KJ, et al. Transcatheter closure of atrial septal defects using the CardioSEAL implant. *Heart* 2000;84:320–326.

46. Rao PS, Berger F, Rey C, et al. Transvenous occlusion of secundum atrial septal defects with 4th generation buttoned device: comparison with 1st-, 2nd,- and 3rd-generation devices. *J Am Coll Cardiol* 2000;36:583–592.

47. Wilson N, Sievert H, Zahn EM, et al. Total world clinical experience with the Helex atrial septal defect occlusion device [Abstract]. *Circulation* 2000;102:588.

48. Rao PS, Sideris EB. Centering-on-demand buttoned device: its role in transcatheter occlusion of atrial septal defects. *J Interv Cardiol* 2001;14:81–89.

49. Rao PS. Summary and comparison of atrial septal closure devices. *Curr Interv Cardiol Rep* 2000;2:367–376.

50. Rao PS, Chandar JS, Sideris EB. Role of inverted buttoned device in transcatheter occlusion of atrial septal defects or patent foramen ovale with right-to-left shunting associated with previously operated complex congenital cardiac anomalies. *Am J Cardiol* 1997;80:914–921.

51. Bohm J, Bittigau K, Kohler F, et al. Surgical removal of atrial septal defect occlusion system-device. *Eur J Cardiothorac Surg* 1997;12:869–872.

52. Gastmann O, Werner GS, Babic UU, et al. Thrombus formation on transcatheter ASD occluder device in a patient with coagulation factor XII deficiency. *Cathet Cardiovasc Diagn* 1998;43:81–83.

53. LaRosse K, Deutsch HJ, Schnabel P, et al. Thrombus formation after transcatheter closure of atrial septal defect. *Am J Cardiol* 1999;84:356–359.

54. Khatchatourov G, Kalangos A, Anwar A, et al. Massive thromboembolism due to transcatheter ASD closure with ASDOS device. *J Invasive Cardiol* 1999;11:743–745.

55. Lambert V, Losay J, Piot JD, et al. Late complications of percutaneous closure of atrial septal defects with Sideris occluder. *Arch Mal Coeur Vaiss* 1997;90:245–251.

56. Bullock AM, Monahem S, Wilkinson JL. Infective endocarditis on an occluder closing an atrial septal defect. *Cardiol Young* 1999;9:65–67.

57. Lock JE, Rome JJ, Davis R, et al. Transcatheter closure of atrial septal defects: experimental studies. *Circulation* 1989;79:1091–1099.

58. Boutin C, Musewe NN, Smallhorn JF, et al. Echocardiographic follow-up of atrial septal defect after catheter closure by double-umbrella device. *Circulation* 1993;88:621–627.

59. Latson LA. Transcatheter closure of atrial septal defects. In: Rao PS, ed. *Transcatheter therapy in pediatric cardiology.* New York: Wiley-Liss, 1993:335–348.

60. Perry SB, Van der Velde ME, Bridges ND, et al. Transcatheter closure of atrial and ventricular septal defects. *Herz* 1993;18:135–142.

61. Lloyd TR, Rao PS, Beekman RH III, et al. Atrial septal defect occlusion with the buttoned device: a multi-institutional U.S. trial. *Am J Cardiol* 1994;73:286–291.

62. Rao PS, Sideris EB. Buttoned device closure of the atrial septal defect. *J Interv Cardiol* 1998;11:467–484.

63. Justo RN, Nykanen DG, Boutin C, et al. Clinical impact of transcatheter closure of secundum atrial septal defects with double umbrella device. *Am J Cardiol* 1996;77:889–892.

64. Prieto LR, Foreman CK, Cheatham JP, et al. Intermediate-term outcome of transcatheter secundum atrial septal defect closure using Bard clamshell septal umbrella. *Am J Cardiol* 1996;78: 1310–1312.

65. Rao PS, Ende DJ, Wilson AD, et al. Follow-up results of transcatheter occlusion of atrial septal defects with buttoned device. *Can J Cardiol* 1995;11:695–701.

66. Zamora R, Rao PS, Lloyd TR, et al. Intermediate-term results of Phase I FDA trial of buttoned device occlusion of secundum atrial septal defects. *J Am Coll Cardiol* 1998;31:674–678.

67. Rao PS, Sideris EB, Rey C, et al. Echo-Doppler follow-up evaluation after transcatheter occlusion of atrial septal defects with the buttoned device. In: Imai Y, Momma K, eds. *Proceedings of the Second World Congress of Pediatric Cardiology and Cardiac Surgery.* Armonk, NY: Futura, 1998:197–200.

68. Latson LA. Comments on Rao PS: Interventional pediatric cardiology: state of the art and future directions. *Pediatr Cardiol* 1998;19:107.

69. Acar P, Saliba R, Bonhoeffer P, et al. Influence of atrial septal defect anatomy in patient selection and assessment of closure with the CardioSEAL device. *Eur Heart J* 2000;21:573–581.

70. Rao PS, Langhough R. Relationship to echographic, shunt flow, and angiographic size to the stretched diameter of the atrial septal defect. *Am Heart J* 1991;123:191–200.

71. Rao PS, Langhough R, Beekman RH, et al. Echocardiographic estimation of balloon-stretched diameter of secundum atrial septal defects for transcatheter occlusion. *Am Heart J* 1992;124:172–175.

72. King TD, Thompson SL, Steiner C, et al. Measurement of atrial septal defect during cardiac catheterization: experimental and clinical trials. *Am J Cardiol* 1978;41:537–542.

73. Zhu W, Cao Q, Rhodes J, et al. Measurement of atrial septal defect size; a comparative study between three-dimensional transesophageal echocardiography and the standard balloon sizing methods. *Pediatr Cardiol* 2000;21:465–469.

74. Gu X, Han Y, Berry J, et al. A new technique for sizing of atrial septal defects. *Cathet Cardiovasc Interv* 1999;46:51–57.

75. Rao PS, Wilson AD, Levy JM, et al. Role of "buttoned" double-disc device in the management of atrial septal defects. *Am Heart J* 1992;123:191–200.

76. Zamora R, Rao PS, Sideris EB. Buttoned device for atrial septal defect occlusion. *Curr Interv Cardiol Rep* 2000;2:167–176.

77. Sideris EB, Sideris SE, Kaneva A, et al. Transcatheter occlusion of experimental atrial septal defects by wireless occluders and patches [Abstract]. *Cardiol Young* 1999;9:92.

12

PFO-STAR FOR CLOSURE OF PATENT FORAMEN OVALE IN PATIENTS WITH PRESUMED PARADOXICAL EMBOLISM

RAINER SCHRÄDER
DIETER FASSBENDER
RUTH H. STRASSER

Paradoxic embolism through a patent foramen ovale (PFO) may be an important cause of unexplained strokes in young adults. Transcatheter occlusion of such atrial defects has recently been used in these patients. In this chapter we will discuss the role of PFO-Star occluder in closing such defects.

DESCRIPTION OF THE DEVICE

The PFO-Star occluder (1) has been developed for the transvenous closure of patent foramen ovale (PFO). Is it introduced through transseptal venous sheaths by means of a modified biopsy forceps, allowing complete retrieval of the device. The sails of the device are made of polyvinyl-alcohol (Ivalon). Ivalon has been used for more than 30 years for closure of patent ductus arteriosus (2–4). No adverse long-term effects of this material have been reported (5,6). The device is manufactured in three different sizes (26, 30, and 35 mm) for both PFOs and atrial septal aneurysms (ASA) (Figures 12.1 and 12.2). Each size is available with a 3-mm or a 5-mm center post for different thicknesses of the atrial septum.

TECHNICAL EVOLUTION
Generation I

Initial devices (Figure 12.3) made for PFO closure were constructed with 2-mm center posts and employed

Rainer Schräder: Professor, Markus-Krankenhaus-CCB, Frankfurt Am Main, Germany
Dieter Fassbender: Herz-und Diabetes-Zentrum, Badoeynhausen, Germany
Ruth H. Strasser: Klinik für Kardiologie, Technische Universität, Dresden, Germany

polypropylene sutures; 22-, 26-, and 30-mm NiTi wires; 2-mm-thick foam Ivalon sails; titanium protective end caps; and a unique system for forceps delivery and retrieval through standard transseptal sheaths (11 to 13F).

Generation II

Second-generation PFO-Star occluders introduced new 3- and 5-mm center posts to accommodate variations in septal thickness. In addition, an improved wire system (wire length, 26 and 30 mm) was developed to increase device flexibility while retaining high tension rates. Thickness of the Ivalon sail was reduced to improve its retrieval and allow the use of smaller delivery sheath sizes (10 to 12F).

Generation III

Third-generation devices are constructed with the left side Ivalon attached on the outside of the frame in order to reduce any potential for clot formation (Figure 12.4). For use in patients with aneurismal septums, a 35-mm device was introduced that provides greater support and structure to the septal tissue, thus reducing mobility. The tension of the wire system was increased by more than 50% and adjusted precisely such that each size has exactly the same tension and spring rate, thus improving the "feel" during deployment. Finally, a method to reinforce the Ivalon was developed to reduce the bulk of the device, allowing smaller delivery sheath sizes (9 to 10F) and further increasing safety and durability.

ANIMAL EXPERIMENTS

Chronic experiments were carried out in lambs (merino mix) under general anesthesia. The animals were intubated and mechanically ventilated during the studies. Catheteri-

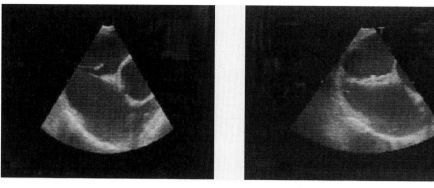

FIGURE 12.1. Transesophageal echocardiographic frame demonstrating a patent foramen ovale prior to **(A)** and following **(B)** closure with a PFO-Star device.

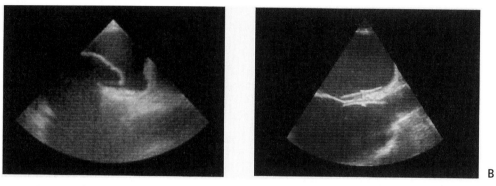

FIGURE 12.2. Atrial septal aneurysm prior to and after occlusion with a PFO-Star device.

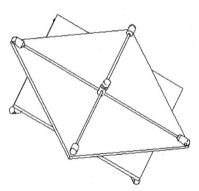

FIGURE 12.3. Diagram of PFO-Star occluder (generation I) showing the 2-mm center post, 4 NiTi wires (for stabilization of the left and right atrial sails) with eight titanium end caps and two Ivalon sails.

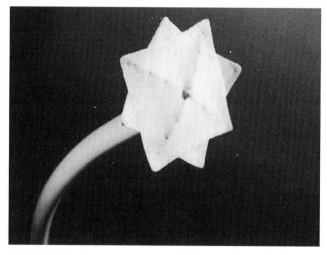

FIGURE 12.4. Photograph of the PFO-Star occluder (generation III) with the left side Ivalon-foam placed on the outside of the frame.

zation was done via cut-down of the right femoral vein using monoplane fluoroscopy. After probing the atrial septum with a guide wire, the PFO was dilated with a 10-mm balloon. The device was then implanted using standard techniques. The animals were recatheterized and then sacrificed 7 to 137 days after implantation. The device and tissue block were harvested for gross (Figure 12.5) and microscopic examination the specimens were fixed in formalin or glutaraldehyde.

METHODS

Patients

Over a period of 44 months (from February 1998 until September 2000), 251 patients with patent foramen ovale (PFO) and at least one documented thromboembolic event have undergone percutaneous PFO closure with the PFO-Star occluder for prevention of recurrence of paradoxical embolism.

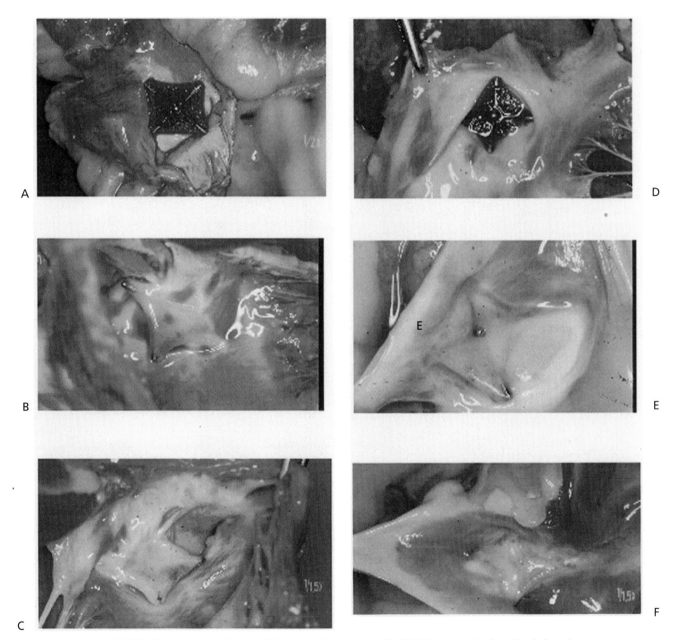

FIGURE 12.5. Gross specimens of lamb's atrial septum with PFO-Star occluder from the left and right atrial side 7, 53, and 137 days following implantation, respectively.

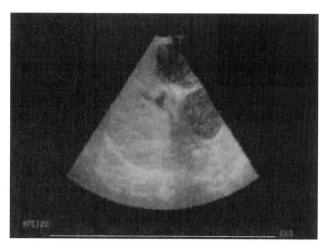

FIGURE 12.6. Transesophageal contrast echocardiography demonstrating spontaneous right-to-left shunt through a patent foramen ovale.

The inclusion criteria were the following:

1. Presence of PFO with or without ASA with spontaneous or provokable right-to-left shunt during contrast transesophageal echocardiography (Figure 12.6).
2. Ischemic stroke or transient ischemic attack (TIA) confirmed clinically by a neurologist and radiologically by either cranial computer tomography or magnetic resonance imaging; or peripheral thromboembolism verified clinically and radiologically.
3. Exclusion of any other identifiable cause for this thromboembolic event.

Initial patient work-up included (a) extracranial Doppler ultrasonography with frequency analysis and B-mode, (b) 12-lead EKG, (c) transthoracic echocardiography, (d) 24-hour Holter EKG, (e) 24-hour blood pressure measurements, and (f) coagulation screening. All patients gave written informed consent before PFO closure.

IMPLANTATION TECHNIQUE

On the day of implantation, patients received one to three standard doses of a second-generation cephalosporin or ampicillin for prophylaxis of bacterial endocarditis. Under local anesthesia, venous access was gained via the right femoral vein. Patients were heparinized with 70 to 100 units unfractioned heparin per kilogram of body weight. Before introduction of the transesophageal echo probe the patients were premedicated with 0.5 to 1.0 mg atropine, 10 mg metoclopramide, and sedatives as required. Some patients, however, did not tolerate the transesophageal echo probe despite the premedication. They were either put under general anesthesia or, in recent months, the implantation was performed without echocardiographic monitoring.

The PFO was crossed with a 5- to 7F multipurpose catheter under fluoroscopic control. The tip of the catheter was placed into the anterior left pulmonary vein, and the position was checked by injection of a small amount of contrast medium. The multipurpose catheter was exchanged for an extra-stiff 0.035-inch exchange wire. In 198 of 251 patients, the stretched diameter of the PFO was measured with a balloon catheter according to standard techniques. Thereafter a 9- to 13F transseptal sheath was introduced into the left atrium using the extra-stiff exchange wire. The selected PFO-Star occluder was connected to the delivery forceps and loaded into a standard 12F sheath. Air bubbles were removed by injecting saline through the side arm of the sheath. With the occluder loaded within its tip, the 12F sheath was inserted through the hemostatic valve into the transseptal sheath. During this maneuver, the side arm was again flushed with saline to prevent air from getting entrapped.

The occluder was then delivered through the transseptal sheath under fluoroscopic as well as transesophageal echocardiographic guidance. The distal sail of the occluder was opened within the left atrium. The delivery forceps with the device attached and the sheath were pulled back as a unit until the fully expanded left atrial sail was in traction against the atrial septum. This was indicated by pulse-synchronous movements of the NiTi wires. While keeping slight tension on the delivery forceps, the sheath was pulled back until the proximal sail of the occluder opened within the right atrium (Figure 12.7A) and the forceps released (Figure 12.7B). Before and after releasing the occluder, the position of the device was checked by right atrial contrast injection through the transseptal sheath (Figure 12.7C). An echocontrast injection (3 g D-galactose bubble-solution injected central venously) was performed immediately after final release of the device to detect residual shunting, if any (Figure 12.8). Usually, patients were discharged from the hospital the next day. Before discharge, the number of white blood cells and C-reactive protein were measured. The position of the device was confirmed by chest x-ray and transthoracic echocardiography.

POSTINTERVENTIONAL TREATMENT

For the prophylaxis of thromboembolic events after device implantation, patients were treated with 75 mg clopidogrel for 6 weeks to 3 months and with 100 mg aspirin for 6 to 12 months. In one center (87 patients), low molecular weight heparin was added to the regimen for the first 3 days after implantation. Standard bacterial endocarditis prophylaxis was recommended for 12 months. Oral anticoagula-

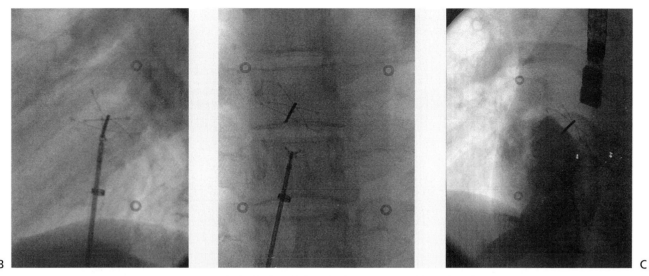

A,B   C

FIGURE 12.7. PFO-Star occluder before **(A)** and after releasing **(B)** with right atrial contrast injection **(C)**.

tion was prescribed in patients with (a) preinterventional deep venous thrombosis, (b) intermittent atrial fibrillation after implantation, (c) coagulation diseases (e.g., APC-resistance, factor V mutation), and (d) device-related thrombus proven by transesophageal echocardiography.

FOLLOW-UP

All patients were followed up prospectively. Outpatient clinical follow-up was performed after 1, 3, 6, and 12 months. Routine transesophageal contrast echocardiography with 3 g D-galactose bubble solution injected into the

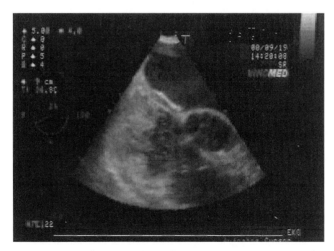

FIGURE 12.8. Transesophageal contrast echocardiography demonstrating complete PFO closure immediately after device implantation.

antecubital vein was performed 3 to 6 months after implantation for detection of residual shunting. Additionally, some patients underwent transesophageal contrast echocardiography for various reasons after 2 to 4 weeks and/or after 1 year. For detection of possible wire fractures, a left-lateral chest x-ray and, in some cases, fluoroscopy were performed routinely after 6 months. Thereafter patients were followed annually either by telephone contact or by their referring physicians. Only one patient was lost for follow-up.

RESULTS

Patient Demographics

There were 127 women and 124 men aged 17 to 79 years (mean age, 46 years). Before PFO closure, they had suffered a total of 338 embolic events, of which 207 (61%) were strokes, 125 (37%) were TIAs, and six (2%) were peripheral embolisms. Individual patients had experienced one to six events with an average of 1.3 events per patient. The incidence of embolic events before PFO closure was 3.4% per year (338 events in 11,526 patient-years). Deep venous thrombosis was found by either phlebography or Doppler ultrasonography with frequency analysis and B-mode in 18 patients (7.1%). Arterial hypertension (controllable with one or two antihypertensive agents) was present in 48 patients (19.1%).

Interventions

General anesthesia was required in 18 patients (7.2%) who did not tolerate the transesophageal echo probe. Recently, device implantation was performed with fluoroscopic guidance only in 13 patients (5.2%). The fluoroscopy time ranged from 3 to 12 minutes (mean, 4 minutes) and the duration of the procedure from 30 to 70 minutes (mean, 40 minutes). In more than 90% of cases the PFO diameter was measured with balloon sizing. PFO diameter ranged from 3 to 21 mm, with an average of 10 mm. An ASA was present in 67 patients (27%).

Generation I devices were used in 38 patients (15%); generation II devices, in 94 patients (38%); and generation III devices, in the remaining 119 patients (47%). The size of the devices used was 22 mm in 9%, 26 mm in 39%, 30 mm in 47%, and 35 mm in 5%. Larger devices were used for PFO with diameters of more than 12 mm or in patients with ASAs. The size of the transseptal sheath used for implantation of the different devices was 9 to 13F. For generation I occluders, the size was 11 to 13F; for generation II, occluders 10 to 12F; and for generation III occluders, 9 to 11F. The average sheath diameter for all procedures was 10.5F. After implantation, residual shunt was detected in 48 patients (19.1%).

Periprocedural Complications (Within 24 Hours)

Device implantation was performed successfully and without complications in 240 of 251 patients (95%). Six patients suffered embolization of air with transient symptoms (ST-segment elevation in five patients and transient neurologic deficit in one patient). In two patients intermittent atrial fibrillation occurred that was treated by means of DC shock in one patient. In one patient a 30-mm generation II device embolized several hours after implantation. The device was retrieved with the forceps from the right renal artery and withdrawn through a 12F sheath via the right femoral artery. In two patients the first device was withdrawn because of misplacement. Subsequently, PFO closure was performed with a second PFO-Star device during the same procedure. There were no myocardial infarctions, strokes, or cardiac tamponade. Bleeding complications did not occur nor was there any need for surgical intervention.

Follow-up

Only one patient was lost for follow-up. All others were followed up from 1 month to 2.7 years. Total follow-up time was 133 patient-years. The mean follow-up interval was 6.3 months. At 6 months' follow-up, residual right-to-left shunting was detected by means of contrast transesophageal echocardiography in 13 patients (5.2%). One device was explanted surgically because of allergic reaction and positive skin test for Ivalon 2 months after implantation. Asymptomatic wire fractures (Figure 12.9) occurred in 15 of 38 generation I devices and in five of 94 generation II devices. No fractures were seen in the remaining patients (Figure 12.10). Thrombus formation (Figure 12.11) on the right

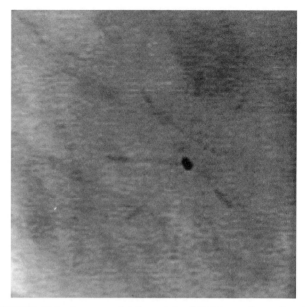

FIGURE 12.9. Fracture of right atrial solid NiTi arm due to bending at the aortic root at 6 months' follow-up (PFO-Star Generation I). The clinical course was uneventful (follow-up, 32 months).

and/or the left atrial side of the occluder was observed in six patients, one with a generation I and five with generation II implants. The thrombus resolved in all patients, and no further clinical events were observed.

Six patients suffered recurrent neurologic symptoms during the follow-up period. One patient, who had a residual shunt, suffered aphasia and hemiparesis during a hypertensive crisis. Cranial CT scan did not show any new defects and the symptoms resolved completely. In the other five

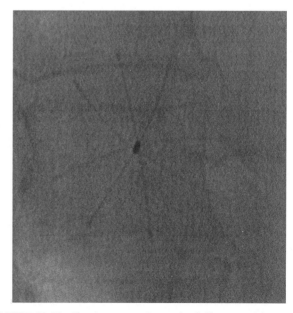

FIGURE 12.10. Fluoroscopy at 6 months' follow-up with normal appearance of stranded NiTi wires (PFO-Star generation III).

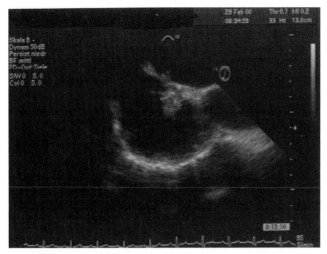

FIGURE 12.11. Thrombus on right atrial side of the device 2 months after implantation. Tunneling of the device because of the softness of stranded NiTi wires (PFO-Star Generation II). The clinical course was uneventful and transesophageal contrast echocardiography revealed no residual shunt and no thrombus after 6 and 12 months, respectively.

patients, no residual shunt was present. One patient had a progredient lesion of the right internal carotid artery as possible cause for a transient ischemic attack. Another patient underwent cerebral angiography after a recurrent ischemic event. An arteriovenous fistula originating from the right medial cerebral artery was detected and the patient underwent neurosurgical ligation with uneventful outcome. In the three other patients, no apparent reason could be detected. None of the remaining 251 patients suffered a stroke.

DISCUSSION

The data presented here reflect the learning curves of three high-volume operators as well as the technical evolution of the device, and this register includes the first cases that have ever been done with this specific technique (7). The feasibility of the technique was improved by technical changes from generation I to generation III of the device, thus reducing technical and clinical complications such as wire fractures and clot formation. The device is fully retrievable before final release, and even in case of embolization, transcatheter retrieval can easily be performed by means of a snare or the forceps. There were only 5% periprocedural (minor) complications. During a follow-up period of 132 patient-years, recurrent cerebral ischemia was prevented in more than 97% of patients. The recurrence rate was 2.3% for transient ischemic attacks, 0 for strokes, and 0 for peripheral thromboembolism.

CONCLUSION

The PFO-Star offers a simple, reliable, and safe method for catheter closure of patent foramen ovale in patients with presumed paradoxical embolism. Currently, no randomized prospective data comparing PFO closure with other therapeutic strategies (e.g., oral anticoagulation, aspirin) are available. It is, however, unlikely that such studies will be completed in the very near future. Until then, all patients undergoing PFO device closure should be monitored prospectively for an unlimited period of time.

ACKNOWLEDGMENT

The authors would like to thank all colleagues and staff members who participated in the interventions and data acquisition: Ingo Esch, Frankfurt, Elisabeth Zadan, Frankfurt, Wolfgang Scholz M.D., Bad Oeynhausen, Klaus Regnen M.D., Dresden, Martin Braun M.D., Heidelberg, and Ralph Grabitz M.D., Ph.D. (Kiel), who performed the animal experiments at the Technical University of Aachen, Germany.

ADDENDUM

Since completion of the manuscript, more than 1,200 patients have been treated with this device. More data has been published by Braun and coworkers (7).

REFERENCES

1. Schräder R, Keppeler P, Rux S, et al. Verschluß des offenen Foramen ovale mit einer neuentwickelten Doppelschirmprothese aus Ivalon und Nitinol (Abstract). *Z Kardiol* 1999;88(Suppl 1):1027.
2. Porstmann W, Wierny L, Warnke H. Der Verschluß des ductus arteriosus persistens ohne Thorakotomie (vorläufige Mitteilung). *Thoraxchirurgie* 1967;15:199–203.
3. Grabitz RG, Schräder R, Sigler M, et al. Retrievable PDA plug for interventional, transvenous occlusion of the patent ductus arteriosus: evaluation in lambs and preliminary clinical results. *Invest Radiol* 1997;32:523–528.
4. Schräder R, Hofstetter R, Faßbender D, et al. Transvenous closure of patent ductus arteriosus with Ivalon plugs: multicenter experience with a new technique. *Invest Radiol* 1999;34:65–70.
5. Wierny L, Plass R, Porstmann W. Transluminal closure of patent ductus arteriosus: long-term results of 208 cases treated without thoracotomy. *Cardiovasc Interv Radiol* 1986;9:279–285.
6. Schräder R. Transcatheter versus surgical closure of patent ductus arteriosus (letter). *N Engl J Med* 1994;330:1014–1015.
7. Braun MU, Fassbender D, Schoen SP, et al. Transcatheter closure of patent foramen ovale in patients with cerebral ischemia. *J Am Coll Cardiol* 2002;39:2019–2025.

PERCUTANEOUS CLOSURE OF PATENT FORAMEN OVALE IN PATIENTS WITH PRESUMED PARADOXICAL EMBOLISM

STEPHAN WINDECKER
BERNHARD MEIER

Recent studies (1,2) indicate that paradoxical embolism through a patent foramen ovale (PFO) may be responsible for unexplained cerebrovascular accidents (CVAs) and transient ischemic attacks (TIAs) in young adults. Long-term anticoagulation, surgical closure, and more recently, transcatheter occlusion (3,4) of the PFO are available treatment options at the present time. This chapter discusses management of such patients with an emphasis on the role of transcatheter occlusion.

PATENT FORAMEN OVALE

Atrial septation involves two overlapping embryologic structures, the right-sided muscular septum secundum and the left-sided fibrous septum primum. The latter grows from the common atrial roof toward the atrioventricular cushions, and apoptosis creates an opening, the ostium secundum. The foramen ovale is an opening in the septum secundum located inferoposteriorly and somewhat offset from the more superior and forward position of the ostium secundum. Together, the foramen ovale and ostium secundum form a one-way channel with the septum primum serving as a flap-valve, allowing for physiologic right-to-left shunting during intrauterine development (Figure 13.1A). The postnatal establishment of the pulmonary circulation with subsequent increase in left atrial pressure result in functional closure of the foramen ovale by apposition of the septum primum against the septum secundum, followed by anatomic closure in the ensuing months (Figure 13.1B).

Autopsy series revealed that a patent foramen ovale (PFO) persists in 20% to 34% of adults with a declining incidence in older age groups, without a gender preference. PFO sizes range from minute to large (mean size, 4.9 mm) (Figure 13.1C) (5). Atrial septal aneurysms (ASA) are amuscular, redundant membranes involving the fossa ovalis or the entire atrial septum. They may be present as an isolated abnormality and are associated with a PFO in approximately 60% of adults (6,7). The prevalence of ASA based on transesophageal screening in a population-based study is approximately 2% (7). Echocardiographic criteria for the ASA are variable but usually require (a) a diameter of the base of the aneurysm >15 mm, and either (b) protrusion of the aneurysmal membrane >10 to 15 mm beyond the plane of the atrial septum or (c) phasic excursion of the aneurysmal membrane >10 to 15 mm in total amplitude during the cardiorespiratory cycle (6–8).

Atrial septal dysmorphogenesis, evident as increased frequency of PFO and ASA, has recently been correlated with heterozygous mutations of the cardiac homeodomain transcription factor *NKX2-5* in mice. This observation provides evidence that the incidence of PFO is a function of genetic factors and that the PFO might be an index of septal dysmorphogenesis encompassing other defects such as ASA, atrial septal defects, and so on (9).

A PFO cannot be detected on clinical grounds, but requires either invasive right heart catheterization with catheter passage of the defect or noninvasive imaging modalities (i.e., transthoracic or transesophageal echocardiography) (10,11). An indirect proof of a PFO can be derived with transcranial Doppler ultrasound (12,13). Multiplane transesophageal contrast echocardiography with Valsalva maneuver is clearly the most sensitive and specific method for noninvasive detection of a PFO. It allows for sizing of the separation between septum primum and secundum, enables the definition of anatomic boundaries, and allows the demonstration of a right-to-

Stephan Windecker: Director, Invasive Cardiology, Swiss Cardiovascular Center Bern, University Hospital, Bern, Switzerland

Bernhard Meier: Professor and Chairman, Cardiovascular Department, Swiss Cardiovascular Center Bern, University Hospital, Bern, Switzerland

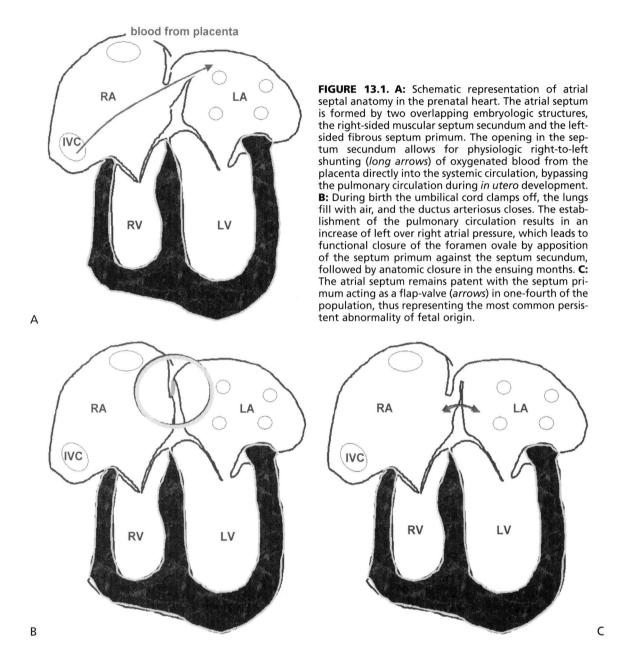

FIGURE 13.1. A: Schematic representation of atrial septal anatomy in the prenatal heart. The atrial septum is formed by two overlapping embryologic structures, the right-sided muscular septum secundum and the left-sided fibrous septum primum. The opening in the septum secundum allows for physiologic right-to-left shunting (*long arrows*) of oxygenated blood from the placenta directly into the systemic circulation, bypassing the pulmonary circulation during *in utero* development. **B:** During birth the umbilical cord clamps off, the lungs fill with air, and the ductus arteriosus closes. The establishment of the pulmonary circulation results in an increase of left over right atrial pressure, which leads to functional closure of the foramen ovale by apposition of the septum primum against the septum secundum, followed by anatomic closure in the ensuing months. **C:** The atrial septum remains patent with the septum primum acting as a flap-valve (*arrows*) in one-fourth of the population, thus representing the most common persistent abnormality of fetal origin.

left shunt by color flow mapping. The shunt may be semi-quantitatively assessed by the number of bubbles crossing from the right to the left atrium after intravenous injection of agitated saline (1). PFO has been increasingly recognized as a potential mediator of disease manifestations such as (a) paradoxical embolism (14), (b) neurologic decompression illness in divers (15,16), (c) refractory hypoxemia due to right-to-left shunt in patients with right ventricular infarction (17) or severe pulmonary disease, and (d) orthostatic desaturation in the setting of the platypnea-orthodeoxia syndrome (18,19), and (e) migraine headaches with aura (20).

PARADOXICAL EMBOLISM

Since the initial description of stroke in a young woman with a PFO by Cohnheim in 1877 (21), the clinical facets of paradoxical embolism encompassing emboli of thrombus (22,23), air, or fat (24) have been well documented. Recently, the PFO was identified as an independent risk factor for mortality (odds ratio of 11) and a complicated in-hospital course (odds ratio, 5.2) in patients with major pulmonary embolism (25). The combination of PFO with stroke of undetermined cause (commonly referred to as cryptogenic) pertains to up to 40% of young stroke patients and has attracted much attention. The mechanism for right-to-left shunting via PFO in patients with paradoxical embolism, right ventricular infarction, or severe pulmonary disease is related to a transient (phase after Valsalva maneuver—for example, during coughing or defecation) or permanent pressure gradient (decreased right ventricular compliance following right ventricular infarction or increased pulmonary artery pressure in case of severe pulmonary disease).

Several case control studies using contrast echocardiography (1,2,11,26,27) established a strong association between the diagnosis of cryptogenic stroke and the presence of PFO in young adults less than 55 years of age, and identified PFO as an independent risk factor for cryptogenic stroke (28). Overell and colleagues (29) recently summarized the currently available evidence in a metaanalysis of case control studies and confirmed a significant association between ischemic stroke and PFO. In patients younger than 55 years, the PFO conferred a relative risk of 3 (95% CI 2 to 4) comparing ischemic stroke with nonstroke control subjects, and a relative risk of 6 (95% CI 4 to 10) comparing cryptogenic stroke with known stroke cause control subjects. In contrast, the association between PFO and ischemic stroke is less well defined for people more than 55 years of age and will require further study. Patients with PFO and cryptogenic stroke also appear to be at risk for recurrent cerebrovascular events, with a yearly stroke rate of 1.2% to 1.9%, and recurrent stroke or transient ischemic attack (TIA) rate of 3.4% to 3.8% (30,31).

Certain morphologic characteristics of PFO as identified by echocardiography appear to predispose patients for paradoxical embolism. Both larger PFO size and a greater degree of right-to-left shunt as assessed by crossing microbubbles (32) signify a higher risk for suffering paradoxical embolism in the presence of PFO. Patients with an atrial septal aneurysm of more than 10 mm excursion appear to be at particularly high risk for thromboembolic complications (6). Thus the relative risk to suffer a thromboembolic event was fourfold higher in patients with PFO and 33 times higher in patients with both PFO and atrial septal aneurysm as compared with controls (26). Similarly, the combination of PFO with an atrial septal aneurysm (ASA) constituted a particularly high-risk situation, with a relative risk of 16 (95% CI 3 to 86) when comparing ischemic stroke with nonstroke control subjects and a relative risk of 17 (95% CI 2 to 134) when comparing cryptogenic stroke with known stroke cause control subjects (age less than 55 years) in the metaanalysis by Overell et al. (29).

Despite a growing body of evidence the diagnosis of paradoxical embolism remains presumptive in the majority of cases, since direct confirmation of a thrombus caught in the PFO is only rarely available. The diagnosis of paradoxical embolism should therefore be entertained in patients with ischemic stroke or systemic embolism in the absence of (a) a left-sided thromboembolic source, (b) the potential for right-to-left shunt, and (c) the detection of thrombus in the venous system or right heart chambers (25). The third criterion is optional, as the thrombi are frequently small and are difficult to document.

TECHNIQUE OF PERCUTANEOUS CLOSURE OF PATENT FORAMEN OVALE

Bridges and colleagues first reported percutaneous PFO closure in a sizeable cohort of patients (3). Table 13.1 summarizes a variety of devices suitable for percutaneous PFO closure. The common construction principle of most devices consists of a double-umbrella design of various sizes closing the PFO by passive countertension against the atrial septal wall. The following description of the implantation procedure is limited to the steps common to most devices. The procedure is performed by transfemoral venous access under local anesthesia. In contrast to percutaneous atrial septal defect closure, transesophageal monitoring is not routinely employed during device implantation. Similarly, measurements of the balloon-stretched diameter are optional, since they only rarely aid in device and size selection. Following administration of 5,000 IU systemic heparin, the PFO is crossed with a 6F (1F = 0.3 mm) Multipurpose catheter under fluoroscopic guidance in the anteroposterior (AP) view. This catheter is exchanged with a device-specific transseptal sheath measuring 8 to 12F. Air in the delivery system is avoided by four measures. First, the dilator of the transseptal sheath is pulled back, while the guidewire remains in the left atrium or a pulmonary vein. This avoids blockage of the end hole and allows the blood to follow the receding dilator. Blood thereby fills the void rather than air sucked in from the outside. Second, the sheath is flushed carefully if necessary while the patient performs a Valsalva maneuver to increase left atrial pressure. Third, the device is introduced into a device-specific loader under water. Fourth, the loader is connected to the transseptal sheath with the device peeking out a few millimeters, while the patient performs a Valsalva maneuver.

The constrained device is then introduced into the transseptal sheath and advanced to the tip of the catheter. First, the left atrial disk of the double umbrella is deployed and gently pulled back against the atrial septum. This and the following maneuvers are best performed under fluoroscopic guidance in a left anterior oblique (LAO) projection with some cranial angulation. To deploy the right atrial disk, tension is maintained on the delivery system, while the delivery sheath is further withdrawn. After a further Valsalva maneuver to produce back bleeding out of the sheath, a right atrial contrast angiography by a hand injection through the side arm of the delivery sheath serves to delineate the atrial septum. Upon verification of a correct position, the device is released from the delivery system. The transseptal sheath is used for a final contrast medium injection. The contrast is followed to also delineate the left

TABLE 13.1. CURRENTLY AVAILABLE PERCUTANEOUS PFO CLOSURE DEVICES

	Amplatzer PFO Occluder	STARFlex Septal Occluder	PFO STAR	Sideris Buttoned Occluder	Helex Septal Occluder
Manufacturer	AGA Medical Corporation	Nitinol Medical Technologies, Inc.	Applied Biometrics, Inc.	Custom Medical Devices	W. L. Gore & Associates, Inc.
Design	Two self-expandable, round, Nitinol disks interconnected by a thin, flexible waist	Double umbrella with eight flexible metal arms covered with Dacron patches connected by a single post	Two square components with four-arm, stainless steel wire cross covered with Dacron patches	Two square components with wire skeleton and polyurethane cover, a counter occluder, and a button loop occluder	Two opposing disks formed by a single Nitinol wire with a patch of polytetra fluoroethylene
PFO dedicated	Yes	No	Yes	No	No
Centering	Noncentering	Self-centering with help of microsprings	Noncentering	Noncentering	Noncentering
Fixation	Passive countertension	Passive countertension	Passive countertension	Sutured counterbutton	Passive and active with locking mechanism
Device size	Right atrial disk 18, 25, 35 mm	23, 33, 40 mm	Umbrella size 22, 26, 30 mm	Umbrella size 15–50 mm	Diameter 15, 20, 25 mm
Delivery Sheath	8–9F	10–11F	10–13F	11–13F	9F
Advantages	Fully retrievable Fully repositionable Easy delivery		Small-profile device	Inexpensive	Small profile Fully retrievable Fully repositionable Retention suture
Disadvantages	Bulky right atrial disk	Not easily repositionable	Not easily repositionable High incidence of air embolism mediated through sheath	Complex multistep implantation procedure Not easily repositionable Spontaneous unbuttoning with device embolization	Potential for wire fracture

The ASDOS and DAS (Angel-Wings Occluder) are no longer available for percutaneous transseptal occlusion procedures.

atrial contour and disk placement (Figure 13.2). Finally, the sheath is removed and hemostasis is achieved by manual compression. Patients may be ambulated within 1 hour of the procedure and discharged the same day.

Occlusion of the PFO is at first by passive countertension of the double umbrella against the atrial septum, which keeps the flap-valve shut. In the days to weeks after implantation, endothelialization will result in complete overgrowth of the device and finally active PFO occlusion. Data derived from animal models suggest that partial endothelial overgrowth occurs at 1 month, and complete endothelialization is present after 3 months, as evidenced by a layer of neoendothelial cells

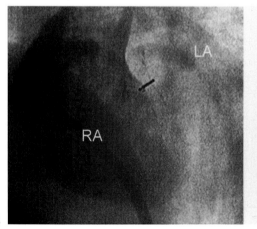
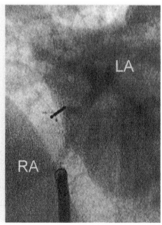

FIGURE 13.2. A: PFO-Star Occluder positioned in a PFO after release from the delivery cable. Right atrial contrast angiography through the transseptal sheath delineates the right-sided atrial septum and confirms correct device position. A short, rigid pin connects the two umbrellas. **B:** The left atrium is opacified during the levophase of right atrial angiography, delineating left-sided atrial septal wall. LA, left atrium; RA, right atrium.

A,B

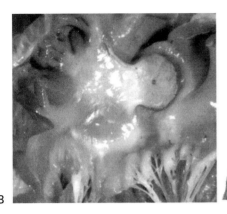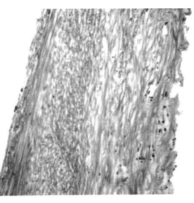

A,B

FIGURE 13.3. A: Postmortem cardiac specimen harvested from a minipig 3 months after implantation of an Amplatzer PFO Occluder revealing complete coverage of the device with neoendocardium. **B:** Microscopic view (160 × magnification) of specimen in (**A**) revealing coverage of both sides of the device with intact neoendocardium. (Both figures were obtained from Han YM, Gu X, Titus JL, et al. New self-expanding patent foramen ovale occlusion device. *Catheter Cardiovasc Interv* 1999; 47:370–376, with permission of Wiley-Liss Publishing Company, New York.) (See Color Figure 13.3.)

continuous with the adjacent atrial septum using scanning electron microscopy (Figure 13.3) (33,34).

Atrial septal aneurysms associated with PFO can also safely be treated percutaneously. It appears that the device not only abolishes the right-to-left shunt, but also immobilizes the previously redundant and mobile septum to some extent. It is our recommendation to choose a larger device size under these circumstances.

CLINICAL RESULTS OF PERCUTANEOUS CLOSURE OF PATENT FORAMEN OVALE

The suggestion that the PFO is a mediator of paradoxical embolism prompted the quest for a therapeutic and preventive strategy in affected patients. There are currently three therapeutic avenues comprising treatment with antiplatelet (aspirin, clopidogrel) or antithrombotic (warfarin) drugs, surgical, or percutaneous PFO closure. To date, no therapy has been evaluated conclusively in this patient population.

Our own experience has been extended to 180 patients implanted with six different atrial septal occluding devices over a 7-year period (35). The procedure was successful in 178 (98%) patients and failed in two. There were a total of ten (6%) periprocedural complications without mortality or long-term sequelae. The underlying mechanisms for the encountered complications were mainly embolization of the device or parts of it, and air embolism during device delivery. Complete closure as assessed by transesophageal contrast echocardiography was achieved in 144 (80%) patients (Figure 13.4). During a mean follow-up period of 1.5 ± 1.6 years (range, 0.1 to 6.5 years; 270 patient-years), 11 recurrent embolic events were encountered in 178

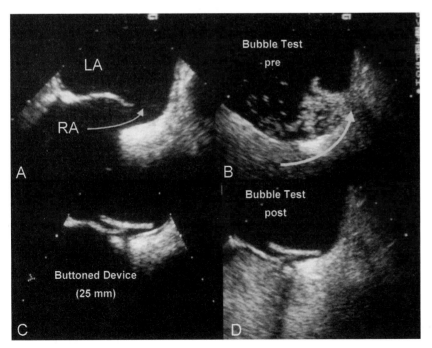

FIGURE 13.4. Contrast transesophageal echocardiography. **A:** Still frame of widely patent foramen ovale prior to percutaneous PFO closure. **B:** Following injection of agitated normal saline into the right antecubital vein, complete opacification of the right atrium with direct transfer of contrast bubbles via PFO into the left atrium. **C:** Still frame of interatrial septum after implantation of a 25-mm Sideris buttoned device. **D:** Following injection of agitated normal saline into the right antecubital vein, there is complete opacification of the right atrium without evidence of a residual right-to-left shunt. LA, left atrium; RA, right atrium.

patients with an implanted device. These comprised one minor ischemic stroke, eight TIAs, and two peripheral emboli. The actuarial freedom from the combined endpoint of recurrent transient ischemic attack, ischemic stroke (CVA), and peripheral embolism was 95% at 1 year, 89% at 2 years, and 89% at 6 years (Figure 13.5). The presence of a postprocedural shunt was a predictor of recurrent thromboembolic events (RR 3.5; 95% CI 1.1 to 11.4; *p* = .04). This not only emphasizes the importance of achieving complete PFO closure, but also suggests that PFO is indeed the mediator of paradoxical embolism in this patient population. In contrast, older age (≥55 years), gender, type and number of prior embolic events, and cardiovascular risk factors did not adversely affect outcome after percutaneous PFO closure. Similarly, the prognosis of patients with PFO and associated ASA was comparable with that without ASA after percutaneous PFO closure, suggesting that this high-risk population may derive a particularly high protective effect from percutaneous PFO closure. Of note, cryptogenic stroke does not imply paradoxical embolism as the sole pathophysiologic mechanism in all patients. Cryptogenic stroke and PFO may coexist independently without causal relation, and in those patients, PFO closure will not reduce the risk of recurrence. This explains the small recurrence rate despite successful PFO closure in our and other series, in addition to the possibility of emboli from the left atrial disc.

Areas of concern have surrounded device-related complications inflicted by large delivery systems, device dislodgment and embolization, structural failure and long-term durability, thrombus formation, inability to reposition or remove the devices, and residual shunts following percutaneous PFO closure. These problems led to the development of newer-generation devices specifically designed for PFO closure as opposed to atrial septal occlusion devices with easier device release, lower embolization potential, and

improved closure mechanism. They have been available for clinical use for 2 years only, and they considerably improved the safety of the procedure and allowed complete closure rates in more than 95% of patients.

OTHER TREATMENT MODALITIES

The risk of recurrent neurologic events during medical treatment with either aspirin (dose, 250 to 500 mg/day) or oral anticoagulation (target INR, 2 to 3) was retrospectively examined in 132 patients with PFO and cryptogenic stroke less than 60 years of age by Mas and colleagues (30). The average annual rate of recurrence was 3.4% for the combined endpoint of TIA and CVA, and 1.2% for CVAs. Patients with both PFO and ASA had an average annual rate of recurrent stroke of 4.4% and were identified as a high-risk group. In the Lausanne Stroke Registry (31), 92 patients with PFO and cryptogenic stroke were treated with aspirin (dosage, 250 to 500 mg daily), and 37 patients were treated with oral anticoagulation (target INR, 2 to 3). The average annual recurrence rate was 3.8% for the combined endpoint of TIA and CVA, and 1.9% for CVA during a follow-up period of 3 years with no significant difference between the two antithrombotic drug regimens. A multicenter study funded by the NIH (PICCS trial) currently investigates the effect of medical treatment on stroke recurrence in such patients by randomly assigning patients to either aspirin or anticoagulant therapy.

Surgical PFO closure was reported by Homma and colleagues in 28 patients with presumed paradoxical embolism (36). Complications consisted of the postpericardiotomy syndrome in five patients (18%) and transient atrial fibrillation in one patient (4%) after the open thoracotomy procedure. One recurrent ischemic stroke and three recurrent TIAs were encountered during clinical follow-up, amounting to an actuarial recurrence rate of 20% at 13 months. In contrast, Ruchat and colleagues (37) observed only one perioperative TIA with no further recurrent embolic events during a mean follow-up of 3 years in 32 patients. Of note, a residual shunt as assessed by transesophageal echocardiography was noted in three patients (9%) after surgery. The largest experience of surgical PFO closure has been reported from the Mayo Clinic (38), where 91 consecutive patients with at least one prior cerebrovascular ischemic event underwent direct suture or patch closure. Complete closure of the defect was documented during intraoperative transesophageal echocardiography in all but one patient. There was no operative mortality, but the morbidity rate was 21%; it consisted of atrial fibrillation in 12%, pericardial drainage for effusion in 4%, exploration for bleeding in 3%, and superficial wound infection in 1% of patients. During follow-up the actuarial freedom from recurrent cerebral events was 93% at 1 year and 83% at 4 years.

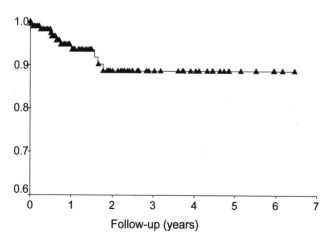

FIGURE 13.5. Actuarial freedom from the combined endpoint of recurrent transient ischemic attacks (TIA), stroke (CVA), and peripheral embolism during follow-up up to 6.5 years.

CONCLUSION

While percutaneous transseptal PFO closure has been shown to be feasible, one must ask whether it should be done. This is the case because (a) the diagnosis of paradoxical embolism is usually presumed and not proved, (b) the risk for stroke recurrence and therefore the benefit of preventive measures is poorly defined, and (c) the outcome of percutaneous PFO closure as compared with medical treatment and surgical PFO closure is unknown (39). Medical treatment with antiplatelet or antithrombotic therapy is simple, ubiquitously available, and relatively cheap. However, with anticoagulant therapy there is a small but definite risk of life-threatening bleeding complications, with an annual rate of intracranial hemorrhage of 0.5% with coumadin (40,41), important drug interactions, a lifelong commitment to therapy at least theoretically, and the need for surveillance of anticoagulation unless platelet inhibitors are selected. Surgical PFO closure is permanent and effective but quite invasive and costly, with inherent periprocedural complications. Percutaneous PFO closure is less invasive than surgery and can be performed with a high success rate (>95%) and low morbidity in patients with presumed paradoxical embolism. Important concerns remain and include thrombus formation on the device surface, embolization of the device, late infections, and arrhythmias. Material fatigue, on the other hand, is hardly an issue, as the device has no mechanical function except for the first few days.

The best therapeutic modality remains unknown at this time. To answer this question, two randomized trials compare medical treatment with antiplatelet or antithrombotic medication against percutaneous PFO closure in patients with paradoxical embolism. (*PC*-trial = *P*atent foramen ovale and *C*ryptogenic embolism. Principal investigator: Bernhard Meier, MD, and Heinrich Mattle, MD, Cardiology and Neurology, University Hospital, Bern, Switzerland. Multicenter, international, randomized study; *PEPSIS*-trial = Paradoxical Embolism Prevention Study in Ischemic Stroke. Principal investigator: Felix Berger, MD, German Heart Center, Berlin, and Ludger Rosin, MD, Neurology, University Hospital Regensburg, Germany. Multicenter, randomized study in Germany.) Until results from these trials become available, the implantation of PFO occlusion devices will remain feasible but should be considered investigational and performed only in appropriately selected and fully informed patients.

REFERENCES

1. Webster MW, Chancellor AM, Smith HJ, et al. Patent foramen ovale in young stroke patients. *Lancet* 1988;2:11–12.
2. Lechat P, Mas JL, Lascault G, et al. Prevalence of patent foramen ovale in patients with stroke. *N Engl J Med* 1988;318:1148–1152.
3. Bridges ND, Hellenbrand W, Latson L, et al. Transcatheter closure of patent foramen ovale after presumed paradoxical embolism. *Circulation* 1992;86:1902–1908.
4. Ende DJ, Chopra PS, Rao PS. Prevention of recurrence of paradoxic embolism: mid-term follow-up after transcatheter closure of atrial defects with buttoned device. *Am J Cardiol* 1996;78:233–236.
5. Hagen PT, Scholz DG, Edwards WD. Incidence and size of patent foramen ovale during the first 10 decades of life: an autopsy study of 965 normal hearts. *Mayo Clin Proc* 1984;59:17–20.
6. Mugge A, Daniel WG, Angermann C, et al. Atrial septal aneurysm in adult patients: a multicenter study using transthoracic and transesophageal echocardiography. *Circulation* 1995;91:2785–2792.
7. Agmon Y, Khandheira BK, Meissner I, et al. Frequency of atrial septal aneurysms in patients with cerebral ischemic events. *Circulation* 1999;99:1942–1944.
8. Hanley PC, Tajik AJ, Hynes JK, et al. Diagnosis and classification of atrial septal aneurysm by two-dimensional echocardiography: report of 80 consecutive cases. *J Am Coll Cardiol* 1985;6:1370–1382.
9. Biben C, Weber R, Kesteven S, et al. Cardiac septal and valvular dysmorphogenesis in mice heterozygous for mutations in the homeobox gene Nkx2-5. *Circ Res* 2000;87:888–895.
10. Di Tullio M, Sacco RL, Venketasubramanian N, et al. Comparison of diagnostic techniques for the detection of a patent foramen ovale in stroke patients. *Stroke* 1993;24:1020–1024.
11. Hausmann D, Mugge A, Becht I, et al. Diagnosis of patent foramen ovale by transesophageal echocardiography and association with cerebral and peripheral embolic events. *Am J Cardiol* 1992;70:668–672.
12. Klotzsch C, Janssen G, Berlit P. Transesophageal echocardiography and contrast-TCD in the detection of a patent foramen ovale: experiences with 111 patients. *Neurology* 1994;44:1603–1606.
13. Di Tullio M, Sacco RL, Massaro A, et al. Transcranial Doppler with contrast injection for the detection of patent foramen ovale in stroke patients. *Int J Card Imaging* 1993;9:1–5.
14. Thompson T, Evans W. Paradoxical embolism. *Quart J Med* 1930;23:135–150.
15. Germonpre P, Dendale P, Unger P, et al. Patent foramen ovale and decompression sickness in sports divers. *J Appl Physiol* 1998;84:1622–1626.
16. Schwerzmann M, Seiler C, Lipp E, et al. Relation between directly detected patent foramen ovale and ischemic brain lesions in sport divers. *Ann Intern Med* 2001;134:21–24.
17. Silver MT, Lieberman EH, Thibault GE. Refractory hypoxemia in inferior myocardial infarction from right-to-left shunting through a patent foramen ovale: a case report and review of the literature. *Clin Cardiol* 1994;17:627–630.
18. Seward JB, Hayes DL, Smith HC, et al. Platypnea-orthodeoxia: clinical profile, diagnostic workup, management, and report of seven cases. *Mayo Clin Proc* 1984;59:221–231.
19. Windecker S, Meier B. Interventional PFO closure: what we see is but the tip of the iceberg. *Catheter Cardiovasc Interv* 2000;50:199–201.
20. Wilmshurst PT, Nightingale S, Walsh KP, et al. Effect on migraine of closure of cardiac right-to-left shunts to prevent recurrence of decompression illness or stroke or for haemodynamic reasons. *Lancet* 2000;356:1648–1651.
21. Cohnheim J. Thrombose und Embolie: Vorlesung über allgemeine Pathologie. In: Handbuch für Aerzte studierende, Berlin, Hirschwald, vol 1, 1877;134:144–145.
22. Caes FL, Van Belleghem YV, Missault LH, et al. Surgical treatment of impending paradoxical embolism through patent foramen ovale. *Ann Thorac Surg* 1995;59:1559–1561.
23. Falk V, Walther T, Krankenberg H, et al. Trapped thrombus in a patent foramen ovale. *Thorac Cardiovasc Surg* 1997;45:90–92.

24. Pell AC, Hughes D, Keating J, et al. Brief report: fulminating fat embolism syndrome caused by paradoxical embolism through a patent foramen ovale. *N Engl J Med* 1993;329:926–929.

25. Konstantinides S, Geibel A, Kasper W, et al. Patent foramen ovale is an important predictor of adverse outcome in patients with major pulmonary embolism. *Circulation* 1998;97:1946–1951.

26. Cabanes L, Mas JL, Cohen A, et al. Atrial septal aneurysm and patent foramen ovale as risk factors for cryptogenic stroke in patients less than 55 years of age. A study using transesophageal echocardiography. *Stroke* 1993;24:1865–1873.

27. De Belder MA, Tourikis L, Leech G, et al. Risk of patent foramen ovale for thromboembolic events in all age groups. *Am J Cardiol* 1992;69:1316–1320.

28. Di Tullio M, Sacco RL, Gopal A, et al. Patent foramen ovale as a risk factor for cryptogenic stroke. *Ann Intern Med* 1992;117:461–465.

29. Overell JR, Bone I, Lees KR. Interatrial septal abnormalities and stroke: a meta-analysis of case-control studies. *Neurology* 2000;55:1172–1179.

30. Mas JL, Zuber M. Recurrent cerebrovascular events in patients with patent foramen ovale, atrial septal aneurysm, or both and cryptogenic stroke or transient ischemic attack. French Study Group on Patent Foramen Ovale and Atrial Septal Aneurysm. *Am Heart J* 1995;130:1083–1088.

31. Bogousslavsky J, Garazi S, Jeanrenaud X, et al. Stroke recurrence in patients with patent foramen ovale: the Lausanne Study. Lausanne Stroke with Paradoxal Embolism Study Group. *Neurology* 1996;46:1301–1305.

32. Homma S, Di Tullio MR, Sacco RL, et al. Characteristics of patent foramen ovale associated with cryptogenic stroke: a biplane transesophageal echocardiographic study. *Stroke* 1994;25:582–586.

33. Han YM, Gu X, Titus JL, et al. New self-expanding patent foramen ovale occlusion device. *Catheter Cardiovasc Interv* 1999;47:370–376.

34. Sharafuddin MJ, Gu X, Titus JL, et al. Transvenous closure of secundum atrial septal defects: preliminary results with a new self-expanding nitinol prosthesis in a swine model. *Circulation* 1997;95:2162–2168.

35. Windecker S, Wahl A, Chatterjee T, et al. Percutaneous closure of patent foramen ovale in patients with paradoxical embolism: long-term risk of recurrent thromboembolic events. *Circulation* 2000;101:893–898.

36. Homma S, Di Tullio MR, Sacco RL, et al. Surgical closure of patent foramen ovale in cryptogenic stroke patients. *Stroke* 1997;28:2376–2381.

37. Ruchat P, Bogousslavsky J, Hurni M, et al. Systematic surgical closure of patent foramen ovale in selected patients with cerebrovascular events due to paradoxical embolism: early results of a preliminary study. *Eur J Cardiothorac Surg* 1997;11:824–827.

38. Dearani JA, Ugurlu BS, Danielson GK, et al. Surgical patent foramen ovale closure for prevention of paradoxical embolism-related cerebrovascular ischemic events. *Circulation* 1999;100(Suppl):II-171–175.

39. Windecker S, Meier B. Percutaneous patent foramen ovale (PFO) closure: it can be done but should it? *Catheter Cardiovasc Interv* 1999;47:377–380.

40. Hirsh J. Oral anticoagulant drugs. *N Engl J Med* 1991;324:1865–1875.

41. Hirsh J, Fuster V. Guide to anticoagulant therapy. Part 2: Oral anticoagulants. *Circulation* 1994;89:1469–1480.

TRANSCATHETER CLOSURE OF ATRIAL SEPTAL DEFECTS WITH RIGHT-TO-LEFT SHUNTS

P. SYAMASUNDAR RAO

Naturally occurring atrial defects (1) or intentionally created fenestrations (2,3) in patients with operated congenital heart defects may cause right-to-left shunt with resultant arterial hypoxemia and consequent polycythemia (4). These atrial defects are also the sites of paradoxical embolism (5,6). Whereas some of these defects may close spontaneously (7), others do not; these result in hypoxemia and pose potential risk for paradoxical embolism, including cerebrovascular accidents. For these reasons, these defects should generally be closed. With the availability of a number of atrial septal defect occluding devices, nonsurgical, transcatheter occlusion appears to be preferred by most cardiologists. This chapter addresses issues related to transcatheter occlusion of such atrial defects.

DEVICES

A number of atrial septal defect occluding devices, currently in clinical trials, as described in Chapter 1, may be useful in occluding atrial septal defects/patent foramina ovale/fenestrations, hereafter referred to as atrial defects (ADs) in this chapter. The use of the clamshell device (USCI Division, CR Bard, Inc., Bellerica, MA) (2,8,9), modified Rashkind's PDA umbrella (USCI Division, CR Bard, Inc., Bellerica, MA) (10), Gianturco coil (Cook, Inc., Bloomington, IN) (7), inverted buttoned device (Custom Medical Devices, Amarillo, TX; Athens, Greece) (1), Amplatzer (AGA Medical Corp., Golden Valley, MN) (11,12), and CardioSEAL (Nitinol Medical Technologies, Inc., Boston, MA) (13) to occlude these ADs has been described.

The clamshell device and Rashkind PDA occluder are no longer in use. The Gianturco coils (Chapter 20), Amplatzer Septal Occluder (Chapter 6), and CardioSEAL (Chapter 7) have been reviewed elsewhere in this book and will not be described here. The inverted buttoned device has not been described in this book and will be briefly reviewed. The regular buttoned device (Chapter 3) consists of a square-shaped occluder for implantation onto the left atrial side of the atrial septum and a rhomboid-shaped, single-strand, counteroccluder that goes onto the right atrial side of the septum and is useful in occluding secundum atrial septal defects (14,15). In patients with right-to-left shunts, however, the device was not effective (16) and therefore its components were reversed or inverted (1,16). In the inverted device (Figure 14.1), the counteroccluder is made up of a single wire covered with a rhomboid-shaped polyurethane foam and goes onto the left atrial side. An 8-mm string loop is attached to its center and has two radiopaque knots (buttons), 4 and 8 mm from the counteroccluder. The occluder, made up of an x-shaped wire skeleton covered with 0.0625-inch polyurethane foam goes onto the right atrial side. A latex piece is sewn to its center and becomes a buttonhole. Hybrid devices can also be utilized; that is, a regular fourth-generation (15) or COD (Chapter 3) occluder on the left atrial side and a square-shaped counteroccluder (1) on the right atrial side.

PROTOCOL

Since none of the devices, at the time of this writing, are approved for general clinical use in the United States, the procedures are generally performed as a part of FDA-approved clinical trials with IDE (investigational device exemption) and IRB (institutional review board) approval. Some devices may be available for use under HDE (humanitarian device exemption). Outside the United States the devices are more readily available and may require IRB approval. The Gianturco coils, however, have been used on

P. **Syamasundar Rao:** Professor of Pediatrics, Medicine, and Cardiology, Department of Pediatrics, University of Texas-Houston Medical School; Director, Division of Pediatric Cardiology, Memorial Hermann Children's Hospital, Houston, Texas

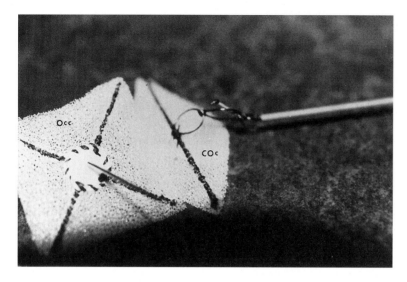

FIGURE 14.1. Photograph of inverted buttoned device. The counteroccluder (COc) is made up of rhomboid-shaped, 0.0625-inch, polyurethane foam mounted on a single, Teflon-coated wire skeleton for implantation onto left side of the atrial septum. An 8-mm string loop is attached to the center of the counteroccluder; it has two radiopaque spring buttons, 4 and 8 mm from the counteroccluder. The occluder (Occ) is made up of an x-shaped Teflon-coated wire skeleton covered with 0.0625-inch polyurethane foam. A rubber piece is sutured into the center of the occluder and becomes a buttonhole.

an off-label basis. Informed consent is, of course, required for use of any device.

PATIENT SELECTION

Two groups of patients are candidates for closure of ADs. The first group of patients is composed of those who had their congenital heart defects treated with either surgical or transcatheter therapy. Typical examples in this group are pulmonary atresia or critical pulmonary stenosis with intact ventricular septum and surgically repaired tetralogy of Fallot, all with residual interatrial communication with right-to-left shunt. The second group consists of patients who had Fontan operation for single-ventricle physiology, such as tricuspid atresia, double inlet left ventricle or hypoplastic left heart syndrome with an intentional fenestration created at the time of Fontan, or residual atrial septal defect, all with right-to-left shunt.

The indications for closure in both groups are a systemic arterial oxygen saturation ≤ 90% or a prior cerebrovascular accident or transient ischemic attack due to paradoxic embolism. Progressive polycythemia secondary to hypoxemia related to right-to-left shunt is also an indication for closure.

Ideally, test occlusion with a balloon catheter should be performed before device closure (1,17,18). Balloon occlusion should be performed under echocardiographic control (Figures 14.2 and 14.3) to ensure that the shunt is abolished (Figure 14.3d). Increase in arterial oxygen saturation can be demonstrated if the AD is completely occluded. A significant fall in cardiac index and systemic oxygen delivery or an increase in right atrial pressure and heart rate

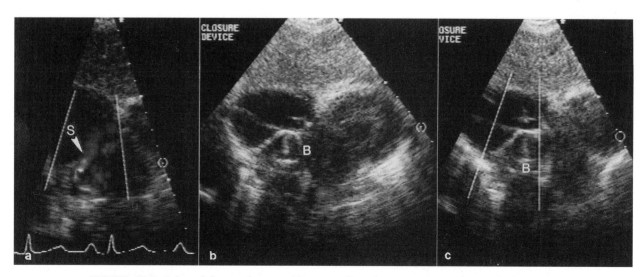

FIGURE 14.2. Selected frames from a video recording demonstrating right-to-left shunt (S) across the atrial defect (**a**). Following occlusion with a balloon (B) (**b**), the shunt is completely abolished (**c**).

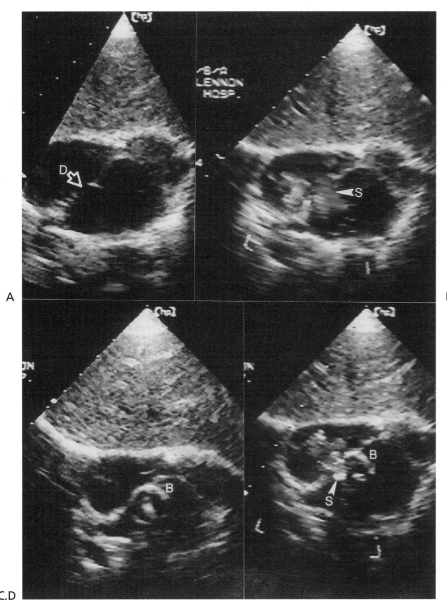

FIGURE 14.3. Selected video frames demonstrating (**A**) the atrial septal defect (D) (*arrow*), (**B**) right-to-left shunts (S) (*arrowhead*) across it, (**C**) inflated balloon (B) across the defect, and (**D**) ineffective occlusion showing residual shunt (S) (*arrowhead*), despite balloon occlusion. (See Color Figures 14.3B and D.)

would suggest that the patient does not tolerate occlusion of ADs and should not undergo device closure of the defect.

Occlusion of ADs following recent surgery appears to adversely affect the cardiac index and systemic oxygen delivery in a larger percentage of patients (18–21) than late occlusion. However, late occlusion (years following surgery) appears to be well tolerated in most patients (1,13,18). Therefore device occlusion of ADs early after surgery in high-risk Fontan patients may not be appropriate, unless there are extenuating circumstances.

DEVICE IMPLANTATION TECHNIQUE

Cardiac catheterization and selective cineangiography to define all the issues related to the particular cardiac defect and residua of prior cardiac surgery should be performed. If other abnormalities such as significant branch pulmonary artery stenosis, residual aortopulmonary shunts or collateral vessels and systemic venous obstruction are present, they should be treated with balloon angioplasty, stent implantation, and coil embolization procedures as appropriate.

Balloon sizing (22–24) of the ADs for selection of the size of the device and test occlusion of the defect, to ensure that the patient tolerates defect closure (1,2,17,18), should then be undertaken. If no significant change in the heart rate, cardiac index, systemic oxygen delivery, and right atrial pressure occurs during a 10- to 15-minute test balloon occlusion, then device closure of ADs is performed.

The technique of device implantation varies from device to device and is described in detail in the other chapters dealing with each device, respectively (Chapters 3 through 8), and will not be reviewed here. Coil implantation technique was described by Summer (7). The diameter of the fenestration was estimated by measuring it from a right atrial cineangiogram. A 0.038-inch Gianturco coil with a loop diameter at least twice the fenestration diameter and of sufficient length to produce four loops was selected for implantation. The tip of the coil delivery catheter was positioned across the fenestration into the pulmonary venous atrium and two coil loops delivered. The catheter was then gently withdrawn into the right or systemic venous atrium and the remaining two loops delivered; thus the coil straddles the fenestration.

The protocols of most of the devices require transesophageal echocardiographic monitoring during implantation and consequently general anesthesia, although we were able implant the inverted buttoned device under precordial echographic monitoring (Figure 14.4) with conscious sedation (1). Administration of heparin before introduction of the delivery sheath for anticoagulation during the procedure and antibiotics (three doses of Ancef) for endocarditis prophylaxis is routinely undertaken in all device protocols. Platelet-inhibiting doses of aspirin or Coumadin for anticoagulation following device implantation are also recommended in all protocols.

Pressure recordings from the right atrium and femoral artery, oxygen saturations from the superior vena cava and from the femoral artery are obtained 15 minutes following device placement to calculate pulmonary-to-systemic flow ratio (Qp:Qs), cardiac index, and systemic oxygen delivery and for comparison with data recorded before device implantation. A right atrial angiogram is then performed. A final transesophageal echocardiogram is also performed before removal of catheters and sheaths.

RESULTS

Several types of devices have been used to occlude ADs causing right-to-left shunt. These results will be reviewed in this section.

Clamshell Device

Rome et al. (25) utilized Rashkind double umbrellas and Lock Clamshell devices to occlude ADs in several patients, but the results were combined with those of secundum atrial septal defects.

Bridges and her associates modified the Fontan operation by creating fenestration in the intraatrial baffle in an attempt to improve outcome in high-risk single-ventricle-physiology patients (2). Seventeen of the 19 survivors were studied in the catheterization laboratory within 20 days of fenestrated Fontan operation, and test occlusion of the fenestration was performed. Eleven of these patients tolerated test occlusion and underwent clamshell device closure at the same sitting (*N* = 10) or 3 months later (*N* = 1). Four patients did not tolerate test occlusion, which was attributed to residual abnormalities. Closure of fenestrations was performed at a later date, following medical and/or transcatheter treatment of residua. Fourteen of these 15 had arterial oxygen saturations of 92% to 93%, and final patient's saturation was 89%, secondary to leak in the inferior baffles. Twelve of these had postclosure Doppler stud-

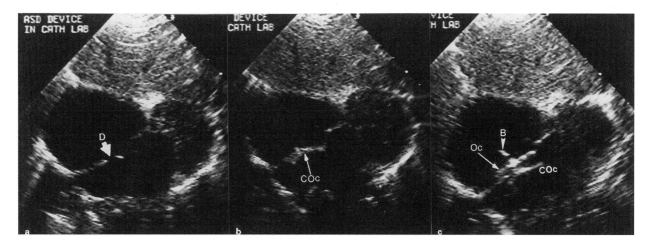

FIGURE 14.4. Selected video frames from two-dimensional echocardiographic subcostal views of the atrial septum recorded during implantation of an inverted buttoned device. **A:** The atrial septal defect (D) is shown. **B:** The counteroccluder (COc) (*arrow*) is positioned on the left atrial side of the septum occluding the defect. **C:** The COc on the left atrial side and the occluder (Oc) (*arrow*), on the right atrial side are shown. Note the button (B) (*arrowhead*), on the right atrial side of the device. (From Rao PS, Chandar JS, Sideris EB. Role of inverted buttoned-device in transcatheter occlusion of atrial septal defects or patent foramen ovale with right-to-left shunting associated with previously operated complex congenital cardiac anomalies. *Am J Cardiol* 1997;80:914–921, with permission.)

ies, which indicated complete closure in ten and trivial residual shunts in two.

Kopf and his associates (8) report on the results of fenestrated Fontan operation in ten patients ages 9 months to 33 years. The fenestrations were 4 to 6 mm in diameter. During postoperative catheterization, test balloon occlusion was performed and six patients judged to tolerate occlusion underwent fenestration closure with a 17-mm clamshell occluder 9 to 16 days after the surgery. The remaining four patients underwent fenestration closure 2 to 6 months after surgery. The systemic arterial oxygen saturation increased from a mean of 86% to a mean of 96%, following fenestration closure. There was no significant change in right atrial mean pressure (11.6 versus 12.0 mm Hg). Data on cardiac indices, Qp:Qs, and systemic oxygen transport were not given. Follow-up for an average of 18 months in seven patients revealed an oxygen saturation of 94% in room air.

Mavroudis et al. (9) performed postoperative cardiac catheterization in 15 of 17 patients undergoing fenestrated Fontan operation at their institution. The fenestration was 2.7 to 5.0 mm (mean, 3.5 mm) in size. Test occlusion of the fenestration was undertaken to evaluate suitability for closure. The clamshell device was implanted in ten patients who tolerated test occlusion. The arterial oxygen saturations increased from 87% ± 1% to 96% ± 0.3% ($p < .05$). Minimal increase in right atrial pressure (11.6 versus 13.4 mm Hg) and slight fall in cardiac index (2.6 versus 2.3 L/min/m^2) occurred. One (10%) clamshell device embolized into the iliac artery, requiring surgical retrieval. No residual shunts were detected by angiography or by color Doppler studies in the remaining patients.

In a recent report, Goff et al. (13) combined the results of 111 clamshell device implantations with those of 70 CardioSEAL device implantations to occlude Fontan fenestrations. These results are discussed in the CardioSEAL section.

Gianturco Coil

Summer and his colleagues (7) utilized Gianturco coils to occlude Fontan fenestration in five patients, 3.5 to 8.3 years of age. The angiographic diameters of the fenestrations varied from 2.6 to 3.2 mm. All implanted coils were of 0.038-inch wire diameter, 8-mm coil loop diameter, and 10-cm-long (four loops) Gianturco coils. The systemic arterial oxygen saturations increased from 74% to 89% before occlusion, to 91% to 96% following coil placement. Angiography in four patients, 10 minutes after the procedure, showed complete occlusion in two patients and residual shunts in two patients. Doppler studies within 24 hours of the procedure revealed residual shunts in two of the five patients. During 1- to 14-month follow-up, residual shunt was present in one (20%) of five patients. No instances of late coil migration, thromboembolic events, hemolysis, or hemodynamic deterioration were observed during follow-up.

Although this method has the advantage of ready availability of the coils and small delivery catheters, the experience is in a limited number of patients. Furthermore, since the mechanism of closure is thrombotic occlusion of the fenestration because of Dacron fibers in the coil, exposed coils on either side of the fenestration may produce clots because of low flow of the Fontan circuit. Because of this concern, results of larger experience with longer duration of follow-up may be required before adoption of this procedure for routine use in closing Fontan fenestration.

Modified Rashkind PDA Occluder

Redington and Rigby (10) modified the Rashkind's PDA umbrella by introducing a bend in each arm of both umbrellas so as to achieve circumferential apposition to adequately close the atrial defects. Eleven patients who had fenestrated Fontan 3 days to 17 weeks previously and one patient with an atrial defect shunting right-to-left late after repair of truncus arteriosus were taken to the catheterization laboratory with intent to occlude. Two procedural failures were observed, one because of obstructed inferior vena cava and the other because of inability to position an 11F sheath. Modified (bent) 17-mm umbrellas were implanted in the remaining ten patients with resultant increase of arterial oxygen saturation from 87% ± 6% to 93% ± 3% ($p < .01$). Follow-up Doppler studies 6 to 12 months later showed complete occlusion in nine (90%) of ten patients.

The concept of introducing bends in the arms of the device to improve device performance is laudable; however, similar bends placed in the clamshell device resulted in fracture of the arms during follow-up, which forced its suspension from use in clinical trials. Because of this, the advisability of introducing such a modification was questioned (26). Furthermore, the Rashkind PDA umbrella is no longer available.

Buttoned Device

During a 17-month period ending August 1996, 12 patients aged 1.6 to 39 years (median, 6.5), with weights of 1.25 to 63 kg (median, 18) underwent buttoned-device occlusion of ADs after repair of pulmonary stenosis/atresia with intact ventricular septum ($N = 5$), modified or fenestrated Fontan operation for tricuspid ($N = 4$), or pulmonary atresia ($N = 1$) or double-inlet left ventricle ($N = 2$) (1). Corrective operations had been performed 1 to 17 years (median, 2) before transcatheter occlusion. The size of the AD varied between 4 and 8 mm (median, 5). Balloon-stretched diameter was 4 to 13 mm with a median of 10 mm.

Temporary balloon occlusion produced an increase in oxygen saturation (82% ± 6% versus 94% ± 4%; $p < .001$) without a change in heart rate or femoral artery pressure. The mean right atrial pressure did not change or increased only by 1 to 2 mm.

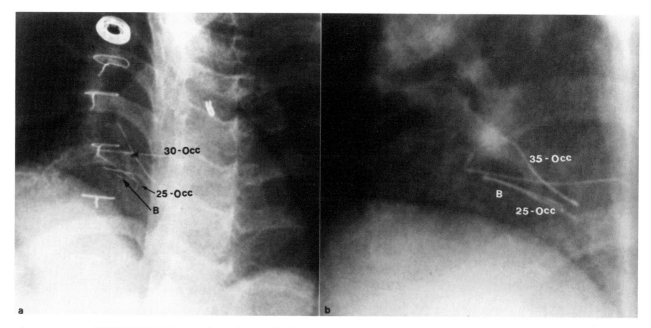

FIGURE 14.5. Selected cineradiographic frames in a left axial oblique view (30 degrees left anterior oblique and 30 degrees cranial) demonstrating 30- and 35-mm occluders (30-Occ and 35-Occ) in the left atrium (**a** and **b** respectively) and the occluder component (25-Occ) of the inverted buttoned device on the right atrial side of the defect. B, radiopaque button. (From Rao PS, Chandar JS, Sideris EB. Role of inverted buttoned-device in transcatheter occlusion of atrial septal defects or patent foramen ovale with right-to-left shunting associated with previously operated complex congenital cardiac anomalies. *Am J Cardiol* 1997;80:914–921, with permission.)

A 25-mm inverted buttoned device was implanted across the defect in nine patients and hybrid devices in three patients (30- or 35-mm occluders of fourth-generation buttoned device on the left atrial side and 25-mm occluder component of the inverted device on the right atrial side) (Figure 14.5). Following device implantation, systemic arterial oxygen saturation (82% ± 7% versus 94% ± 3%; $p < .001$) (Figure 14.6) and Qp:Qs (0.62 ± 0.15 versus 0.95 ± 0.07; $p < .001$) increased without a change in heart rate or cardiac index (3.5 ± 0.7 versus 3.1 ± 0.7 L/min/m²; $p > .1$). Increase in systemic venous oxygen saturation (62% ± 7% versus 71% ± 5%; $p < .001$) was observed but arteriovenous differences in oxygen content (45 ± 18 versus 48 ± 17 mL/L; $p > .1$) and systemic oxygen delivery (573 ± 119 versus 594 ± 140 mL/min/m²) did not change. Mean right atrial pressure did not change (10.8 ± 3.5 versus 10.9 ± 4.3 mm; $p > .1$) after device deployment. Echo-Doppler studies on the morning following device placement revealed no residual shunt in seven (Figure 14.7) and trivial shunt in five.

Follow-up data 6 to 18 months (median, 12) after this procedure revealed improved symptomatology. The oxygen saturations were 92% ± 3% by pulse oximetry (Figure 14.6). Echo-Doppler studies revealed no residual shunts in ten patients, trivial in one, and small to moderate in the final patient. The patient with 86% arterial oxygen saturation underwent a second device implantation 2 years after the

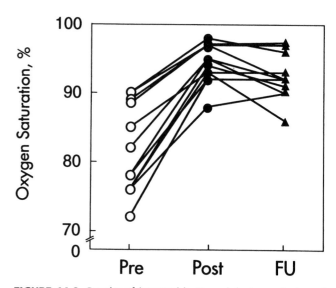

FIGURE 14.6. Results of inverted buttoned-device occlusion of right-to-left atrial shunts. Systemic arterial oxygen saturations before (Pre) and immediately after (Post) device implantation across the atrial septum demonstrating increase in the saturation. At follow-up (FU) of 6 to 18 months (median, 12), the saturations remained high ($p < .01$). (From Rao PS, Chandar JS, Sideris EB. Role of inverted buttoned-device in transcatheter occlusion of atrial septal defects or patent foramen ovale with right-to-left shunting associated with previously operated complex congenital cardiac anomalies. *Am J Cardiol* 1997;80:914–921, with permission.)

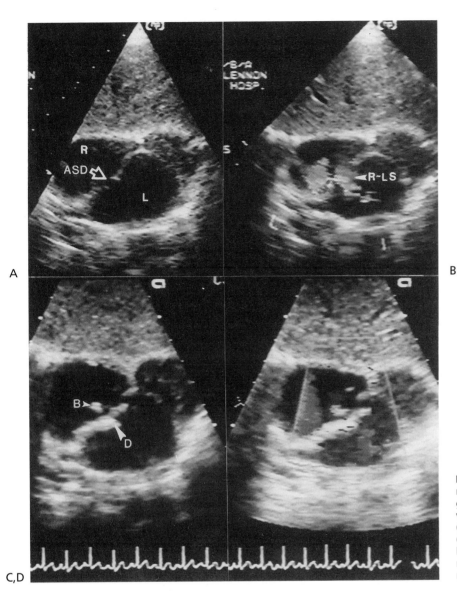

FIGURE 14.7. Selected frames from video recordings of two-dimensional echocardiographic studies from subcostal four chamber views demonstrating the atrial septal defect (ASD) (*arrow*), in (**A**) with right-to-left shunt (R~LS) (*arrowhead*) in (**B**). Following inverted button device (**D**) placement (**C**), the shunt is no longer seen (**D**). B, button; L, left atrium; R, right atrium. (See Color Figures 14.7B and D.)

first procedure with resolution of the residual shunt. None of the patients with fenestrated Fontan had a residual shunt.

In the US multicenter FDA Phase II clinical trial (27), there were 242 buttoned-device implantations. Of these, 31 were ADs with right-to-left shunt; most of these were fenestrated Fontans. Inverted or hybrid buttoned devices were used to occlude these ADs. The oxygen saturation increased from 84% ± 6% to 93% ± 3% ($p < .01$). Detailed follow-up data for this subgroup are not available for review.

Based on the available data, it is concluded that inverted or hybrid buttoned-device occlusion of right-to-left shunt ADs is feasible, safe, and effective in relieving arterial hypoxemia.

Amplatzer Septal Occluder

Tofeig et al. (11) utilized Amplatzer for occlusion of fenestrations created at the time of modified Fontan operation in children ages 5 to 10 years. All patients tolerated test occlusion. The device was implanted successfully at the first attempt in all patients. The arterial oxygen saturations rose from 91% ± 1% to 97% ± 0.2% ($p < .01$). Right atrial angiography revealed small residual shunt in one patient and trivial residual shunt in the remaining four patients. However, echo-Doppler studies 1 and 3 months later revealed complete occlusion in all five patients. Arterial oxygen saturations by pulse oximetry were 92% to 98%.

Cowley et al. (13) also utilized Amplatzer to occlude Fontan fenestrations. Thirteen patients 2.0 to 19.5 years of age (median, 3.2) who had fenestrated lateral tunnel Fontan 0.6 to 4.8 years (median, 1.7) years previously underwent closure. Femoral venous route was used in nine children and transhepatic access was necessary in four children because of femoral vein occlusion ($N = 3$) or infrahepatic interruption of the inferior vena cava ($N = 1$). Successful device implantation was achieved in all 13 patients.

Increase in arterial oxygen saturation (89% ± 5% versus 96% ± 0.06%; *p* < .001) and Qp:Qs (0.77 ± 0.12 versus 0.97 ± 0.06; *p* < .001) occurred without a change in right atrial (baffle) pressure or systemic arterial pressure. The cardiac index decreased by 25% ± 16% (*p* < .001). Severe tricuspid valve regurgitation was noted 2 days after the procedure in one patient and required surgical explantation of the device. Follow-up 1.2 to 9.4 months (mean, 10.4) revealed no residual shunts by transthoracic Doppler study. Oxygen saturation by pulse oximetry was 95% ± 3% (range, 89% to 98%) in nine patients in whom such data are available. The authors conclude that Amplatzer offers an effective method of transcatheter occlusion of Fontan fenestrations (12).

CardioSEAL Device

Goff and her associates (14) examined clinical outcome of transcatheter closure of ADs in fenestrated Fontan patients. Of the 181 patients who had device closure, 154 patients had a single fenestration closed. Clamshell device was implanted in 91 patients and CardioSEAL in 63 patients. In the clamshell group, the age at the time of procedure was 1.3 to 22 years (median, 4.4), and the devices were implanted 0.2 to 35 months (median, 5) after the fenestrated Fontan operation. They were thereafter followed for 0.4 to 10.3 years (median, 6.1). CardioSEAL closure of the fenestration was undertaken 6 to 84 months (median, 33) after Fontan at an age of 3.1 to 43 years (median, 8.9). Follow-up data were available 0.5 to 2.4 years (median, 1.7) after device closure. For the entire group systemic arterial oxygen saturation increased from 88% ± 6% to 92% ± 5% (*p* < .001) following device placement. There was a slight but significant decrease in cardiac index (3.1 ± 1.0 versus 2.7 ± 1.1 L/min/m²; *p* < .001) and increase in mean right atrial pressure (13 ± 3 versus 15 ± 4 mm Hg; *p* < .001). At late follow-up 0.4 to 10.3 years (median, 3.4), the arterial oxygen saturations were 94%. During this time, clinical deterioration was observed in seven (4.5%) patients, including death (*N* = 2), Fontan revision (*N* = 3), protein-losing enteropathy (*N* = 1), and ascites (*N* = 1). Twenty-one (14%) patients developed new arrhythmias and two (1.3%) had cerebrovascular incidents. In the remaining patients, however, decreased use of anticongestive medications and improvement in height and weight percentiles occurred. The authors conclude the device closure of fenestrations is a successful clinical strategy in the management of Fontan patients with single-ventricle physiology.

Other Devices

Transcatheter closure of right-to-left shunt ADs has also been reported with the Das Angel Wing device (28), but this report did not separately examine the results of closure of right-to-left shunt ADs. While it is theoretically possible to occlude right-to-left shunt ADs with ASDOS and Helex devices, no reports of such occlusion have been published.

APPLICABILITY TO ADULT SUBJECTS

Device closure of residual ADs with right-to-left shunt in adult subjects following prior cardiac surgery is as effective as in children. Indeed, most studies quoted in the foregoing presentation include a number of adult subjects, and no specific or additional problems were encountered in the adult patients.

DISCUSSION

Residual atrial septal defects may be present following transcatheter or surgical treatment of a number of cardiac defects. If there is significant right-to-left shunt causing hypoxemia, the defects should be closed. Either prior paradoxical embolism or increased risk for development of such emboli also warrants closure. The majority of the devices that are currently in clinical trials appear to be suitable for closing these atrial defects. Test occlusion should be performed before transcatheter closure. In the absence of significant decrease in cardiac index, systemic venous saturation or systemic oxygen delivery, or an increase in right atrial pressure, the defect may be closed. If the test occlusion is not feasible, other features, such as right ventricular size and function, should be carefully evaluated in the pulmonary atresia/stenosis group before embarking on the closure of ADs (1).

Fenestrations created at the time of Fontan operation, while helpful in the immediate postoperative period, do cause arterial hypoxemia and become the seat of paradoxical embolism. All these fenestrations should eventually be closed. Whereas early (shortly after surgery) closure has been advocated in the past, recent data (1,13) suggest that late (>6 to 12 months) closure is advisable. Patients whose fenestrations close spontaneously need not undergo an additional procedure. Also, hemodynamic adjustment to the Fontan circulation should have taken place by that time. Residual abnormalities such as branch pulmonary artery stenoses, obstruction in the Fontan pathway, residual surgical shunts, or collateral vessels should be relieved appropriately before closing the fenestration. Certainly, test occlusion should be performed to ensure that significant fall in cardiac index or significant increase in the right atrial pressure does not occur. Again, most of the devices that are currently in clinical trials are suitable for closing the fenestration. Availability of device and trained personnel in the use of the device are main prerequisites for selection of a particular device. It is also possible that a particular device is more suitable for a clinical situation than another device. This is likely to be explored in greater detail when multiple devices are available for use by the cardiologist. Consideration of the cost of the device may also eventually enter into the decision-making.

With the advent of staged cavopulmonary connection with bidirectional Glenn initially followed by diversion of inferior vena caval flow into the pulmonary artery via an extra cardiac conduit, the necessity of routinely fenestrating the Fontan is questioned (29). Fenestrations may be required in only highly selected high-risk patients in whom the risk factors could not be completely eliminated. With this development fewer fenestrations will be created and consequently fewer closures would be required.

Recent studies (13) suggest favorable late clinical outcome following closure of a fenestrated Fontan.

CURRENT STATUS

At the time of this writing, for general clinical use in the United States, the FDA approves none of the devices described in this chapter. Recently, the CardioSEAL was approved by the FDA under humanitarian device exemption (HDE) for occlusion of Fontan fenestrations. More recently Amplatzer device is approved by the FDA (13). Most of the devices are, however, available outside the United States and can be used after IRB approval, based on local regulations.

SUMMARY AND CONCLUSION

Surgically created or residual ADs causing right-to-left shunt with consequent hypoxemia and risk for development of paradoxical embolism should be closed if test occlusion data suggest that closure is tolerated. A number of atrial septal occluding devices have been successfully used to close the ADs. Improvement in arterial oxygen saturation along with no substantial change in cardiac index or right atrial pressure have been demonstrated if the occlusion is undertaken 6 months or later following the "corrective" surgery or intervention. Clinical outcome studies suggest that patients accrue clinical benefits during follow-up after device closure of the residual atrial defects.

REFERENCES

1. Rao PS, Chandar JS, Sideris EB. Role of inverted buttoned-device in transcatheter occlusion of atrial septal defects or patent foramen ovale with right-to-left shunting associated with previously operated complex congenital cardiac anomalies. *Am J Cardiol* 1997;80:914–921.
2. Bridges ND, Lock JE, Castaneda AR. Baffle fenestration with subsequent transcatheter closure: modification of Fontan operation for patients with increased risk. *Circulation* 1990;82:1681–1689.
3. Laks H, Pearl JM, Haas GS, et al. Partial Fontan advantages of an adjustable interatrial communication. *Ann Thorac Surg* 1991; 52:1084–1095.
4. Rao PS. Pathophysiologic consequences of cyanotic heart disease. *Indian J Pediatr* 1983;50:479–487.
5. DuPlessis AJ, Chang AC, Wessel DL, et al. Cerebrovascular accidents following Fontan operation. *Pediatr Neurol* 1995;12: 230–236.
6. Wilson DG, Wisheart JD, Stuart AG. Systemic thromboembolism leading to myocardial infarction and stroke after fenestrated total cavopulmonary connection. *Br Heart J* 1995;73:483–485.
7. Sommer R, Recto M, Golinko R, et al. Transcatheter coil occlusion of surgical fenestration after Fontan operation. *Circulation* 1996;94:249–252.
8. Kopf GS, Kleinman CS, Hijazi ZM, et al. Fenestrated Fontan with delayed catheter ASD closure: improved results in high-risk patients. *J Thorac Cardiovasc Surg* 1992;103:1039–1047.
9. Mavroudis C, Zales VR, Backer CL, et al. Fenestrated Fontan with delayed catheter closure: effects of volume loading and baffle fenestration on cardiac index and oxygen delivery. *Circulation* 1992;86(Suppl):II-85–II-92.
10. Redington AN, Rigby ML. Transcatheter closure of interatrial communication with a modified umbrella device. *Br Heart J* 1994; 72:372–377.
11. Tofeig M, Walsh K, Chan C, et al. Occlusion of Fontan fenestrations using the Amplatzer Septal Occluder. *Heart* 1998;79: 368–370.
12. Cowley CG, Badran S, Gaffney D, et al. Transcatheter closure of Fontan fenestrations using the Amplatzer Septal Occluder: initial experience and follow-up. *Catheter Cardiovasc Interv* 2000;51: 301–304.
13. Goff DA, Blume ED, Gauvreau K, et al. Clinical outcome of fenestrated Fontan patients after closure: the first 10 years. *Circulation* 2000;102:2094–2099.
14. Rao PS, Sideris EB, Hausdorf G, et al. International experience with secundum atrial septal defect occlusion by the buttoned device. *Am Heart J* 1994;128:1022–1035.
15. Rao PS, Berger F, Rey C, et al. Results of transvenous occlusion of secundum atrial septal defects with the fourth generation device: comparison with first, second and third generation devices. *J Am Coll Cardiol* 2000;36:583–592.
16. Rao PS, Ende DJ, Wilson AD, et al. Follow-up results of transcatheter occlusion of atrial septal defects with buttoned device. *Can J Cardiol* 1995;11:695–701.
17. Van der Hauwaert LG, Michaelsson M. Isolated right ventricular hypoplasia. *Circulation* 1971;44:466–471.
18. Bridges ND, Lock JE, Mayer JE, et al. Cardiac catheterization and test occlusion of the interatrial communication after fenestrated Fontan operation. *J Am Coll Cardiol* 1995;25:1712–1717.
19. Hijazi ZM, Fahey JT, Kleinman CS, et al. Hemodynamic evaluation before and after closure of fenestrated Fontan: an acute study of changes in oxygen delivery. *Circulation* 1992;88:196–202.
20. Harke B, Kuhn MA, Jarmakani JM, et al. Acute hemodynamic effects of adjustable atrial septal defect closure in the lateral tunnel Fontan procedure. *J Am Coll Cardiol* 1994;23:1671–1677.
21. Kuhn MA, Jarmakani JM, Laks H, et al. Effect of late post-operative atrial septal defect closure on hemodynamic function in patients with lateral tunnel Fontan procedure. *J Am Coll Cardiol* 1995;26:259–265.
22. King TD, Thompson SL, Steiner C, et al. Measurement of atrial septal defect during cardiac catheterization: experimental and clinical trials. *Am J Cardiol* 1978;41:537–542.
23. Rao PS, Langhough R. Relationship of echocardiographic, shunt flow, angiographic size to the stretched diameter of the atrial septal defect. *Am Heart J* 1991;122:505–508.
24. Rao PS, Langhough R, Beekman RH, et al. Echocardiographic estimation of balloon stretched diameter of secundum atrial septal defects for transcatheter occlusion. *Am Heart J* 1992;124:172–175.
25. Rome JJ, Keane JF, Perry SB, et al. Double umbrella closure of atrial defects: initial clinical applications. *Circulation* 1990;82: 751–758.

26. Rao PS, Sideris EB. Transcatheter occlusion of cardiac defects (Letter). *Br Heart J* 1995;73:585–586.

27. Chandar JS, Rao PS, Lloyd TR, et al. Atrial septal defect closure with 4th generation buttoned device: results of US multicenter FDA Phase II clinical trial. (Abstract). *Circulation* 1999;100 (Suppl):I-708.

28. Das GS, Harrison JK, O'Laughlin MP. The Angel Wing Das devices for atrial septal defect closure. *Curr Interv Cardiol Rep* 2000;2:78–85.

29. Thompson LD, Petrossion E, McElhinney DB, et al. Is it necessary to routinely fenestrate an extracardiac Fontan? *J Am Coll Cardiol* 1999;34:539–544.

Catheter Based Devices: For the Treatment of Non-coronary Cardiovascular Diseases in Adults and Children. Edited by P. Syamasundar Rao and Morton J. Kern, Lippincott Williams & Wilkins, Philadelphia © 2003.

15

PLATYPNEA-ORTHODEOXIA SYNDROME: TRANSCATHETER MANAGEMENT

SAAD R. BITAR
P. SYAMASUNDAR RAO

Burchell et al. first described the platypnea-orthodeoxia syndrome (POS) in 1949 (1). It is a relatively uncommon but serious symptom complex, including arterial hypoxemia, usually seen in elderly subjects. Its exact incidence is still undetermined. Fewer than 100 cases have been described in the literature so far (2–4). POS is characterized by increased dyspnea in the upright position and is relieved by assuming the recumbent position, thus the term *platypnea,* in contrast with *orthopnea* (breathing difficulty which is partly or completely relieved by sitting or standing) that is commonly seen in patients with cardiac disorders. It is associated with development of or an accentuation of hypoxemia in the upright position, thus the term *orthodeoxia,* which may be confirmed by arterial blood gas analysis or pulse oximetry. This unusual presentation may contribute to underdetection of this syndrome. This chapter will discuss the etiology, diagnosis, and management, with particular attention to transcatheter treatment.

ETIOLOGY

The POS has been described in association with several pulmonary disorders such as postpneumonectomy (5,6) or lobectomy (7), as well as obstructive lung disease (8). In these cases the syndrome is probably related to the displacement of the interatrial septum, as will be discussed later. It is also seen in patients with anatomic pulmonary vascular shunts such as pulmonary arteriovenous malformations (8). The amount of blood going though those communications is increased in the upright position, especially if they are located in the lower lobes. POS is also described in patients with advanced liver disease as part of the hepatopulmonary syndrome (8,9). The proposed mechanism is decreased metabolism of several vasodilators due to diseased liver leading to pulmonary vasodilatation. It has been described in association with recurrent pulmonary emboli (3,10) due to the presence of significant ventilation perfusion mismatch and in patients with amiodarone lung toxicity (11,12).

Nevertheless, this syndrome is more frequently seen in patients with or without pulmonary disease secondary to intracardiac shunt via a patent foramen ovale (PFO) that is exaggerated in the upright position. These patients usually have normal right heart pressures and tend to be older (2–4,13).

Given the high prevalence (25% to 30%) of patency of the foramen ovale in otherwise normal hearts (14–16), the potential for development of right-to-left shunt exists. The dilemma is whether the mere presence of PFO would lead to the development of this syndrome. Apparently, other coexisting factors may contribute to such shunting but are poorly understood. There are several proposed mechanisms (10), including the horizontal displacement of the interatrial septum as seen in patients after pneumonectomy (4,17), elongated ascending aorta or ascending aortic aneurysms (18–20), and severe thoracic skeletal abnormalities (21,22). This displacement may also be an age-related change without associated abnormality. This leads to preferential blood flow from the inferior vena cava via the patent foramen ovale into the left atrium, with intermittent right-to-left shunting that is exaggerated in the upright position. This phenomenon does not require increased right atrial pressure; a proposed mechanism is the instantaneous pressure difference between the right and left atria (23–25), despite normal mean right atrial pressure.

Other proposed mechanisms include persistent Eustachian valve causing the redirection of flow (26) as well

Saad R. Bitar: Clinical Assistant Professor of Medicine, Department of Internal Medicine, Saint Louis University; Director, Coronary Care Unit, Department of Medicine, Division of Cardiology, Saint Louis University Hospital, Saint Louis, Missouri

P. Syamasundar Rao: Professor of Pediatrics, Medicine, and Cardiology, Department of Pediatrics, University of Texas-Houston Medical School; Director, Division of Pediatric Cardiology, Memorial Hermann Children's Hospital, Houston, Texas

as decreased right atrial compliance (10,27–29) that may even be due to injury such as that produced by Swan-Ganz catheter placement (10).

Rarely, the syndrome has also been seen without any associated abnormalities (3,23,30).

DIAGNOSIS

The unique feature of POS, incapacitating dyspnea, which improves in the recumbent position, in the absence of overt pulmonary disease should raise the possibility of this syndrome. Documentation of hypoxemia by either arterial blood gas analysis or pulse oximetry is usually the first clue of this syndrome. Lack of improvement of hypoxia by supplemental oxygen indicates the presence of a fixed right-to-left shunt.

The next step is to document dynamic change of arterial oxygen saturation between the upright and recumbent positions, which is usually associated with the development of hypocapnea and tachypnea in the upright position, which is consistent with the subjective complaint of breathlessness. This may be elaborately investigated by performing shunt fraction calculations in the upright and supine positions as well as continuous arterial blood gas analysis or by simple pulse oximetry in the supine and upright positions.

The presence of intracardiac shunting at the level of the PFO may be documented by injection of intravenous agitated saline (bubble study) during echocardiography (3). The contrast echocardiography should be performed in both the supine and upright positions, perhaps with the use of a tilt table (3,21) to demonstrate the orthostatic nature of the bubble passage to the left side. This may be further demonstrated during transesophageal echocardiography, which also allows for further delineation of the atrial septal anatomy and the frequently coexisting atrial septal aneurysms.

Other suggested diagnostic testing includes cardiac catheterization with special attention for demonstrating left-sided saturation step-down between the pulmonary veins and left atrium/ventricle and/or peripheral artery. This saturation step-down can be further exaggerated in the catheterization lab in the upright position or with the Valsalva maneuver (30). Cardiac catheterization is also helpful to directly measure pulmonary artery pressures and in demonstrating other associated cardiac abnormalities that may require therapy. Magnetic resonance imaging (6,31) and angiography (3) may also be helpful in establishing the diagnosis.

THERAPY

The use of opiates to alleviate the symptoms of breathlessness (32) may not be effective in treatment of POS. Such a therapy for treatment of POS has been suggested (32), but no data to substantiate such recommendation have been provided. Supplemental oxygen is usually ineffective, and the symptoms are frequently incapacitating (10,32). Treatment is largely dependent upon the associated pathophysiologic abnormalities. Management of patients in whom the syndrome is related to intrapulmonary shunt should be directed to the specific etiology, such as elimination of pulmonary arteriovenous malformations (surgically or by embolization) or treatment of coexisting disorders such as hepatopulmonary syndrome in which liver transplantation is usually effective in alleviating the syndrome. In some patients, symptoms of POS are precipitated or accentuated by hypovolemia. In such patients, correction of hypovolemia improves symptomatology (33,34). When loculated pericardial effusion is responsible for POS, drainage of effusion is likely to relieve POS (35).

For the purpose of this chapter, further discussion will be limited to the treatment of POS due to intracardiac shunting at the level of the foramen ovale. Surgical closure of the PFO, the recommended treatment option (3,5,7,21,23,36,37), is technically simple and remains the standard. It should be considered particularly if the patient requires surgical intervention for other reasons, such as ascending aortic aneurysm or coronary artery disease. In the absence of coexisting disorders requiring cardiac surgery, transcatheter closure appears to be an effective management option (22,31,38–40).

Landzberg and colleagues first reported transcatheter closure of PFO for the treatment of POS in 1995 using a clamshell device (22). They treated eight patients from three different institutions. Following device placement, reduction in right-to-left atrial shunt along with increase in oxygen saturation occurred in each patient. Significant complications occurred in three patients; device embolization required transcatheter retrieval in two patients and nonsustained ventricular arrhythmia in another. Two patients died during follow-up, 2 and 3 months after device implantation, respectively, secondary to underlying cancer. Cerebrovascular accident resulting in death occurred in a third patient 11 months after the procedure. Symptoms of POS improved in the remaining five living patients. A buttoned device was used by Godart et al. (38) to occlude the PFO in a 67-year-old patient with POS. They used a hybrid device (regular buttoned device on the left atrial side plus a square-shaped counteroccluder on the right atrial side). Relief of platypnea and orthodeoxia was noted during a follow-up for a 6-month period. We implanted regular ($N = 2$) and hybrid ($N = 8$) buttoned devices in ten patients, ages 71 ± 9 years, to treat POS (39). Most of them had multiple comorbidities. Eight patients had normal pulmonary artery pressures and all had successful device implantation. In all patients there was significant improvement of oxygen saturations in the upright position (Figure 15.1) as well as contrast bubble crossover immediately after the procedure. Over a follow-up period (mean, 12 months), one patient required a second procedure for incomplete closure during our early experience. Transthoracic echocardiographic studies were performed in all patients, and interarterial shunts were seen

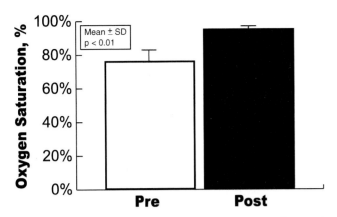

FIGURE 15.1. Bar graph demonstrating improvement (*p* < .010) in oxygen saturation in upright position following buttoned device closure of patent foramen ovale in patients suffering from platypnea-orthodeoxia syndrome. (From Rao PS, Palacios IF, Bach RG, et al. Platypnea-orthodeoxia: management by transcatheter buttoned device implantation. *Cath Cardiovasc Intervent* 2001;54:77–82, with permission.)

only in two, with acceptable oxygen saturation of more than 92% by oximetry in the upright position. Waight and colleagues also recently reported on successful PFO closure in four patients using the Amplatzer device for similar patients with remarkable improvements in oxygen saturations and symptomatology (40). Godart et al. reported a series of 11 patients who were treated with transcatheter closure using several devices [Buttoned device (*N* = 5), CardioSEAL (*N* = 2) and Amplatzer PFO Occluder (*N* = 4)] with successful results in ten of 11 patients with complete or near complete resolution of shunt by the end of the procedure (31). Only six of the 11 patients were thought to have POS. Complications (*N* = 4) included supraventricular tachycardia in two, successfully treated medically; death in one on the day following the procedure, which was secondary to sepsis unrelated to the device placement; and cerebrovascular accident in one, which resolved within 1 month of the procedure. During follow-up (up to 30 months), no or trivial residual shunts were documented by contrast echocardiography in nine out of ten patients (31).

In summary, clamshell (22), buttoned (31,38,39,41), Amplatzer (31,40), and CardioSEAL (31) devices have been used successfully in occluding PFOs to treat POS. The clamshell device is no longer in use, but its successor, CardioSEAL, the buttoned device, and Amplatzer are in clinical trials. The hybrid version of the buttoned device (Chapter 14) (41), modified version of the Amplatzer, the Amplatzer PFO Occluder (42), and PFO-Star (Chapter 12) are specifically designed to occlude PFOs. Other devices, namely, ASDOS, Das Angel Wings, and Helex, though not reported to have been used in the management of POS, may be useful in PFO occlusion in POS. The protocols, procedures, and methods of implantation of these devices are described in detail in the preceding chapters in this book, and the reader is referred to these chapters for details pertaining to device implantation.

Closure of the PFO is clearly indicated to relieve the symptoms of patients with POS. These patients usually have significant comorbidities that would make them high-risk surgical candidates. Transcatheter closure using a variety of devices (e.g, hybrid buttoned device, Amplatzer PFO Occluder) is a safe, effective, and less invasive alternative to surgical closure. This procedure can be done with either transthoracic or transesophageal echocardiographic guidance and requires an average 1-day stay in the hospital. Pending FDA approval of these devices for general use, transcatheter closure will probably become the treatment of choice for closure of PFO causing POS syndrome.

SUMMARY AND CONCLUSION

Platypnea-orthodeoxia syndrome is a unique clinical entity, uncommon but probably underdetected. It is characterized by arterial hypoxemia in the upright position (orthodeoxia) associated with dyspnea and hypocapnea (platypnea). Both symptoms are relieved in the supine position. POS is usually associated with thoracic, pulmonary, or aortic pathology, although it is seen rarely without any discernible abnormalities. Posture-related right-to-left shunting across the PFO is seen in a large proportion of these patients. Although surgical closure currently remains the standard for PFO closure, several transcatheter devices have been used to occlude them successfully, with marked improvement of symptoms in most patients at low morbidity and virtually no mortality. After FDA approval of these devices, transcatheter closure will probably become the method of choice for closing PFO in patients with POS, as they are frequently at high surgical risk due to advanced age and comorbidities. Prior to such approval, the transcatheter option is available only at institutions participating in clinical trials with investigational device exemption.

REFERENCES

1. Burchell HB, Helmholz HF Jr, Wood EH. Reflex orthostatic dyspnea associated with pulmonary hypertension. *Am J Physiol* 1949;159:563–564.
2. Winters WL, Cortes F, McDonough M, et al. Venoarterial shunting from inferior vena cava to left atrium in atrial septal defect with normal heart pressures: report of two cases. *Am J Cardiol* 1967;19:293–300.
3. Seward JB, Hayes DL, Smith HC, et al. Platypnea-orthodeoxia: clinical profile, diagnostic work-up, management, and report of seven cases. *Mayo Clin Proc* 1984;59:221–231.
4. Cheng TO. Platypnea-orthodeoxia syndrome: etiology, differential diagnosis, and management. *Catheter Cardiovasc Interv* 1999;47:64–66.
5. Bakris NC, Siddiqi AJ, Fraser CD, et al. Right-to-left interatrial shunt after pneumonectomy. *Ann Thorac Surg* 1997;63:198–201.
6. Mercho N, Stoller JK, White RD, et al. Right-to-left interatrial

shunt causing platypnea after pneumonectomy: a recent experience and diagnostic value of dynamic magnetic resonance imaging. *Chest* 1994;105:931–933.

7. Smeenk FW, Postmus PE. Interatrial right-to-left shunting developing after pulmonary resection in the absence of elevated right-sided heart pressures: review of literature. *Chest* 1993;105:528–531.

8. Robin ED, Lamon D, Horn BR, et al. Platypnea related to orthodeoxia caused by true vascular lung shunts. *N Engl J Med* 1976;294:941–943.

9. Byrd RP, Jr, Lopez OS, Joyce BW, et al. Platypnea, orthodeoxia and cirrhosis. *J Ky Med Assoc* 1992;90:189–192.

10. Robin ED, McCauley RF. An Analysis of platypnea-orthodeoxia syndrome including a "new" therapeutic approach (Editorial). *Chest* 1997;112:1449–1451.

11. Papiris SA, Maniati MA, Manussakis MN, et al. Orthodeoxia in amiodarone-induced acute reversible pulmonary damage. *Chest* 1994;105:965–966.

12. Iskander S, Raible DG, Brozena SC. Acute alveolar hemorrhage and orthodeoxia induced by intravenous amiodarone. *Catheter Cardiovasc Interv* 1999;47:61–63.

13. Sorrentino M, Resnekov L. Patent foramen ovale associated with platypnea and orthodeoxia. *Chest* 1991;100:1157–1158.

14. Scammon RE, Norris EH. On the time of the postnatal obliteration of the fetal blood passages (foramen ovale, ductus arteriosus, ductus venosus). *Anat Rec* 1918;15:165–180.

15. Patten BM. The closure of the foramen ovale. *Am J Anat* 1931;48:19–44.

16. Hagen PT, Scholz DG, Edwards WD. Incidence and size of patent foramen ovale during the first 10 decade of life: an autopsy study of 965 normal hearts. *Mayo Clin Proc* 1984;59:17–20.

17. Springer RM, Gherorghiade M, Chakko CS, et al. Platypnea and interatrial right-to-left shunting after lobectomy. *Am J Cardiol* 1983;51:1802–1803.

18. Tan KL, Robinson TD, Celermajer DS, et al. Intermittent hypoxaemia without orthodeoxia due to right-to-left shunting related to an elongated aorta. *Respirology* 1999;4:291–293.

19. Faller M, Kessler R, Chaouat A, et al. Platypnea-orthodeoxia syndrome related to an aortic aneurysm combined with an aneurysm of the atrial septum. *Chest* 2000;118:553–557.

20. Laybourn KA, Martin ET, Cooper RAS, et al. Platypnea and orthodeoxia: shunting associated with an aortic aneurysm. *J Thorac Cardiovasc Surg* 1997;113:955–956.

21. Popp G, Melek H, Garnett AR, Jr. Platypnea-orthodeoxia related to aortic elongation. *Chest* 1997;112:1682–1684.

22. Landzberg MJ, Sloss LJ, Faherty CE, et al. Orthodeoxia-platypnea due to intracardiac shunting: relief with transcatheter double umbrella closure. *Catheter Cardiovasc Diagn* 1995;36:247–250.

23. Nazzal SB, Bansal RC, Fitzmorris SJ, et al. Platypnea-orthodeoxia as a cause of unexplained hypoxemia in an 82-yr-old female. *Catheter Cardiovasc Diagn* 1990;19:242–245.

24. Levin AR, Spat MS, Bionic JP, et al. Atrial pressure-flow dynamics in atrial septal defects (secundum type). *Circulation* 1968;3:476–488.

25. Rao PS. Left-to-right atrial shunts in tricuspid atresia. *Br Heart J* 1983;49:345–349.

26. Bashour T, Kabbani S, Saalouke M, et al. Persistent Eustachian valve causing severe cyanosis in atrial septal defect with normal right atrial pressure. *Angiology* 1983;34:79–83.

27. Joffe HS. Effect of age on pressure-flow dynamics in secundum atrial septal defect. *Br Heart J* 1984;5:469–472.

28. Galve E, Angel J, Evangelista A, et al. Bidirectional shunt in uncomplicated atrial septal defect. *Br Heart J* 1984;51:480–484.

29. Ciafone RA, Avoerty JM, Weintraub RM, et al. Cyanosis in uncomplicated atrial septal defect with normal right cardiac and pulmonary arterial pressures. *Chest* 1978;74:596–599.

30. Mills TJ, Seward JB, McGoon MD, et al. Platypnea-orthodeoxia; assessment with a unique cardiac catheterization procedure. *Catheter Cardiovasc Diagn* 1986;12:100–102.

31. Godart F, Rey C, Prat A, et al. Atrial right-to-left shunting causing severe hypoxemia despite normal right-sided pressures. Report of 11 consecutive cases corrected by percutaneous closure. *Eur Heart J* 2000;21:483–489.

32. Robin ED, Burke CM. Risk-benefit analysis in chest medicine: single-patient randomized clinical trial: opiates for intractable dyspnea. *Chest* 1986;90:888–892.

33. Wranne B, Tolagen K. Platypnea after pneumonectomy caused by a combination of intracardiac right-to-left shunt and hypovolemia: relief of symptoms on restitution of blood volume. *Scand J Thorac Cardiovasc Surg* 1978;12:129–131.

34. LaBresh KA, Pietro DA, Coates EO, et al. Platypnea syndrome after left pneumonectomy. *Chest* 1981;79:605–607.

35. Adolph EA, Lacy WO, Hermoni Y, et al. Reversible orthodeoxia and platypnea due to right-to-left intracardiac shunting related to pericardial effusion. *Ann Intern Med* 1992;116:138–139.

36. Burchell HB. An introduction to the clinical applications of oximetry. *Proc Staff Meet Mayo Clin* 1950;25:377–384.

37. Khouzaie T, Bussor JR. A rare cause of dyspnea and arterial hypoxemia. *Chest* 1997;112:1681–1682.

38. Godart F, Porte HL, Rey C, et al. Post pneumonectomy interatrial right-to-left shunt: successful percutaneous treatment. *Ann Thorac Surg* 1997;64:834–836.

39. Rao PS, Palacios IF, Bach RG, et al. Platypnea-orthodeoxia: management by transcatheter buttoned device implantation (Abstract). *J Am Coll Cardiol* 2000;35:199A.

40. Waight DJ, Cao Q-L, Hijazi AM. Closure of patent foramen ovale in patients with orthodeoxia-platypnea using the Amplatzer devices. *Catheter Cardiovasc Interv* 2000;50:195–198.

41. Rao PS, Palacios IF, Bach RG, et al. Platypnea-orthodeoxia: management by transcatheter buttoned device implantation. *Catheter Cardiovasc Interv* 2001;54:77–82.

42. Han Y, Gu X, Titus JL, et al. New self-expanding patent foramen ovale occlusion device. *Catheter Cardiovasc Interv* 1999;47:370–376.

16

ROLE OF THREE-DIMENSIONAL ECHOCARDIOGRAPHIC RECONSTRUCTION IN TRANSCATHETER OCCLUSION OF ATRIAL SEPTAL DEFECTS

ANIRBAN BANERJEE
HITENDRA T. PATEL
NATESA G. PANDIAN

The success of transcatheter closure of any cardiac defect is largely dependent upon understanding the anatomy of the defect and its contiguous structures. Secundum atrial septal defect (ASD) is a deficiency in the septum primum in the floor of the fossa ovalis. However, the size, the number of defects, and the location of the defect within the atrial septum vary from patient to patient. Most modern transcatheter devices designed to close ASDs have a double-disk configuration, requiring approximately a 4-mm rim of atrial septal tissue around the defect to anchor the device. The elements outlined above need to be determined precisely for successful transcatheter closure and to avoid residual shunts.

Two-dimensional (2D) echocardiography is the principal diagnostic modality utilized in the diagnosis and characterization of ASDs. Angiography and fluoroscopy have proven to be inadequate, and transesophageal 2D echocardiography (TEE) plays a pivotal role in the deployment of various transcatheter ASD closure devices (1,2). However, 2D echocardiographic images provided by TEE often fail to provide the spatial relationship of the ASD to various parts of the atrial septum itself and to the structures surrounding the atrial septum. To overcome this shortcoming of 2D echocardiography, an experienced examiner utilizes an array of 2D images acquired sequentially by the ultrasound machine, to mentally create a three-dimensional (3D) image. Thereafter the examiner tries to portray this mentally constructed 3D image to his colleagues using anatomic descriptors. Traditionally, this technique of mental reconstruction has been used in various imaging modalities that utilize 2D tomographic images (e.g., echocardiography, computerized tomography scan, and magnetic resonance imaging). More recently, it has been utilized successfully in transcatheter deployment of various ASD devices. However, it would be truly advantageous to actually see this mentally reconstructed image on a screen, thereby allowing visualization of the atrial septum and its defect *en face*. The advent of 3D reconstruction of tomographically acquired 2D images brought this to fruition, allowing examiners to actually see an *en face* view of the atrial septum (3).

In adult patients the first attempt to visualize the atrial septum and its defects was made by Belholvalek et al. (3), who performed it by using a TEE probe held in a custom-made frame rotated by a stepper motor. These investigators were the first to show images of ASDs and that of a Clamshell device occluding the ASD. This was followed by a study evaluating ASDs in pediatric patients (4). In pediatric patients a specially designed TEE probe was utilized to obtain transthoracic images. The transducer was moved

Anirban Banerjee: Associate Professor, Division of Pediatric Cardiology, Tufts University School of Medicine; Director of Pediatric Echocardiography, Division of Pediatric Cardiology, Tufts-New England Medical Center, Boston, Massachusetts

Hitendra T. Patel: Pediatric Cardiologist, Department of Cardiology, Children's Hospital Oakland, Oakland, California

Natesa G. Pandian: Director, Cardiovascular Imaging and Hemodynamic Laboratory, Tufts-New England Medical Center, Boston, Massachusetts

along the chest wall from the inferior to the superior margin of the heart, by a stepper motor creating parallel tomographic "slices" of the cardiac image. This helped in obtaining *en face* views of ASDs in children. For the first time such studies made it possible to see the circumferential rims surrounding the ASD, in a single plane and pointed out a potential superiority of 3D imaging over 2D imaging during device closure of ASDs.

Three-dimensional echocardiography has been utilized to evaluate the size and shape of ASDs, in both *in vitro* and *in vivo* models. In an *in vitro* porcine heart model, several types of ASDs were created artificially (5). These hearts were suspended in a water bath and excellent 3D echocardiographic images of the various types of ASDs were obtained. Subsequently, anatomic views were obtained by removing the right atrial free wall. These 3D images closely resembled actual anatomic views of the ASDs and the adjoining anatomic landmarks (i.e., inferior and superior vena cavae and tricuspid valve). Most important, ASD sizes obtained by 3D imaging showed an excellent correlation ($r > 0.9$) with anatomic measurement of ASD sizes (5). *In vivo*

studies in humans have also shown a good correlation between maximal ASD diameter measured by 3D echocardiography and during surgery (6). Subsequent studies performed in patients showed a poorer correlation between 3D reconstructions and direct surgical measurements (7). This can be explained by the vastly different physiologic states of the heart during these measurements. During 3D reconstruction, the heart was filled with blood and was beating, whereas during surgical measurements the heart was devoid of blood and in diastolic arrest, making it a flabby and stretchable organ.

Magni et al. were the first to utilize 3D echocardiography in the assessment of ASD closure by the Das Angel Wings device (8). The rim surrounding the ASD may be arbitrarily classified into four segments: superior anterior (SA), inferior anterior (IA), superior posterior (SP), and inferior posterior (IP) (Figure 16.1). Three-dimensional echocardiography provides excellent images of all four rims of the atrial septum surrounding the ASD. However, it is often difficult to visualize the IP rim in its entirety by 2D echocardiography. Since 3D reconstruction is depen-

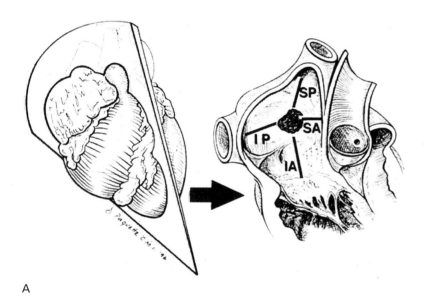

A

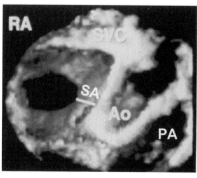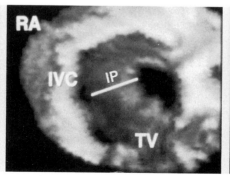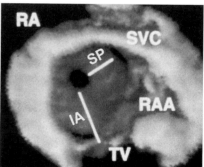

B   C   D

FIGURE 16.1 A: Schematic diagram depicting the *en face* view of the atrial septum. It shows the secundum ASD and the surrounding septal rims. IA, inferior anterior; IP, inferior posterior; SA, superior anterior; SP, superior posterior. **B:** Three-dimensional reconstruction showing *en face* view of the atrial septum and a secundum ASD. It includes the ascending aorta (AO) and the SA rim behind the aorta. PA, pulmonary artery. **C:** Three-dimensional cut plane includes the inferior vena cava (IVC) and the IP rim. **D:** Cut plane depicts the SP and IA rims of the atrial septum as well as the tricuspid valve (TV), right atrial appendage (RAA), and superior vena cava (SVC). (From Magni G, Hijazi ZM, Pandian NG, et al. Two- and three-dimensional transesophageal echocardiography in patient selection and assessment of atrial septal defect closure by the new Das-Angel Wings device: initial clinical experience. *Circulation* 1997; 96:1722–1728, with permission.)

dent on optimal images of 2D slices, the full length of the IP rim is not seen adequately by 3D echocardiography as well. On the other hand, the segment of the rim that is much better visualized by 3D echocardiography than by 2D TEE is the SA rim (part of the rim separating the ASD from the posterior aortic wall). The whole SA rim is often in a slightly different plane than its counterpart, the SP rim. This may result in noninclusion of a portion of the SA rim in 2D images. Therefore in instances where 2D echocardiography has deemed the SA rim to be inadequate (<4 mm), 3D reconstruction has invariably shown this rim to be of adequate length (9). This has resulted in inclusion of previously excluded patients for device closure.

ADVANTAGES OF 3D ECHOCARDIOGRAPHY

ASD Shape

Three-dimensional echocardiography has demonstrated a significant variability in the shape of secundum ASDs. Only about half of them are round in shape. The rest show a more complex configuration, oval, racquet-shaped or multiple (9). The various shapes are best depicted in *en face* views generated by 3D reconstruction.

ASD Size

An accurate assessment of the size of the ASD is a prerequisite for successful device closure. Traditionally, the balloon-stretched dimension (BSD) has been regarded as the gold standard for selection of the device size. BSD has been measured by withdrawing a sizing balloon across the ASD and measuring the maximal dimension of the balloon just before it pops into the right atrium. However, several studies have reported that the BSD overestimates the size of the ASD measured by 3D imaging (8,9). It has been proposed that BSD is perhaps an artificial measurement resulting from overstretching of the ASD. Oblique passage of the balloon through the ASD may also contribute to the overestimation of the size of the ASD (10). Therefore more recently, balloon occlusion diameter (BOD) has been used for device selection. For this measurement a fully inflated balloon is pulled against the ASD until it eliminates all flow across the ASD, as detected by color Doppler. The segment of the balloon occluding the ASD acts as a plug, without popping through it. Measurement of this segment of the balloon provides us with the BOD, which is smaller than the BSD on an average by 1.98 mm (11). When balloon "occlusion" rather than balloon "stretching" was used to size the ASD, an excellent correlation ($r = 0.98$) was noted between BOD and the maximal diameter of ASD measured by 3D echocardiography (11). Further studies may demonstrate that the 3D diameter is more accurate and should be used as the new gold standard for device selection.

En Face View of ASD Device

For ASD devices that have a square configuration (e.g., Angel Wings and CardioSEAL devices), 3D reconstruction allows *en face,* simultaneous visualization of the four corners, as well as of the four margins of either right or left atrial disks (Figure 16.2). Such views are difficult to obtain by 2D echocardiography. For more echogenic devices such as the Amplatzer device, *en face* views of the device can be noted by TEE. However, when the device is seen in this view by TEE, the atrial septum is also in an *en face* position. Two-dimensional imaging does not allow a full-face view of the atrial septum. This is an inherent limitation of 2D echocardiography, which only allows structures such as septa and valves to be visualized "in profile." Therefore the spatial relationship of the ASD device with the atrial septum and neighboring structures such as ascending aorta or vena cavae cannot be depicted adequately by TEE. An experienced echocardiographer overcomes this shortcoming by mentally constructing a 3D image from the various 2D slices obtained by TEE. However, at times it is difficult to project this mentally reconstructed picture into the minds of others. In contrast, 3D reconstruction is capable of showing both the device and the atrial septum *en face*. Hence it depicts the relative position of the device along the septum on a single screen. This allows the mental picture of the echocardiographer to be actually visualized by others. We conclude that the spatial relationship between the device, the atrial septum and the contiguous structures, can only be established by 3D reconstruction. Moreover, such *en face* views can be obtained not only from the right atrial side, but also from the left atrial side. Such right and left atrial *en face* views are equivalent to anatomic views obtained by "unroofing" of the corresponding atrial free wall, and they provide valuable insight regarding device position (Figures 16.3 and 16.4).

Mechanism of Residual Shunt

When a residual shunt is noted after deployment of an ASD device, it is sometimes difficult by 2D imaging to determine the exact mechanism responsible for the residual shunt. Consequently, this lack of understanding may lead to acceptance of suboptimal device positions. Three-dimensional echocardiography often helps in shedding additional

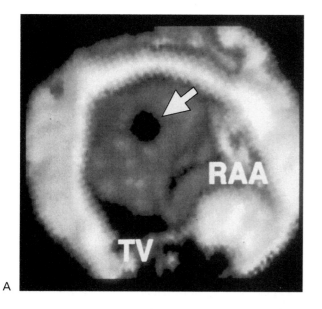

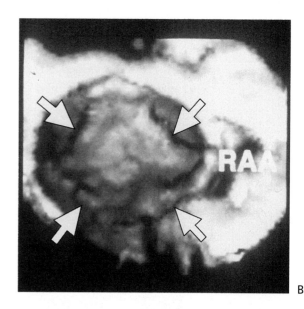

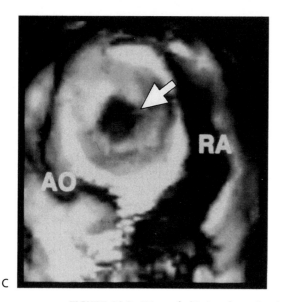

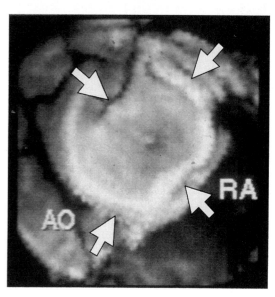

FIGURE 16.2. "Unroofed" view from the right atrium showing 3D image of (**A**) secundum ASD and (**B**) normally positioned Das Angel Wings device. The *arrows* point to the four sides of this square device. **C:** Similar unroofed view of the atrial septum and the ASD from the left atrial side. **D:** *En face* view of the Angel Wings device from the left atrium. The *arrows* point to the four sides of the device, which have a corrugated appearance, due to the sewing of the fabric along the wire frames of this device. (From Magni G, Hijazi ZM, Pandian NG, et al. Two- and three-dimensional transesophageal echocardiography in patient selection and assessment of atrial septal defect closure by the new Das-Angel Wings device: initial clinical experience. *Circulation* 1997;96:1722–1728, with permission.)

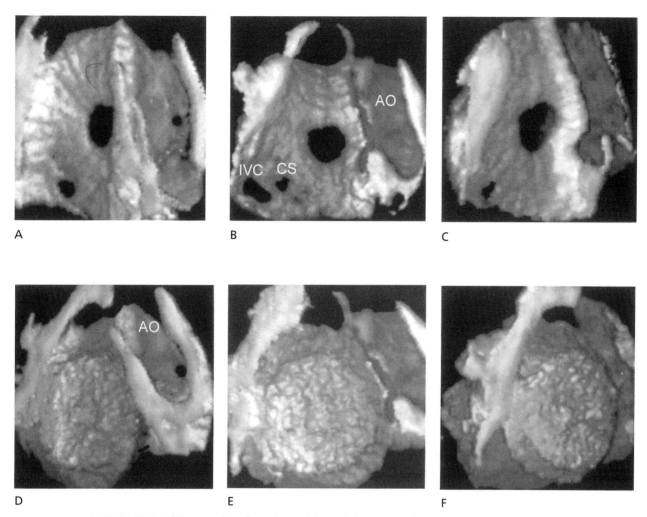

FIGURE 16.3. Oblique and *en face* views of the atrial septum and secundum ASD viewed from the right atrium before **(A, B, C)** and after **(D, E, F)** closure with an Amplatzer Septal Occluder. AO, ascending aorta; CS, coronary sinus; IVC, inferior vena cava.

light on the etiology of residual shunts. For example, in square devices such as the Angel Wings device it is often difficult to say by TEE exactly which corner of the device has prolapsed through the ASD to produce the configuration noted on TEE. Three-dimensional imaging provides a better understanding as to which corner has indeed prolapsed (Figure 16.5) (8,9). At other times the wings of square devices may fold on themselves to produce an abnormal triangular appearance that cannot be fully appreciated by TEE (Figure 16.6).

Multiple ASDs

The region of the fossa ovalis may have multiple fenestrations, characterized by a main defect accompanied by multiple smaller, accessory defects (9,12). Despite successful closure of the main defect, failure to recognize these additional accessory defects by 2D echocardiography has resulted in residual left-to-right shunting across the atrial septum even after device closure (1). When multiple openings were present, TEE failed to detect the exact number of smaller (<2 mm) openings in 25% of cases, that were subsequently detected by 3D imaging (13). We feel that 3D echocardiography is clearly superior to 2D echocardiography in accurately demonstrating the number, shapes, and particularly distances between the various openings in a convenient single view.

Three-dimensional imaging may play a vital role in pre-selection of patients with multiple defects for double device

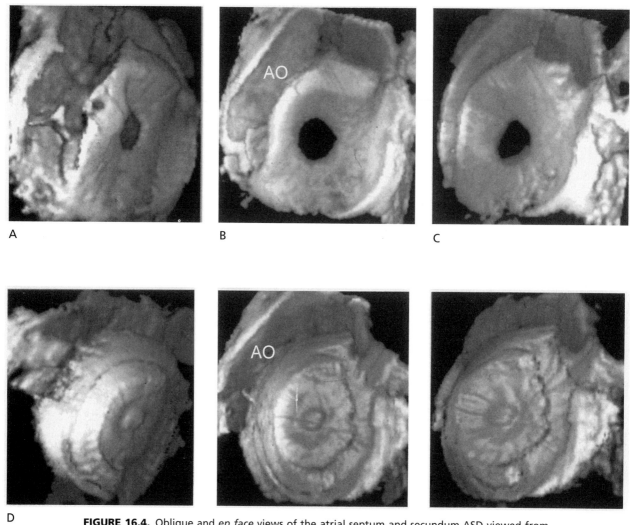

FIGURE 16.4. Oblique and *en face* views of the atrial septum and secundum ASD viewed from the left atrium before **(A, B, C)** and after **(D, E, F)** closure with an Amplatzer Septal Occluder. AO, ascending aorta.

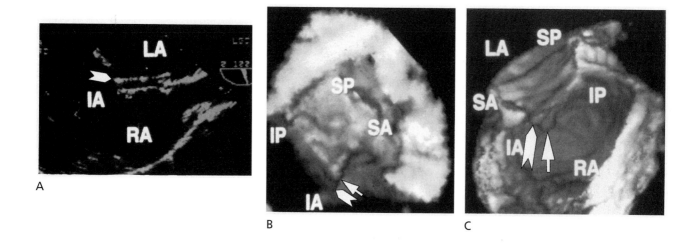

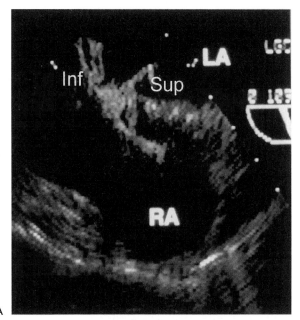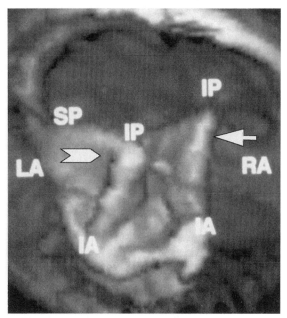

FIGURE 16.6. A: Bicaval 2D view of TEE shows that both inferior parts of the left- and right atrial wings have folded away from the atrial septum. **B:** Three-dimensional reconstruction demonstrates the folding of the wings more clearly. The *notched arrow* depicts the left atrial wing and shows that its SP, IP, and IA corners have folded inward toward each other. The SA corner has folded toward the IA corner, changing the shape of the left atrial wing from a square to a triangle. The normal *arrow* depicts the right atrial wing and shows prolapse of its IA corner into the left atrium. (From Magni G, Hijazi ZM, Pandian NG, et al. Two- and three-dimensional transesophageal echocardiography in patient selection and assessment of atrial septal defect closure by the new Das-Angel Wings device: initial clinical experience. *Circulation* 1997;96:1722–1728, with permission.)

closure. The criteria for using two Amplatzer devices are as follows: (12,13).

1. Adequate size of the atrial septum. Dimension of atrial septum in the plane aligning the defects should be adequate to accommodate two devices and should approach the sum of, larger device size + 7 mm + smaller device size + 5 mm. Usually a larger Amplatzer device has a left sided rim of 7 mm and a smaller device has a rim of 5

mm, which form the basis of this formula. For all practical purposes this can only be performed in older children (>20 kg).
2. Distance between main defect and accessory orifices of more than 7 mm.
3. Accessory orifice of more than 2 mm.

In a recent study, two Amplatzer ASD devices have been used to close more than one ASD in the same patient (12).

FIGURE 16.5. A: Bicaval 2D view of TEE shows the inferior part of the left atrial wing *(notched arrow)* of an Angel Wings device that has prolapsed across the ASD into the right atrium. It is difficult to say from this 2D image exactly which corner of this square wing has prolapsed. LA, left atrium; RA, right atrium **B:** Three-dimensional reconstruction shows that the IA corner *(notched arrow)* of the left atrial wing is displaced into the right atrium. The normal *arrow* depicts the IA corner of the right atrial wing. **C:** Oblique 3D image depicts IA corner *(notched arrow)* of left atrial wing prolapsed into the RA. Adjacent to it is the IA corner *(normal arrow)* of the right atrial wing. See Figure 16.1 for other abbreviations. (From Magni G, Hijazi ZM, Pandian NG, et al. Two- and three-dimensional transesophageal echocardiography in patient selection and assessment of atrial septal defect closure by the new Das-Angel Wings device: initial clinical experience. *Circulation* 1997;96:1722–1728, with permission.)

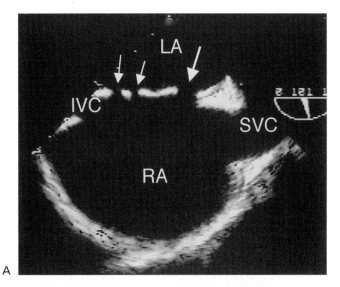

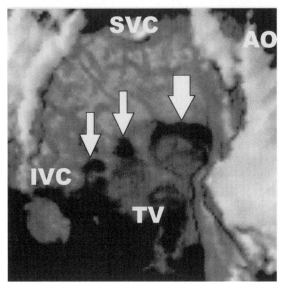

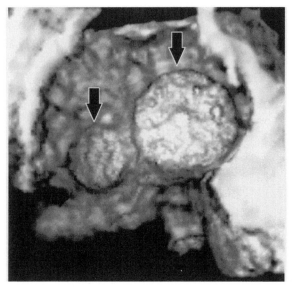

FIGURE 16.7. A: Bicaval 2D view of TEE shows a main defect *(larger white arrow)* and two smaller defects *(smaller white arrows)* in the atrial septum. **B:** Three-dimensional reconstruction shows the *en face* view of the three defects. **C:** Two Amplatzer devices *(black arrows)* are shown *en face*. The larger device closed the main defect and the adjacent one. The smaller device was deployed to close the more remote defect. TV, tricuspid valve. For other abbreviations see previous figures.

During deployment of two devices, 3D echocardiography provides better understanding of the spatial relationship of multiple devices and the orifices (Figure 16.7).

SHORTCOMINGS OF 3D ECHOCARDIOGRAPHY

The drawback of 3D echocardiography is the time taken for reconstruction of the image and the high level of expertise needed to generate these images. Even with the advent of faster computers and in the most experienced hands, it takes approximately 5 minutes for acquisition and postprocessing and 15 minutes to reconstruct the images that provide full understanding of the atrial septal anatomy prior to closure. Presently, 3D reconstructions are performed off-

line. New technology for on-line 3D reconstruction is just starting to emerge. This will make it an appealing imaging modality in the catheterization laboratory.

EVOLVING ADVANCES AND FUTURE DIRECTIONS

Multidimensional imaging for guiding procedures such as ASD closure is likely to see further developments. Speed of acquisition should improve, and with faster image processing, 3D usage will be even more practical in the interventional laboratory. Real-time 3D echocardiography is an exciting new area of cardiac imaging. By recording a volumetric data set of the entire heart and with on-line 3D reconstruction, one can appreciate the dynamic morphology of all cardiac chambers while an interventional procedure is being performed. At the present time, real-time 3D echocardiography is applicable only to transthoracic imaging. Development of a TEE probe equipped for real-time 3D imaging would be the next logical step. An alternate approach is 3D imaging with the use of intracardiac ultrasound catheters. Currently available intracardiac ultrasound catheters are either too big or too limited in imaging depth. The development of smaller intracardiac ultrasound catheters with adequate imaging depth could make the ultrasound guidance easier and more practical. Such catheters would avoid the use of transesophageal probes that interfere with fluoroscopic images during the interventional procedure. Another exciting prospect is that of solid modeling of the heart and its lesions. By using the digital images obtained from a 3D dataset, one can produce an exact physical replica of the human heart. This could have uses in detailing the geometry of the cardiac lesions and in designing corrective devices. With all its versatility, 3D imaging has the potential for becoming a routine modality for guiding interventional procedures in the future.

ACKNOWLEDGMENT

We wish to acknowledge the dedication and hard work of our former fellows, Drs. Wei Zhu and Giuseppina Magni, in generating the 3D images depicted in this chapter. We also wish to thank Ms. Santhini Ramasamy for her excellent graphic skills.

REFERENCES

1. Banerjee A, Bengur AR, Li J, et al. Echocardiographic characteristics of successful deployment of the Das Angel Wings atrial septal defect closure device: initial multicenter experience in the United States. *Am J Cardiol* 1999;83:1236–1241.

2. Hellenbrand WE, Fahey JT, McGowan FX, et al. Transesophageal echocardiographic guidance of transcatheter closure of atrial septal defect. *Am J Cardiol* 1990;66:207–213.

3. Belohlavek M, Foley D, Gerber TC, et al. Three-dimensional ultrasound imaging of the atrial septum: normal and pathologic anatomy. *J Am Coll Cardiol* 1993;22:1673–1678.

4. Marx GR, Fulton DR, Pandian NG, et al. Delineation of site, relative size and dynamic geometry of atrial septal defects by real-time three-dimensional echocardiography. *J Am Coll Cardiol* 1995;25:482–490.

5. Magni G, Cao QL, Sugeng L, et al. Volume-rendered, three-dimensional echocardiographic determination of the size, shape, and position of atrial septal defects: validation in an *in vitro* model. *Am Heart J* 1996;132:376–381.

6. Franke A, Kuhl HP, Rulands D, et al. Quantitative analysis of the morphology of secundum-type atrial septal defects and their dynamic change using transesophageal three-dimensional echocardiography. *Circulation* 1997;96(Suppl):II-323–II-327.

7. Dall'Agata A, McGhie J, Taams MA, et al. Secundum atrial septal defect is a dynamic three-dimensional entity. *Am Heart J* 1999;137:1075–1081.

8. Magni G, Hijazi ZM, Pandian NG, et al. Two- and three-dimensional transesophageal echocardiography in patient selection and assessment of atrial septal defect closure by the new Das-Angel Wings device: initial clinical experience. *Circulation* 1997;96: 1722–1728.

9. Acar P, Saliba Z, Bonhoeffer P, et al. Influence of atrial septal defect anatomy in patients selection and assessment of closure with the CardioSEAL device; a three-dimensional transesophageal echocardiographic reconstruction. *Eur Heart J* 2000; 21:573–581.

10. Rao PS, Langhough R. Relationship of echocardiographic shunt flow and angiographic size to the stretched diameter of the atrial septal defect. *Am Heart J* 1991;122:505–508.

11. Zhu W, Cao Q-L, Rhodes J, et al. Measurement of atrial septal defect size: a comparative study between three-dimensional transesophageal echocardiography and the standard balloon sizing methods. *Pediatr Cardiol* 2000;21:465–469.

12. Cao Q, Radtke W, Berger F, et al. Transcatheter closure of multiple atrial septal defects. Initial results and value of two- and three-dimensional transesophageal echocardiography. *Eur Heart J* 2000;21:941–947.

13. Banerjee A, Cao Q, Zhu W, et al. Echocardiographic characteristics of transcatheter closure of multiple atrial septal defects: a multicenter experience. *J Am Soc Echocardiogr* 1999;12:802B.

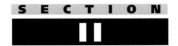
TRANSCATHETER OCCLUSION OF PATENT DUCTUS ARTERIOSUS

17

HISTORY OF TRANSCATHETER PATENT DUCTUS ARTERIOSUS CLOSURE DEVICES

P. SYAMASUNDAR RAO

Since the description of successful surgical ligation of patent ductus arteriosus (PDA) by Gross and Hubbard (1) in 1939, surgery has been used extensively in the treatment of PDA. Surgical treatment has been shown to be safe and effective with only occasional complications. However, cardiologists have been attempting to develop less invasive, transcatheter methodology to occlude the PDA. The pioneering efforts of Porstmann (2–4), Rashkind (5,6), and their associates paved the way to the development of a number of transcatheter methods of PDA closure. This chapter reviews historical development of transcatheter PDA closure technology.

Based on our own reviews (7–9) and those of others (10,11), as well as an extensive literature search, historical developments of transcatheter occlusion of PDA are tabulated (Tables 17.1 and 17.2). The sequence of listing is primarily determined by priority of publication. Table 17.1 lists devices/methods that have been utilized in human subjects, whereas Table 17.2 shows devices that have undergone testing in *in vitro* and/or animal experimental models but have not reached the stage of human clinical trials.

PORSTMANN IVALON PLUG

Porstmann and his associates were the first to develop and utilize the transcatheter technique to occlude PDA (2–4). The device consists of conical-shaped Ivalon foam plastic plug, prepared based on the shape and size of the ductus visualized on the lateral view of an aortogram. Initially, a guide wire (0.04 mm) loop from the femoral artery, aorta, ductus, pulmonary artery, right ventricle, right atrium, and inferior vena cava to the femoral vein was established. The Ivalon prosthesis was inserted over the guide wire into the

femoral artery via a tubular applicator. The plug was advanced with a catheter, still over the guide wire, and rammed into the aortic ampulla of the PDA. Following confirmation of closure of the ductus by various methods, including aortography, the guide wire loop was withdrawn from the femoral vein. Heparin was used during the proce-

TABLE 17.1. TRANSCATHETER PDA DEVICES THAT HAVE UNDERGONE HUMAN CLINICAL TRIALS

Authors (Ref)	Year	Description of the Devices
Porstmann et al. (2,3)	1967	Conical-shaped Ivalon foam plug
Rashkind and Cuaso (5)	1979	Polyurethane foam-covered single umbrella with miniature hooks
Rashkind (6)	1983	Two opposing polyurethane-covered umbrellas
Saveliev et al. (12,13)	1984, 1988	Polyurethane foam plug, Botallo-occluder
Sideris et al. (14)	1990	Two polyurethane foam discs attached to each other with elastic thread
Rao et al. (15,16)	1991	Square-shaped polyurethane occluder and rhomboid-shaped counter-occluded attached to each other *in vivo* by buttoning
Bridges et al. (17)	1991	Clamshell ASD device
Cambier et al. (18)	1992	Gianturco coil
Le et al. (19)	1993	Duct-occlude pfm
Cambier et al. (20)	1993	Cook detachable coil
Uzun et al. (21)	1996	Flipper detachable coil
Grifka et al. (22)	1996	Gianturco-Grifka Sac
Grabitz et al. (23)	1997	Polyvinyl alcohol foam plug mounted on titanium core pin
Masura et al. (24)	1998	Amplatzer duct-occluder
Rao et al. (25)	1999	Folding plug buttoned device
Sideris et al. (26)	2001	Wireless PDA devices

ASD, atrial septal defect; PDA, patent ductus arteriosus.

P. Syamasundar Rao: Professor of Pediatrics, Medicine, and Cardiology, Department of Pediatrics, University of Texas-Houston Medical School; Director, Division of Pediatric Cardiology, Memorial Hermann Children's Hospital, Houston, Texas

TABLE 17.2. EXPERIMENTALLY USED PDA CLOSURE DEVICES

Authors (Ref)	Year	Description of Device
Mills and King (27)	1976	Dumbbell-shaped plug
Leslie et al. (28)	1977	Cylindrical Ivalon sponge plug tied securely to a stainless steel umbrella
Warnecke et al. (29)	1986	Detachable silicone double-balloon
Magal et al. (30)	1989	Conical nylon sack filled with segments of modified guide wire with a 1.5-cm-long flexible wire cross bar attached to the distal end of the sack
Echigo et al. (31)	1990	Temperature–shape changeable, shape–memory polymer (polynorbornene)
Nazarian et al. (32)	1993	Butterfly vascular stent plug
Pozza et al. (33)	1995	Conical-shaped stainless steel wire mesh
Liu et al. (34, 35)	1993, 1996	Thermal shape–memory nickel–titanium coil
Grabitz et al. (36)	1996	Miniaturized duct-occluder pfm

PDA, patent ductus arteriosus.

dure. The device and materials used and various steps of the procedure were described in explicit detail in their 1971 review in the *Radiological Clinics of North America* (4). Animal experimentation was undertaken initially to develop and refine the method. Porstmann and associates' first clinical cohort consisted of 62 patients. Successful catheter closure was accomplished in 56 (90%) of these patients. In the remaining six (10%) patients, it was not technically feasible to implant the Ivalon plug. Successful closure required that the ductus be conical in shape and that the femoral artery diameter be larger than the plug required to close the ductus. There was no mortality, and the morbidity was minor. During a follow-up period of up to 4.5 years, no recurrences were observed. Because of the large applicator (16 to 22F) necessary to insert the plug into the femoral artery, only five patients less than 10 years of age were among Porstmann's initial 62 patients (4). In a later publication (37), Porstmann's group reported a larger experience involving 208 patients, ages 5 to 62 years. Successful Ivalon plug closure of the ductus was accomplished in 95% of patients. Follow-up evaluation by auscultation and phonocardiography revealed no recanalization. Slippage of the Ivalon plug in 23 (11%) of 197 patients and arterial complications in 16 (8%) of 197 patients were also observed. Several other groups of workers in Europe and Japan adopted this technique and reported varying success rates (38–46). By 1985, the Porstmann's method was used in 800 patients, as estimated by Wierney et al. (37). Some modifications of the technique introduced by Porstmann and Wierney (37,47)

and other workers (38–46) have resulted in use of this technique in children down to 4 years of age. Although Porstmann's method has been known for more than three decades, it has not been widely adopted, presumably because of complexity of the procedure, the requirement of a large-caliber applicator to introduce the plugs, and the need for the transarterial route.

EXPERIMENTALLY ATTEMPTED DUCTAL CLOSURE DEVICES

Most devices that follow their design are tested in animal experimental models and then in human trials. However, several devices have been used in experimental models, but did not undergo human application, for a number of reasons. These devices (Table 17.2) will be reviewed in this section.

Mills and King (27) utilized a dumbbell-shaped plug and a Dacron-covered umbrella to occlude experimentally created PDAs in dogs. Successful closure was achieved in five (50%) of ten dogs in which they attempted device deployment. All five successful PDA closures remained occluded 6 months later. The authors sought to develop a safe procedure to treat a number of problematic PDAs through improvements in miniaturization.

Leslie and his colleagues (28) attempted to occlude surgically created aortopulmonary shunts in 13 mongrel dogs with Ivalon sponge plugs sutured onto stainless steel umbrellas. In ten (77%) of the experiments, they successfully occluded the shunt. They concluded that their technique has potential for use in patients with small and long PDAs.

Warnecke and her associates (29) designed a 5- and 6F triple-lumen catheter with a detachable silicone double balloon at its tip. This device was used to occlude experimentally created PDAs in beagles. Successful closure was accomplished in 15 (71%) of 21 experimental subjects. The authors believe that their method has advantages over other methods and that their technique may be suitable for children with PDA.

Megal et al. (30) employed Nylon sack with a crossbar filled with segments of guide wire to occlude vascular channels in mongrel dogs. The device was successfully deployed in all ten dogs with complete occlusion of the recipient vessel. Follow-up arteriograms revealed that complete occlusion was maintained. The authors concluded that the device is far from ideal and that additional research is needed to evaluate stability of the device.

Echigo et al. (31) designed an occluder device made up of temperature-shape changeable shape-memory polymer (polynorbornone). The device can be inserted transvenously across the PDA. Injection of hot (45°C) water via catheter causes expansion of the device, thus occluding the PDA. *In vitro* PDA model was used to test the device, which demonstrated feasibility of the method. *In vivo* testing in piglets was said to be in progress (31). The conclusion was that the technique might have clinical application.

Nazarian et al. (32) tested four variations of vascular stent plugs. Each type had a different type of constriction of the stent. The butterfly device was tested in occluding surgically created aortopulmonary Gore-Tex shunts, simulating PDAs. Of the ten attempts, three (30%) devices were misplaced. Shunt occlusion by color Doppler was demonstrated by 1 to 2 days. Mild hemolysis was present in two dogs in which serum haptoglobin was measured. The authors conclude that the balloon-expandable vascular plugs show promise but that modification of the delivery system is necessary to reduce the incidence of misplacement of the device.

Pozza and his colleagues (33) described a self-expanding, conically shaped stainless steel wire mesh device with four hooks at its base to secure the device in the ductus and with a screw thread at the apex for attachment to a long delivery stylet for closure of PDA. The device was deployed through a 6F delivery system to occlude aortopulmonary Gore-Tex shunts (simulating PDA) in 20 mongrel dogs. The device was deployed in 18 animals but was in secure position in 13. Complete occlusion was demonstrated in 60 minutes in eight dogs (44%). By 1 week 12 dogs (67%) were completely occluded, and by 3 months there was 93% occlusion. The authors state that further design modifications are being considered before embarking on clinical trials.

Liu et al. utilized a thermal shape-memory nickel-titanium occlusion coil to test its effectiveness in *in vitro* (34) models and in *in vivo* (35) experimental PDA models. Of the ten attempted implantations, the coil was successfully implanted in eight (80%) on first attempt. Complete occlusion of PDA model was demonstrated by angiography at 24 hours after the procedure in seven (70%) of ten mongrel dogs. In full occlusions, complete thrombosis of the coiled segment was demonstrated at necropsy, while only partial thrombosis was found in partially occluded vessel. Thrombus formation was not detected at any other site. They concluded that shape-memory coil delivered via 7F sheath is effective in occluding small-diameter PDA models.

Grabitz et al. (36) employed a miniaturized version of duct-occlude (19) to evaluate its efficacy in neonatal piglet PDAs. The device is a biconical, double-disk coil made up of shape-memory metal wire designed to cause mechanical and thrombotic closure of PDA. The device is delivered via 3F catheter. The device was implanted successfully in all piglet PDAs, which were maintained patent either by stents (*N* = 6) or by balloon angioplasty (*N* = 7). The ductus was completely occluded within 1 hour of the procedure in 13 (87%) piglets. No device dislodgments were noted. Angiography 16 to 73 days after the procedure showed complete occlusion in all piglets. The authors concluded that the device was effective in occluding experimental neonatal PDAs in piglets and the results warrant clinical trials in neonates.

RASHKIND'S HOOKED PROSTHESIS

Rashkind designed a single polyurethane foam-covered umbrella with miniature hooks (fish hooks) to occlude the PDA (5,6). The prosthesis was attached to the delivery system by a simple eye pin and sleeve mechanism. The entire device could be loaded into a 6F sheath and introduced via the femoral artery. In the experimental calf model, there was a 100% rate of success. Of the 20 patients with intent to occlude, the device was implanted successfully in 17 (85%). In two, the device was not implanted because the ductus was too large by balloon sizing. In the third, the prosthesis embolized into a peripheral pulmonary artery. Eight (47%) of the 17 patients had complete closure. In the remaining patients with incomplete closure, uneventful surgical closure was accomplished. In two of these in whom the device was embolized into the pulmonary artery branches, the device was successfully retrieved via a catheter snare. Rashkind (6) concluded that while the results are encouraging, they are not adequate.

RASHKIND PDA OCCLUDER SYSTEM

Following experimental and clinical experience with the hooked prosthesis (6,48), Rashkind observed (a) difficulty in manipulating/repositioning the prosthesis once extruded from the catheter delivery system, (b) high incidence of incomplete closures, (c) improper implantation, and (d) prosthesis embolization. Therefore he redesigned the system into a double-disk, nonhooked device (6,48). The device consisted of two opposing umbrellas made up of polyurethane foam disks mounted on three stainless steel arms attached to a central spring mechanism. A knuckle and sleeve mechanism was introduced to lock the device at the time of loading and unlock it following implantation. Two sizes were manufactured, 12 and 17 mm in diameter. The device is delivered into the ductus transvenously in contradistinction to transarterial device delivery required with Porstmann's Ivalon plug and Rashkind's single-disk hooked device. Implantation of the devices required 8- and 11F sheaths, respectively, for 12- and 17-mm devices, although front-loading modification (49) allowed device delivery via smaller sheaths.

Experimental testing in animal models in 19 calves and swine revealed successful implantation in all (48). Postmortem examination of an occluded ductus demonstrated sealing of aortic and pulmonary ends of the ductus with heavy tissue in growth. In five animals where the device was intentionally released into a branch pulmonary artery, the device tended to rest on the side of the vessel and to become embedded into the vessel wall without complete occlusion of the vessel (48). In another experimental study in 12 piglets, nine (75%) successful implantations and closures were observed (50). Four complications occurred and included device embolization into the left pulmonary artery ($N = 1$) or femoral artery ($N = 1$), torn pulmonary valve cusp ($N = 1$), and misplacement of the device on a pulmonary valve cusp ($N = 1$) (50).

Rashkind (6), in his initial experience with eight patients, found three (38%) PDAs too large to attempt closure, four (50%) successful closures, and one (13%) incomplete closure. In a multicenter FDA protocol organized by Rashkind (48), successful closure was reported in 94 (64%) of 146 patients. Device embolization in 19 (15%) and significant residual shunts in 15 (10%) were also observed. With experience the results improved in the latter part of the study. Successful closure rates increased to 78% and the device embolization rate decreased to 10% of patients. Subsequently, the device underwent clinical trials performed by these (48) and other investigators (51–58). Successful implantations were reported in 72% to 81% patients. Detailed analysis of differing outcomes (59) suggested lack of influence of age and weight of the patient as well as the institution where the procedure was performed. However, improvement over time (47% in 1982 to 83% in 1987) and lower ductal occlusion rates with increasing PDA sizes (87% in PDAs of 1.5 to 2.5 mm versus 47% in PDAs of 4.1 to 9.0 mm minimal ductal diameters) was observed (59). Further discussion of the Rashkind PDA occluder may be found in the next chapter.

BOTALLO-OCCLUDER

Saveliev, Prokubovski, Verin, and their associates, beginning in the early 1980s, conceived, developed, and used transcatheter occlusion with a polyurethane device and named it the Botallo-Occluder (12,13,60,61). The device consists of a conical polyurethane foam plug mounted on a stainless steel frame that can be compressed for loading into a delivery sheath. The thinner pulmonary end contains a simple bolt-and-nut, attach–release mechanism to which the stainless steel delivery stylet is screwed. The devices are made in four sizes: 8, 10, 12, and 14 mm in diameter at the aortic end. These devices can be delivered via 10-, 12-, 14-, and 16F sheaths, respectively. During a 10-year period preceding 1991, 307 patients 2 to 43 years of age underwent catheterization with intent to occlude. The device was implanted in 273 (89%) patients; the remaining 34 (11%) patients were considered not suitable candidates for closure for varied reasons. Device embolization or misplacement occurred in ten (4%) patients. Seven underwent surgery and three had larger devices placed successfully. Eight (3%) patients had residual shunts, four required surgery, and four

were considered to have insignificant shunt. The authors stated that their results improved in their more recent experience; in the last 100 cases, there were only one embolization and two incomplete closures. Although the results look good, the requirement for a large delivery sheath is a drawback. No further reports have been published. Apparently, the device is not currently in use (*personal communication,* Dr. V. E. Verin, December 2000).

BUTTONED DEVICE

A self-adjustable buttoned device was developed by Sideris and his coworkers (14). The device consisted of two polyurethane foam disks, each mounted on a single wire skeleton, attached to each other by an elastic thread. The device was delivered transarterially via a 6F sheath. Successful device implantation and occlusion of PDA were demonstrated in all 11 piglets in which they attempted the procedure. This device was modified, incorporating the principles of the atrial septal defect occlusion device (62), and its feasibility, safety, and effectiveness in occluding PDA were tested initially in limited clinical trials (15,16,63). The device consists of an occluder, counteroccluder, and delivery system. The occluder consists of an x-shaped, Teflon-coated stainless steel wire covered with 0.0625-inch-thick polyurethane foam and can be folded for introduction into a 7F sheath. An-8 mm string loop is attached to the center of the occluder, which has two knots (buttons) 4 and 8 mm from the occluder. Radiopaque material is incorporated into the proximal (farthest from the occluder) knot. The counteroccluder consists of a single-strand Teflon-coated stainless steel wire skeleton covered with a rhomboid-shaped polyurethane foam. A latex piece sutured into its center becomes a buttonhole. Fifteen- and 20-mm devices are manufactured. For larger PDAs, larger devices used for atrial septal defect closure may be used (25,26). The occluder and the counteroccluder are positioned across the ductus, introduced transvenously (16). If the ductus is short, the counteroccluder is advanced across both buttons, and if the PDA is long, buttoning across only the proximal radiopaque button is adequate, thus the name *adjustable buttoned device* (16). In more recent clinical trials (25,64) both knots are made radiopaque with spring buttons. Immediate (15,16,25,63, 64) and follow-up (25,64) results in children (15,16,25) and adults (63,64) indicate excellent results. To decrease the prevalence of residual shunts at implantation, a folding plug was incorporated over the button loop (25,26). Most recent innovations include introduction of wireless PDA devices, namely, detachable balloon and transcatheter patch devices for occlusion of large PDAs (26). Detailed discussion of all buttoned devices will be presented in chapters to follow.

CLAMSHELL OCCLUDER

Because of failure to achieve successful occlusion of large PDAs (>4 mm) with the Rashkind PDA occluder, Bridges and her associates employed the Bard clamshell septal umbrella to occlude large PDAs (17). Fourteen patients 0.7 to 30.4 years of age with minimal ductal diameters of 4.5 to 14 mm underwent the procedure. One device migrated into the descending aorta, which was retrieved with a snare and the PDA was closed with a larger device. Complete closures in two (14%), trivial shunts in three (21%), and small shunts in nine (64%) were observed by angiography. At follow-up 1 day to 6 months, complete closure in 11 (79%) and trivial residual shunts in three (21%) were observed. The authors concluded that the clamshell device provides effective occlusion of large PDA not amenable to other transcatheter closure methods. No further experience with this device was reported. The device was removed from further use in clinical trials because of arm fractures observed in the atrial septal defect device during follow-up.

GIANTURCO COIL

Cambier and coworkers were the first to report transcatheter closure of small PDA with Gianturco coils (18). These coils were originally described in 1975 (65) and were used to occlude renal arteries. They have undergone some changes over the years and are now commercially available for clinical use. They are made up of stainless steel wire with thrombogenic Dacron fibers attached to them and are available in a variety of wire diameters, helical decimeters, and lengths. In Cambier's initial experience with occluding very small (≤2.5 mm) PDA in four patients, there were three (75%) successful closures. In the fourth patient with a minimal ductal diameter of 2.5 mm, the coil embolized into the left pulmonary artery, requiring transcatheter retrieval. Subsequent experience from initial investigators and others, extensively referenced and tabulated elsewhere (8,9), has been generally encouraging. Since the first description by Cambier's group (18) a number of modifications and refinements have been undertaken and include snare-assisted coil implantation (66), antegrade coil placement (67), multiple coil delivery (67), bioptome-assisted coil deployment (68), temporary balloon occlusion of the ductus on the aortic (69), or pulmonary artery (70) side during coil deposition, five-loop coil design (71), increased wire diameter to 0.052-inch (72), coil delivery via a tapered-tip catheter (73,74), and coil implantation without the use of heparin (75). At the time of this writing, Gianturco coil occlusion is the preferred method for closure of very small and small PDAs at most institutions around the world (76). The technique and results of this method of PDA closure will be described in detail in chapter 20 of this book and therefore will not be further dealt with here.

DUCT-OCCLUD

Lê (19,77), Neuss (78), and their colleagues developed a new stainless steel coil without Dacron fibers, which evolved into the currently used Duct-Occlud system. A standard device and a reinforced device are available. In the standard device, a 0.028-inch stainless steel wire coil is configured into an hourglass shape. The diameter of the distal (aortic) end is larger than the proximal (pulmonary) end. In the reinforced device, a thicker (0.032-inch) double-strand wire is used, the windings are stiffer, it has a cone shape, and the proximal windings are wound in a reversed direction. A movable hollow wire mounted onto the proximal part of core wire along with stainless steel pins attached to it serves to control the delivery of the device and can be detached following implantation. The standard device is delivered transvenously via 4F catheter, whereas the reinforced device requires a 5F catheter.

Surgically created aortopulmonary Gore-Tex grafts (77) in neonatal piglets in whom stents were implanted into ductus to keep it open (78) and neonatal lambs whose PDAs were kept open by balloon dilataion (79) served as animal models to test the device. Successful implantation of the coil in most experiments and full occlusion of most PDAs demonstrated feasibility and effectiveness of the device. Studies in human subjects (80) revealed successful device deployment in 44 (86%) of 51 patients; three (5.8%) device embolizations occurred. Complete occlusion was demonstrated by color flow Doppler in 40 (91%) of 44 patients. The authors concluded that this detachable coil system compares favorably with other catheter-directed methods, and the small delivery system is useful for use in young children. Other studies describing further details of its use will be discussed in chapter 22.

DETACHABLE COILS

Whereas the Gianturco coil has been successfully used in occlusion of PDA, lack of controlled delivery and ability to retrieve and reposition the coil are impossible. Therefore detachable coils have been developed. Two different designs have been undertaken. The first type of detachable coil has a mechanism in which the notch of the stretched coil winding interlocks with the bead at the end of the core wire in the delivery catheter (20). Once the coil is positioned appropriately, it can be released by the handle at the proximal (outside the patient) end of the delivery catheter. The system (Cook detachable coil) was tested in 11 newborn lamb and goat models, and the results revealed successful delivery of 0.038-inch coils at the intended vascular site, including PDAs without embolization. However, the system requires a 5- or 6F catheter for delivery. Although systematic studies to close human PDAs have not been published, the device has been used successfully to occlude aortopulmonary surgical shunts (81). The second design is also a Gianturco coil, but with an added short, threaded extension at its proximal end. This is attached to the distal end of the delivery wire, which provides for control delivery and retrieval when required. Following implantation at the desired location, the delivery wire is unscrewed from the coil, thus releasing the coil. This is also called the "Flipper" detachable coil. The initial reported experience (21) was in 43 patients. Embolization into the pulmonary artery occurred in three (7%) patients in the catheterization laboratory and in two (5%) after reaching the ward. Complete occlusion of the PDA was achieved in the catheterization laboratory in 26 (60%) patients. By next morning, the occlusion rate increased to 72%, which increased to 86% by 3 months. A number of other reports followed, which will be reviewed in a separate chapter on detachable coils.

GIANTURCO-GRIFKA VASCULAR OCCLUSION DEVICE

The Gianturco-Grifka vascular occlusion device (GGVOD), consisting of a flexible nylon sac and an occluding wire (22), may have been a further modification of Megal's nylon sac with a crossbar (30), which has been experimented with in the late 1980s. The GGVOD is manufactured in 3-, 5-, 7-, and 9-mm sizes, all of which can be deployed via 8F sheaths. In an acute animal model, the feasibility of implantation into subclavian, renal, and carotid arteries was demonstrated (82). Device embolizations have not occurred and there was complete occlusion of the vessel into which the GGVOD was implanted. In a second series of experiments (82) aortopulmonary Gore-Tex shunts were created, which were occluded with GGVOD. During a 2- to 6-month follow-up, complete closure of the shunt was observed, along with good endothelialization. Clinical use in human subjects followed (22,83). Of the 32 PDAs measuring 2.6 to 6.9 mm (median, 4.1), occluded with GGVOD, 20 (62%) had complete closure; 12 (38%) had minute residual shunt through the neck of the sack. Complete occlusion was demonstrated in 29 (91%) by 24 hours and in 31 (97%) by 1 month after implantation. The remaining patient was found to have complete occlusion by 8 months. The authors conclude the GGVOD has become another important tool in the transcatheter armamentarium (83). A more detailed discussion of this device is included in chapter 23 in this book.

POLYVINYL ALCOHOL FOAM PLUG

Grabitz et al. (23) utilized polyvinyl alcohol (Ivalon R) foam plug mounted on a titanium core pin with Nitinol legs at both ends (four at the aortic end and two at the pulmonary end) to occlude PDAs in lambs. In all 11 lambs the device was successfully implanted across the ductus. However, in only three (27%) of 11 was the ductus completely closed on aortography. At a mean of 112 days, the ductus was demonstrated closed by aortography in seven (64%) of 11 lambs. In subsequent clinical studies in 16 patients, ages 13 to 72 years (mean, 43), with PDAs ranging in size from 3 to 6.5 mm (mean, 5), 8- to 16-mm-diameter foam plugs were implanted via 10- to 16F sheaths. Successful device deployment was possible in 15 (94%) patients. In the remaining patient, the foam plug embolized into the left pulmonary artery but was retrieved with a snare. Complete occlusion was documented in 14 (88%) of 16 patients by Doppler studies performed on the day of procedure. In the remaining two, the residual shunts spontaneously closed at 12 and 24 months after device placement, respectively. In a later multicenter clinical study of 100 patients, Schräder et al. (84) reported successful device placement in 88% patients at first attempt. Malposition ($N = 12$) or embolization ($N = 3$) occurred in 15 patients, but the device was retrieved in all but one. Following a second or third attempt, the overall device placement was successful in 98% of patients. Complete occlusion by aortography and color Doppler was demonstrated in 85% of patients; the larger the ductus, the greater the percentage of residual shunt. During follow-up no late complications were encountered, but reintervention to close residual shunt by another device ($N = 1$), coils ($N = 2$), and surgery ($N = 1$) was undertaken. Complete closure was achieved in 89% of patients at a median follow-up of 16 months. The authors concluded that their system is a valuable addition to other methods of treatment of PDA and that technical modifications are necessary to reduce the prevalence of residual shunts. This device has some similarities with Porstmann's Ivalon plug and the Botallo Occluder, although the authors have not acknowledged this.

AMPLATZER DUCT OCCLUDER

Musura and his associates (24) were the first to report clinical use Amplatzer Duct Occluder. The device is constructed with 0.004-inch-thick Nitinol wire mesh, mushroom in shape and self-expandable in design. The devices are 7 mm long; the aortic end is 2 mm larger than the pulmonary end. A thin retention disk is located on the aortic side, 4 mm larger than the aortic diameter of the device. A recessed screw is built into the pulmonary end for connection to the delivery wire. Polyester fibers are sewn into the device to induce thrombosis after implantation. The devices, depending on the size of the device, can be delivered via 6- to 8F sheaths. In the initial, experimental phase, the device was tested to occlude surgically created aortopulmonary shunts in 19 dogs (85). Device misplacement occurred in one (5%) dog. In the remaining 18, complete closure was documented in 39% in 30 minutes, 71% in 1 week, 82% in 1 month, and 92% in 3 months after implantation. When a comparison between the devices filled with and without polyester was made, there were higher occlusion rates with polyester-filled devices. The authors concluded that the device has advantages because of the small delivery system, ease of placement, ability to self-center, facility with which it is repositioned, and fact that the polyester-filled prosthesis produces immediate shunt closure.

The device was used in clinical trials in 24 patients (24) 0.4 to 48 years of age (median, 3.8). Successful implantation was accomplished in 23 (96%) patients. Angiography immediately following closure revealed complete closure in seven (30%). The remaining 16 had foaming through the device (N = 14) or a small residual shunt (N = 2). Color Doppler studies on the morning following the procedure revealed complete occlusion in all 23 patients. The authors concluded that transvenous closure of PDA with the new device is an effective therapy for patients with minimal ductal diameters of up to 6 mm. A number of studies were performed subsequently and will be reviewed in chapter 24.

FOLDING-PLUG BUTTONED DEVICE

The results of buttoned-device occlusion (25) revealed residual shunts in 40% of patients at implantation. Most of these closed during follow-up. During the follow-up those patients who did not have complete closure at implantation are at risk for endocarditis until closure. To decrease the residual shunt rate, a plug of polyurethane was incorporated over the buttoned loop of the device; this decreased the residual shunts (25,26). Further discussion will be presented in the chapter dealing with the buttoned device.

WIRELESS PDA DEVICES

To avoid wire-related problems and to increase the ability to close large (huge) PDAs, detachable balloons and transcatheter patches were developed (Chapter 9) (26). The data in animal models and preliminary data in human subjects (Chapter 9) (26) appear encouraging.

SUMMARY AND CONCLUSION

Historical aspects related to the development of transcatheter-delivered devices to occlude PDAs were reviewed in this chapter. A number of devices have been developed since the first description of transcatheter closure of PDA by Porstmann in the late 1960s. Some are tested in *in vitro* and in *in vivo* animal models, and others have been tried in human subjects. Design, redesign, testing and retesting, and further refinement have been the case with most devices. Gianturco coils and Gianturco-Grifka sac are the only two types of PDA closure devices that are currently available for routine clinical use. The remaining devices have not received approval from the appropriate regulatory authority but are available for use at institutions participating in clinical trials with a particular device. It is hoped that some of these will receive approval in the near future and become available for use.

REFERENCES

1. Gross RE, Hubbard JP. Surgical ligation of a patent ductus arteriosus: a report of first successful case. *JAMA* 1939;112:729–731.
2. Porstmann W, Wierny L, Warnke H. Der Verschluß des Ductus arteriosus persistens ohne Thorakotomie (Vorläufige, Mitteilung). *Thoraxchirurgie* 1967;15:109–203.
3. Porstmann W, Wierney L, Warnke H. Closure of persistent ductus arteriosus without thoracotomy. *German Med Monthly* 1967; 12:259–261.
4. Porstmann W, Wierny L, Warnke H, et al. Catheter closure of patent ductus arteriosus: 62 cases treated without thoracotomy. *Radiol Clin North Am* 1971;9:203–218.
5. Rashkind WJ, Cuaso CC. Transcatheter closure of a patent ductus arteriosus: successful use in a 3.5-kg infant. *Pediatr Cardiol* 1979;1:3–7.
6. Rashkind WJ. Transcatheter treatment of congenital heart disease. *Circulation* 1983;67:711–716.
7. Rao PS. Historical aspects of therapeutic catheterization. In: Rao PS, ed. *Transcatheter therapy in pediatric cardiology*, Mt. Kisco, NY: Futura, 1993:1–6.
8. Rao PS, Sideris EB. Transcatheter closure of patent ductus arteriosus: state of the art. *J Invasive Cardiol* 1996;8:278–288.
9. Rao PS. Transcatheter occlusion of patent ductus arteriosus: which method to use and which ductus to close? (Editorial). *Am Heart J* 1996;132:905–909.
10. Rashkind WJ, Tait MA, Gibbon RJ, Jr. Interventional cardiac catheterization in congenital heart disease. *Int J Cardiol* 1985;7: 1–11.
11. Sandhu SK, King TD. Historical aspects of transcatheter closure of the patent ductus arteriosus. *Curr Interv Cardiol Rep* 2000;2: 361–366.
12. Saveliev VS, Prokubovski VI, Kolody SM, et al. Interventional radiology: new directions in prophylaxis and treatment of surgical disease. *Khirurgiia (Mosk)* 1984;8:113–117.
13. Prokubovski, Kolody SM, Saveliev SV, et al. Transluminal closure of the patent ductus arteriosus with transvenous approach: alternative to surgery. *Grad Khirurgiia* 1988;1:42–47.
14. Sideris EB, Sideris SE, Ehly RL. Occlusion of patent ductus arteriosus in piglets by a double disk self-adjustable device (Abstract). *J Am Coll Cardiol* 1990;15:240A.
15. Rao PS, Wilson AD, Sideris EB, et al. Transcatheter closure of patent ductus arteriosus with buttoned device: first successful clinical application in a child. *Am Heart J* 1991;121:1799–1802.
16. Rao PS, Sideris EB, Haddad J, et al. Transcatheter occlusion of

patent ductus arteriosus with adjustable buttoned device: initial clinical experience. *Circulation* 1993;88:1119–1126.

17. Bridges ND, Perry SB, Parness I, et al. Transcatheter closure of a large patent ductus arteriosus with the clamshell septal umbrella. *J Am Coll Cardiol* 1991;18:1297–1302.

18. Cambier PA, Kirby WC, Wortham DC, et al. Percutaneous closure of small (<2.5 mm) patent ductus arteriosus using coil embolization. *Am J Cardiol* 1992;69:815–816.

19. Lê TP, Neuss MB, Redel DA, et al. A new transcatheter occlusion technique with retrievable double disk shaped coils: first clinical results in occlusion of patent ductus arteriosus. *Cardiol Young* 1993;3:I-38.

20. Cambier PA, Stajduhar KC, Powell D, et al. Improved safety of transcatheter vascular occlusion utilizing a new retrievable coil device. *J Am Coll Cardiol* 1994;23:359A.

21. Ozun O, Hancock S, Parsons JM, et al. Transcatheter occlusion of the arterial duct with Cook detachable coils: early experience. *Heart* 1996;176:269–273.

22. Grifka RG, Vincent JA, Nihill MR, et al. Transcatheter patent ductus arteriosus closure in an infant using Gianturco-Grifka device. *Am J Cardiol* 1996;15:78:721–723.

23. Grabitz RG, Schräder R, Sigler M, et al. Retrievable patent ductus arteriosus plug for interventional transvenous occlusion of the patent ductus arteriosus: evaluation in lambs and preliminary clinical results. *Invest Radiol* 1997;32:523–528.

24. Masura J, Walsh KP, Thanopoulos B, et al. Catheter closure of moderate-to-large-sized patent ductus arteriosus using new Amplatzer Duct Occluder; immediate and short-term results. *J Am Coll Cardiol* 1998;31:1878–1882.

25. Rao PS, Kim SH, Choi J, et al. Follow-up results of transvenous occlusion of patent ductus arteriosus with the buttoned device. *J Am Coll Cardiol* 1999;33:820–826.

26. Sideris EB, Rao PS, Zamora R. The Sideris' buttoned devices for transcatheter closure of patent ductus arteriosus. *J Interv Cardiol* 2001;14:239–246.

27. Mills NL, King TD. Non-operative closure of left-to-right shunts: *J Thorac Cardiovasc Surg* 1976;72:371–378.

28. Leslie J, Lindsay W, Amplatz K. Nonsurgical closure of patent ductus arteriosus: an experimental study. *Invest Radiol* 1977;12:142–145.

29. Warnecke I, Frank J, Hohle R, et al. Transvenous double-balloon occlusion of the persistent ductus arteriosus: an experimental study. *Pediatr Cardiol* 1986;5:79–84.

30. Magal C, Wright KC, Duprat G, et al. A new device for transcatheter closure of patent ductus arteriosus: a feasibility study in dogs. *Invest Radiol* 1989;24:272–276.

31. Echigo S, Matsuda T, Kamiya T, et al. Development of a new transvenous patent ductus arteriosus occlusion technique using a shape memory polymer. *ASAIO Trans* 1990;36:M195–198.

32. Nazarian GK, Qian Z, Vladaver Z, et al. Evaluation of a new vascular occlusion device. *Invest Radiol* 1993;28:1165–1169.

33. Pozza CH, Gomes MR, Qian Z, et al. Transcatheter occlusion of patent ductus arteriosus using a newly developed self-expanding device. *Invest Radiol* 1995;30:104–109.

34. Liu C, Shiraishi H, Yanagisawar M. Effectiveness of patent ductus arteriosus occlusion coil: *in vitro* study. *Jichi Med Schl J* 1993;16:57–65.

35. Liu C, Shiraishi H, Kikuchi Y, et al. Effectiveness of a thermal shape-memory patent ductus arteriosus occlusion coil. *Am Heart J* 1996;131:1018–1023.

36. Grabitz RG, Neuss MB, Coe JY, et al. A small interventional device to occlude persistently patent ductus arteriosus in neonates: evaluation in piglets. *J Am Coll Cardiol* 1996;28:1024–1030.

37. Wierny L, Plass R, Portsmann W. Transluminal closure of patent

ductus arteriosus: long-term results of 208 cases treated without thoracotomy. *Cardiovasc Interv Radiol* 1986;9:279–285.

38. Takamiya M. Ductus closure without thoracotomy. *Jpn J Thorac Surg* 1973;26:749–753.

39. Sato K, Masaoki F, Kozuka T, et al. Transfemoral plug closure of patent ductus arteriosus: experience with 61 consecutive cases. *Circulation* 1975;31:337–341.

40. Kitamura S, Sato K, Naito Y, et al. Plug closure of patent ductus arteriosus by transfemoral catheter method: a comparative study with surgery and a new technical modification. *Chest* 1976;70:631–635.

41. Furukawa S, Toriedo M, Nakayama T, et al. Catheter closure of patent ductus arteriosus without thoracotomy. *Kyobu Geka* 1977;30:673–677.

42. Naito Y, Shirakura R, Matsudo Y, et al. Plug closure of patent ductus arteriosus without thoracotomy: experience in 50 consecutive patients with technical improvements. *Kyobu Geka Gakkai Zasshi* 1977;25:1270–1277.

43. Shimizu Y, Miyamoto T, Horiguchi Y, et al. . [A comparative study with surgical division and plug closure for patent ductus arteriosus (author's transl)]. *Nippon Kyobu Geka Gakkai Zasshi* 1978;26:1093–1104.

44. Bussmann WD, Sievert H, Kaltenbach M, et al. Transfemoraler Verschlusse des Ductus arteriosus persistens. *Dtsch Med Wochenschr* 1984;35:1322–1326.

45. Schrader R. Eine neue methode zum verschlub des persisteirenden ductus arteriosus (Botall). *Herz* 1995;20:146–154.

46. Schrader R, Kadel C, Cieslinski G, et al. Nonthoracotomy closure of persistent ductus arteriosus beyond age 60 years. *Am J Cardiol* 1993;72:1319–1321.

47. Portstmann W, Wierny L. Percutaneous transfemoral closure of patent ductus arteriosus: an alternative to surgery. *Semin Roentgenol* 1981;16:95–102.

48. Rashkind WJ, Mullins CE, Hellenbrand WE, et al. Nonsurgical closure of patent ductus arteriosus: clinical application of the Rashkind PDA occluder system. *Circulation* 1987;75:583–592.

49. Perry SB, Lock JE. Front-loading of double-umbrella devices, a new technique for umbrella delivery for closing cardiovascular defects. *Am J Cardiol* 1992;70:917–920.

50. Lock JE, Bass JL, Lund G, et al. Transcatheter closure of patent ductus arteriosus in piglets. *Am J Cardiol* 1985;55:826–829.

51. Wessel DL, Keane JF, Parness I, et al. Outpatient closure of the patent ductus arteriosus. *Circulation* 1988;77:1068–1071.

52. Dyck JD, Benson LN, Smallhorn JF, et al. Catheter closure of the persistently patent ductus arteriosus. *Am J Cardiol* 1988;62:1089–1092.

53. Latson LA, Hofschire PJ, Kugler JD, et al. Transcatheter closure of patent ductus arteriosus in pediatric patients. *J Pediatr* 1989;115:549–553.

54. Khan MA, Mullins CE, Nihill MR, et al. Percutaneous catheter closure of the ductus arteriosus in children and young adults. *Am J Cardiol* 1989;64:218–221.

55. Hellenbrand WI, Mullins CE. Catheter closure of congenital cardiac defects. *Cardiol Clin* 1989;7:351–368.

56. Nykanen DG, Hayes AM, Benson LN, et al. Transcatheter patent ductus arteriosus occlusion: application in the small child. *J Am Coll Cardiol* 1994;23:1666–1670.

57. Gatzoulis MA, Rigby ML, Redington AN. Umbrella occlusion of persistent arterial duct in children under two years. *Br Heart J* 1994;72:364–377.

58. Report of the European Registry. Transcatheter occlusion of persistent arterial duct. *Lancet* 1992;340:1062–1066.

59. Gray DT, Walker AM, Fyler DC, et al. Examination of the early "learning curve" for transcatheter closure of patent ductus arte-

riosus using the Rashkind occluder. *Circulation* 1994;90:II-36–II-42.

60. Saveliev VS, Prokubovski VI, Kolody SM, et al. Patent ductus arteriosus: transcatheter closure with a transvenous technique. *Radiology* 1992;186:341–344.

61. Verin VE, Saveliev SV, Kolody SM, et al. Results of transcatheter closure of patent ductus arteriosus with the Batalloccluder. *J Am Coll Cardiol* 1993;22:1509–1514.

62. Sideris EB, Sideris SE, Fowlkes JP, et al. Transvenous atrial septal occlusion in piglets using a "buttoned" double disk device. *Circulation* 1990;81:312–318.

63. Lochan R, Rao PS, Samal AK, et al. Transcatheter closure of patent ductus arteriosus with an adjustable buttoned device in an adult patient. *Am Heart J* 1994;127:941–943.

64. Rao PS, Kim SH, Rey C, et al. Results of transvenous buttoned device occlusion of patent ductus arteriosus in adults. *Am J Cardiol* 1998;82:827–829.

65. Gianturco C, Anderson JH, Wallace S. Mechanical device for arterial occlusion. *Am J Roentgenol* 1975;124:428–435.

66. Sommer RJ, Guitierrez A, Lai WW, et al. Use of preformed Nitinol snare to improve transcatheter coil delivery in occlusion of patent ductus arteriosus. *Am J Cardiol* 1994;74:836–839.

67. Hijazi ZM, Geggel RL. Results of antegrade transcatheter closure of patent ductus arteriosus using single or multiple Gianturco coils. *Am J Cardiol* 1994;74:925–929.

68. Hays MD, Hoyer NH, Glasow PF. New forceps delivery technique for coil occlusion of patent ductus arteriosus. *Am J Cardiol* 1996;77:209–211.

69. Berdjis F, Moore JW. Balloon occlusion delivery technique for closure of patent ductus arteriosus. *Am Heart J* 1997;133:601–604.

70. Dalvi B, Goyal V, Narula D, et al. A new technique using temporary balloon occlusion for transcatheter closure of patent ductus arteriosus with Gianturco coils. *Cathet Cardiovasc Diagn* 1997;41:51–62.

71. Rao PS, Balfour IC, Chen S. Effectiveness of 5-loop coils to occlude patent ductus arteriosus. *Am J Cardiol* 1997;80:1498–1501.

72. Owada CY, Teitel DF, Moore P. Evaluation of Gianturco coils for closure of large (>3.5 mm) patent ductus arteriosus. *J Am Coll Cardiol* 1997;30:1859–1862.

73. Kuhn MA, Latson LA. Transcatheter embolization coil closure of patent ductus arteriosus–modified delivery for enhanced control during coil positioning. *Catheter Cardiovasc Diagn* 1995;36:288–290.

74. Prieto LR, Latson LA, Dalvi B, et al. Transcatheter coil embolization of abnormal vascular connections using a new type of delivery catheter for enhanced control. *Am J Cardiol* 1999;83:981–983.

75. Liang CD, Wu CJ, Fang CY, et al. Retrograde transcatheter occlusion of patent ductus arteriosus and preliminary experience in Gianturco coil technique without heparinization. *J Invasive Cardiol* 2000;13:31–35.

76. Rao PS. Coil occlusion of patent ductus arteriosus (editorial). *J Invasive Cardiol* 2000;13:36–38.

77. Lê TP, Neuss MB, Kirchhoff AH, et al. Transkatheter verchluss von persistierendem Ductus arteriosus mit Spiralfedern. Eine tier experimentelle studies mit Schafen (abstract). *Z Kardiol* 1993;82:71.

78. Neuss MB, Coe JY, Tio F, et al. Occlusion of neonatal patent ductus arteriosus with a simple retrievable device: a feasibility study. *Cardiovasc Interv Radiol* 1996;19:170–173.

79. Grabitz RG, Freudenthal F, Sigler M, et al. double-helix coil for occlusion of large patent ductus arteriosus: evaluation in a chronic lamb model. *J Am Coll Cardiol* 1998;31:677–683.

80. Tometzki A, Redel DA, Wilson N, et al. Total UK multi-center experience with a novel arterial occlusion device (Duct Occlud). *Heart* 1996;76:520–524.

81. Moore JW, Ing FF, Drummond D, et al. Transcatheter closure of surgical shunts in patients with congenital heart disease. *Am J Cardiol* 2000;85:636–640.

82. Grifka RG, Mullins CE, Gianturco C, et al. Initial studies using the Gianturco-Grifka vascular occlusion device in a canine model. *Circulation* 1995;91;1840–1846.

83. Grifka RG. Transcatheter PDA closure using the Gianturco-Grifka vascular occlusion device. *Curr Interv Cardiol Rep* 2001;3:174–182.

84. Schräder R, Hofstetter R, Fabbernder D, et al. Transvenous closure of patent ductus arteriosus with Ivalon plugs: multicenter experience with a new technique. *Invest Radiol* 1999;34:65–70.

85. Sharafuddin MJA, Gu X, Titus JL, et al. Experimental evaluation of a new self-expanding patent ductus arteriosus occluder in a canine model. *J Vasc Interv Radiol* 1996;7:877–887.

Catheter Based Devices: For the Treatment of Non-coronary Cardiovascular Diseases in Adults and Children. Edited by P. Syamasundar Rao and Morton J. Kern, Lippincott Williams & Wilkins, Philadelphia © 2003.

18

RASHKIND DEVICE

SHAKEEL A. QURESHI

Catheter closure of the patent arterial duct has been attempted since 1967, when Porstmann et al. reported on the technique using an Ivalon (polyvinyl alcohol) plug (1). Although this technique appeared to be effective, its disadvantage was that, because of the large profile, a femoral arteriotomy was required for the placement of a large sheath. Furthermore, it was a complicated technique necessitating the establishment of an arteriovenous guide-wire circuit. Both of these disadvantages restricted its use to adolescent and adult patients. Subsequently, attempts were made to close the arterial duct with other devices. These included detachable silicone double balloons, nylon sacs filled with pieces of guide wire, and modified single-disk devices intended for closing atrial septal defects. It was not until 1979 that Rashkind and Cuaso reported the use of a device, which consisted of an umbrella with stainless steel hooks covered with foam (2). From this evolved the Rashkind double-umbrella device (3), which did not have any hooks (USCI, Billerica, MA).

In the 1980s for almost a whole decade, the technique of catheter closure of the arterial duct using the Rashkind double-umbrella device became very popular throughout the world, after the initial experimental assessment (4). Most centers performing interventional techniques became involved with this procedure. However, it was superseded in the early 1990s by other, simpler and cheaper techniques. Therefore the technique and the results of the Rashkind double-umbrella device are discussed here for mainly historical reasons, as very few centers use it nowadays and the device is no longer being manufactured.

RASHKIND DOUBLE-UMBRELLA DEVICE

The Rashkind device consists of two opposing disks made from polyurethane foam. The devices are available in 12-

and 17-mm-diameter disks. The foam is mounted on a small metal frame with three-arm spring wire disks for the 12-mm device and four-arm spring wire disks for the 17-mm device (Figure 18.1A). Each arm is made from 0.005-inch stainless steel for the 12-mm device and 0.010-inch for the 17-mm device. The arms of each disk are attached to a central spring mechanism in such a way that the arms are 120 degrees to each other for the 12-mm device and 90 degrees to each other for the 17-mm device. Each arm is rounded at the outer edge to prevent damage to the vessel with which it may come into contact. The arms of the opposing umbrellas are offset in such a way that each of the six arms is 60 degrees apart for the 12-mm device and 45 degrees apart for the 17-mm device. Both the disks are joined at the center by a metal hinge. When the device is opened, the arms spring at right angles to the catheter shaft and resemble two umbrellas opposing each other (Figure 18.1B). Both the metal frames/umbrellas are joined in the middle by a metal hinge.

The device delivery system consists of a fine central core wire inside a coiled-spring delivery guide wire, which in turn is enclosed in a delivery catheter (Figure 18.2). The distal end of the spring guide wire is welded to a sleeve, through which passes the central core wire. Molded to the end of the delivery catheter is a stainless steel tubular delivery pod, which is 8 or 11F in size.

The whole device can be folded into the delivery pod, but to do this, a plastic loader has to be used first to fold the device before pulling it inside the pod. The delivery pod is 8F for the loading of the 12-mm umbrella device and 11F for the 17-mm device. The tip of the central core wire ends in a knuckle, which can be attached to the eyelet built into the center of one of the umbrellas. The eyelet and the knuckle attachment system allows the device to be folded initially into the clear plastic loader. Once folded inside the loader, the delivery pod and catheter are advanced over the spring guide wire into the loader (Figure 18.3). The folded umbrella device can then be pulled into the delivery pod safely for a controlled delivery into the delivery sheath. At the other end of the delivery catheter is a back-bleed assembly through which the delivery catheter can be flushed and

Shakeel A. Qureshi: Senior Lecturer, Department of Congenital Heart Disease, Guy's, King's & St. Thomas Medical Schools; Consultant Pediatric Cardiologist, Department of Congenital Heart Disease, Guy's Hospital, London, United Kingdom

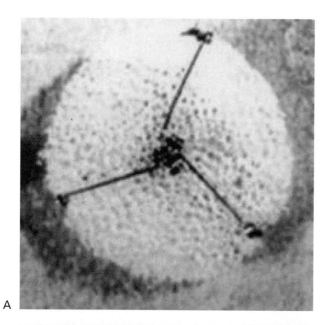

A

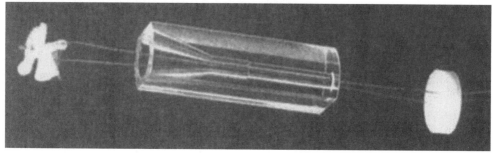

B

FIGURE 18.1. A: Rashkind 12-mm double-umbrella device. **B:** Rashkind umbrella device with its plastic loader.

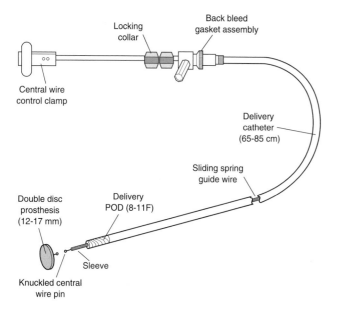

FIGURE 18.2. Rashkind patent ductus arteriosus double umbrella with all the components of the system.

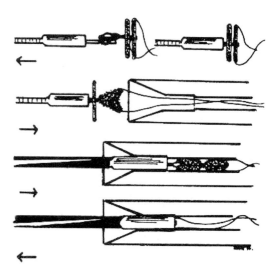

FIGURE 18.3. Method of loading the Rashkind umbrella device into the plastic loader and then onto the delivery catheter.

de-aired. Proximal to this is a locking collar that can be tightened to lock the spring guide wire that prevents inadvertent movements of the delivery pod. Further proximally, there is a wing-shaped control clamp that controls the movement of the knuckle on the inner core wire. This clamp can be activated to attach the device to the knuckle and the sleeve as well as to finally release the device.

TECHNIQUE

Although the procedure can be performed in babies weighing 5 or 6 kg, the technique is much easier when used in children weighing more than 8 to 10 kg. It should certainly not be used in premature babies. Care is given to using a sterile technique and the patient is given antibiotics before and after the procedure. Local anesthesia with sedation may be used, although it is preferable to perform this under general anesthesia.

The technique is precluded if the inferior vena cava is occluded or if there is azygos continuation of the inferior vena cava. The procedure can be accomplished in many ways (4,5). It can be performed using a single femoral vein for both the angiography and the device implantation. Both the femoral veins can be used, one for the delivery of the device and the other for a transseptal puncture for angiography in the left ventricle or the ascending aorta. Both the femoral vein and the femoral artery may be used, the vein for the device implantation and the artery for evaluative angiography before, during, and after the implantation of the device.

If the femoral arterial and venous sheaths are placed, a 4- or 5F sheath in the artery is usually sufficient for angiography. Using a pigtail or NIH catheter placed in the distal aortic arch, an aortogram is performed to define the size, anatomy, and landmarks of the arterial duct. The lateral projection is the most useful and the most frequently used projection, as the important landmark of the anterior border of the tracheal shadow defining the pulmonary arterial end of the duct is easily identified. A multipurpose or an end-hole catheter is advanced in the right heart for hemodynamic assessment. The catheter is manipulated from the main pulmonary artery through the arterial duct into the descending aorta. Although on most occasions, the catheter crosses the duct easily from the pulmonary arterial end, occasionally a straight-tipped guide wire may be needed to cross the duct, and once the guide wire is placed in the abdominal aorta, the catheter is passed over this wire.

A 0.035-inch exchange length ordinary guide wire or Amplatz guide wire is passed through the catheter and positioned in the lower thoracic or upper abdominal aorta. A Mullins transseptal sheath has to be passed over this guide wire. It is preferable to use a sheath with a hemostatic valve mechanism, as this will prevent blood loss during the manipulation of the device. The size of the Mullins sheath depends on the size of the arterial duct, which will determine the size of the umbrella device to be implanted. Gen-

erally, for a duct less than 3 to 3.5 mm at its minimum dimension (usually at the pulmonary arterial end), a 12-mm double-umbrella device is selected, and for ducts larger than this up to about 8 mm, a 17-mm device is selected. The appropriate Mullins sheath (65- or 75-cm length) is advanced over the guide wire until both the dilator and the sheath have crossed the arterial duct and are positioned in the upper thoracic aorta just below the ampulla of the arterial duct. The guide wire and the dilator are withdrawn, keeping the sheath in place, taking care not to push the sheath inadvertently, as this would cause the unprotected sheath to kink in the right ventricular outflow tract. The kinked sheath could in turn prevent the passage of the umbrella device, necessitating the removal of the whole assembly in order to start the procedure again. If it is not possible to cross the duct from the pulmonary artery end, then a catheter is placed via the femoral artery in the duct ampulla and a guide wire is used to cross the duct. Once this is accomplished, using a snare to capture the guide wire in the pulmonary artery, an arteriovenous guide wire circuit can be established and a catheter or a Mullins sheath is passed from the femoral vein to cross the duct (5).

Once the sheath is in the correct position and the whole system is flushed, the previously selected Rashkind double-umbrella device, loaded into the delivery pod, is passed through the hemostatic valve on the Mullins sheath. The pod is advanced up to the inferior vena caval junction with the right atrium (Figure 18.4). It is preferable to avoid passing the pod round the curve of the right atrium to the pulmonary

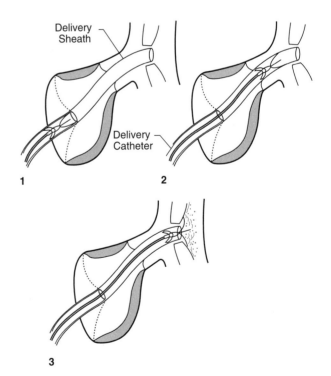

FIGURE 18.4. Drawings of the steps in the technique for the delivery of the device through the femoral venous approach.

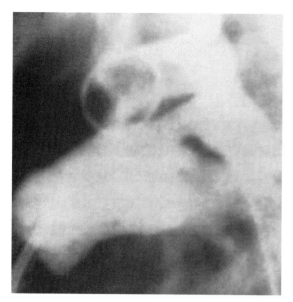

FIGURE 18.5. An aortogram in left lateral projection showing a large patent ductus arteriosus.

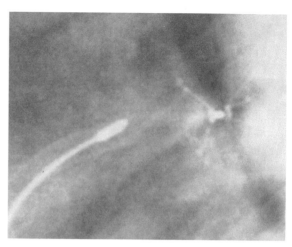

FIGURE 18.7. The double-umbrella device has now been released after opening the proximal arms in the pulmonary artery. Note that the knuckle has been withdrawn inside the sheath.

artery, as the rigid length of the pod may cause the sheath to kink. By unlocking the locking collar, the spring guide wire is advanced so that the umbrella device is pushed out of the pod into the Mullins sheath. The device is then advanced round the curves of the right heart until the distal umbrella is fully extruded out of the sheath in the distal aorta (Figures 18.5 and 18.6). The locking collar is locked to avoid the inadvertent deployment of the proximal umbrella in the aorta. The sheath and the delivery catheter are withdrawn slowly as one unit until the arms of the distal umbrella start to flex and the hinge point of the umbrellas is at the level of the pulmonary arterial end of the duct (usually at the anterior border of the trachea in the lateral projection). This posi-

tioning and a reduction in the movement of the arms of the distal umbrella help to confirm that the distal umbrella is engaged in the ampulla of the duct. At this point, while maintaining the device in position by holding the delivery catheter still, the Mullins sheath is slowly and smoothly withdrawn over the delivery catheter so that the proximal umbrella is fully deployed. An aortogram is repeated in the lateral projection to ensure the correct positioning of the fully deployed device. The release mechanism is now activated using the wing-shaped control clamp (Figure 18.7). The delivery catheter and the sheath are withdrawn well away from the device. If it appears as if the knuckle is caught in the fabric of the umbrella, it is safer to keep this in position, advance the Mullins sheath up to the device, and then gently pull the knuckle and the spring wire back into the sheath or alternatively retract the sleeve instead of advancing the knuckle for activating the release mechanism (6). After release of the device, an aortogram is repeated to check for the amount of residual flow, if any (Figure 18.8).

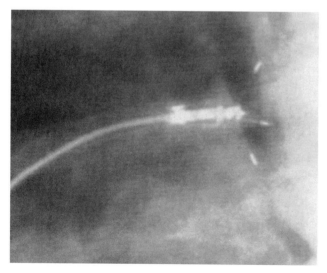

FIGURE 18.6. The distal arms of the double umbrella have been opened in the descending aorta, and the whole assembly is pulled to engage the ampulla of the ductus arteriosus. The proximal umbrella arms are still inside the 11F delivery sheath.

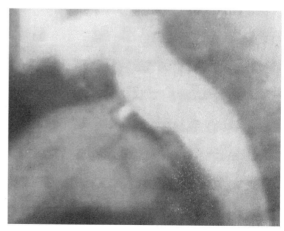

FIGURE 18.8. Aortogram in the lateral projection shows a significant leak after 17-mm Rashkind device.

RESULTS

Over the years, as the Rashkind double-umbrella device was increasingly used around the world, it became clear, not surprisingly, that the device was unsuitable for the variety of patent arterial ducts that are encountered clinically (7–10). One limiting factor was the size of the arterial duct; a duct larger than 7 to 8 mm could not be closed safely or effectively. Another factor that influenced the results was the morphology of the duct. While the device could be placed successfully in all the variety of ducts, it did not necessarily lead to complete occlusion (8,11,12). The technique of device implantation was fairly complex and thus initially involved a potentially important learning curve. Not all the operators were comfortable with the technique. The device was expensive. Consequently, if it embolized and had to be retrieved, implantation of another device to close the duct became prohibitively expensive, especially in the developing countries. Furthermore, if the duct was incompletely occluded, a further procedure to close the duct added to the expense. Thus it was not surprising that other devices, such as controlled-release coils, were evaluated in the early 1990s and have become part of the routine management of catheter closure of the arterial duct.

Successful Implantation and Residual Flow

In most of the series in the literature, the Rashkind double-umbrella device was implanted in the arterial duct in more than 90% of the cases. However, angiographic occlusion at the end of the procedure occurred in just over half of the patients. Within the next 4 to 6 weeks, complete occlusion had occurred in another 10% to 20% of the cases, resulting in complete occlusion in about 70% of cases. Although the murmur arising from the duct had disappeared, more thorough evaluation by color Doppler echocardiography revealed a much higher incidence of residual flow. (4,7–10). These residual shunts were more frequently seen after closure with the 17-mm device (8,12).

In a large multicenter registry established in Europe involving 686 patients, the Rashkind umbrella device was successfully implanted at the first attempt in 642 (94%) of the patients (11). At the latest follow-up, 71% of all the patients entered into the registry had complete occlusion of the ductus arteriosus with a single device. Kaplan-Meier analysis showed a complete occlusion rate of 82% at 1 year after device implantation. In patients with residual leaks, 41 had a second Rashkind umbrella device implanted; complete occlusion occurred in 37. Thus the actuarial rate of complete occlusion after one or two devices was 95% at 30 months after the very first procedure. In this registry there were two early deaths, both in patients with associated ventricular septal defects. Complications such as embolization of the device were encountered in 2.4% of patients, and hemolysis occurred in 0.5% of the patients. The embolized

devices were retrieved by transcatheter techniques in a third of the patients; in the remainder, the devices were retrieved surgically, at which time the duct was surgically ligated.

In a series of 190 patients in whom implantation of an umbrella device was attempted, the rate of residual shunting was 34% at 1 year, 19% at 2 years, and 11% at 40 months, indicating ongoing closure with time, but still quite a high rate of residual flow (13). Other smaller series were reported earlier, and subsequently (8,14). In a series of 40 patients, two devices embolized and surgical retrieval was performed. Angiography immediately at the end of the procedure showed a residual shunt in 32% of the patients. At the latest follow-up, 21% of the patients had a residual leak. This series also alerted us to the possibility of probable endarteritis (reported in one patient) and mild stenosis of the left pulmonary artery (also in one patient).

It became clear over the years of use of the Rashkind umbrella device that residual shunting was a major concern (8,11). Various operators used different methods to reduce the incidence of residual shunting. These included soaking of the device in thrombin solution or balloon-tamponading the device by pushing the arms of the device against the duct with a balloon from either the aortic end or the pulmonary arterial end (7). These did not have any beneficial effects (15). In a study of 117 consecutive patients, this method did not produce higher rates of complete occlusion (15). Some other rare events were reported. After previously documented complete occlusion following umbrella device implantation, reopening of the arterial duct occurred (16). Thrombus formation detected by echocardiography has been reported within 6 hours of the procedure (17). This was treated by intravenous heparin infusion with resolution of the thrombus. It is surprising that this complication did not occur more frequently, and if it did, it has certainly been underreported.

The rate of residual flow during the follow-up period in different studies varies between 5% and 20%. When residual leaks persisted beyond 1 or 2 years, this was dealt with in various ways. A second umbrella device was implanted using a similar technique to the initial implant (Figure 18.9). This resulted in high closure rates approaching 95% (18,19). In other cases, coils or other devices have been used to close small residual leaks (20).

Device Embolization

Embolization of the device may occur either immediately after release of the device or within 24 hours after the procedure. The device may embolize to either the systemic or the pulmonary circulation. On some occasions, the device was retrieved surgically; however, on most occasions, the device could be retrieved by catheter means using snares, baskets, or grasping forceps. Once trapped by a snare, the device has to be retracted fully into the Mullins sheath before withdrawal of the whole assembly through the right heart structures (4,9). The device usually embolized because it was undersized

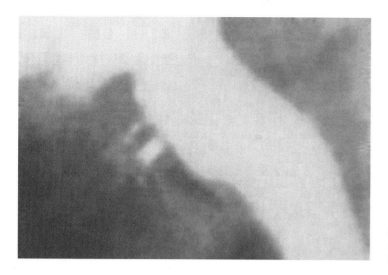

FIGURE 18.9. Aortogram after the implantation of a second Rashkind umbrella device a year later showing complete occlusion of the ductus.

in comparison with the size of the duct. This error occurred either during the measurement of the dimensions of the duct or because the duct may have developed spasm leading to an underestimation of the dimension of the duct.

Hemolysis

Another important complication encountered with device implantation is hemolysis. This occurs when there is significant high-velocity flow through or around the device. Sometimes hemolysis is mild and settles with conservative treatment with reduction of residual flow. If there is persistent hemolysis, then this can be dealt with by implantation of a further device or coils to diminish or stop the flow, by surgical removal of the device and occlusion of the duct, or by oversewing on the device. Although hemolysis has been encountered in a small proportion of patients, it can present with difficulties of clinical management, especially when it is severe. Hemolysis tends to occur when there is a large residual leak with a high-velocity jet through or around the umbrella device placed in the arterial duct. In some patients, the device has been removed surgically and the duct ligated (21). In others, implantation of another device resulted in the resolution of the hemolysis (22–25). Other authors have reported leaving the umbrella device *in situ* and oversewing the arterial duct (26). It is interesting to note that evidence of mild or subclinical intravascular hemolysis can occur after catheter closure of a patent arterial duct, whether it is closed with an umbrella device or with coils (27).

Device Protrusion

Increased Doppler flow velocities have been encountered at the origin of the left pulmonary artery, which may occur when a large 17-mm device is implanted in a small child weighing less than 6 to 8 kg. Follow-up studies have shown no progression in the velocities in these patients (28). One study investigated the possible effects of protrusion of the device into the aorta or the pulmonary artery. It was found that the device may protrude on occasion in the aorta or the pulmonary artery, and in some but not all the patients, it may cause turbulence of blood flow on color Doppler echocardiography. Both protrusion and turbulence of blood flow may resolve during the follow-up (29,30). Residual shunting may be due to a mismatch between the size of the duct and the device or the shape of the duct or suboptimal position of the device (30).

USE IN ADULT PATIENTS

The Rashkind umbrella device can be used in adult patients to close the arterial duct also, although if the duct is too large, then alternative devices or techniques may be needed. Furthermore, in some patients the duct may also be calcified, making surgery more difficult to perform. Although complete closure may be achieved with a single device, because the duct tends to be larger, residual flow and hemolysis may require additional procedures (31). In one case, two umbrella devices were implanted simultaneously in an adult patient with a 9-mm-diameter arterial duct (32).

USE IN SMALL INFANTS

Although the device was recommended for use in predominantly older children weighing more than 8 to 10 kg, it was used also in smaller children. In these smaller children, the device could be front-loaded in such a way that the 12-mm device could be passed through a 6F Mullins transseptal sheath and the 17-mm device through an 8F sheath. With this modification a device was successfully implanted in 25 of 29 (86%) infants under the age of 2 years (33). The rate of residual leak was similar to the studies in older children, confirming that irrespective of the age or size of the patient, there was a similar incidence of residual leaks.

In its time the Rashkind double-umbrella device established an important role for itself in closing patent arterial ducts. There were limitations to the technique. Nevertheless, the improvement in the results seemed to correlate more with the application of this technique to patients with smaller arterial ducts, increasing operator experience, increasing experience of the center, and more judicious selection of the patients (34). It is worth emphasizing the contribution made by the device in advancing the knowledge of the anatomy of the arterial duct and in the development of subsequent devices.

REFERENCES

1. Porstmann W, Wierny L, Warneke H. Der vershluss des ductus arteriosus persistens ohne thorakotomie. *Thoraxchirurgie* 1967; 15:199–203.
2. Rashkind WJ, Cuaso CC. Transcatheter closure of patent ductus arteriosus: successful use in a 3.5 kilogram infant. *Pediatr Cardiol* 1979;1:3–8.
3. Rashkind WJ. Transcatheter treatment of congenital heart disease. *Circulation* 1983;67:711–716.
4. Rashkind WJ, Mullins CE, Hellenbrand WE, et al. Nonsurgical closure of the patent ductus areteriosus: clinical application of the Rashkind PDA Occluder System. *Circulation* 1987;75:583–592.
5. Benson LN, Dyck J, Hecht B. Technique for closure of the small patent ductus arteriosus using the Rashkind occluder. *Catheter Cardiovasc Diagn* 1988;14:82–84.
6. Bjornstad PG. Wire trapping in Rashkind's patent ductus arteriosus occluder: its etiology and how it may be avoided. *Cardiovasc Interv Radiol* 1995;18:203–204.
7. Wessel DL, Keane JF, Parness I, et al. Outpatient closure of the patent ductus arteriosus. *Circulation* 1988;77:1068–1071.
8. Dyck JD, Benson LN, Smallhorn JF, et al. Catheter occlusion of the persistently patent ductus arteriosus. *Am J Cardiol* 1988;62: 1089–1092.
9. Latson LA, Hofschire PJ, Kugler JD, et al. Transcatheter closure of patent ductus arteriosus in pediatric patients. *J Pediatr* 1989; 115:549–553.
10. Ali Khan MA, Mullins CE, Nihill MR, et al. Percutaneous catheter closure of the ductus arteriosus in children and young adults. *Am J Cardiol* 1989;64:218–221.
11. Anonymous. Transcatheter occlusion of persistent arterial duct. Report of the European Registry. *Lancet* 1992;340:1062–1066.
12. Musewe NN, Benson LN, Smallhorn JS, et al. Two-dimensional echocardiographic and colour-Doppler evaluation of ductal occlusion with the Rashkind prosthesis. *Circulation* 1989;80: 1706–1710.
13. Hosking MCK, Benson LN, Musewe N, et al. Transcatheter closure of the persistent patent ductus arteriosus: forty months follow-up and prevalence of residual shunting. *Circulation* 1991;84: 2312–2317.
14. Arora R, Kalra GS, Nigam M, et al. Transcatheter occlusion of patent ductus arteriosus by Rashkind umbrella device: follow-up results. *Am Heart J* 1994;128:539–541.
15. Vitiello R, Benson L, Musewe N, et al. Factors influencing the persistence of shunting within 24 hours of catheter occlusion of the ductus arteriosus. *Br Heart J* 1991;65:211–212.
16. Galal O, Abbag F, Fadley F, et al. Reopening of an arterial duct after total occlusion with Rashkind's double umbrella device. *Catheter Cardiovasc Diagn* 1994;33:132–134.
17. De Moor M, Abbag F, al Fadley F, et al. Thrombosis on the Rashkind double umbrella device: a complication of PDA occlusion. *Catheter Cardiovasc Diagn* 1996;38:186–188.
18. Abbag F, Galal O, Fadley F, et al. Re-occlusion of residual leaks after transcatheter occlusion of patent ductus arteriosus. *Eur J Pediatr* 1995;154:518–521.
19. Huggon IC, Tabatabaei AH, Qureshi SA, et al. Use of a second transcatheter Rashkind arterial duct occluder for persistent flow after implantation of the first device: indications and results. *Br Heart J* 1993;69:544–550.
20. De Moor M, Al Fadley F, Galal O. Closure of residual leak after umbrella occlusion of the patent arterial duct, using Gianturco coils. *Int J Cardiol* 1996;56:5–9.
21. Ladusans EJ, Murdoch I, Franciosi J. Severe haemolysis after percutaneous closure of a ductus arteriosus (arterial duct). *Br Heart J* 1989;61:548–550.
22. Hayes AM, Redington AN, Rigby ML. Severe haemolysis after transcatheter duct occlusion: a non-surgical remedy. *Br Heart J* 1992;67:321–322.
23. Murakami H, Tsuchihashi K, Tomita H, et al. Combined use of detachable coil against persistent mechanical hemolysis after transcatheter occlusion using Rashkind umbrella device in adult patient with patent ductus arteriosus. *Heart Vessels* 1997;12:49–51.
24. Cheung YF, Leung MP, Chau KT. Early implantation of multiple spring coils for severe haemolysis after incomplete transcatheter occlusion of persistent arterial duct. *Heart* 1997;77:477–478.
25. Wang LH, Wang JK, Mullins CE. Eradicating acute hemolysis following transcatheter closure of ductus arteriosus by immediate deployment of a second device. *Catheter Cardiovasc Diagn* 1998; 43:295–297.
26. Chisholm JC, Salmon AP, Keeton BR, et al. Persistent hemolysis after transcatheter occlusion of a patent ductus arteriosus: surgical ligation of the duct over the occlusion device. *Pediatr Cardiol* 1995;16:194–196.
27. Jamjureeruk V, Kirawittaya T, Ningsnondh V. Mild or subclinical intravascular haemolysis subsequent to transcatheter occlusion of the patent arterial duct. *Cardiol Young* 1999;9:58–62.
28. Fadley F, Al Halees Z, Galal O, et al. Left pulmonary artery stenosis after transcatheter occlusion of the persistent arterial duct. *Lancet* 1993;341:559–560.
29. Ottenkamp J, Hess J, Talsma MD, et al. Protrusion of the device: a complication of catheter closure of patent ductus arteriosus. *Br Heart J* 1992;68:301–303.
30. Magee AG, Stumper O, Burns JE, et al. Medium-term follow-up of residual shunting and potential complications after transcatheter occlusion of the ductus arteriosus. *Br Heart J* 1994;71:63–69.
31. Bonhoeffer P, Borghi A, Onorato E, et al. Transfemoral closure of patent ductus arteriosus in adult patients. *Int J Cardiol* 1993;39: 181–186.
32. Sievert H, Moor T, Ensslen R, et al. Transcatheter closure of oversized persistent ductus arteriosus by simultaneous delivery of two Rashkind umbrella devices. *Catheter Cardiovasc Diagn* 1995;36: 251–254.
33. Gatzoulis MA, Rigby ML, Redington AN. Umbrella occlusion of persistent arterial duct in children under two years. *Br Heart J* 1994;72:364–367.
34. Gray DT, Walker AM, Fyler DC, et al. Examination of the early "learning curve" for transcatheter closure of patent ductus arteriosus using the Rashkind occluder. *Circulation* 1994;90:II-36–II-42.

19

BUTTONED DEVICE

P. SYAMASUNDAR RAO

Following the description by Gross and Hubbard of surgical ligation of patent ductus arteriosus (PDA) in 1938 (1), surgery has become the standard therapy in the management of PDA. Although safety and efficacy of surgical therapy have been demonstrated, cardiologists have been trying to develop less invasive techniques of PDA closure. Porstmann (2,3) and Rashkind (4,5) pioneered such efforts. Since the first demonstration of Porstmann and his associates (2,3) of the feasibility of transcatheter closure of PDA, a number of transcatheter methods, reviewed in Chapter 17 (6), have been described. After experimental studies in animal models (7) and clinical application in a limited number of human subjects (8–10), the buttoned device (Custom Medical Devices, Athens, Greece, and Amarillo, TX) has undergone clinical trials in a large number of patients (11,12). This chapter describes the buttoned device and various modifications that it underwent in the 1990s and discusses the immediate and follow-up results of their implantation to treat PDA.

THE DEVICES

The device has been described in detail elsewhere (9,11,12). It is made up of three components: the occluder, the counteroccluder, and the delivery system.

The *occluder* is made up of x-shaped, Teflon-coated, stainless steel wire skeleton covered with 0.0625-inch polyurethane foam (Figure 19.1). When wires of the occluder are folded, it can be introduced into a 7F sheath. Following the delivery to the implantation site, the occluder assumes the original square-shaped configuration. An 8-mm-long string loop is connected to the center of the occluder; the loop incorporates two knots (buttons) 4-mm apart. In the original design (9) radiopaque material was incorporated into the proximal button (farthest from the

occluder) and the distal button (closer to the occluder) was not radiopaque. But, in the more recent devices (11,12) both knots (buttons) were made radiopaque, in a manner similar to that employed for the fourth generation atrial septal devices (13).

The *counteroccluder* is made up of a single-strand Teflon-coated stainless steel wire skeleton covered with a rhomboid-shaped 1/16-inch polyurethane foam. A latex piece is sewn in the center of the counteroccluder and becomes a buttonhole.

The *delivery system* has several components: (a) a delivery wire, a Teflon-coated 0.035-inch guide wire (Cook, Inc., Bloomington, IN); (b) a folded 0.008-inch nylon thread passing through the delivery wire, after having its core removed (this nylon thread also passes through the loop attached to the occluder); (c) a 6- or 7F pusher catheter used to advance the occluder and the counteroccluder through the sheath, respectively; and (d) a 7F long blue Cook sheath (Cook, Inc.) with a radiopaque marker at the tip.

This device was originally named the *adjustable buttoned device* (9) because buttoning with both buttons could be undertaken for short ducti and buttoning with only the proximal (farthest from the occluder) button was believed to be adequate for a long ductus. Here, however, it will be called the *regular* buttoned device.

Device Sizes

The device size is measured by the diagonal length of the device or the length of the counteroccluder. Fifteen- and 20-mm devices are manufactured for PDA closure. Generally, 15-mm devices are considered adequate for young children and small PDAs, whereas 20-mm devices are useful in adults and larger PDAs. In very large PDAs, 25-mm and larger atrial septal occluder devices (13) may be utilized.

Infant Buttoned Device

To utilize this device in infants and young children, the delivery sheath size had to be reduced from 7 to 6F. There-

P. Syamasundar Rao: Professor of Pediatrics, Medicine, and Cardiology, Department of Pediatrics, University of Texas-Houston Medical School; Director, Division of Pediatric Cardiology, Memorial Hermann Children's Hospital, Houston, Texas

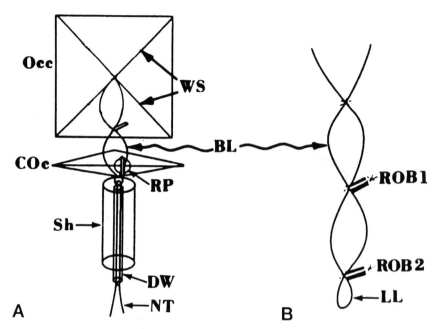

FIGURE 19.1. A: A cartoon of the buttoned device used for occlusion of patent ductus arteriosus. The occluder (Occ) is made up of 0.0625-inch polyurethane foam covering an x-shaped Teflon-coated wire skeleton (WS) connected to a button loop (BL). A folded nylon thread (NT) passes through the lower loop (LL) of the BL following its passage through the delivery wire (DW) after having its core removed. The counteroccluder (COc) is made up of rhomboid-shaped polyurethane foam covering a single-strand Teflon-coated wire. A rubber piece (RP) is sutured into its center, forming the buttonhole. The sheath (Sh) tip is shown, which is either 7 or 8F, through which the folded occluder would pass. **B:** Magnified view of the BL showing radiopaque spring buttons (ROB). The top part is connected to the occluder in the middle and the NT goes through the LL. In the initial design (9) only ROB 2 was radiopaque. (From Rao PS, Kim SH, Rey C, et al. Results of transvenous buttoned device occlusion of patent ductus arteriosus in adults. *Am J Cardiol* 1998;82:827–829, with permission.)

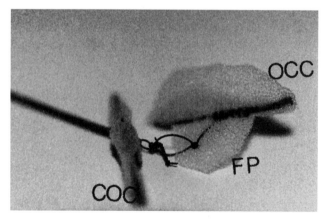

FIGURE 19.2. Photograph of an infant buttoned device. Basic design of the device is similar to the buttoned device described in the preceding sections except that the occluder (Occ) has a single wire (instead of two wires in an x-shaped pattern) covered with polyurethane foam and a folding plug (FP) sutured onto the button loop of the occluder. COc, counteroccluder. (From Rao PS, Sideris EB. Transcatheter closure of patent ductus arteriosus: state of the art. *J Invasive Cardiol* 1996;8:278–288, with permission.)

fore the occluder component of the regular buttoned device was replaced with a single-strand, Teflon-coated stainless steel wire skeleton covered with rhomboid-shaped polyurethane foam and was named the *infant buttoned device* (14,15). At the same time, a folding plug made up of polyurethane foam covering the button loop was incorporated into the device design (Figure 19.2). The occluder goes into the aorta, the plug in the ductal lumen, and the counteroccluder in the pulmonary artery. The devices are manufactured in two different sizes: 15 and 20 mm. The 15-mm infant buttoned device can be delivered through a 6F sheath, whereas the 20-mm devices require a 7F sheath.

Folding-Plug Device

Preliminary analysis of data (16) of the regular buttoned device revealed a high residual shunt rate at implantation. Because of this, the device was modified by incorporating a polyurethane foam plug over the button loop of the regular

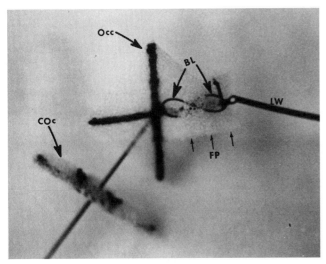

FIGURE 19.3. Photograph of the modified folding-plug buttoned device showing the occluder (Occ), counteroccluder (COc), and polyurethane folding plug (FP) covering *(arrows)* the button loop (BL). The device is similar to the regular buttoned device except for FP. LW, loading wire. (From Rao PS, Kim SH, Choi J, et al. Follow-up results of transvenous occlusion of patent ductus arteriosus with the buttoned device. *J Am Coll Cardiol* 1999;33: 820–826, with permission.)

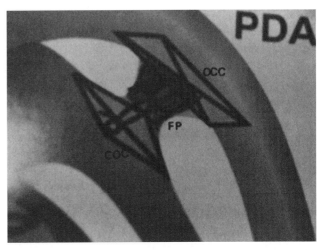

FIGURE 19.4. A cartoon of the folding-plug device across the patent ductus arteriosus (PDA) with the occluder (Occ) at the aortic end of the ductus counteroccluder (COc) in the pulmonary artery (PA) and the folding plug (FP) in the ductus. (From Sideris EB, Rao PS. Buttoned device occlusion of patent ductus arteriosus. *Curr Interv Cardiol Rep* 2001;3:71–79, with permission.)

A radiopaque thread is sewn onto the patch so that it can be localized and retrieved, if necessary. Deflated balloons with the patch on them can be introduced via a sheath for delivery to the implantation site.

PROTOCOL/CLINICAL TRIALS

Buttoned-device implantations were performed under a protocol approved by the US Food and Drug Administration (FDA) with an investigational device exemption (IDE). Approval of the Institutional Review Board (IRB) at each of the participating hospitals was also obtained before the implantation of this device. Additional procedures were followed, as per the local regulations in the international trials. Informed consent was obtained from the parents or patients as appropriate.

buttoned device (Figure 19.3). The occluder will go onto the aortic end of the PDA; the foam plug, into the ductus; and the counteroccluder, into the pulmonary artery (Figure 19.4) (17). The device is referred to as the *folding-plug buttoned device* (12). The devices are manufactured in several sizes: 15, 20, 25, and 30 mm.

Wireless Devices

Since all PDA devices contain wire components, complications related to wire frames are likely. Therefore wireless devices were conceived (18). The device consists of two latex balloons mounted on a wire (Figure 19.5). A polyurethane foam patch is mounted on the distal balloon.

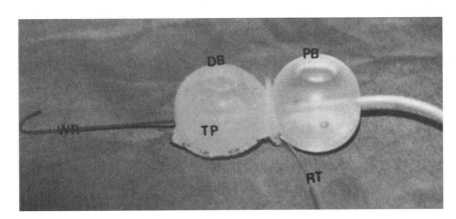

FIGURE 19.5. Photograph of transcatheter patch supported by two balloons over a wire (WR). The transcatheter patch (TP) is mounted on the distal balloon (DB) and connected to a retrieval thread (RT). PB, proximal balloon. (From Sideris EB, Rao PS. Sideris' buttoned device for transcatheter closure of patent ductus arteriosus. *J Interv Cardiol* 2001;14:239–246, with permission.)

The results of a number of international and FDA-approved clinical trials (11,12,14,19,20) with the buttoned device have been published using these protocols.

PATIENT SELECTION

Both children and adults with clinical (continuous murmur) and echocardiographic and Doppler features of PDA were recruited into the study. The silent PDAs were not offered the procedure. Otherwise, no patients were excluded because of size and shape of the ductus. Patients with associated defects were not excluded unless the patient required surgical intervention for the associated defect. Patients with ductal dependent lesion or those who developed irreversible pulmonary vascular obstructive disease are not included.

DEVICE IMPLANTATION TECHNIQUE

The procedure is generally performed while the patient is sedated with an intramuscular injection of a sedative mixture (Demerol, Phenergan, and Thorazine) supplemented with intermittent doses of medazolam and fentanyl as required. Some investigators use general anesthesia. Initially, right and left heart catheterization is performed to confirm the clinical diagnosis and to exclude any associated defects. Heparin (100 U/kg) is administered immediately following insertion of the arterial catheter, and additional doses are given to maintain activated clotting times between 200 to 250 seconds. Aortography is performed in posteroanterior (more recently, 30 degrees right anterior oblique) and lateral projections to evaluate the size and shape of the ductus. This is either via a retrogradely introduced catheter or via an anterogradely introduced balloon angiographic (Berman) catheter by balloon occlusion angiography (21). The minimal ductal diameter is measured and the shape is characterized. The PDA occlusion studies began before the publication of Krichenko's paper (22); therefore that classification was not employed in this review.

A 5F multi-A$_2$ catheter (Cordis, Miami, FL) is introduced via the femoral vein and advanced from the main pulmonary artery into the descending aorta via the ductus arteriosus. When necessary, a 0.035-inch straight Benston guide wire (Cordis, Miami, FL) is utilized to facilitate catheterization of the ductus. This guide wire is then exchanged with a 0.035-inch, exchange length, J-shaped, extra-stiff Amplatz wire (Cook, Bloomington, IN) and the multi-A$_2$ catheter removed. A 7- or 8F long blue Cook sheath (Cook, Inc.) with a radiopaque tip is advanced into the descending aorta.

The occluder component of the device is folded and introduced into the sheath. The occluder is advanced with the pusher catheter supplied by the manufacturer. The occluder is delivered into the descending aorta, where the occluder assumes its original square-shaped configuration.

It is slowly pulled against the tip of the sheath and the entire system is withdrawn as one unit until the occluder is anchored onto the aortic end of the ductus. Test aortography is performed to visualize the position of the occluder and, if necessary, is repositioned to achieve optimal results. The tip of the delivery sheath is withdrawn into the main pulmonary artery and the pusher catheter is removed out of the patient while maintaining the position of occluder. The sheath is then clamped.

The counteroccluder is threaded over the delivery wire with the help of the needle provided by the manufacturer and is introduced into the sheath. The system is flushed and the sheath is unclamped. The counteroccluder is advanced over the delivery wire, but within the sheath, with the pusher catheter and is delivered into the main pulmonary artery.

Then buttoning is done by slowly advancing the counteroccluder over the delivery wire while applying gentle traction on the occluder with the delivery wire. As the buttonhole of the counteroccluder passes over the buttons attached to the occluder, a gentle "tug" is felt by the operator. This procedure is performed while monitoring the device position on lateral fluoroscopy. The radiopaque component of the counteroccluder should be beyond the radiopaque buttons (i.e., between the buttons and occluder). If the ductus is short, buttoning across both buttons is recommended. If the ductus is long, buttoning across one button (proximal) may be adequate. Additional aortography is optional at this juncture.

The delivery wire is cut and withdrawn, followed by cutting and removal of the nylon thread, thus releasing the device. During these two maneuvers, the tip of the sheath is gently apposed against the device so that excessive tension is not applied on the device, thus preventing inadvertent withdrawal of the occluder across the ductus.

Postimplantation aortography is performed to document the device position and residual shunt. Three doses of cefazolin (25 mg/kg/dose, maximum 1 g) are administered for bacterial endocarditis prophylaxis. Platelet-inhibiting doses (5 to 10 mg/kg/day) of aspirin are given for a 6-week period.

RESULTS

As alluded in the preceding sections, a number of alterations have been introduced subsequent to initial use of the buttoned device. The results of the regular buttoned device and its modification will be described separately.

REGULAR BUTTONED DEVICE
Description of the Subjects

A total of 284 patients was taken to the catheterization laboratory with intent to occlude the ductus, during a 6-year period ending August 1996 at 21 institutions around the world (12). The number of subjects undergoing buttoned-device closure of ductus varied from three to 79 at each institution, with a median of six.

The patient's ages were 4 months to 92 years, with a median of 7 years. Seventy-seven (27%) patients were more than 16 years of age. Their weights varied between 5 and 90 kg, with a median of 19 kg.

Size and Shape of the Ductus

The size of the ductus is judged based on the shunt across it and the minimal ductal diameter measured on the lateral view. The data on pulmonary-to-systemic flow ratio (Qp:Qs) are available in 169 patients and varied between 1.2 and 4.8, with a mean of 1.8 ± 0.6. The narrowest ductal diameters varied between 1 and 15 mm, with a median of 4 mm. Ten PDAs were larger than 10 mm and 20 measured more than 8 mm.

The ducti were conical in shape in 164, tubular in 56, short in 29, and of miscellaneous shapes in 25. The remaining ten were residual shunts after prior Rashkind device placement.

Devices Used

Fifteen-mm devices were implanted in 140 patients, and 20-mm devices were implanted in 115. These devices were delivered through 7F sheaths. Larger devices were used in the remaining patients: 25 mm in 15, 30 mm in six, 35 mm in two, and miscellaneous sizes in six. These devices were implanted across the ductus via 8F sheaths.

Immediate Results

Devices were successfully deployed at first attempt in 278 (98%) of 284 patients taken to the catheterization laboratory with intent to close. The unsuccessful implantations will be dealt with in the "Complications" section. Two of these patients had a larger device implanted at the same sitting.

Following device deployment, the Qp:Qs decreased from 1.8 ± 0.6 to 1.09 ± 0.19 ($p < .001$). Complete occlusion by angiography performed 15 minutes after device delivery was present in 168 (60%) of 280 patients. Examples of device position are shown in Figures 19.6 to 19.8. Doppler echocardiography performed within 24 hours of device deployment revealed effective occlusion [defined as no ($N = 167$) or trivial ($N = 79$) residual shunt] in 246 (88%) of 280 patients. Detailed statistical analysis revealed that there was no relationship between minimal ductal diameters and the shape of the ductus, on the one hand, and effective occlusion, on the other. In all ten patients with prior Rashkind device, there was complete occlusion of the ductus. Continuous murmur of the ductus disappeared in all but four (1.4%) patients.

Residual shunts (as defined in ref. 12), judged to be trivial in 79 and small in 34, were present in 113 (40%) of 280

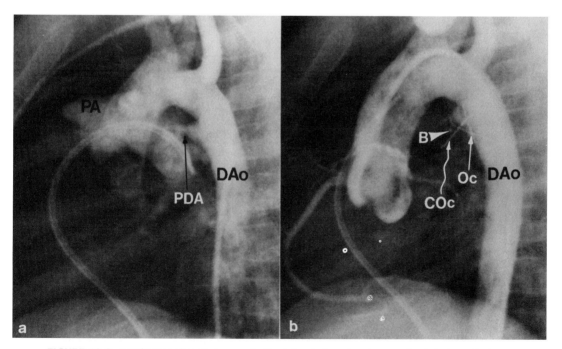

FIGURE 19.6. Aortic root cineangiogram in the lateral view showing a patent ductus arteriosus (PDA) (*arrow*) before closure (**a**). After device implantation, there was no opacification of PDA, but the ductal ampulla was seen. The occluder (Oc) (*straight arrow*), counteroccluder (COc) (*curved arrow*), and radiopaque button (B) (*arrowhead*) are shown (**b**). DAo, descending aorta; PA, pulmonary artery. (From Rao PS, Sideris EB, Haddad J, et al. Transcatheter occlusion of patent ductus arteriosus with adjustable buttoned device: initial clinical experience. *Circulation* 1993;88: 1119–1126, with permission.)

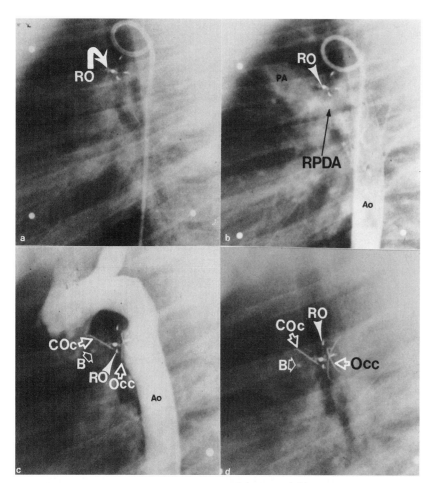

FIGURE 19.7. Selected cineradiographic frame showing Rashkind patent ductus arteriosus occluder (RO) device (*curved arrow*) (**a**), 1 year after its implantation. Aortogram (**b**) showed significant residual shunt (RPDA) (*arrow*) across the ductus with opacification of the pulmonary artery (PA). After occlusion of the residual ductus with a buttoned device (**c**), no residual shunt is seen. The occluder (Occ) (*arrow*) of the buttoned device in the aorta (Ao), counteroccluder (COc) (*arrow*), and button (B) (*arrow*) in the PA are visualized. **d:** Radiographic components of both the Rashkind (*arrowhead*) and buttoned devices (*arrows*) are shown. (From Rao PS, Sideris EB, Haddad J, et al. Transcatheter occlusion of patent ductus arteriosus with adjustable buttoned device: initial clinical experience. *Circulation* 1993;88:1119–1126, with permission.)

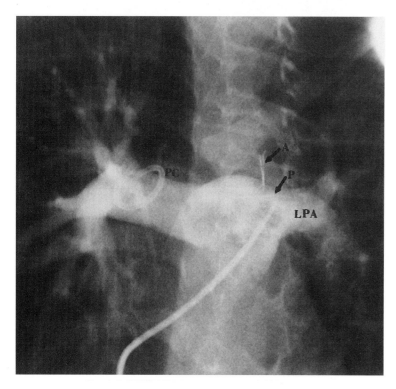

FIGURE 19.8. Main pulmonary arteriographic frame following buttoned-device implantation. Note that there was no evidence for left pulmonary artery (LPA) obstruction. A, occluder component of the device (*top arrow*); P, counteroccluder (*bottom arrow*); PG, end of the pig-tail catheter in the aorta. (From Rao PS, Sideris EB. Transcatheter closure of patent ductus arteriosus: state of the art. *J Invasive Cardiol* 1996;8:278–288, with permission.)

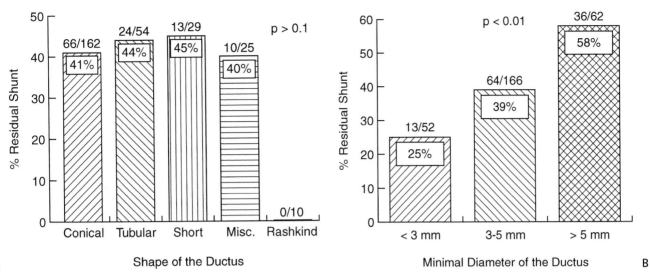

FIGURE 19.9. A: Relationship of residual shunt by echo-Doppler within 24 hours of the procedure with the shape of the ductus; note that there is no significant ($p > .1$) relationship. **B:** Relationship of residual shunt with the size of the ductus is shown. Note higher incidence of residual shunts with larger ducti. (From Rao PS, Kim SH, Choi J, et al. Follow-up results of transvenous occlusion of patent ductus arteriosus with the buttoned device. *J Am Coll Cardiol* 1999;33: 820–826, with permission.)

patients. The presence of residual shunt did not correlate with ductal shape (Figure 19.9A). However, minimal ductal diameter plays a role in determining the prevalence of residual shunt (Figure 19.9B); the larger the ductus, the greater ($p < .001$) the probability for a residual shunt.

Complications

Device implantation was unsuccessful in six (2%) of the 284 patients. The device pulled through the ductus either during implantation or while disconnecting the delivery wire. In three of these six, the device was retrieved with a snare. In two of these, a larger device was implanted successfully at the same sitting. The third patient was sent to elective surgical closure at the discretion of the primary cardiologist. The final three patients underwent surgical retrieval of the device along with ductal ligation, again at the discretion of the primary cardiologist. No additional complications occurred.

Follow-up

Clinical examination, chest x-ray, and echocardiographic studies were performed 1 day and 1, 6, and 12 months after device deployment and yearly thereafter. Follow-up data were available for analysis in 234 (86%) of 280 patients 1 to 60 months (median, 24) after device implantation.

Follow-up Results

Reinterventions were performed in seven (2.5%) patients to treat residual shunts. Four patients had elective surgical lig-

ation, as per the wishes of the primary cardiologists. Two of these also had evidence for hemolysis that resolved following surgery. In the remaining three patients, the residual shunts were closed by placement of coil ($N = 2$) or by a second buttoned device ($N = 1$), all with success. Actuarial reintervention-free rates are depicted in Figure 19.10.

Chest x-rays revealed the stable position of the device, and no wire fractures were noted. No evidence for late

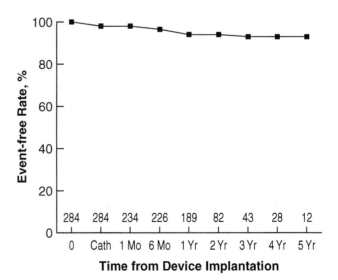

FIGURE 19.10. Graph showing actuarial reintervention-free rates following transvenous buttoned device closure of patent ductus arteriosus. (From Rao PS, Kim SH, Choi J, et al. Follow-up results of transvenous occlusion of patent ductus arteriosus with the buttoned device. *J Am Coll Cardiol* 1999;33:820–826, with permission.)

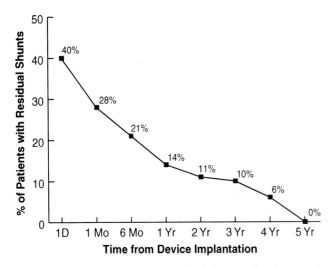

FIGURE 19.11. Resolution of residual shunts after buttoned-device closure of patent ductus arteriosus. (From Rao PS, Kim SH, Choi J, et al. Follow-up results of transvenous occlusion of patent ductus arteriosus with the buttoned device. *J Am Coll Cardiol* 1999;33:820–826, with permission.)

Transvenous occlusion is feasible, and relatively small sheaths are adequate for device delivery. The ductus can be closed irrespective of the size (small or large), shape (conical, tubular, or AP window type), and length (short or long). Results during follow-up confirm the favorable immediate results. Modification of the device to reduce the size of the delivery sheath and to decrease or eliminate residual shunts at implantation is necessary.

APPLICABILITY TO ADULT SUBJECTS

The results of PDA occlusion in adult subjects are generally similar to those reported in children, with occasional exceptions, and have been summarized elsewhere (11). Since the initial report of use in an adult subject (10), the device has undergone a multiinstitutional study (11). During a 40-month period ending August 1996, 77 patients 16 to 19 years of age underwent transvenous buttoned-device closure. The indications, patient selection, and protocol for buttoned-device closure are similar to those described earlier.

The mean age of the patients was 34 ± 16 years (range, 16 to 92 years). There were 48 women and 19 men. Their weights were 29 to 92 kg, with a median of 52 kg.

The size of the PDA at its narrowest diameter was 2 to 15 mm, with a median of 5 mm. Eleven were larger than 8 mm and six were larger than 10 mm. The Qp:Qs was 1.9 ± 0.5, with a range of 1.3 to 3.3. The shape of the PDA was characterized as conical in 45 (58%), tubular in 17 (22%), short in nine (12%), and miscellaneous in three (4%). Three (4%) patients had a prior Rashkind device occlusion but had significant residual shunt.

Fifteen- to 35-mm devices have been used for PDA occlusion; 21 were 15 mm, 42 were 20 mm, eight were 25 mm, and three each were 30 and 35 mm. These devices were implanted via 7F (*N* = 21) or 8F (*N* = 56) sheaths.

embolization of the device or its components, or clinical thromboembolic events were noted.

Doppler echocardiographic studies revealed gradual reduction of the residual shunt rate (Figure 19.11). None of the echocardiographic studies showed evidence for thrombus or vegetation on the device. Also, there was no evidence for obstruction in the descending aorta or in the left pulmonary artery.

DISCUSSION

The preceding data suggest that occlusion of the ductus with the buttoned device is feasible, safe, and effective.

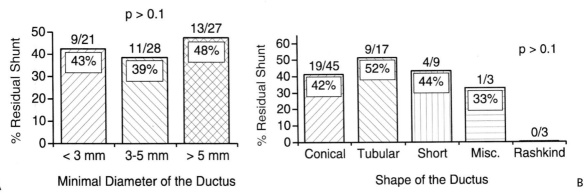

FIGURE 19.12. **A:** Relationship of residual shunt with the size of the patent ductus arteriosus in adult subjects. Note that there is no significant (*p* > .1) difference. **B:** Relationship between ductal shape and percentage of residual shunt; again, there is no significant (*p* > .1) difference. (From Rao PS, Kim SH, Rey C, et al. Results of transvenous buttoned device occlusion of patent ductus arteriosus in adults. *Am J Cardiol* 1998;82:827–829, with permission.)

The devices were placed successfully in all but one patient. The Qp:Qs decreased from 1.9 ± 0.5 to 1.1 ± 6.2 (*p* < .001) following device implantation. Continuous murmur of PDA was no longer heard in any of the 76 patients whose devices were successfully deployed.

Doppler echocardiographic studies performed within 24 hours of the procedure revealed effective occlusion [defined as trivial (*N* = 27) or no (*N* = 43) residual shunt] in 70 (92%) of 76 patients. Small shunts (*N* = 6) were present in the remaining patients. Ductal size and shape had no correlation with effective occlusion.

Complete occlusion was seen in 43 (67%) patients, whereas residual shunts are present in 33 (43%) patients. Neither the ductal shape nor size had any influence on the residual shunt rate (Figure 19.12).

In a single patient (1.3%), the device slipped through the ductus during buttoning and was transcathetered. Elective surgical ligation of the PDA was undertaken successfully, at the discretion of the treating cardiologist.

Follow-up protocol was similar to the previously described group. Follow-up data were available for review in 61 (80%) patients. The follow-up period lasted from 1 to 48 months, with a median of 24 months. Reintervention to treat residual shunts was required in two (3.5%) patients. The residual shunt in one patient was treated by coil placement. In the second patient with evidence for hemolysis, the primary cardiologist opted for surgical ligation, which successfully ended both the residual shunt and hemolysis. Thromboembolism, vegetation, and wire fractures were not observed during the follow-up period. Residual shunts gradually decreased with time (Figure 19.13).

Thus these data on adult subjects are similar to the entire cohort (12) with the exception of influence of ductal size on the percentage of residual shunt. The data demonstrate feasibility, safety, and effectiveness of buttoned-device occlusion of PDA in adults.

INFANT BUTTONED DEVICE

Although the feasibility, safety, and effectiveness of the regular buttoned device were well established by the preceding studies (9,11,12), the device delivery sheath (7F) was too bulky to employ routinely in small infants. In an attempt to extend its use to small infants, the device was redesigned so that it could be implanted through a 6F sheath. Replacing the square-shaped occluder with a single-strand occluder and incorporation of foam plug over the button loop (Figure 19.2) were such design modifications.

The infant buttoned device underwent clinical trials in seven centers (14,15,23,24). Forty-eight devices were implanted, and preliminary analysis of the data revealed the following: Minimal PDA diameters varied between 2 and 5 mm, with a median of 3.5 mm. Complete closure of the ductus by Doppler echocardiography was seen in 39 (81%) of 48 patients. No immediate complications were encountered. During follow-up, implantation of a second device to treat significant residual shunt was required in two (4%) patients. In the remaining patients the residual shunts disappeared.

Subclinical aortic perforation was observed by one group of investigators (25). When this was brought to the device manufacturer's attention, further use of infant buttoned devices was suspended (24). The investigators at the remaining six centers were notified of this concern with the recommendation that careful follow-up of the infant buttoned-device implantations be undertaken. However, it should be noted that the investigators using infant buttoned devices are impressed with the simplicity of device implantation, lack of embolizations, minimal metal content, and effectiveness of the device. Although the use of the infant device remains suspended, a final decision on its use will be made after collection and analysis of detailed follow-up data on all infant buttoned-device implantations.

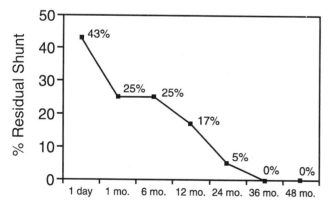

FIGURE 19.13. Residual shunts at varying time periods following device implantation in adult subjects showing gradual reduction of residual shunt. (From Rao PS, Kim SH, Rey C, et al. Results of transvenous buttoned device occlusion of patent ductus arteriosus in adults. *Am J Cardiol* 1998;82:827–829, with permission.)

FOLDING-PLUG BUTTONED DEVICE

Despite an 88% rate of effective occlusion, residual shunt was seen in 40% of patients following regular buttoned-device implantation, although the residual shunts decreased and disappeared with time. However, the indications for closure for many of these PDAs is prevention of bacterial endocarditis. Therefore these patients are at risk for bacterial endocarditis before complete resolution of the shunt. Thus it would seem logical to modify the device to effect complete closure of the ductus at the time

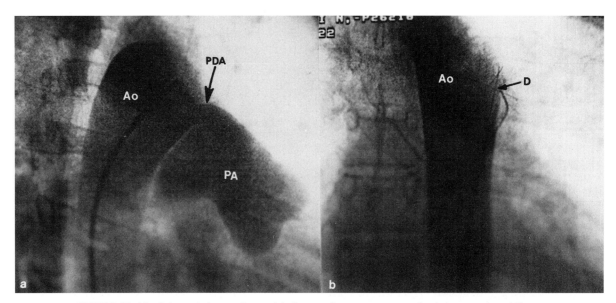

FIGURE 19.14. Selected cineangiographic frames from aortograms in right anterior oblique view before (**a**) and 15 minutes following (**b**) transvenous implantation of a folding plug buttoned device across a patent ductus arteriosus (PDA) demonstrating a large PDA in **a,** which is completely occluded following device (D) placement (**b**). Ao, aorta; PA, pulmonary artery. (From Rao PS, Kim SH, Choi J, et al. Follow-up results of transvenous occlusion of patent ductus arteriosus with the buttoned device. *J Am Coll Cardiol* 1999;33:820–826, with permission.)

of initial implantation of the device. Accordingly, polyurethane foam was incorporated over the button loop of the regular buttoned device; this modified device is named the *folding-plug buttoned device* (Figures 19.3 and 19.4). The device is currently in clinical trials internationally as well as in an FDA-approved US trial with IDE.

The preliminary data of the first 20 patients will be reviewed. The patients' ages varied between 3 and 39 years. Their weights were 4 to 70 kg, with a median of 12 kg. The minimal PDA diameter was 3 to 12, with a median of 7 mm. Fifteen- to 25-mm devices were used and delivered across the ductus via 7- and 8F sheaths. Excellent angiographic improvement was observed (Figure 19.14). Doppler echocardiography within 24 hours after device placement revealed complete occlusion in 17 (85%) of 20 patients. Trivial residual shunt was present in the remaining three (15%) patients. Follow-up data from 3 to 24 months revealed complete closure in 19 (95%) patients. No reinterventions were required during the short period of follow-up. No immediate complications were seen, nor were any observed during follow-up.

The data, though preliminary, indicate that full occlusion rates improved (Figure 19.15) without increasing any adverse effect following incorporation of the folding plug. A larger experience with a longer follow-up is necessary to confirm these encouraging observations.

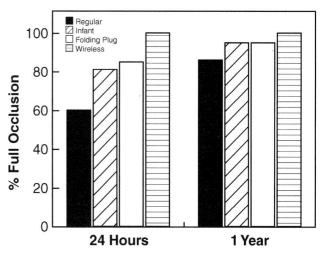

FIGURE 19.15. Bar graph showing complete occlusion rates with different types of buttoned devices. Twenty-four-hour occlusion rate of 60% with regular buttoned device improved both with infant and folding-plug device to 81% and 85%, respectively. This is presumably related to the folding plug over the button loop in both these devices. With transcatheter patch device, there was 100% occlusion, although the number of subjects is small (*N* = 4). Similarly, 1-year occlusion rate improved from 86% with regular buttoned device to 95% with plug devices to 100% with patch device. (From Sideris EB, Rao PS. Sideris' buttoned device for transcatheter closure of patent ductus arteriosus. *J Interv Cardiol* 2001;14:239–246, with permission.)

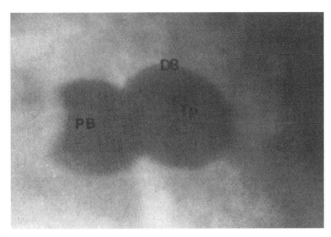

FIGURE 19.16. Selected cineradiographic frame in lateral view showing occlusion of a 22-mm patent ductus arteriosus with a 23-mm double balloon supporting a transcatheter patch. DB, distal balloon; PB, proximal balloon. (From Sideris EB, Rao PS. Sideris' buttoned device for transcatheter closure of patent ductus arteriosus. *J Interv Cardiol* 2001;14:239–246, with permission.)

WIRELESS DEVICES

Wireless PDA devices were conceived after animal experimentation and preliminary clinical experience with occlusion of atrial septal defects with detachable balloons (18,20) and transcatheter patches (8,26) suggested the feasibility of such devices. Subsequently, clinical trials were undertaken (24).

The protocol is similar to the implantation of the other buttoned devices except that balloon sizing of large PDAs is required. The device requires a 9- to 11F sheath for delivery and implantation. Initially, the distal balloon is inflated (1 to 2 mm larger than the balloon diameter of the PDA) in the descending aorta slightly distal to the ductal attachment. The entire system (inflated balloon and sheath) is withdrawn so that the distal balloon is wedged into the ductal lumen. The proximal balloon on the pulmonary end of the ductus is then inflated (Figure 19.16). Aortography to ensure the correct position of the device and to demonstrate ductal occlusion is performed. The device delivery wire is fixed in the groin and left *in situ* for 48 hours. Then the balloons are deflated and withdrawn; the patch remains in the ductus.

In all four patients with a large PDA, there was full occlusion. The PDA remained completely occluded at the last follow-up (24).

CURRENT STATUS

The folding-plug buttoned device is currently under FDA-supervised clinical trials with IDE and is available for use at the institutions participating in clinical trials. Outside the United States it is available for clinical use with approval by local IRBs, as per local regulations. The PDA patch device is available outside the United States at institutions participating in clinical trials. Application for IDE is pending with FDA and will not be available in the United States until the IDE is approved.

SUMMARY AND CONCLUSION

In this chapter transvenous occlusion of ductus arteriosus with regular buttoned device, infant buttoned device, folding-plug buttoned device and transcatheter patch was described.

The results of the regular buttoned device demonstrate feasibility, safety, and effectiveness in occluding PDA. All types and sizes of the ductus can be occluded transvenously. Attempts to reduce the size of the delivery sheath resulted in the design of the infant buttoned device. Although the results are encouraging, a report of subclinical aortic perforation by one of the participating centers resulted in suspension of use of infant buttoned device pending further study of the remaining cases. Because of the high incidence of residual shunts at implantation, folding-plug modification of the buttoned device was introduced. Preliminary results suggest marked reduction of residual shunts at implantation both immediately after implantation and during follow-up. This device should be useful in occluding moderate-sized to large PDAs. The folding-plug modification is currently undergoing international and FDA-supervised clinical trials with IDE. The experience with transcatheter patch occlusion of the PDA is extremely limited. Further experience with this device is needed to make any definitive conclusions.

REFERENCES

1. Gross RE, Hubbard JP. Surgical ligation of a patent ductus arteriosus: a report of first successful case. *JAMA* 1939;112:729–731.
2. Portsmann W, Wierny L, Warnke H. Der Verschluss des Ductus arteriosus persistens ohne Thorakotomie (1, Miffeilung). *Thoraxchirurgie* 1967;15:109–203.
3. Portsmann W, Wierny L, Warnke H, et al. Catheter closure of patent ductus arteriosus: 62 cases treated without thoracotomy. *Radiol Clin North Am* 1971;9:203–218.
4. Rashkind WJ, Cuaso CC. Transcatheter closure of a patent ductus arteriosus: successful use in a 3.5 kg infant. *Pediatr Cardiol* 1979;1:3–7.
5. Rashkind WJ. Transcatheter treatment of congenital heart disease. *Circulation* 1983;67:711–716.
6. Sandhu SK, King TD. Historical aspects of transcatheter closure of the patent ductus arteriosus. *Curr Interv Cardiol Rep* 2000;2:361–366.
7. Sideris EB, Sideris SE, Ehly RL. Occlusion of patent ductus arteriosus in piglet by a double disk self-adjustable device (Abstract). *J Am Coll Cardiol* 1990;15:240A.
8. Rao PS, Wilson AD, Sideris EB, et al. Transcatheter closure of patent ductus arteriosus with buttoned device; first successful

clinical application in a child. *Am Heart J* 1991;121: 1799–1802.

9. Rao PS, Sideris EB, Haddad J, et al. Transcatheter occlusion of patent ductus arteriosus with adjustable buttoned device: initial clinical experience. *Circulation* 1993;88:1119–1126.

10. Lochan R, Rao PS, Samal AK, et al. Transcatheter closure of patent ductus arteriosus with an adjustable buttoned device in an adult patient. *Am Heart J* 1994;127:941–943.

11. Rao PS, Kim SH, Rey C, et al. Results of transvenous buttoned device occlusion of patent ductus arteriosus in adults. *Am J Cardiol* 1998;82:827–829.

12. Rao PS, Kim SH, Choi J, et al. Follow-up results of transvenous occlusion of patent ductus arteriosus with the buttoned device. *J Am Coll Cardiol* 1999;33:820–826.

13. Rao PS, Berger F, Rey C, et al. Results of transvenous occlusion of secundum atrial septal defect with the fourth generation buttoned device: comparison with first, second and third generation devices. *J Am Coll Cardiol* 2000;36:583–592.

14. Sideris EB, Rey C, de Lezo JS, et al. Infant buttoned device for the occlusion of patent ductus arteriosus: early clinical experience (Abstract). *Cardiol Young* 1996;6:56.

15. Rao PS, Sideris EB. Transcatheter closure of patent ductus arteriosus: state of the art. *J Invasive Cardiol* 1996;8:278–288.

16. Rao PS, Sideris EB, Haddad J, et al. Follow-up results of transvenous occlusion of patent ductus arteriosus with the adjustable buttoned device. *Proceedings of the Second World Congress of Pediatric Cardiology and Cardiac Surgery.* Societas Cardiol Pediat Japonica, Honolulu, Hawaii, 1997:257.

17. Sideris EB, Rao PS. Buttoned device occlusion of patent ductus arteriosus. *Curr Interv Cardiol Rep* 2001;3:71–79.

18. Sideris EB, Sideris SE, Toumanides S, et al. From disk devices to transcatheter patches: the evolution of wireless heart defect occlusion. *J Interv Cardiol* 2001;14:211–214.

19. Sideris EB, Rey C, de Lezo JS, et al. Occlusion of large patent ductus arteriosus by buttoned devices with incorporated folding plugs. *Proceedings of the Second World Congress of Pediatric Cardiology and Cardiac Surgery.* Societas Cardiol Pediat Japonica, Honolulu, Hawaii, 1997:258.

20. Sideris EB, Chiang CW, Zhang JC, et al. Transcatheter correction of heart defects by detachable balloon buttoned devices: a feasibility study. *J Am Coll Cardiol* 1999;23:526A.

21. Rao PS. Descending aortography with balloon inflation: a technique for evaluating the size of the patent ductus arteriosus in infants and children with large proximal left-to-right shunt. *Br Heart J* 1985;54:527–532.

22. Krichenko A, Benson L, Burrows P, et al. Angiographic classification of the isolated persistently patent ductus arteriosus and implications for percutaneous catheter occlusion. *Am J Cardiol* 1989;63:887–889.

23. Rao PS, Sideris EB. Infant buttoned device. *Catheter Cardiovasc Interv* 2000;50:125–126.

24. Sideris EB, Rao PS. Sideris' buttoned device for transcatheter closure of patent ductus arteriosus. *J Interv Cardiol* 2001;14: 239–246.

25. Wilson NJ, Occleshaw EJ, O'Donnell, et al. Subclinical aortic perforation with the infant double-button patent ductus arteriosus occluder. *Catheter Cardiovasc Interv* 1999;48:296–298.

26. Sideris E, Sideris S, Poursanov M, et al. Transcatheter patch correction of atrial septal defects: experimental validation and early clinical experience (Abstract). *Cardiol Young* 2000;10:13.

20

GIANTURCO COILS

DOUGLAS J. SCHNEIDER
JOHN W. MOORE

Stainless steel coils have been used extensively for vascular occlusion since Gianturco's initial description in 1975 (1). Their original applications were for control of hemorrhage, occlusion of tumor vascular supply, and nonsurgical treatment of arteriovenous malformations (1–3). In 1981, transcatheter Gianturco coil occlusion of systemic to pulmonary artery collateral arteries was reported in a patient with pulmonary atresia (4). Subsequently, this technique became the procedure of choice to obliterate undesirable systemic to pulmonary artery collaterals in patients with congenital heart disease (5,6). With the first report of transcatheter coil occlusion of the patent ductus arteriosus (PDA) in 1992 (7), the clinical applications of this device were expanded to include occlusion of the PDA. Using an enlarging inventory of coil sizes and various modifications of the delivery technique, clinical investigators subsequently improved the efficacy and the safety of the procedure, while extending the range of PDA sizes feasible for occlusion. At the present time, due to the high efficacy, very low morbidity, and economic efficiency of transcatheter PDA occlusion with Gianturco coils, the procedure has replaced surgery as the procedure of choice for small to medium-sized PDA.

DEVICE

Standard Gianturco Coils

The original stainless steel coils described by Gianturco in 1975 were essentially guide wires with the core removed, shaped into a helical conformation, with strands of wool attached to one end (1). Despite the proliferation of a wide variety of coil shapes and sizes for a large number of vascular occlusion applications, the design of the standard

Gianturco coil (Cook Cardiology, Bloomington, IN) has been modified only slightly since that time (2,3). The coil consists of primary and secondary windings of stainless steel wire, with strands of Dacron fiber attached along most of the length (Figure 20.1).

The steel wire (0.004 to 0.008 inch in diameter, depending on the final coil size) is wound in a tight helical configuration to form straight segments, which resemble coreless guide wires with diameters of 0.015, 0.021, 0.028, or 0.043 inch. These segments are then shaped into coils with secondary loops ranging from 2 to 20 mm. A rounded bead (diameter equal to the diameter of the primary windings) is welded to one end of the coil, and Dacron strands are embedded at regular intervals along the coil, from the beaded end to within about 1 cm of the nonbeaded end. The coils are packaged in straight steel sleeves, which have a black band at one end to indicate the direction of loading, such that the beaded end of the coil is loaded into the delivery catheter first.

The diameter of the primary windings and adjacent Dacron determine the functional diameter of the coils from

Douglas J. Schneider: Associate Professor of Pediatrics, Drexel University School of Medicine, Philadelphia, Pennsylvania; Director, Cardiac Catheterization Laboratory, St. Christopher's Hospital for Children, Peoria, Illinois

John W. Moore: Professor of Pediatrics, Department of Pediatrics, The David Geffen School of Medicine at UCLA; Director, Cardiac Catherization Laboratory, Mattel Children's Hospital at UCLA, Los Angeles, California

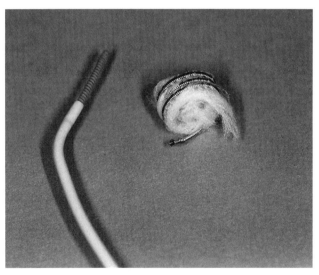

FIGURE 20.1. Gianturco coil, delivery catheter, and pusher wire.

the standpoint of the minimum delivery catheter lumen size into which the coils will fit. Standard Gianturco coils are available in functional diameters of 0.025, 0.035, 0.038, and 0.052 inch. The smaller coils are more pliable and conforming than the stiffer, larger coils. A given coil size is described by the functional diameter of the primary windings and Dacron, the length of the coil (with the secondary loops straightened out), and the diameter of the secondary coil loops. For example, a 38–8–5 coil has a functional diameter 0.038 inch, straightened length of 8 cm, and secondary loop diameter of 5 mm. The number of secondary coil loops is determined by the length of the coil and the diameter of the loops, mathematically expressed by the equation number of loops = length of coil ÷ (π × diameter of loops). The 38–8–5 coil, therefore, has about five loops.

Detachable Coil Modifications

To improve control of delivery and retrievability, modifications of the Gianturco coil have resulted in two widely available "detachable" delivery systems. One system uses a screw mechanism, and the other uses an interlocking bead mechanism. These systems are described in more detail later.

PATIENT SELECTION

There is general agreement that clinically apparent PDA should be closed to eliminate the adverse hemodynamic effects and risk of endarteritis, regardless of which method of intervention is used. The issue of the clinically silent PDA discovered incidentally by color flow Doppler remains controversial.

Since the initial success in coil occlusion of small PDA (minimum diameter < 2.5 mm) (7), the patient population suitable for PDA coil occlusion has expanded to include patients with moderate and in some cases large PDA (8). The likelihood of successful coil occlusion depends not only on the minimum PDA diameter, but also on the size and configuration of the entire ductus (9,10), quantity of shunt flow (8), and relative sizes of the PDA and descending aorta (8,11). Essentially, there must be sufficient space within the ductus to accommodate sufficient coil mass to achieve occlusion without causing obstruction in the aorta or pulmonary artery. In addition, the geometry of the ductus must be such that stable anchoring of the coil is feasible and hemodynamic forces will not lead to migration of the coil. There are no established patient selection criteria for coil occlusion of the PDA. In general, excluding small babies, most PDA less than 5 mm in diameter can be successfully coil occluded, whereas many PDA larger than 5 mm are candidates for other devices or for surgery.

Although there have been reports of PDA coil occlusion in infants as small as 2.3 kg (12,13) and our experience includes successful coil occlusion of the PDA in a 1.9-kg premature infant using the umbilical artery, experience in small babies is limited. Because of the relatively large diameter and short course of many PDA in premature neonates, combined with the overall small size of these patients, PDA coil occlusion is technically challenging. There are as yet no established criteria for patient selection for PDA coil occlusion in this patient population, and studies are needed.

In addition to many patients with native PDA, coil occlusion is the procedure of choice for occlusion of residual PDA shunts after previous surgical ligation or transcatheter device placement (14–19), including those with residual shunting after previous coil deployment (20).

PDA coil occlusion may be performed in combination with other interventions, such as coarctation angioplasty (21) during a single catheterization.

DEVICE IMPLANTATION TECHNIQUE

The original reports of PDA coil occlusion described delivery of the coil across the PDA utilizing an end-hole catheter passed across the PDA from the aorta (retrograde approach), with the coil extruded as the catheter was withdrawn through the ductus (7,9,10,22). Although this method continues to be a basic and widely employed technique, many technical modifications have evolved as experience with PDA coil occlusion has accumulated. No single technique is superior to others in every situation, and it is important to have more than one approach in one's armamentarium to appropriately manage the many variations in PDA anatomy.

Basic Technique

After right and left heart catheterization with standard heparinization (100 U/kg), including aortography in the anterio-posterior (or 30 degrees right anterior oblique) and straight lateral projections, the hemodynamics and PDA anatomy are analyzed. The minimum PDA diameter, PDA length, and aortic ampulla diameter are measured. Successful PDA occlusion depends largely on selection of the proper coil size. For most small to moderate-sized PDA, 0.038-inch coils are preferred. In larger patients with moderate-sized PDA and significant shunts, 0.052-inch coils are often preferred because of increased stiffness and bulk, which result in greater stability and higher occlusiveness. In patients with very small PDA, it may be necessary to use the less bulky 0.035-inch coils, as they can be delivered through smaller catheters. Various strategies have been advocated for selection of coil length and secondary loop diameter. In general, a coil is selected such that the secondary loop helical diameter is at least twice the minimum PDA diameter and less than or equal to the diameter of the aortic ampulla. We prefer to use a coil with the largest diameter that will fit within the aortic ampulla, often significantly greater than twice the minimum PDA diameter. Others have advocated using smaller-diameter coils, even less than two times the minimum PDA diameter, so that the coil may attain a more compact configuration and thereby possibly greater occlusiveness (23). Coil length should be chosen so that there will be a minimum of three to four loops. Some investigators have recommended coils with a total of five loops to increase the likelihood of complete closure with a single coil and to decrease the possibility of coil migration (24–26).

Although there are no data to confirm benefit, most operators administer prophylactic antibiotics (e.g., cefazolin 50 mg/kg) before coil deployment. One small study (27) demonstrated no infectious complications without antibiotics in 32 consecutive patients, but larger studies have not been reported. Depending on the coil size chosen, an appropriate-size end-hole catheter (such as a Judkins right coronary artery catheter) is advanced across the PDA into the main pulmonary artery over a standard straight-tip guide wire. The catheter lumen should accommodate a maximum guide wire diameter equal to the effective diameter of the primary coil windings and Dacron. For example, for 0.038-inch coils a catheter that accommodates a maximum guide wire diameter of 0.038 inch should be used. If the lumen is significantly larger than the coil, then the coil and fibers can bunch up, or the pusher wire may overlap with the coil and wedge tightly, resulting in difficulty advancing the coil through the catheter.

The coil is loaded into the catheter by inserting the introducer sleeve into the hub and advancing a guide wire (which is the same diameter as the coil and catheter lumen) through the introducer, which is then pulled out of the hub and off the wire. The coil is advanced through the catheter until one-half to three-quarters of a loop protrudes from the end of the catheter into the main pulmonary artery. The entire unit is pulled back until the extruded portion of the coil contacts the pulmonary artery end of the PDA, using the lateral angiogram image and tracheal shadow for guidance. The coil deforms slightly when it contacts the vascular wall. The catheter is gradually withdrawn through the PDA while the coil is held steady as needed by the guide wire, effectively "unsheathing" the catheter off the coil. When a sufficient length of coil is extruded from the catheter in the aortic ampulla, loops of coil begin to form. The coil is gradually advanced out of the catheter as the catheter is withdrawn into the aorta, and the loops will retract into the aortic ampulla once the entire coil is out of the catheter. Care should be taken to avoid advancing additional coil into the pulmonary artery. If the proximal coil loops protrude significantly into the aorta, they may be gently repositioned into the ampulla using the tip of the delivery catheter (28).

Some operators prefer the venous (anterograde) approach, in which the delivery catheter is passed across the PDA from the pulmonary artery (12,29). An advantage of this approach is that aortography can be performed using the arterial access during coil positioning. It may be difficult to cross very small PDA from the pulmonary artery, but larger PDA can be crossed without difficulty. The first portion of coil is extruded into the aorta and pulled back with the catheter into the aortic ampulla. All but one loop of the coil is then extruded into the aortic end of the PDA. The catheter is then pulled back into the pulmonary artery, where the last loop of coil is delivered.

If the coil position is unsatisfactory, the coil may be repositioned or removed using a loop snare or biopsy forceps. If the coil position is satisfactory, aortic angiography is repeated after 10 to 15 minutes to allow thrombus formation within the coil. Although small residual shunts often close over time (13,30,31), many persist (10). For this reason most operators advocate placing additional coils as necessary to achieve complete occlusion or only trace residual shunting (13,23,32). As many as nine coils have been implanted in a PDA (13). In general, subsequent coils are smaller than the first coil, often delivered through a 4F catheter after the PDA is recrossed retrograde using a soft-tip guide wire, taking care to avoid dislodgment of the previously placed coil or coils. Aortic angiography is repeated, and additional coils are placed as needed. PDA with larger minimum diameters are more likely to require multiple coils (33). Selection of the correct initial coil size and optimal positioning decreases the need for subsequent additional coils (23–25).

Modifications of Delivery Technique

Several modifications of delivery technique have been developed to reduce the risk of coil embolization and to improve the precision of coil placement. These techniques enhance control of coil positioning and in many cases simplify the task of coil retrieval. Although additional equipment adds cost to the procedure, reduced need for retrieval of migrated coils and potentially higher complete closure rates due to better coil-positioning capability may compensate for higher equipment costs.

As noted, more than one coil may be required for complete closure of moderate-sized PDA. As an alternative to sequential delivery using a single catheter, some operators deliver two coils simultaneously in moderate-sized PDA. Two delivery catheters are placed across the PDA (12,34). Both catheters may be advanced anterograde using two venous sheaths, or they may be "criss-crossed" with one anterograde and the other retrograde. The coils are delivered sequentially or simultaneously. This technique obviates the need to recross the PDA with a catheter after the first coil has been deployed, potentially decreasing the risk of unfavorably altering the position of an initial coil. The additional advantage of simultaneous delivery is that the coils intertwine while they are delivered, resulting in more stability with less likelihood of migration. In small patients, a single larger coil may protrude significantly into the aorta or pulmonary artery; simultaneous delivery of two smaller coils may be preferable (35). Another reported technique to deliver two coils simultaneously is to deliver both coils through a single long 6F sheath (36).

Use of a balloon catheter to support the coil during delivery adds control in coil deployment, enhancing the ability to place the coil in a desirable position and decreasing the likelihood of coil migration or having extra loops protrude into the pulmonary artery (37). The technique we

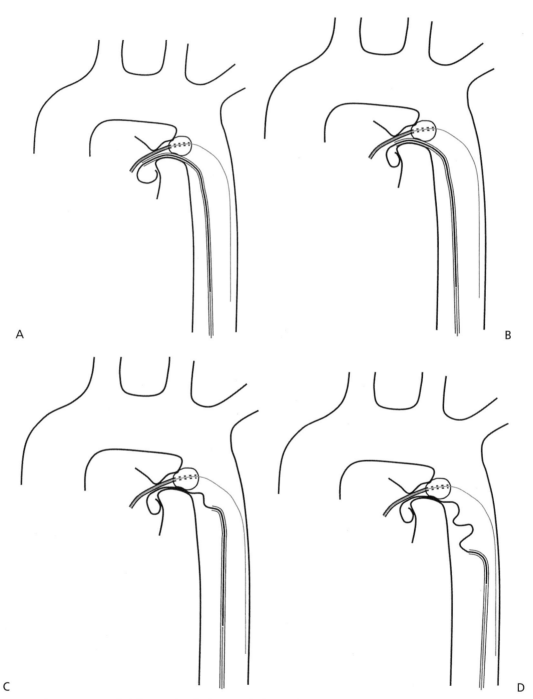

FIGURE 20.2. Coil delivery using balloon occlusion technique. **A:** With wedge catheter balloon inflated and pulled back into PDA, one-half to two-thirds of a coil loop is extruded into the pulmonary artery from the delivery catheter. **B:** Delivery catheter and coil pulled back as a unit until coil deforms slightly from contact with pulmonary artery wall. **C:** Delivery catheter withdrawn out of PDA, with wedge catheter balloon holding coil position stable. **D:** As catheter is pulled back off the coil, secondary loops begin to form in the aorta.

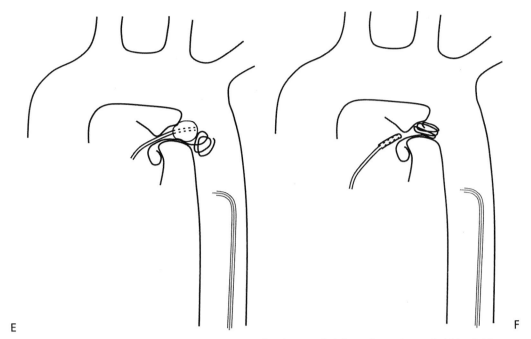

E   F

FIGURE 20.2. *(continued)* **E:** The coil is completely extruded from the catheter, held in stable position by wedge catheter balloon. **F:** Wedge catheter withdrawn into main pulmonary artery when deflated, allowing aortic end of coil to configure within the ampulla.

prefer for occlusion of most PDA involves delivering the coil from a catheter placed across the PDA retrograde from the aorta while supporting the coil firmly in the aortic ampulla with a wedge catheter advanced through the PDA anterograde from the pulmonary artery (Figure 20.2). The balloon is inflated in the aorta and pulled back into the aortic end of the PDA, and tension is held during delivery of the coil from the retrograde catheter. Once the aortic loops are extruded from the catheter, the balloon is gradually deflated and withdrawn into the pulmonary artery, and the aortic coil loops retract into the aortic ampulla. If the coil size has been properly selected, the risk of coil migration is very small. The mechanical pressure of the balloon against the coil and the elimination of flow through the PDA by the balloon contribute to stabilizing coil position during delivery. A variation of this technique is to occlude the PDA and support the coil with a wedge catheter balloon on the pulmonary artery side of the ductus (38,39). Forward pressure ("pushing") on the wedge catheter, which is supported and directed into the PDA by a guide wire through its lumen into the descending aorta, results in occlusion of PDA flow and support of the coil as it is delivered. With this method the coil attains its position within the aortic ampulla before release, and some operators leave the balloon inflated for several minutes before deflation so that developing thrombus might further stabilize the coil. The guide wire is withdrawn through the ductus into the wedge catheter before the balloon is deflated.

Snare-assisted coil delivery is the preferred method for PDA occlusion by some operators. The coil is delivered from the arterial approach and is snared by a loop snare after its first portion is extruded from the catheter. In the original report of this technique, the coil tip was snared in the pulmonary artery and supported there during delivery of the remainder of the coil on the aortic side (23,40). Another variation is to snare the coil tip in the aorta and extrude the entire coil from the delivery catheter before pulling it back into the PDA with the snare until the desired position is achieved (41). The snare allows control and stability during coil delivery, and it provides a means for retrieval of poorly positioned coils. One potential pitfall is that the snare may become entangled in the coil's Dacron fibers, occasionally making release difficult (41).

A third technique for stabilization of coils during delivery involves use of a 3F biopsy forceps to grasp the beaded end of the coil, allowing for the possibility of repositioning the coil or easy retrieval before release (42–44). This method is particularly useful with 0.052-inch coils, as these are more difficult to retrieve with a snare. The beaded end of the coil needs to be pulled or stretched slightly away from the body of the coil using a hemostat, allowing for closure of the biopsy forceps jaws around the bead. Back loading is possible using either a long 14F needle or a cutoff 4F sheath. Delivery may be accomplished via either the anterograde or retrograde approach. The 0.052-inch coils may be delivered through a 6F right coronary guide catheter or a long 4F sheath. A 5F right coronary guide catheter may be used for delivery of 0.038-inch coils. The biopsy forceps and snare techniques have been combined to provide "bidirectional" control of coils and may be useful in situations where there is high flow through a relatively short, large PDA (45).

Another technique modification that provides retrievability and improved control of positioning is the use of a modified end-hole catheter (46). The tip of the catheter is reshaped with heat such that the end-hole is smaller, leading to significant tension when the coil is protruded. The force required to completely extrude the coil is easily achieved with the pusher wire, but sufficient to hold the coil firmly during delivery and to allow retrieval of the coil through an arterial or venous sheath even after most of the coil is extruded out of the catheter.

Detachable Coil Systems

Two controlled delivery systems designed for Gianturco coils are now available. One is the Detachable Embolization Coil (Cook Cardiology, Bloomington, IN), which attaches the coil to a positioning catheter via a mechanism that interlocks a stretched-coil winding ("notch") with a bead on the end of a catheter core wire (47,48). When the core wire bead is retracted into the positioning catheter tip, it holds the coil end firmly in the catheter tip by interlocking with the coil at the "notch." The handle at the other end of the positioning catheter has a mechanism that extrudes the core wire bead from the end of the catheter, releasing the coil. The coils, available in 0.035- and 0.038-inch sizes, are made with smaller-diameter stainless steel or platinum wire and twice as many Dacron strands, which are half as long as those on the standard Gianturco coils. Because the coils are made with smaller wire than the standard coils, they are less bulky and have less occlusiveness than standard Gianturco coils. For this reason many operators avoid using these coils as the primary coil for PDA occlusion. However, the Detachable Embolization Coils offer significant advantages as additional (second or third) coils in partially occluded PDA.

The Flipper Detachable Embolization Coil Delivery System (Cook Cardiology, Bloomington, IN) utilizes a screw mechanism for attachment and detachment. The positioning wire to which the coil attaches has a core mandrel, which advances through the primary windings of the coil during loading. The coil is delivered through an end-hole catheter with a diameter of 0.041 inch, and detachment is accomplished by rotating the positioning wire to unscrew the connection. This system has been used extensively in Europe and Asia (15,49–54) and is now available in the United States.

RESULTS

Many series reporting results of PDA coil occlusion have been published since the initial description of this procedure in 1992. After the early reports, experience with the procedure in many centers led to improvements in coil selection and delivery techniques, resulting in high closure rates and fewer coil migrations, despite the fact that patient selection gradually expanded to include larger PDA and smaller patients. Efficacy of transcatheter coil occlusion of the PDA may be defined in several ways, including the ability to successfully implant the coil or coils, clinical success (absence of residual continuous murmur), absence of residual shunt by angiography, and absence of residual shunt by Doppler. Because many patients with initially trace or small residual shunts progress to complete closure during follow-up without further intervention, and because recurrence of shunting after apparent early complete closure has been documented (13,31,55), follow-up data are essential to evaluate the effectiveness of this technique. Although the significance of "silent" residual shunts in the absence of hemolysis is controversial, we believe that complete closure by Doppler at 6- to 12-month follow-up should be the standard for successful occlusion of PDA.

Immediate Results

Table 20.1 summarizes results from many of the reported series of PDA coil occlusion (9,13,22,30,56–61). Study group sizes range from the relatively small initial reports to the large multicenter registries in the United States and Europe. The most extensive data set is the PDA registry, which involved almost 1,400 procedures in the 64 participating centers. The rate of successful implantation was high in this group of studies, ranging from 89% to 100%, with an average of 96%. The primary reasons for unsuccessful implantation were that the PDA was too large or too small, and these numbers are clearly affected by patient selection and operator experience.

In patients in whom successful coil implantation was achieved, clinical closure (defined as absence of residual PDA murmur and other signs of hemodynamically important shunt) was 97% in the PDA registry data. This finding is probably related to the fact that the PDA registry represents data primarily from the early experience, between 1992 and 1996. Most recent series report 100% clinical closure. Residual shunting, then, represents almost exclusively "silent" residual PDA.

Immediate PDA closure rates are evaluated by angiography (Figure 20.3) a few minutes after coil implantation and/or by Doppler echocardiography within the first 24 hours. In the studies listed in Table 20.1, immediate angiographic complete closure was reported in 58% to 97% of cases, with an average of 71%. Centers whose protocols promote delivery of additional multiple coils until complete angiographic closure is achieved demonstrate higher rates of immediate complete closure (32,60). Given the fact that Doppler echocardiography may be more sensitive than angiography in detecting very small residual shunts, the

TABLE 20.1. RESULTS OF PDA COIL OCCLUSION

Investigators, Year	Total Patients	Successful Implantation	Immediate Angiographic Complete Closure	Complete Occlusion Within 24 Hours	Complete Occlusion at Follow-up*	Follow-up Time
Lloyd et al., 1993 (22)	24	92%	75%			
Moore et al., 1994 (9)	30	96%	80%		90%	6 mo
Shim et al., 1996 (30)	75		58%		85%	10 mo
PDA Registry† 1992–96	1,366	96%	73%	84%	93%	1 yr
Alwi et al., 1997 (58)	211	97%	60%	77%	93%	1 yr
Ing et al., 1999 (23)	104	100%	70%		95%	2–16 mo
Goyal et al., 1999 (13)	84	98%	65%	71%	88%	1 yr
Hofbeck et al.,‡ 1999 (59)	317	89%	62%	82%	95%	2 yr
Patel et al., 1999 (60)	149	98%	97%	97%	98%	6 mo
ERCCAD§ 1999 (61)	567	95%		82%	98%	8 mo

*Without second procedure.
†64 centers, mostly in the United States.
‡Seven centers in Europe.
§European Registry for Catheter Closure of the Arterial Duct, 42 centers (includes 56 patients with DuctOcclud device).

data in Table 20.1 demonstrate clearly that within the first 24 hours there is progression to complete closure in many patients. In the listed studies, the average complete occlusion rate at 24 hours was 82%. Factors associated with incomplete closure include larger PDA size (10), shorter PDA length (9), larger shunt ratio (8), and larger ratio of PDA diameter to aortic diameter (47).

Complications

Serious complications of PDA coil occlusion are rare. There are no reported cases of procedure-related death, infection, or stroke. In the PDA registry, 96% of cases were free of any complications. Most complications were minor and not associated with sequelae, and were essentially the same as

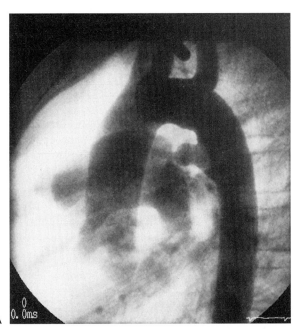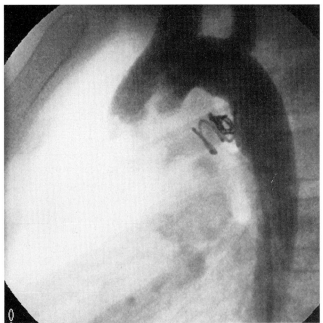

FIGURE 20.3. Angiograms of PDA coil occlusion. **A:** Lateral angiogram with injection in aorta demonstrating PDA anatomy before coil occlusion. **B:** Lateral angiogram with injection in aorta after occlusion using two Gianturco coils

those encountered in routine cardiac catheterization. Issues pertaining specifically to potential adverse effects of PDA coil occlusion include migration of coils to pulmonary or systemic arteries, disturbance of flow in the left pulmonary artery and/or aorta, and hemolysis.

The reported incidence of coil migration to the pulmonary or systemic arteries has been up to 14% when data from the early experience are included. Because of the emergence of technique modifications and detachable systems, the incidence has decreased. Furthermore, in most cases a migrated coil can be retrieved using a loop snare or biopsy forceps. In patients with migrated coils that were not retrieved, there have been only rare reported adverse effects. In one patient infrarenal IVC thrombosis occurred because of an unretrieved coil (62). Rare complications have occurred during attempts to retrieve migrated coils, including vascular injury to an iliac artery that required surgery (13) and entanglement of a coil in the tricuspid valve apparatus that necessitated surgery (63,64). Use of a long sheath allows the operator to avoid pulling an exposed coil through the heart, and should prevent coil entanglement in the tricuspid valve apparatus (65). Flow disturbance in the proximal left pulmonary artery from the pulmonary artery coil loops has been reported in many series. Doppler echocardiography may demonstrate turbulent flow and increased velocity approaching or exceeding 2 m/sec, and these findings are generally mild and often resolve over time (66,67). Two-dimensional echocardiographic images are often misleading in that they may suggest significant obstruction that is not confirmed by other methods, including pressure recordings, angiography, lung perfusion scans, and/or pulse Doppler (35,67). Clinically significant left pulmonary artery obstruction is rare. However, cases of significant LPA obstruction have been reported (8,13,58,62,) and this complication is associated with the use of larger (62) and multiple (68) coils in smaller patients. Obstruction of the aorta is an extremely rare complication of PDA coil occlusion (69). Poor position of the coil in the aorta during or after deployment mandates repositioning or removal. A small amount of coil projecting into the aortic lumen is not problematic (5), however, and careful hemodynamic and angiographic assessment is important.

Hemolysis has been reported in several patients with significant residual shunting, primarily early in the experience (70–74). Complete resolution of hemolysis results from elimination of the residual shunt by placement of additional coils. One reported case had resolution of hemolysis without reintervention despite persistence of significant residual shunting (75).

No long-term adverse effects of stainless steel coils in the body have been reported. Studies and postmortem pathologic evaluations have shown that at 6 months there is organized thrombus, fully covered by endothelium, with minimal inflammation or tissue reaction (76,77).

Follow-up

Follow-up data demonstrate that many patients with small residual shunts in the immediate postprocedure period progress to complete closure without further treatment, as demonstrated in Table 20.1. In the 6-month to 1-year follow-up period, complete closure rates were 85% to 98%, with an average of 93%. Interestingly, there are reports of PDA reopening after previous demonstration of complete closure (13,31,55,78), although most series report no instances of reopening. The shorter (type B) morphology was identified as a potential risk factor (78). One proposed mechanism is vasomotor reactivity of the PDA, with relaxation leading to alteration in the coil position and subsequent recurrence of shunting. Another is retraction of the clot. We believe that differences in coil selection strategies and positioning technique may account for the inconsistency of this finding among various investigators.

Late migration of coils to the pulmonary arteries has also been reported (63,79), but this is an extremely rare event. These instances likely occurred within the first few days after implant, before the thrombus was firmly organized. In one case thrombolytic therapy was being administered for loss of lower-extremity pulse after the procedure (79). It is likely that coil size and positioning are also factors in these rare occurrences.

APPLICABILITY IN ADULT SUBJECTS

Because surgical treatment for PDA in adult patients carries higher risk than in infants and children, coil occlusion of the small to moderate PDA in adults is the procedure of choice. In general, larger coils are preferred, often 0.052-inch coils. The procedure is essentially no different from that in children and infants, and results have been similar (34,80,81).

CURRENT STATUS

Gianturco coils and their controlled delivery systems are available worldwide and are widely employed for PDA occlusion. The devices are FDA approved in the United States for vascular occlusion but are not FDA approved for the indication of PDA occlusion. Nevertheless, the exceptional results of Gianturco coil occlusion of the PDA over a decade of clinical practice have made Gianturco coil occlusion of the PDA the *de facto* standard treatment for small to moderate-sized PDA.

CONCLUSION

Since the introduction of Gianturco coil occlusion, transcatheter coil occlusion has become the treatment of choice for small to moderate-sized PDA. Compared with surgical treatment, PDA occlusion with coils is associated with less morbidity and is cheaper (82–84). Serious complications have been extremely rare. Several modifications of the delivery technique have been developed, and detachable coil systems are now available. These techniques and delivery systems have enabled operators to improve coil position and to prevent most coil embolizations. At the present time, among properly selected patients, operators may achieve PDA closure rates approaching 100% with essentially no morbidity and no mortality.

REFERENCES

1. Gianturco C, Anderson JH, Wallace S. Mechanical devices for arterial occlusion. *Am J Roentgenol* 1975;124:428–435.
2. Anderson JH, Wallace S, Gianturco C, et al. "Mini" Gianturco stainless steel coils for transcatheter vascular occlusion. *Radiology* 1979;132:301–303.
3. Chuang VP, Wallace S, Gianturco C. A new improved coil for tapered-tip catheter for arterial occlusion. *Radiology* 1980;135:507–509.
4. Szarnicki R, Krebber HJ, Wack J. Wire coil embolization of systemic-pulmonary artery collaterals following surgical correction of pulmonary atresia. *J Thorac Cardiovasc Surg* 1981;81:124–126.
5. Verma R, Lock BG, Perry SB, et al. Intraaortic spring coil loops: early and late results. *J Am Coll Cardiol* 1995;25:141–149.
6. Perry SB, Radtke W, Fellows KE, et al. Coil embolization to occlude aortopulmonary collateral vessels and shunts in patients with congenital heart disease. *J Am Coll Cardiol* 1989;13:100–108.
7. Cambier PA, Kirby WC, Moore JW. Percutaneous closure of the small (less than 2.5 mm) patent ductus arteriosus using coil embolization. *Am J Cardiol* 1992;69:815–816.
8. Owada CY, Teitel DF, Moore P. Evaluation of Gianturco coils for closure of large (≥3.5 mm) patent ductus arteriosus. *J Am Coll Cardiol* 1997;30:1856–1862.
9. Moore JW, George L, Kirkpatrick SE, et al. Percutaneous closure of the small patent ductus arteriosus using occluding spring coils. *J Am Coll Cardiol* 1994;23:759–765.
10. Shim D, Beekman RH. Transcatheter management of patent ductus arteriosus. *Pediatr Cardiol* 1998;19:67–71.
11. Berdjis B, Moore JW. Coil occlusion of patent ductus arteriosus. *Prog Pediatr Cardiol* 1996;6:137–147.
12. Hijazi ZM, Geggel RL. Results of antegrade transcatheter closure of patent ductus arteriosus using single or multiple Gianturco coils. *Am J Cardiol* 1994;74:925–929.
13. Goyal VS, Fulwani MC, Ramakantan R, et al. Follow-up after coil closure of patent ductus arteriosus. *Am J Cardiol* 1999;83:463–466.
14. De Moor M, Al Fadley F, Galal O. Closure of residual leak after umbrella occlusion of the patent arterial duct, using Gianturco coils. *Int J Cardiol* 1996;56:5–9.
15. Uzun O, Hancock S, Parsons JM, et al. Transcatheter occlusion of the arterial duct with Cook detachable coils: early experience. *Heart* 1996;76:269–273.
16. Podnar T, Masura J. Transcatheter occlusion of residual patent ductus arteriosus after surgical ligation. *Pediatr Cardiol* 1999;20:126–130.
17. Dalvi B, Vora A, Narula D, et al. Coil occlusion of a residual ductus arteriosus remaining after implantation of a buttoned device. *Catheter Cardiovasc Diagn* 1996;39:52–54.
18. Hijazi ZM, Geggel RL, Al-Fadley F. Transcatheter closure of residual patent ductus arteriosus shunting after the Rashkind occluder device using single or multiple Gianturco coils. *Catheter Cardiovasc Diagn* 1995;36:255–258.
19. Moore JW, George L, Kirkpatrick SE. Closure of residual patent ductus arteriosus with occluding spring coil after implant of a Rashkind occluder. *Am Heart J* 1994;127:943–945.
20. Moore JW. Repeat use of occluding spring coils to close residual patent ductus arteriosus. *Catheter Cardiovasc Diagn* 1995;35:172–175.
21. Ing FF, McMahon WS, Johnson GL, et al. Single therapeutic catheterization to treat coexisting coarctation of the aorta and patent ductus arteriosus. *Am J Cardiol* 1997;79:535–537.
22. Lloyd TR, Fedderly R, Mendelsohn AM, et al. Transcatheter occlusion of patent ductus arteriosus with Gianturco coils. *Circulation* 1993;88:1412–1420.
23. Ing FF, Sommer RJ. The snare-assisted technique for transcatheter coil occlusion of moderate to large patent ductus arteriosus: immediate and intermediate results. *J Am Coll Cardiol* 1999;33:1710–1718.
24. Rao PS, Balfour IC, Chen S. Effectiveness of five-loop coils to occlude patent ductus arteriosus. *Am J Cardiol* 1997;80:1498–1501.
25. Ino T, Nishimoto K, Akimoto K, et al. Is transcatheter closure of patent ductus arteriosus using multiple coils feasible? *Am J Cardiol* 1995;76:637.
26. Rao PS, Balfour IC, Jureidini SB, et al. Five-loop coil occlusion of patent ductus arteriosus prevents recurrence of shunt at follow-up. *Catheter Cardiovasc Interv* 2000;50:202–206.
27. Hoyer MH, Marvin WH, Fricker FJ. Prophylactic use of antibiotics unnecessary during coil closure of patent ductus arteriosus. *Catheter Cardiovasc Interv* 1999;47:141.
28. Rothman A, Lucas VW, Sklansky MS, et al. Percutaneous coil occlusion of patent ductus arteriosus. *J Pediatr* 1997;130:447–454.
29. Hijazi ZM, Lloyd TR, Beekman RH, et al. Transcatheter closure with single or multiple Gianturco coils of patent ductus arteriosus in infants weighing ≤ 8 kg: retrograde versus antegrade approach. *Am Heart J* 1996;132:827–835.
30. Shim D, Fedderly RT, Beekman RH, et al. Follow-up of coil occlusion of patent ductus arteriosus. *J Am Coll Cardiol* 1996;28:207–211.
31. Uzun O, Dickinson D, Parsons J, et al. Residual and recurrent shunts after implantation of Cook detachable duct occlusion coils. *Heart* 1998;79:220–222.
32. Zellers TM, Wylie KD, Moake L. Transcatheter coil occlusion for the small patent ductus arteriosus (<4 mm): improved results with a "multiple coil-no residual shunt" strategy. *Catheter Cardiovasc Interv* 2000;49:307–313.
33. Hijazi ZM. Transcatheter coil closure of patent ductus arteriosus in small children: does approach really matter? *Catheter Cardiovasc Diagn* 1998;44:309.
34. Laird JR, Slack MC, Gurczak P, et al. Spring coil embolization of a patent ductus arteriosus in an adult. *Cardiovasc Interv Radiol* 1995;18:259–261.
35. Evangelista JK, Hijazi ZM, Geggel RL, et al. Effect of multiple coil closure of patent ductus arteriosus on blood flow to the left lung as determined by lung perfusion scans. *Am J Cardiol* 1997;80:242–244.
36. De Wolf D, Verhaaren H, Matthys D. Simultaneous delivery of two patent arterial duct coils via one venous sheath. *Heart* 1997;78:201–202.
37. Berdjis F, Moore JW. Balloon occlusion delivery technique of closure of patent arteriosus. *Am Heart J* 1997;133:601–604.
38. Dalvi B, Goyal V, Narula D, et al. New technique using tempo-

rary balloon occlusion for transcatheter closure of patent ductus arteriosus with Gianturco coils. *Catheter Cardiovasc Diagn* 1997; 41:62–70.

39. Dalvi B, Nabar A, Goyal V, et al. Transcatheter closure of patent ductus arteriosus in children weighing < 10 kg with Gianturco coils using the balloon occlusion technique. *Catheter Cardiovasc Diagn* 1998;44:303–308.

40. Sommer RJ, Gutierrez A, Lai WW, et al. Use of preformed Nitinol snare to improve transcatheter coil delivery in occlusion of patent ductus arteriosus. *Am J Cardiol* 1994;74:836–839.

41. Weber HS, Cyran SE. Transvenous "snare-assisted" coil occlusion of patent ductus arteriosus. *Am J Cardiol* 1998;82:248–251.

42. Hays MD, Hoyer MH, Glasow PF. New forceps delivery technique for coil occlusion of patent ductus arteriosus. *Am J Cardiol* 1996;77:209–211.

43. Grifka RG, Jones TK. Transcatheter closure of large PDA using .052-inch Gianturco coils: controlled delivery using a bioptome catheter through a 4 French sheath. *Catheter Cardiovasc Interv* 2000;49:301–306.

44. Hays MD. Anterograde coil closure of patent ductus arteriosus using a modified bioptome delivery technique. *Catheter Cardiovasc Interv* 2000;50:191–194.

45. Ing FF, Recto MR, Saidi A, et al. A method providing bidirectional control of coil delivery in occlusions of patent ductus arteriosus with shallow ampulla and Pott's shunts. *Am J Cardiol* 1997;79:1561–1563.

46. Kuhn MA, Latson LA. Transcatheter embolization coil closure of patent ductus arteriosus-modified delivery for enhanced control during coil positioning. *Catheter Cardiovasc Diagn* 1995;36: 288–290.

47. Cambier PA, Stajduhar KC, Powell D, et al. Improved safety of transcatheter vascular occlusion utilizing a new retrievable coil device. *J Am Coll Cardiol* 1994;23:359A.

48. Johnston TA, Stern HJ, O'Laughlin MP. Transcatheter occlusion of the patent ductus arteriosus: use of the retrievable coil device. *Catheter Cardiovasc Interv* 1999;46:434–437.

49. Akagi T, Hashino K, Sugimura T, et al. Coil occlusion of patent ductus arteriosus with detachable coils. *Am Heart J* 1997;134: 538–543.

50. Podnar T, Masura J. Percutaneous closure of patent ductus arteriosus using special screwing detachable coils. *Catheter Cardiovasc Diagn* 1997;41:386–391.

51. Celiker A, Qureshi SA, Bilgic A, et al. Transcatheter closure of patent arterial ducts using controlled-release coils. *Eur Heart J* 1997;18:450–454.

52. Rosenthal E, Qureshi SA, Reidy J, et al. Evolving use of embolisation coils for occlusion of the arterial duct. *Heart* 1996;76: 525–530.

53. Tometzki AJ, Arnold R, Peart I, et al. Transcatheter occlusion of the patent ductus arteriosis with Cook detachable coils. *Heart* 1996;76:531–535.

54. Celiker A, Bilgic A, Alehan D, et al. Transcatheter closure of patent ductus arteriosus using controlled-release coils. *Acta Paediatr Jpn* 1996;38:500–505.

55. Tomita H, Fuse S, Akagi T, et al. Coil occlusion for patent ductus arteriosus in Japan. *Jpn Circ J* 1997;61:997–1003.

56. Lloyd TR, Beekman RH, Moore JW, et al. The PDA coil registry: report of the first 535 procedures. *Circulation* 1995;92(Suppl I): 380.

57. Lloyd TR, Beekman RH, Moore JW, et al. The PDA coil registry: 250 patient-years of followup. *J Am Coll Cardiol* 1996;27:34A.

58. Alwi M, Kang LM, Samion H, et al. Transcatheter occlusion of native persistent ductus arteriosus using conventional Gianturco coils. *Am J Cardiol* 1997;79:1430–1432.

59. Hofbeck M, Bartolomaeus G, Buheitel G, et al. Safety and efficacy of interventional occlusion of patent ductus arteriosus with detachable coils: a multicentre experience. *Eur J Pediatr* 2000; 159:331–337.

60. Patel HT, Cao QL, Rhodes J, et al. Long-term outcome of transcatheter coil closure of small to large patent ductus arteriosus. *Catheter Cardiovasc Interv* 1999;47:457–461.

61. Tynan M, Huggon I, Rosenthal E, et al. Coil occlusion of the arterial duct. *J Interv Cardiol* 1999;12:73–77.

62. Hijazi ZM, Geggel RL. Transcatheter closure of patent ductus arteriosus using coils. *Am J Cardiol* 1997;79:1279–1280.

63. Hijazi A, Mazhar R, Bricelj B, et al. Embolization of Gianturco coil into the pulmonary artery requiring emergency surgical intervention. *Tex Heart Inst J* 1999;26:300–302.

64. Fulwani MC, Vajifdar B, Tendolkar AG, et al. Coil entrapment in the tricuspid valve apparatus requiring surgical removal: an unusual complication of transcatheter closure of patent ductus arteriosus. *Indian Heart J* 1999;51:77–79.

65. Mullins CE. Editorial commentary in: embolization of Gianturco coil into the pulmonary artery requiring surgical intervention. *Tex Heart Inst J* 1999;26:300–302.

66. Carey LM, Vermilion RP, Shim D, et al. Pulmonary artery size and flow disturbances after patent ductus arteriosus coil occlusion. *Am J Cardiol* 1996;78:1307–1310.

67. Stromberg D, Pignatelli R, Rosenthal GL, et al. Does ductal occlusion with the Gianturco coil cause left pulmonary artery and/or descending aorta obstruction? *Am J Cardiol* 1999;83:1229–1235.

68. Galal MO, Von Sinner W, al-Fadley F, et al. Radiographic characteristics of Cook detachable and Gianturco coils as well as clinical results of transcatheter closure of the patent ductus arteriosus. *Z Kardiol* 1999;88:1006–1014.

69. Moore JD, Shim D, Mendelsohn AM, et al. Coarctation of the aorta following coil occlusion of a patent ductus arteriosus. *Catheter Cardiovasc Diagn* 1998;43:60–62.

70. Shim D, Wechsler DS, Lloyd TR, et al. Hemolysis following coil embolization of a patent ductus arteriosus. *Catheter Cardiovasc Diagn* 1996;39:287–290.

71. Henry G, Danilowicz D, Verma R. Severe hemolysis following partial coil-occlusion of patent ductus arteriosus. *Catheter Cardiovasc Diagn* 1996;39:410–412.

72. Tomita H, Fuse S, Akagi T, et al. Hemolysis complicating coil occlusion of patent ductus arteriosus. *Catheter Cardiovasc Diagn* 1998;43:50–53.

73. Wang LH, Wang JK, Mullins CE. Eradication acute hemolysis following transcatheter closure of ductus arteriosus by immediate deployment of a second device. *Catheter Cardiovasc Diagn* 1998; 43:295–297.

74. Kapoor A, Radhakrishnan S, Shrivastave S. Severe intravascular haemolysis following coil occlusion of patent ductus arteriosus. *Indian Heart J* 1996;48:173–174.

75. Lee C, Hsieh K, Huang T, et al. Spontaneous resolution of hemolysis after partial coil occlusion of ductus arteriosus. *Pediatr Cardiol* 1999;20:371–372.

76. Sigler M, Handt S, Seghaye MC, et al. Evaluation of *in vivo* biocompatibility of different devices for interventional closure of the patent ductus arteriosus in an animal model. *Heart* 2000;83:570–573.

77. Lloyd RJ, Sinman R, Sharratt GP, et al. Transvenous closure of patent ductus arteriosus in a sick 2780 g infant. *Can J Cardiol* 1996;12:300–302.

78. Daniels CJ, Cassidy SC, Teske DW, et al. Reopening after successful coil occlusion for patent ductus arteriosus. *J Am Coll Cardiol* 1998;31:444–450.

79. Huang T, Hsieh K, Lee C. Late coil migration due to thrombolysis after successful implantation of a coil for persistent ductus arteriosus. *Catheter Cardiovasc Interv* 2000;50:334–336.

80. Ing FF, Mullins CE, Rose M, et al. Transcatheter closure of the patent ductus arteriosus in adults using the Gianturco coil. *Clin Cardiol* 1996;19:875–879.

81. Oishi T, Okamoto M, Sueda T, et al. Transcatheter coil embolization of large-size patent ductus arteriosus in adult patients: usefulness and problems. *Jpn Circ J* 1999;63:994–998.
82. Prieto LR, DeCamillo DM, Konrad DJ, et al. Comparison of cost and clinical outcome between transcatheter coil occlusion and surgical closure of isolated patent ductus arteriosus. *Pediatrics* 1998;101:1020–1024.
83. Singh TP, Morrow WR, Walters HL, et al. Coil occlusion versus conventional surgical closure of patent ductus arteriosus. *Am J Cardiol* 1997;79:1283–1285.
84. Fedderly RT, Beekman RH, Mosca RS, et al. Comparison of hospital charges for closure of patent ductus arteriosus by surgery and by transcatheter coil occlusion. *Am J Cardiol* 1996;77:776–779.

Catheter Based Devices: For the Treatment of Non-coronary Cardiovascular Diseases in Adults and Children. Edited by P. Syamasundar Rao and Morton J. Kern, Lippincott Williams & Wilkins, Philadelphia © 2003.

21

DETACHABLE COILS

NARAYANSWAMI SREERAM
SING-CHIEN YAP

The detachable coil (Cook Cardiology, Bloomington, IN) has gained widespread acceptance for patent ductus arteriosus (PDA) occlusion outside the United States. The detachable coil is a Gianturco coil modified so that it is attached to a delivery wire. This allows improved control over positioning of the coil across the PDA and full retrievability up to the point of release of the coil from the delivery wire. The major advantages of the detachable coil are that, compared with the umbrella devices, the coil and delivery wire are small enough to be accommodated within a 4F end-hole catheter, allowing the coil to be used via the arterial or venous approach. In addition, compared with the standard (nondetachable) Gianturco coil, optimal positioning of the coil can be more easily achieved, particularly as the coil is fully retrievable even after extrusion from the delivery catheter and until detachment from the delivery wire. In theory, any size of PDA may be occluded, although this may necessitate the use of multiple coils for the larger ducts. The procedure can be safely performed in infants of more than 2 kg body weight. Ductal diameter and morphology do not appear to play an important role when considering the use of detachable coils for PDA occlusion. In the reported series, PDAs with a minimum diameter of 5 mm have been successfully occluded using multiple coils. The only relative contraindication would be the neonate with a large symptomatic PDA in whom it may be anticipated that multiple coils would be needed. In this situation, the risk of potential stenosis of one or another branch pulmonary artery from the bulk of the coils in the pulmonary arterial side would weigh in favor of surgical ligation of the PDA.

DEVICE DESCRIPTION

The detachable coil is a stainless steel coil with a covering of Dacron wool fibers (Figure 21.1A). The coils that are specif-

ically for use to occlude PDAs are available in three standard diameters: 3, 5, and 8 mm. For each diameter, different coil lengths are also available, with the result that the deployed coil can have three, four, or five loops (turns). The delivery wire is hollowed, with a central mandrel, which can be passed into the central lumen of the coil (Figure 21.1B). The helical screw on the proximal end of the coil can then be locked onto an opposing screw on the delivery wire by making a series of clockwise turns (Figure 21.1C). The central mandrel maintains the coil in a straight position during insertion and advancement of the coil to the tip of the delivery catheter (Figures 21.1D and 21.1E). Once the coil is advanced to the tip of the delivery catheter, which is positioned to straddle the duct, the mandrel is withdrawn. The coil can then be extruded, allowing the loops to form in the vascular tree (Figures 21.1F and 21.1G). The coil can be delivered using either an anterograde (venous) or retrograde (arterial) approach. When the arterial approach is used, the coil is extruded from the delivery catheter so that the first loop is formed on the pulmonary arterial side of the PDA. The catheter, with the partially extruded coil, is then withdrawn into the ampulla of the PDA, and the remaining loops form on the aortic side of the duct. Detachment of the coil is achieved by making several anticlockwise turns on the delivery wire. Until this maneuver is performed, the coil is fully retrievable. When a venous approach is used, coil deployment is performed in the reverse order. The bulk of the coil (most turns) is allowed to form on the aortic side of the duct, and the last loop on the pulmonary arterial side.

CHOICE OF COIL

The duct is crossed in the anterograde or retrograde direction using a 4- or 5F catheter with a single end-hole, and a large (0.038-inch diameter) central lumen (William Cook Europe, Bjaeverskov, Denmark or Microvena Corporation, White Bear Lake, MN), over a standard 0.035-inch-diameter guide wire. Initial coil diameters are generally chosen as follows: if the minimum diameter of the PDA is <2 mm, a

Narayanswami Sreeram: Director, Division of Cardiology, Wilhelmina Children's Hospital, University Medical Center, Utrecht, the Netherlands
Sing-Chien Yap: Division of Cardiology, Wilhelmina Children's Hospital, University Medical Center, Utrecht, the Netherlands

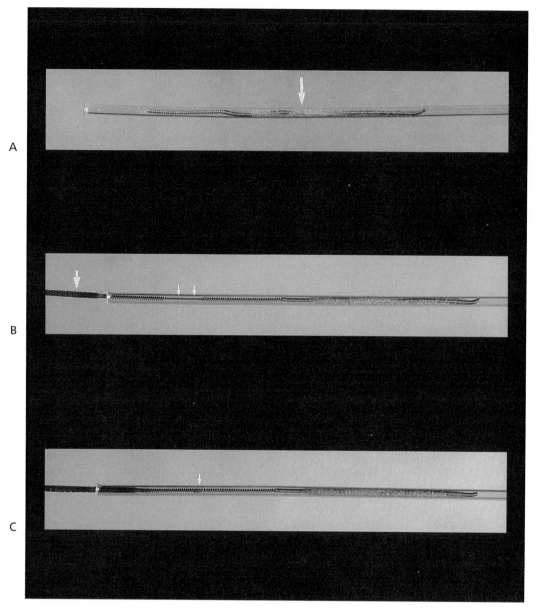

FIGURE 21.1. A: The coil *(arrow)* is delivered by the manufacturer, preloaded in a hollow plastic sleeve. **B:** The hollow delivery wire *(single arrow)*, with the central mandrel *(double arrows)*, is advanced into the plastic sleeve, so that the mandrel passes through the central lumen of the coil. This allows the helical screw of the coil to be locked onto the opposing screw on the delivery wire, by making a series of turns manually. The locking procedure has been completed in **(C)**; *(arrow* marks where the screws interlock).

5-mm-diameter coil is implanted. If the minimum PDA diameter is >2 mm, an 8-mm diameter coil is chosen. The number of loops (and therefore the length of the coil used) is determined by the length and morphology of the PDA. The shape and length of the duct have little effect on coil size. In general, for shorter ducts a shorter length coil (three or four loops) is used. The aim is to implant the coil in such a way that the minimum amount (usually one loop) of the coil is on the pulmonary arterial side of the PDA. The

remaining loops are formed in the PDA and on the aortic side.

SINGLE VERSUS MULTIPLE COILS

The issue of whether a single or multiple coil should be used is largely subjective. After the first coil has been satisfactorily positioned and detached, repeat aortography may

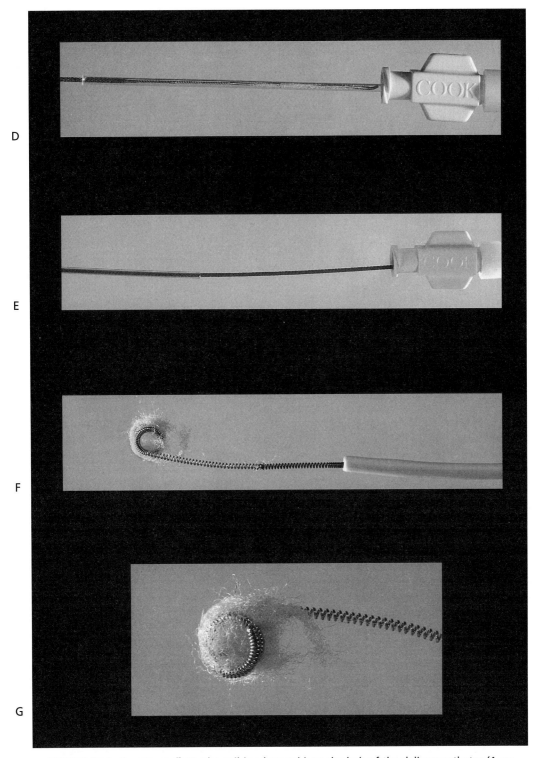

FIGURE 21.1. *(continued)* D: The coil is advanced into the hub of the delivery catheter (4- or 5F diameter). The plastic sleeve *(arrow)* can then be withdrawn **(E)**, and the coil can be advanced further to its delivery site. When the mandrel is withdrawn and the coil is extruded from the delivery catheter, it assumes the required number of turns **(F)**. At this point the coil is still fully retrievable, as the spring remains locked to the delivery wire. A close-up view of a released coil is shown in **(G)**.

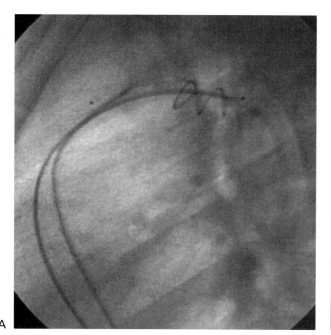
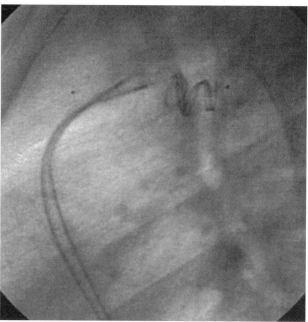

A   B

FIGURE 21.2. A: One coil has already been deployed via an anterograde approach in the PDA. The duct has been recrossed with a second delivery catheter containing the second coil. **B:** The second coil is deployed in the duct. The first coil can now be released, and if necessary, a third coil can be introduced, while keeping the second coil still attached to its delivery wire.

be performed to assess the degree of residual shunting. Alternatively, on-table echocardiography may provide a comparable assessment of the degree of shunting. In our practice, we use the presence of a residual murmur (especially if continuous) as an indication for further coil implantation. This is based on the (not unreasonable) premise that the aim of therapy is complete occlusion of the PDA. Accordingly, we have placed multiple coils in the PDA to ensure that there is no residual shunt, even if in most patients it is likely that small residual shunts presenting immediately after use of a single coil may disappear at later follow-up. The second (and subsequent) coil can be positioned in one of several ways. In some patients we have used a combined arterial and venous approach, crossing the duct with two delivery catheters and deploying the two coils simultaneously and allowing the two coils to interlock. Another technique is to deploy the first coil but not to release it from the delivery wire. The duct is then crossed with a standard 0.035-inch guide wire and 4F delivery catheter, and the second coil is deployed (Figures 21.2A and 21.2B). If a third coil is deemed necessary, the first coil can be released, keeping the second coil attached to the delivery wire, and the process can be repeated (Figure 21.3). The simplest way, however, is to release the first coil and recross the duct with a guide wire and catheter, and proceed to fur-

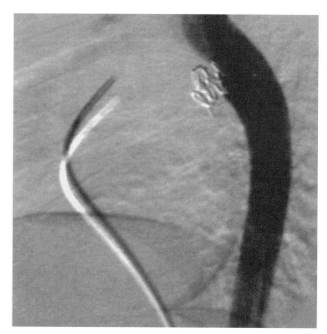

FIGURE 21.3. The final angiographic result (aortogram) after insertion of three coils in this patient, confirming that there is no residual shunt.

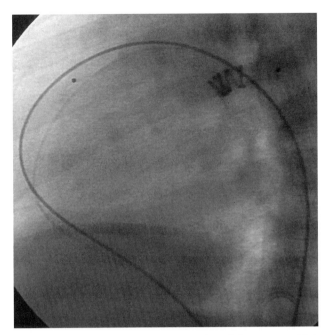

FIGURE 21.4. Alternative technique for delivering multiple coils. The first coil is appropriately deployed and released. The duct is then recrossed with a 0.035-inch guide wire *(arrow)*, to facilitate introduction of the second coil delivery system.

ther coil deployment (Figure 21.4). The risks of coil displacement or embolization during this maneuver appear to be surprisingly low.

RESULTS

Occlusion Rates

In the early results reported for detachable coil occlusion of the PDA, immediate occlusion occurred in 60% of patients, increasing to 72% within 24 hours of the procedure and 86% 3 months later (1). Shunts that persist beyond 3 months after initial coil occlusion are unlikely to close spontaneously and may require further coil implantation. Most patients received a single coil. The immediate occlusion rates may be improved substantially if a more aggressive approach is taken, using multiple coils to abolish any shunt deemed more than trivial on angiography, color Doppler echocardiography, or cardiac auscultation after deployment of the first coil. Tometzki et al. reported 89% complete occlusion at 24 hours after the procedure, increasing to 98% by 6 months after the procedure (2). In a smaller series of patients, Sreeram et al. reported a 100% occlusion rate with a protocol of using additional coils if the PDA could be crossed with a 0.035-inch guide wire and 4F catheter after implantation of the first coil (3). However, this may be unnecessarily aggressive, as it has been demon-

strated both for Gianturco coil and for detachable coil closures that the prevalence of residual shunts tend to diminish with time.

For residual ductal shunting following a previous surgical ligation or previous implantation of an umbrella device, the results of detachable coil occlusion are similarly encouraging. In the series of Tometzki et al., of 25 patients with residual ductal shunting following a previous procedure, occlusion rates were 88% at 24 hours, increasing to 96% at 6-month follow-up.

Our current policy is to undertake detachable coil closure of any residual shunt persisting at 1 year after initial occlusion.

Complications

Immediate Complications

The major immediate complication is coil embolization, usually to one or the other lung. This is more likely to occur when a small coil (e.g., a 5-mm-diameter coil for a PDA with a minimum diameter of >2 mm) is used. An additional risk factor is the length of coil (and therefore the number of turns) deployed on the pulmonary arterial side of the PDA. As a rule, this should be kept to a minimum (usually a half turn or a single turn is sufficient). If a longer length of coil protrudes into the pulmonary artery, then the coil is likely to be unstable and is best retrieved into the delivery catheter. Embolized coils can be removed in a relatively straightforward fashion. The safest technique is to position an 8F long sheath in the pulmonary trunk or branch pulmonary artery to which the coil has embolized. A gooseneck snare (Microvena Corporation, White Bear Lake, MN) can then be used to retrieve the coil into the long sheath and remove it. This also avoids pulling the exposed coil back through the pulmonary or tricuspid valves.

Short-Term Complications

As with other occlusion devices, persistent intravascular hemolysis has occasionally been reported in patients with residual shunts following coil occlusion (4). The therapy for this condition is occlusion of the residual shunt with a second coil.

Long-Term Complications

Recurrent Shunts Following Successful Initial Occlusion

Uzun et al. have reported recurrent shunts after apparently successful coil occlusion of the PDA (4). In most instances the new shunt was detectable by color Doppler echocardiography within 24 hours of coil occlusion, although in two patients in their series recurrence of ductal shunting was noted 1 month after initial occlusion. A significant proportion of recurrent shunts observed within 24 hours of the procedure tend to resolve spontaneously. The most likely explanation for this event is minor degrees of movement of the coil/s in the first hours following implantation. In patients in whom recurrent shunting is observed beyond a month after the procedure, recanalization of the PDA, as has been described following surgical ligation (5) or the use of other devices (6), cannot be excluded. Further coil occlusion procedures may be necessary in some of these patients.

Acquired Obstruction of a Branch Pulmonary Artery

Branch pulmonary arterial stenosis following device occlusion of the PDA is a well-recognized sequela. This was initially reported for the Rashkind double-umbrella device. Although it was most likely to occur when a large (17-mm) device was used in a small-body-weight (<10 kg) patient (7), this complication has also been reported with the smaller (12 mm) umbrella device (8), and following the use of multiple (nondetachable) Gianturco coils for PDA occlusion (9). In the only comparable study reported following the use of detachable coils, decreased perfusion to the left lung (defined as <40% of total lung flow) was reported in a single patient, who previously had a 17-mm Rashkind umbrella device implanted (3). Coil protrusion into the pulmonary trunk and left pulmonary artery as assessed by cross-sectional echocardiography is a relatively common finding. This is more commonly observed when multiple coils are used. When three or more coils are used, coil protrusion into the left pulmonary artery always occurs. Coil protrusion is also associated with higher peak velocities in the affected branch pulmonary artery on spectral Doppler echocardiography. However, although patients with coil protrusion and higher Doppler velocities in the left pulmonary artery tended to have lower values for left lung perfusion, this was not significantly different when compared with patients without evidence of coil protrusion and with normal Doppler velocities in the left pulmonary artery (43.7% ± 1.7% in the multiple coil/coil protrusion group versus 44.8% ± 1.6% in patients without coil protrusion). Another important outcome of this study was the absence of correlation between peak left pulmonary artery Doppler velocities and left lung perfusion.

COSTS

The detachable coil represents a considerable saving in the cost of PDA occlusion when compared with either the umbrella device or surgery (10). The average cost of all disposables used for a PDA occlusion procedure is between US $450 and $500.

FDA STATUS

The manufacturer informs us that the detachable Cook coil is FDA approved. The MRI-compatible version of these coils still does not have FDA approval.

CONCLUSION

The detachable Cook coil may be the safest and one of the least expensive catheter device for PDA closure currently available (11).

REFERENCES

1. Uzun O, Hancock S, Parsons JM, et al. Transcatheter occlusion of the arterial duct with Cook detachable coils: early experience. *Heart* 1996;76:269–273.
2. Tometzki AJP, Arnold R, Peart I, et al. Transcatheter occlusion of the patent ductus arteriosus with Cook detachable coils. *Heart* 1996;76:531–534.
3. Sreeram N, Tofeig M, Walsh KP, et al. Lung perfusion studies after detachable coil occlusion of persistent arterial duct. *Heart* 1999;81:642–645.
4. Uzun O, Dickinson D, Parsons J, et al. Residual and recurrent shunts after implantation of Cook detachable duct occlusion coils. *Heart* 1998;79:220–222.
5. Sorensen KE, Kristensen BO, Hansen OK. Frequency of occurrence of residual ductal flow after surgical ligation by colour-flow mapping. *Am J Cardiol* 1991;67:653–654.
6. Bjornstad PG, Smevik B. Recanalization of the arterial duct after initial total occlusion with the Rashkind umbrella. *Cardiol Young* 1995;5:98–99.
7. Nykanen DG, Hayes AM, Benson LN, et al. Transcatheter patent ductus arteriosus occlusion: application in the small child. *J Am Coll Cardiol* 1994;23:1666–1670.
8. Dessy H, Hermus JPS, van den Heuvel F, et al. Echocardiographic and radionuclide pulmonary blood flow patterns after transcatheter closure of patent ductus arteriosus. *Circulation* 1996;94:126–129.
9. Evangelista JK, Hijazi ZM, Geggel RL, et al. Effect of multiple coil closure of patent ductus arteriosus on blood flow to the left lung as determined by lung perfusion scans. *Am J Cardiol* 1997;80:242–244.
10. Gray DT, Fyler DC, Walker AM, et al. Clinical outcomes and costs of transcatheter as compared with surgical closure of patent ductus arteriosus. *N Engl J Med* 1993;329:1517–1523.
11. Rigby ML. Editorial. Closure of the arterial duct: past, present, and future. *Heart* 1996;76: 461–462.

Catheter Based Devices: For the Treatment of Non-coronary Cardiovascular Diseases in Adults and Children. Edited by P. Syamasundar Rao and Morton J. Kern, Lippincott Williams & Wilkins, Philadelphia © 2003.

22

DUCT-OCCLUD

TRONG-PHI LÊ
MALTE B. NEUSS
FRANZ FREUDENTHAL

The first transcatheter device for closure of the patent ductus arteriosus (PDA) was a plug of polyvinyl alcohol foam described by Porstmann et al. (1) in 1966. Subsequently, a double-umbrella device was utilized by Rashkind (2). This device was used around the world. Over the years other devices have been designed and investigated (3–6).

Gianturco coil occlusion of PDA was described in the early 1990s (7) and gained importance as it became apparent that the Rashkind device (USCI Bard, Billerica, MA) had significant disadvantages. The Rashkind device could not be used in small patients and had significant problems, including protrusion into the pulmonary artery (8) or the aorta and a high rate of residual shunts. Gianturco coils (Cook, Bloomington, IN) (9) were used in the initial reported series (7,10) of coil occlusion of the PDA. They could be implanted via small-caliber catheters, preventing damage of vessels used for access and thus allowing use in very small patients. However, significant risk of inadvertent embolization due to lack of control and retrievability existed. In addition, poor maneuverability of the Gianturco coil may result in suboptimal coil positioning, such as protrusion of coils into the left pulmonary artery or the descending aorta, and hemolysis.

To achieve better-controlled deployment of the Gianturco coil, several modified delivery techniques were developed. These include use of snares (11,12), forceps (13), tapered-tip catheters (14), and balloon occlusion catheters (15). Safe use of coils for PDA occlusion requires a reliable retrieval mechanism.

Neuss designed a new retrievable, stainless steel coil in 1990 (Neuss, personal communication). In contrast to the Gianturco coil, this coil did not contain Dacron fibers. By 1991, Neuss and his coworkers had succeeded in fully controlled deployment of this new retrievable coil to occlude renal arteries in sheep (16). Additional modifications of the Neuss coil with various coil configurations and sizes resulted in the currently used Duct-Occlud Occlusion System (Pfm, Cologne, Germany). In this chapter we describe the Duct-Occlud device and delivery system, the method of device selection, the technique of device implantation, and the clinical results available to date.

THE DUCT-OCCLUD DEVICE

Since its initial use in 1992, the Duct-Occlud system has been modified several times. However, the main technical principles have remained unchanged. The Duct-Occlud PDA Occlusion System consists of a coil with core wire and pusher assembly, the coil positioner grip, and the implantation catheter. Two different devices are currently available: the standard Duct-Occlud coil and the reinforced Duct-Occlud coil. Both devices are manufactured in a number of sizes with a known axial length and different proximal and distal loop diameters. The central portion of all devices has a diameter of less than 2.5 mm.

The standard device is made of a 0.17-mm stainless steel wire and has primary windings and secondary coil loops. Primary windings are made around a straight core wire producing a highly flexible, straight tension spring with an internal diameter of 0.37 mm and an outer diameter of 0.72 mm (0.028 inch). This spring is wound around a fixture with an hourglass shape and is shock-heated. This process forms permanent secondary coil loops. The standard device has an asymmetric hourglass shape, which has a distal diameter larger than the proximal diameter (Figure 22.1).

The reinforced device is produced by a similar process, using a thicker (0.20-mm) wire that is double-stranded on the distal end for the length of two or more secondary loops, depending on the distal diameter of the coil. The primary windings have a slightly larger outside diameter (0.80 mm, or 0.032 inch). Because of the double-stranded structure of the distal portion, these windings are substantially "stiffer" than the single-stranded loops of either the stan-

Trong-Phi Lê: Consultant, Department of Pediatric Cardiology, University Hospital of Hamburg, Hamburg, Germany; Chief, Department of Pediatric Cardiology, Central Hospital links der Weser, Bremen, Germany

Malte B. Neuss: German Heart Center Berlin, Augustenburger Platz, Berlin, Germany

Franz Freudenthal: Fellow, Department of Radiology, Technical University of Aachen, Pauwelsstr, Germany

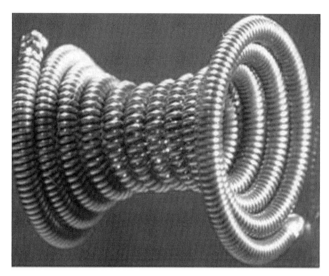

FIGURE 22.1. The standard Duct-Occlud device has a biconical shape. The primary spring is wound on a core wire, which is shock-heated to produce an hourglass shape.

dard or the reinforced device. The reinforced coil is cone-shaped because the proximal windings are wound in reverse direction (Figure 22.2). The axial length of the reinforced coil is therefore shorter than the standard coil with corresponding distal loop diameter, making the device more compact than the standard version.

The coil is mounted in a straightened profile on the distal end of a 0.35-mm Nitinol core wire that has two circumferential grooves (for the standard device) and a forged prominence (for the reinforced device) at its tip. The proximal primary windings of the coil are designed to catch the restraint of the core wire. In this manner, the proximal 5

mm of the coil is attached to the core wire. For coil detachment the pusher assembly has to overcome an attachment force of 4 to 12 N, according to the stiffness of the coil being used.

The pusher assembly is a moveable hollow wire co-mounted on the proximal part of the core wire. The pusher assembly is single-stranded and has the same outer diameter as the coil. Stainless steel pins are attached to the proximal ends of the core wire and the pusher assembly. The pins allow the core wire to be stabilized while the pusher assembly is advanced over the core wire, pushing the device off the core wire following implantation.

The coil positioner grip is a disposable stainless steel device that allows controlled coil delivery and detachment (Figure 22.3). The positioner grip consists of a stainless steel bar with an engraved millimeter scale. It consists of a stop-lock and two sliding carriages that hold the pins of the pusher assembly and the core wire. The devices are implanted via 4F (for the standard device) and 5F (for the reinforced device) end-hole polytetrafluoroethylene (Teflon) catheters with hockey-stick configurations and radiopaque distal tip markers.

PATIENT SELECTION

Small to moderate-sized PDAs are selected for closure with this method. Patients are excluded if the PDA is considered too large or if the pulmonary vascular resistance is elevated. Patients who require open-chest surgery for indications other than PDA are also excluded. The delivery system of the Duct-Occlud device is small enough for use in all ages, but a minimum weight of 3 kg is recommended.

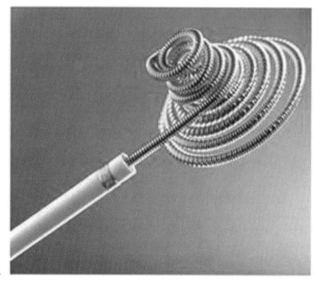

A

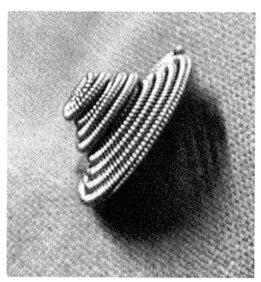

B

FIGURE 22.2. The (**A**) reinforced and (**B**) reverse Duct-Occlud device have a double-stranded primary spring in the distal loops. The proximal loops are wound the reverse direction, giving the device a monoconical shape.

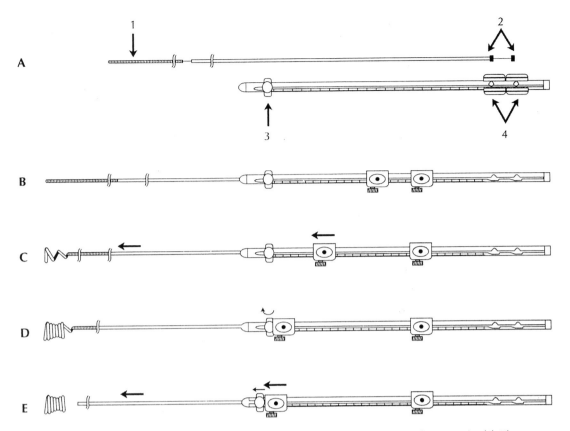

FIGURE 22.3. Coiled position grip. **A:** *Upper panel:* The coil stretched over the core wire (1). The pins (2) of the core wire and the pusher are at the other end of the delivery system. *Bottom panel:* The prepared coil positioning grip with the stop-lock (3) and the two sliding carriages (4). **B:** The coil delivery system is mounted into the positioning grip. **C:** The sliding carriage of the pusher assembly is moved forward to extrude the coil. **D:** The stop-lock is loosened when the coil is ready for detachment. **E:** The sliding carriage of the pusher and the stop-lock are moved to the end of the grip to detach the coil.

IMPLANTATION PROCEDURE

Confirmation of the clinical diagnosis is made by Doppler echocardiographic examination. The implantation procedure may be performed under general anesthesia or conscious sedation. Heparin for anticoagulation and antibiotics for endocarditis prophylaxis are usually administered.

A lateral aortogram is performed prior to coil implantation to delineate the anatomy and size of the PDA. Four French pigtail graduated marker catheter (OccluMarker, Pfm, Cologne, Germany) placed in the proximal descending aorta facilitates the calibration procedure and allows precise measurement of PDA. The narrowest PDA diameter, aortic ampulla diameter, and axial PDA length are measured. The narrowest PDA diameter (D_1) and the aortic ampullar diameter (D_2) are measured perpendicularly to the PDA axis. The length (L) is defined as the distance between D_1 and D_2 (Figure 22.4). These spatial dimensions of the PDA are useful in selecting an appropriate-sized coil. Selection of the Duct-Occlud device is based on the following considerations: (a) the largest device loop is equal to or slightly larger than D_2; (b) D_1 is smaller than 4 mm; and (c) the configured length of the device is equal to or shorter than L. We suggest a reinforced device in larger patients with significant PDA or if D_1 is greater than 1.5 mm.

If the PDA can easily be crossed from the pulmonary artery, transvenous occlusion is recommended. Otherwise, the transarterial approach is used. Figure 22.5 demonstrates the key steps of the transvenous procedure. The tip of the implantation catheter is positioned in the descending aorta and the coil delivery system is advanced to its tip. Approximately 80% to 90% of the coil is then pushed off the core wire into the descending aorta using the positioner grip. Before this the pigtail catheter in the descending aorta should be pulled away from the implantation catheter to prevent coil entanglement. By advancing the delivery system through the implantation catheter, the coil is configured in the descending aorta. The remaining proximal portion of the coil, still stretched over the core wire, is retained in the tip of the implantation catheter. The entire system (catheter, core wire, and pusher) is carefully withdrawn until the configured portion of the coil enters the ductal ampulla. Then the tip of the implantation catheter is pulled back into the narrowest part of the PDA. The remaining loops are pushed off the core wire by moving the pusher carriage close to the stop-lock on the positioner grip. By very carefully advancing the delivery system while withdrawing the

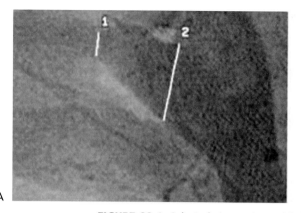

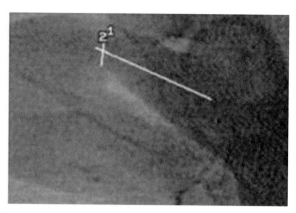

FIGURE 22.4. Selected cineangiographic frames in a lateral row demonstrating key measurements of the patent ductus arteriosus for occlusion using Duct Occlud. **A:** (1) Minimal diameter; (2) diameter of the ampulla. **B:** (3) Length of the ductus.

implantation catheter into the pulmonary artery simultaneously, one or two loops are delivered on the pulmonary side. This final step of the implantation procedure is the most difficult maneuver. It is suggested that this maneuver is performed by using the operator's left hand to pull the implantation catheter at the introducing sheath while the right hand pushes the delivery system simultaneously. The pulmonary loops are considered important because they provide an anchor for the coil in the PDA. In addition, they may absorb the detachment force, preventing movement of the coil toward the aorta during detachment. An aortogram is performed to confirm the position of the device. If the position or size of the coil is sub-

optimal, it can be retrieved and repositioned or exchanged. If it is found to be in a good position, the coil is detached from the retrieval mechanism by loosening the stop-lock and sliding the pusher carriage all the way toward the tip of the positioner grip. A final aortogram is performed to document coil position and PDA occlusion. Figure 22.6 shows three typical examples of PDA occlusion using the standard Duct-Occlud.

In very large PDAs simultaneous implantation of two or more devices may be performed to achieve complete occlusion. The devices may be implanted transvenously from the pulmonary artery side, or one device transvenously and the other by a transarterial approach (Figure 22.7). However,

FIGURE 22.5. Stages of the implantation procedure (left to right). **A:** Lateral cineangiographic row of patent ductus arteriosus (PDA). **B:** The delivery system crossed the PDA from the pulmonary side. **C:** The coil is configured in the descending aorta and retracted into the ductus lumen. **D:** One proximal loop is positioned on the pulmonary side of the PDA. The junction of the coil to the pusher is now moved outside the implantation catheter. The coil is ready for release. **E:** Angiogram a few minutes after coil detachment.

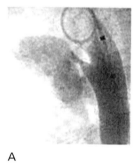

A

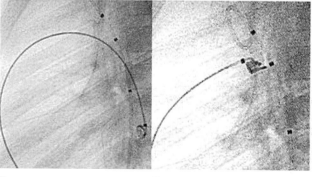

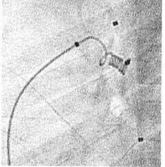

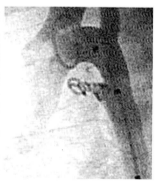

B   C   D   E

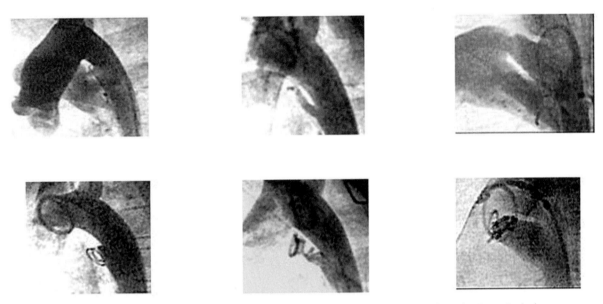

FIGURE 22.6. Typical examples of patent ductus arteriosus occlusion using the Duct-Occlud device. Angiogram before (upper row) and after coil occlusion (bottom row). *Left:* type B ductus. *Middle:* Small type E ductus. *Right:* Large type E ductus.

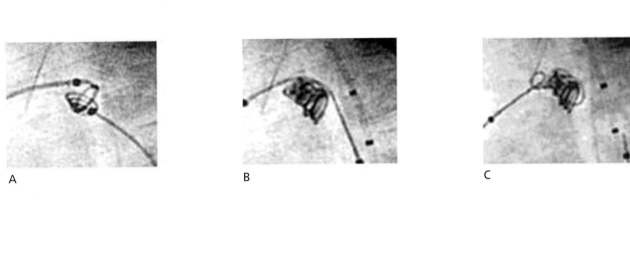

A   B   C

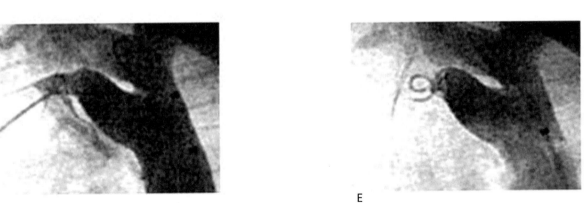

D   E

FIGURE 22.7. Simultaneous implantation of two Duct-Occlud devices to close a large PDA. **A, B:** Coils advanced from the pulmonary and aortal side are configured step by step inside the ductus lumen. **C:** The "aortal" coil is released; the "pulmonary" coil is still attached to the delivery system. **D:** The PDA is almost completely closed before the "pulmonary" coil being released.

this technique requires experience and manual dexterity of the operator. The Pfm Company does not recommend simultaneous placement of two devices because of the considerable potential for complications.

The patient is observed in the hospital for several hours. Follow-up includes an early (within 24 hours of implantation) and a late (6 months after implantation) echocardiogram to evaluate coil position and hemodynamics. If there is no residual shunt, antibiotic prophylaxis for subacute bacterial endocarditis is not required more than 6 months after implantation.

RESULTS

Animal Studies

The first Duct-Occlud feasibility study was undertaken in 1992 (16). A PDA model was created using 4- and 6-mm Gore-Tex (W. L. Gore, Flagstaff, AZ) tubes in five sheep weighing 10 to 20 kg. Device implantation was carried out using the aortic approach within hours (in four cases) or 7 days (in one case) after creation of artificial PDA. In four animals, the coil implantation was successful without complications. The coil was safely deployed, repositioned, and detached (Figure 22.8). The artificial PDA was completely occluded within a few minutes. In one animal the coil was suboptimally implanted with three loops protruding into the pulmonary artery. During coil retrieval, sutures of the artificial PDA tore, causing bleeding and the eventual death of the sheep. A coil was well endothelialized in one animal, who was sacrificed 20 months after implantation (Figure 22.9).

In another animal study the Duct-Occlud device was evaluated in neonatal piglets weighing between 1.4 and 2.1 kg (17). The ductus arteriosus was kept open by transvenous delivery of Palmaz coronary stainless steel stents (Johnson & Johnson, Skillman, NJ). Two weeks later, after confirming persistent patency, a miniaturized version of the standard device was implanted via an anterior jugular vein cut down in 13 animals. Sixteen to 73 days after coil implantation, piglets were restudied by cardiac catheterization and sacrificed. After 16 days all PDAs were closed by angiography. Coils within the PDA were engulfed by a histiocytic foreign-body reaction. Coils exposed to the bloodstream had partial or complete coverage by a thin endothelial layer. The extent of the endothelial coverage was dependent on the time from implantation as well as the degree of protrusion into the aortic or pulmonary artery lumen.

The reinforced device has been evaluated in a chronic lamb model (18). In eight neonatal lambs the PDA was dilated using a pediatric valvuloplasty catheter (balloon diameter, 6 to 8 mm; Dr. Osypka, GmbH, Grenzach, Germany) on the first day of life. The ductus was dilated for 10 minutes. The angioplasty procedure was repeated on postpartum day 5 or 6, and an angiogram was performed to verify a minimum inner diameter greater than 5 mm. Four to 53 days after the last angioplasty, coil occlusion of the PDA was carried out transvenously. At the time of coil implantation, the PDA was tubular in shape, with an average minimal inner diameter of 6.3 mm (range, 5.2 to 7.8 mm). PDA length ranged between 6.5 and 15 mm (mean, 10 mm). The stiffer distal loops of the device were deployed in the descending aorta and pulled into the aortic ampulla of the

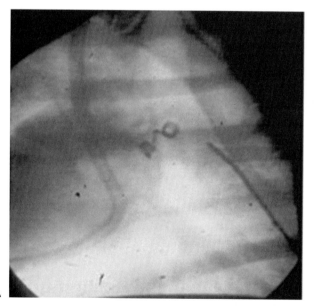 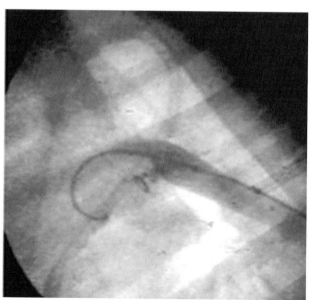

A   B

FIGURE 22.8. Coil implanted in an artificial PDA (sheep) with proper configuration.

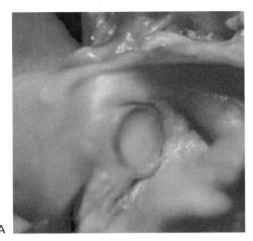

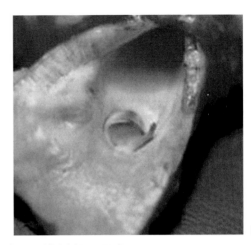

FIGURE 22.9. Pathologic specimens 20 months after occlusion of an artificial (Gore-Tex) patent ductus arteriosus using the aortic access. **A:** The coil is well adapted to the aortal wall. Its funnel is filled by organized thrombus and the coil is completely embedded into the endothelium. **B:** The proximal loop of the coil is positioned close to the wall of the pulmonary artery. The slightly protruding tip of the coil is covered by a thin layer of endothelium.

duct. The remaining loops were released within the duct. In one animal with a very large PDA, two coils were implanted simultaneously using a crossover technique from the aorta and the pulmonary artery.

One animal was prematurely sacrificed 1 day after coil implantation due to recurrent arterial bleeding at the femoral puncture site. In another animal the placement of a second coil was necessary to close a significant residual leak 3 months after primary implantation. In the remaining animals a final angiogram taken 7 to 181 days after coil implantation confirmed complete occlusion of the PDA. Postmortem macroscopic examination showed excellent coil position with no protrusion into the aorta or the pulmonary artery. The coils were partially or completely covered by an endothelial layer, depending on the time since implantation.

Human Studies

The European Duct-Occlud Study is the largest clinical experience with the Duct-Occlud device thus far reported (19). The initial cases were performed in 1993 (20). The experience extends through July 1997 and includes clinical data from 29 centers in 10 countries. The study encompasses 514 patients who underwent 522 catheterizations. In this European multicenter study the standard device was primarily used.

Patient characteristics included an average weight of 20.0 kg (range, 3.2 to 87.4 kg) and an average age of 64 months (range, 1 to 681 months). PDAs measured mean D_1, 1.6 mm (range, 0.1 to 5 mm); mean D_2, 5.6 mm (range, 1.0 to 18 mm); and mean L, 7.4 mm (range, 1.0 to 24 mm). Mean pulmonary to systemic blood flow ratio was 1.4. PDA angiographic characteristics: hourglass (type A),

39%; tunnel (type C or E), 42%; and window (type B), 6%, as per Krichenko's classification (21). Fourteen patients had surgical ligation; 32 patients had a Rashkind device implanted; and ten patients had a Gianturco coil implanted.

PDA access was achieved via a venous route in 90% of patients. The remaining 10% had their PDAs closed via the transarterial route. A total of 365 Duct-Occlud devices was implanted in the 349 patients. The procedure was terminated without a device placement in 48 (9%) of 512 patients. Sixteen (4.3%) standard devices embolized after detachment. In these patients the PDAs were moderate in size and had high flow. The embolized devices were retrieved by transcatheter techniques in 13 cases. In the remaining three cases the coils were left in a peripheral pulmonary artery. Other complications included pulse loss or weakness ($N = 9$), severe groin hematoma ($N = 8$), and entanglement in valve structures ($N = 3$). Entanglement was the most important complication, requiring surgical removal of the device in one patient. The reinforced device was introduced late in 1996. Only 17 reinforced devices were deployed in this study. Late migration of the device into the pulmonary artery was reported in one patient after 1-year follow-up with severe residual leak. This device was surgically removed.

Long-term follow-up data are relatively limited in the study. Complete PDA occlusion (within 24 hours of device placement) was observed in 268 patients (58%). In patients with more than 1 month of follow-up (311 patients), there is a 94.5% complete occlusion rate. According to the ductal shape the highest occlusion rate (97%) was achieved in elongated PDA (type E).

Results of other multicenter registries are similar to those of the European multicenter study (22–24). Tometzki et al.

(22) published a six-center British study in 1996. Implantation of the Duct-Occlud device was feasible in 44 (86%) of 51 cases with PDA. The minimal ductal diameters ranged from 1.0 to 4.3 mm (mean, 2.1 mm). In the remaining seven (14%) patients the PDA was judged too large for the device and Rashkind devices were used. In 39 patients Duct-Occlud was implanted via the transvenous route. In five patients the device was deployed retrogradely. Embolization of the Duct-Occlud device occurred in three cases (5.8%). In one patient the device embolized hours after placement and a second procedure was required for removal. In one patient the device could not be retrieved from a distal branch of the right pulmonary artery and was left in place. In another patient a 3-mm fragment of the device got entangled in the tricuspid apparatus. The patient had another device successfully deployed, and at the 12-month follow-up the fragment remained *in situ* with no evidence of tricuspid valve regurgitation. In 40 (91%) of the 44 patients in whom the Duct-Occlud device was used, complete occlusion at 24 hours could be demonstrated on color flow Doppler echocardiography. There has been one late recanalization through the center of the device, noted 6 months after device placement.

In another multicenter trial, reported by Oho et al. (23) in 1998, the Duct-Occlud was used in 35 patients aged 0.5 to 27.2 years (median, 7.6 years). The minimal ductal diameter was 2.0 ± 0.7 mm (range, 1.0 to 3.3 mm). Pulmonary–systemic flow ratio (Qp:Qs) was 1.3 ± 0.3 (range, 1.0 to 2.2). The devices were successfully implanted in 32 (91%) patients. Of 31 patients who were followed 6 months after the procedure, 26 (84%) had no residual shunt and five (16%) had a trivial residual shunt. One patient had infective endocarditis 1 month after the procedure but recovered completely. There were no incidences of coil embolization, hemolysis, late coil migration, or obstruction of the pulmonary artery or the aorta.

The multicenter study performed in the United States was published in February 2001 (24). The results of this phase I Food and Drug Administration–approved clinical trial were similar to those of the preceding studies. The Duct-Occlud device showed a relatively low percentage of complete closure within 24 hours of implantation. The occlusion rate of 94% after 12 months was equivalent to the results of other clinical studies with the Duct-Occlud device.

In the human studies mentioned earlier, the standard devices were mainly used. In this setting the standard device was very effective in the occlusion of elongated PDA (type E) and of PDA with a minimal diameter smaller than 2.0 mm. The complete occlusion rate was more than 95% within 1 month of coil implantation. In larger PDA of type A or in window-type PDA it was often difficult to place the standard device safely. As a result, the feasibility of coil implantation using the standard Duct-Occlud device in such cases was poor and the incidence of residual leak was

significantly higher than that seen in Krichenko-type E PDAs.

The reinforced Duct-Occlud device was introduced at the end of 1996 (25). To demonstrate its effectiveness in comparison with the standard device, results of PDA occlusion using the reinforced device are analyzed separately. Data of 172 cases, in which implantation procedures of the reinforced device have been performed, are available (unpublished data of the Pfm Company) for review. The implantation procedures were carried out at 26 international centers between October 1997 and February 2000. The average age of the patients was 75 months (range, 1 to 900 months). The average minimal ductal diameter was 2.5 mm (range, 1.0 to 5.2 mm). The distribution of the PDA shapes was type A, 54%; type B, 10%; and type C or E, 36%.

In six (3.5%) cases the anatomy of the PDA was unfavorable (i.e., too large or distensible) and Duct-Occlud was not implanted. In six (3.5%) other cases the device was improperly positioned and therefore removed immediately after detachment using a catheter technique. In the remaining 166 cases device implantation was successful. The transvenous route was used in all cases. In one case, the PDA was very distensible and stretched considerably, so that 50% of the device migrated into the pulmonary artery within 24 hours of placement. The residual leak remained significant 7 days after coil placement; therefore surgical ligation and device removal were performed. In one case the reinforced device could not be detached and hemopericardium occurred during device manipulation. Surgical intervention was successfully performed, and the patient suffered no further complications. In seven patients with very large type A PDA, two coils were simultaneously implanted using a crossover technique from the aorta and the pulmonary artery. In five of seven cases, one reinforced and one standard device were used; in two cases both devices were reinforced. In one patient with trisomy-21 and slightly elevated pulmonary resistance, embolization of the device in the descending aorta was discovered 3 months after implantation. Surgical removal of this device was necessary. The complete occlusion rate within 24 hours demonstrated on color flow Doppler echocardiography was 65%. Within 3 months of coil implantation, however, a complete closure rate was noted to be 97%.

Recanalizations, significant flow disturbances in the aorta or in the pulmonary artery, and hemolysis have not been reported.

Using the reinforced device type A PDA with a significantly larger minimal diameter, D_1 can be closed successfully. Figure 22.10 demonstrates a typical PDA occlusion using the reinforced Duct-Occlud device. The most important difference between the standard and the reinforced device is the relationship of occlusion rates to the particular shapes of the ductus. Using the reinforced coil, the occlusion rate within 6 months after implantation in type A duc-

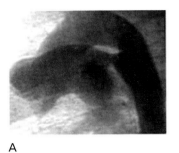

A

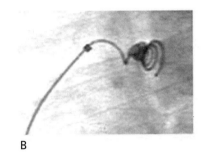

B

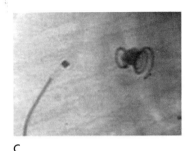

C

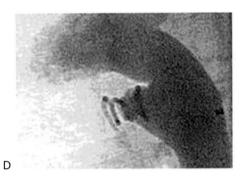

D

FIGURE 22.10. Occlusion of patent ductus arteriosus (PDA) using the reinforced Duct-Occlud device (left to right). **A:** Angiographic frame of a medium-sized PDA of type A. **B:** The coil is positioned in the duct. Note the compact mid-portion of the coil due to the reverse loops. The pulmonary loop is configured prior to coil detachment. **C:** After coil release the pulmonary loop adapted well to the vessel wall. **D:** The coil is optimally placed with compact configuration within the duct. Complete occlusion a few minutes after detachment.

tus increased from 80% (using the standard coil) to 97%. In type B ductus the occlusion rate improved from 30% to 65%. Because of its stiffer distal loops, the reinforced device can be seated more securely. This fact explains the low incidence of device embolization or migration after placement. The enhanced stiffness of the reinforced device, however, causes more friction within the delivery catheter and requires stronger retrieval mechanism. For this reason, detachment of the reinforced device may be difficult.

DISCUSSION

The occluding principles of coils are based on flow reduction and subsequent thrombosis. Consequently, the immediate occlusion rate is relatively low using the Duct-Occlud systems. Within hours or days, however, the occlusion rate increases to about 95%. Using the Duct-Occlud device, it is crucial to insert a sufficient quantity of thrombogenic material inside the ductal lumen. The configured structure of the Duct-Occlud devices resembles the shape of the PDA. The choice of the appropriate device for the respective PDA seems sometimes to be sophisticated. If the spatial dimensions of the ductus could be filled with device material as much as possible, complete occlusion is very likely. On the pulmonary side, only one or two coil loops are required to anchor the device safely. The narrowest portion of the device is positioned within the ductal lumen and not at the smallest diameter of the PDA. Before detaching the device the operator should ensure deposition of at least one loop in the pulmonary artery so that the detachment force of 4 to 12 N can be absorbed by the cranial wall of the pulmonary artery, preventing potential risk of device embolization toward the aorta.

The greater flexibility of the standard Duct-Occlud device allows it to tamponade the ductal lumen. On the other hand, its flexible structure increases the possibility of device embolization. The standard Duct-Occlud device is recommended for use in elongated PDA or in PDA of type A with a minimal diameter of less than 2 mm. Transvenous access is preferable if the PDA can easily be crossed from the pulmonary artery. In smaller PDAs the aortic route should be chosen instead of creating an arteriovenous loop, which could be very time-consuming.

The reinforced Duct-Occlud device is suitable to close medium-sized or large PDA (D_l 2 to 4 mm) if the ductal shape is favorable. The risk of device embolization is low because of the enhanced stiffness of the distal coil loops. The compact configuration with the reversed proximal loops facilitates insertion of sufficient thrombogenic material even in short (type B) PDA. The reversed proximal loops enable a compact configuration of the device. Consequently, more thrombogenic material can be inserted into even short (type B) PDA. It is our recommendation that the reinforced Duct-Occlud not be implanted from the arterial side, because large PDA may easily be crossed from the pulmonary side and the distal stiff loops may stretch the minimal diameter, complicating safe placement. If the PDA is very large and the Duct-Occlud device does not appear stable inside the ductal lumen, a multiple-coil technique may be considered to fix the device and to place more thrombogenic coils in the PDA. In such cases a crossover technique from the aorta and from the pulmonary artery may be safer than unilateral access.

Compared with free Gianturco and Cook detachable coils, multiple coils are less necessary with Duct-Occlud. The incidence of device embolization during or after placement is lower (26–30). In the vast majority, PDA can be effectively closed using one device. Because the Duct-Occlud device is detached by a pushing force and not by rotating the delivery system, the position of the device inside the duct usually remains unchanged after device detachment. The most interesting advantage of the Duct-Occlud system compared with all other devices, however, is the apparent absence of hemolysis, even with persistent residual leaks (31–38). The incidence of device protrusion into the aorta or into the pulmonary artery is extremely low. Complications requiring surgical interventions are also rare. Device entanglement in the right ventricle or right atrium has occurred only in the initial experience with the Duct-Occlud systems. There have been no procedure-related deaths.

The delivery system of the Duct-Occlud device must be mounted on the positioner grip before the implantation procedure. Because some operators found this step complicated, a disposable Duct-Occlud occlusion system was developed and is currently available. This system simplifies the implantation procedure.

CURRENT STATUS

The Duct-Occlud system is available in the United States at institutions participating in FDA-supervised clinical trials with Investigational Device Exemption (IDE). The Nit-Occlud PDA occlusion system is a further improvement of the Duct-Occlud coil system. Nit-Occlud received the CE mark (European approval) in March 2001. Like the Duct-Occlud coil, the Nit-Occlud is designed for PDA closure with one coil only. The main differences are a stronger, more compact coil shape that can be well controlled; a new enforced release mechanism, which avoids early coil release; and easy handling with a premounted system. The Nit-Occlud device comes in three versions, "flex," the flexible coil for small PDA up to approximately 2 mm; "medium," the reinforced coil for PDA sizes between 1.5 and 5.0 mm (smallest diameter); and "stiff," the very stiff coil for large and short ductus or for adult patients. The new system has been used in about 80 cases successfully for all types of PDA up to 5 mm. Data analysis is under way.

CONCLUSION

The Duct-Occlud system is safe and effective for occlusion of PDA with a diameter of up to 4 mm. Larger PDAs, especially type B PDA, may not be suitable for closure using the currently available stainless steel Duct-Occlud system. A coil device made of nickel–titanium (Nit-Occlud, Pfm,

Cologne, Germany) has been developed for PDAs larger than 4 mm and is now in the initial stages of clinical testing.

ACKNOWLEDGMENTS

We thank Professor D. A. Redel (Director of the Department of Pediatric Cardiology, University of Bonn, Germany) for his useful advice and the Pfm Company (Cologne, Germany) for technical support.

REFERENCES

1. Porstmann W, Wierny L, Warnke H. Closure of ductus arteriosus persistens without thoracotomy. *Radiol Diagn Berlin* 1968;9:168–169.
2. Rashkind WJ, Cuaso CC. Transcatheter closure of patent ductus arteriosus: successful use in a 3.5 kilogram infant. *Pediatr Cardiol* 1979;1:3–7.
3. Warnecke I, Frank J, Hohle R, et al. Transvenous double-balloon occlusion of the persistent ductus arteriosus: an experimental study. *Pediatr Cardiol* 1984;5:79–84.
4. Magal C, Wright KC, Duprat G, et al. A new device for transcatheter closure of the patent ductus arteriosus: a feasibility study in dogs. *Invest Radiol* 1989;24:272–274.
5. Bridges ND, Perry SB, Parness I, et al. Transcatheter closure of a large patent ductus arteriosus with the Clamshell septal umbrella. *J Am Coll Cardiol* 1991;18:1297–1302.
6. Rao PS, Wilson AD, Sideris EB, et al. Transcatheter closure of patent ductus arteriosus with buttoned device: first successful clinical application in a child. *Am Heart J* 1991;121:1799–1802.
7. Cambier PA, Kirby WC, Wortham DC, et al. Percutaneous closure of the small (<2.5 mm) patent ductus arteriosus using coil embolization. *Am J Cardiol* 1992;69:815–816.
8. Ottenkamp J, Hess J, Talsma MD, et al. Protrusion of the device: a complication of catheter closure of patent ductus arteriosus. *Br Heart J* 1992;68:301–303.
9. Lloyd TR, Fedderly R, Mendelsohn AM, et al. Transcatheter occlusion of patent ductus arteriosus with Gianturco coils. *Circulation* 1993;88:1412–1420.
10. Gianturco C, Anderson JH, Wallace S. Mechanical devices for arterial occlusion. *Am J Roentgenol* 1975;124:428–435.
11. Sommer RJ, Gutierrez A, Lai WW, et al. Use of preformed Nitinol snare to improved transcatheter coil delivery in occlusion of patent ductus arteriosus. *Am J Cardiol* 1994;74:836–839.
12. Ing FF, Sommer RJ. The snare-assisted technique for transcatheter coil occlusion of moderate to large patent ductus arteriosus: immediate and intermediate results. *J Am Coll Cardiol* 1999;33:1710–1718.
13. Hays MD, Hoyer MH, Glasow PF. New forceps delivery technique for coil occlusion of patent ductus arteriosus. *Am J Cardiol* 1996;77:209–211.
14. Kuhn MA, Latson LA. Transcatheter embolization coil closure of patent ductus arteriosus—modified delivery for enhanced control during coil positioning. *Catheter Cardiovasc Diagn* 1995;36:288–290.
15. Berdjis F, Moore JW. Balloon occlusion delivery technique for closure of patent ductus arteriosus. *Am Heart J* 1997;133:601–604.
16. Lê TP, Neuss MB, Kirchhoff AH, et al. Transkatheterverschluss von persistierendem Ductus arteriosus mit Spiralfedern. Eine

tierexperimentelle Studie mit Schafen [abstract]. *Z Kardiol* 1993; 82:71.

17. Neuss MB, Coa JY, Tio F, et al. Occlusion of the neonatal patent ductus arteriosus with a simple retrievable device: a feasibility study. *Cardiovasc Interv Radiol* 1996;19:170–175.

18. Grabitz RG, Freudenthal F, Sigler M, et al. Double-helix coil for occlusion of large patent ductus arteriosus: evaluation in a chronic lamb model. *J Am Coll Cardiol* 1998;31:677–683.

19. Redel DA and European Duct Occlud Study Members. Results of the European Duct Occlud MultiCenter Study using the spiral coil for ductal occlusion. *Second World Congress of Pediatric Cardiology and Cardiovascular Surgery*, Societas Cardiol Pediat Japonica, Honolulu, Hawaii, 1997, 226.

20. Le TP, Neuss MB, Redel DA, et al. A new transcatheter occlusion technique with retrievable double-disk shaped coils: first clinical results in occlusion of patent ductus arteriosus [abstract]. *Cardiol Young* 1993;3:I-38.

21. Krichenko A, Benson I, Burrows P, et al. Angiographic classification of the persistently ductus arteriosus and implications for percutaneous catheter occlusion. *Am J Cardiol* 1989;63:877–880.

22. Tometzki A, Redel DA, Wilson N, et al. Total UK multi-centre experience with a novel arterial occlusion device (Duct Occlud). *Heart* 1996;76:520–524.

23. Oho S, Ishizawa A, Koike K, et al. Transcatheter occlusion of patent ductus arteriosus with a new detachable coil system (Duct Occlud): a multicenter clinical trial. *Jpn Circ J* 1998;62: 489–493.

24. Moore JW, DiMeglio D, Javois AP, et al. Results of the Phase I Food and Drug Administration clinical trial of Duct-Occlud device occlusion of patent ductus arteriosus. *Catheter Cardiovasc Interv* 2001;52:74–78.

25. Lê TP, Neuss MB, Freudenthal F, et al. The closure of PDA by means of DuctOcclud coils: a report on a single-institutional experience in view of the continual development of an interventional closure method [abstract]. *Catheter Cardiovasc Interv* 1999;47:121.

26. Hijazi ZM, Geggel RL. Transcatheter closure of patent ductus arteriosus using coils. *Am J Cardiol* 1997;79:1279–1280.

27. Galal O, de Moor M, Fadley F, et al. Problems encountered during introduction of Gianturco coils for transcatheter occlusion of the patent arterial duct. *Eur Heart J* 1997;18:625–630.

28. Celiker A, Qureshi SA, Bilgic A, et al. Transcatheter closure of patent arterial ducts using controlled-release coils. *Eur Heart J* 1997;18:450–454.

29. Janorkar S, Goh T, Wilkinson J. Transcatheter closure of patent ductus arteriosus with the use of Rashkind occluders and/or Gianturco coils: long term follow-up in 123 patients and special reference to comparison, residual shunts, complications and technique. *Am Heart J* 1999;138:1176–1183.

30. Patel HT, Cao QL, Rhodes J, et al. Long-term outcome of transcatheter coil closure of small to large patent ductus arteriosus. *Catheter Cardiovasc Interv* 1999;47:457–461.

31. Ladusans EJ, Murdoch I, Franciosi J. Severe haemolysis after percutaneous closure of a ductus arteriosus (arterial duct). *Br Heart J* 1989;61:548–550.

32. Kapoor A, Radhakrishnan S, Shrivastava S. Severe intravascular haemolysis following coil occlusion of patent ductus arteriosus. *Indian Heart J* 1996;48:173–174.

33. Shim D, Wechsler DS, Lloyd TR, et al. Hemolysis following coil embolization of a patent ductus arteriosus. *Catheter Cardiovasc Diagn* 1996;39:287–290.

34. Henry G, Danilowicz D, Verma R. Severe hemolysis following partial coil-occlusion of patent ductus arteriosus. *Catheter Cardiovasc Diagn* 1996;39:410–412.

35. Uzun O, Veldtman GR, Dickinson DF, et al. Haemolysis following implantation of duct occlusion coils. *Heart* 1999;81: 160–161.

36. Jamjureeruk V, Kirawittaya T, Ningsnondh V. Mild or subclinical intravascular haemolysis subsequent to transcatheter occlusion of the patent arterial duct. *Cardiol Young* 1999;9:58–62.

37. Wilson NJ, Occleshaw CJ, O'Donnell CP, et al. Subclinical aortic perforation with the infant double-button patent ductus arteriosus occluder. *Catheter Cardiovasc Interv* 1999;48:296–298.

38. Godart F, Rodés J, Rey C. Severe haemolysis after transcatheter closure of a patent arterial duct with the new Amplatzer duct occluder. *Cardiol Young* 2000;10:265–267.

Catheter Based Devices: For the Treatment of Non-coronary Cardiovascular Diseases in Adults and Children. Edited by P. Syamasundar Rao and Morton J. Kern, Lippincott Williams & Wilkins, Philadelphia © 2003.

23

GIANTURCO-GRIFKA VASCULAR OCCLUSION DEVICE

RONALD G. GRIFKA

Transcatheter interventional procedures for the treatment of congenital and postoperative cardiovascular defects have evolved into an important therapeutic option (1,2). One area that has been researched widely and applied clinically is transcatheter closure of abnormal vascular communications. Transcatheter occlusion devices have been used for many cardiovascular defects, including the patent ductus arteriosus (PDA) (3,4). A number of occlusion devices have been used. However, each device has limitations, including large delivery sheaths, complicated device design, and incomplete occlusion. In an effort to overcome these deficiencies, we developed a new device.

DEVICE

In 1989, we began developing the Gianturco-Grifka vascular occlusion device (GGVOD) (Cook Inc., Bloomington, IN) (5,6). The GGVOD consists of two main components, a flexible nylon sack (henceforth *sack*) and an occluding wire. The sack is attached to an end-hole catheter. A modified spring guide wire is advanced through the end-hole catheter into the sack. Once inside the sack, the wire coils, which fills the sack and occludes the vessel. Then the coil-filled sack is released from the catheter.

The sack is constructed from two circular pieces of tightly woven medical-grade nylon. The edges of the two nylon pieces are thermally sealed, affording a circular sack enclosure (Figure 23.1A). The sack is attached to the sack catheter, which is a 4.5F end-hole catheter with an everted flare on the distal end (Figure 23.1B). The sack is form-fitted tightly over the flared catheter end and is secured by a radiopaque metal tie string. The 4.5F sack catheter is placed inside a 5.5F end-hole "release catheter"; the release catheter is 2 cm shorter than the sack catheter. The release catheter is used to "push" the sack off the sack catheter (Figure 23.1).

The sack and catheters are delivered to the vessel through a modified 8F transseptal sheath; this sheath is supplied with the device.

The device has two separate wires, a floppy filler wire and a stiff pusher wire. The filler wire is a standard 0.025-inch stainless steel spring guide wire that has three modifications. The stiff inner core is removed. There is a J curve on the distal end, and the proximal end has a smooth, spherical ball. The pusher wire is a stiffer wire, which has a smooth, spherical ball on its distal end. The balls on the ends of these two wires overlap and are contained within a thin plastic catheter. As long as the balls are overlapped and inside the plastic catheter, the wires are attached to each other, allowing them to move as one wire. This overlapping wire position allows the interventionalist to advance the

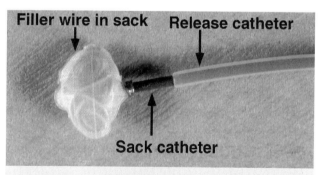
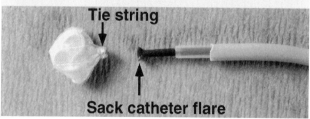

FIGURE 23.1. A: The sack is made from two pieces of thermally sealed nylon that are fitted tightly over the flared end of the sack catheter. There is a radiopaque metal tie-string on the proximal end of the sack. The filler wire is inserted into the sack. **B:** The wire-filled sack has been pushed off the flared end of the sack catheter.

Ronald G. Grifka: Associate Professor of Pediatrics, Baylor College of Medicine; Director, Cardiac Catheterization Laboratory, Texas Children's Hospital, Houston, Texas.

stiff pusher wire, which pushes the floppy filler wire into the sack. Once inside the sack, the filler wire coils, serving two functions: (a) filling the sack, thus occluding the vessel lumen, and (b) providing transmural pressure to maintain the sack position in the vessel. After all the filler wire is pushed into the sack, the sack should be fixed in a stable position in the vessel. Then the pusher and filler wires are separated. The proximal end of the pusher wire has a handle with finger holes (Figure 23.2). The handle is extended approximately 10 mm, pushing the overlapping ends of both wires out of the plastic catheter, allowing the wires to separate. The pusher wire is removed. At this point the sack is filled with the filler wire, but the sack remains attached to the sack catheter. To release the sack, the release catheter is advanced several millimeters up against the sack and held firmly in this position. By pulling the sack catheter with a slow, steady pulling motion (not a rapid jerk, as used for a septostomy procedure), the everted flare on the sack catheter is pulled through the neck of the sack, releasing the sack.

The GGVOD design allows the sack to be repositioned prior to separating the two wires. After pushing the filler wire into the sack, but before the wires are separated, an angiogram is performed to assess device position and vessel occlusion. If the sack position is suboptimal, the filler wire can be pulled out of the sack and the sack repositioned; then the filler wire can be reinserted into the sack. The filler wire can be removed and reinserted numerous times, until the optimal sack position is obtained. If the sack does not attain the optimal position or does not occlude the vessel, the filler wire can be pulled out of the sack and the sack can be pulled back into the sheath and replaced with a different-sized GGVOD (all through the same 8F sheath).

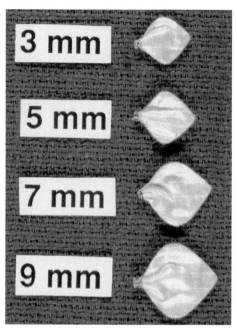

FIGURE 23.3. The GGVOD is available in four sizes; 3, 5, 7, and 9 mm. The sack size should be 1 to 1.5 mm larger than the vessel to be occluded at the site where the sack is implanted.

To have a GGVOD that will allow a wide range of blood vessel diameters to be occluded, the GGVOD is manufactured in four sizes: 3, 5, 7, and 9 mm (Figure 23.3). All four GGVOD sizes are delivered through the 8F long sheath. Each size GGVOD has a single filler wire of a specific length that completely fills the sack. For the device to maintain its position in the vessel, the device must provide sufficient transmural pressure against the vessel wall. To generate sufficient transmural pressure, the device size should be 1.0 to 1.5 mm larger than the diameter of the blood vessel, at the site the vessel is occluded. For example, if a PDA has a narrowing at the main pulmonary artery (MPA) insertion that measures 3.7 mm but the mid-portion of the PDA (where the sack device is placed) measures 5.9 mm, a 7-mm sack device should be implanted. This is a crucial point that must not be overlooked; the GGVOD size should be 1.0 to 1.5 mm larger than the PDA at the exact site that the sack is implanted.

PATIENT SELECTION

The ideal PDA for using the GGVOD is type C, D, or E (long, tubular vessels), as described by Krichenko et al. (7) (Figure 23.4). However, we have occluded a PDA type A-1 with a generous aortic ampulla. The very short, so-called window ductus (type B) should *not* be attempted with this device. There is not enough vessel length against which the sack is in contact with the vessel. Thus, there is insufficient transmural pressure to maintain the sack position. To min-

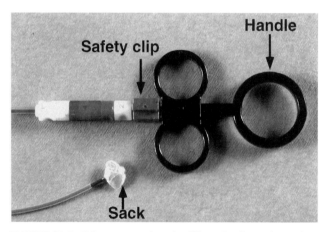

FIGURE 23.2. When separating the filler wire from the pusher wire, a thumb is placed in the handle large ring, and the index and middle fingers are inserted into the two smaller rings. By extending the fingers from the thumb, this pushes the overlapping balls apart on the wires, separating the wires. There is a safety clip *(arrow)* that must be removed before separating the wires; this prevents accidental release of the wires during the procedure.

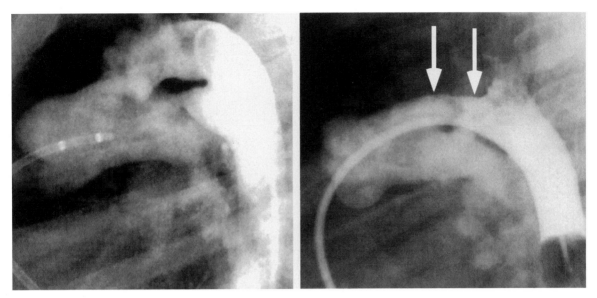

FIGURE 23.4. Lateral angiograms displaying different-shaped patent ductus arteriosus (PDAs). The conically shaped PDA with a narrowing on the pulmonary orifice *(left)* is ideal for occlusion with a Gianturco coil. The long, tubular PDA *(right)* is easily occluded with a GGVOD. Note that the optimal site for GGVOD placement is not just any site of the PDA, but is the segment *between* the *arrows*.

imize the possibility of sack embolization, the minimal length of vessel needed is 1.5 to 2.0 times the sack diameter. For example, if a PDA minimum diameter is 3.8 mm and a 5-mm GGVOD is implanted, the PDA length should be 7.5 to 10 mm. As more experience is gained with the device, shorter vessels may be pursued (lengths of 1.3 to 1.5 times the sack diameter). In several large vessels ≥10-mm diameter), we have simultaneously implanted two sacks side by side, with or without a Gianturco embolization coil placed between the sacks (8). The patient needs to be big enough to have an 8F sheath placed in the femoral vessel. We have implanted the device in an infant as small as 3.2 kg without any vascular problems.

DEVICE IMPLANT TECHNIQUE

To implant the GGVOD in a PDA, we routinely use the prograde (transvenous) approach. We always place a short sheath in the femoral artery to insert a pigtail catheter to perform angiograms during PDA device implant. In several patients, we have used the retrograde (arterial) approach to implant the device; a liberal amount of lidocaine was administered around the femoral artery before and after sheath insertion.

A short sheath (5 to 7F) is placed in the femoral vein. An end-hole catheter is advanced prograde through the right heart, into the MPA, across the PDA, into the descending aorta. A 0.038-inch Teflon-coated exchange length wire is placed through the catheter, into the descending aorta. The catheter and short sheath are removed, leaving the exchange wire in place. The 8F long sheath and dilator (which come

with the GGVOD) are advanced over the wire, into the descending aorta. The radiopaque band on the distal end of the sheath simplifies visualization of the sheath end. The wire and dilator are removed, leaving the sheath in the descending aorta. Because of the wire and catheter exchanges, we use extreme caution throughout the procedure, making sure not to introduce air into the vascular system, clearing the sheath after every catheter removal. While flushing the sheath, the GGVOD is advanced through the sheath, into the descending aorta. The sack is filled with approximately 35% to 45% of the filler wire (the wire makes three or four loops in the sack), to distend the sack. The partially filled sack is pulled back slowly into the PDA. An angiogram is performed, using the retrograde pigtail catheter, to assess device position in the PDA; if the sack is not in the optimal position, it is repositioned. When the sack is well positioned, the remainder of the wire is inserted into the sack. Again, an angiogram is performed to assess device position. The device is repositioned as many times as needed, to obtain optimal position, confirmed by an angiogram. With the sack in optimal position and completely filled with wire, the filler wire is separated from the pusher wire. Finally, the sack is released ("pushed off") from the sack catheter.

Several technical points that facilitate successful GGVOD implant deserve mentioning. We have occluded a large PDA (minimum diameter 5 mm) in children as small as 3.2 kg. The patient needs to be big enough to have an 8F sheath placed in the femoral vein (or femoral artery if the retrograde approach is used). We have implanted the device in infants as small as 3.2 kg using the femoral vein without any vascular problems. When implanting a GGVOD, remember to advance approximately 35% to 45% of the filler wire into the sack in the aorta; then slowly pull the sack into the PDA. With the partially filled sack positioned in the optimal PDA location, insert the remainder of the filler wire. It is important to have the sack in the optimal PDA position because the final 30% to 40% of the filler wire is inserted into the sack. This allows the filler wire to press the sack firmly against the PDA wall, at the optimal position, ensuring that the device will maintain its position after it is released. If the sack is filled completely with wire and then pulled back into the PDA, it will not generate an evenly distributed amount of transmural pressure against the PDA wall, making the device more likely to embolize.

If the vessel is a conical shape, the sack may need to be more than 1.0 to 1.5 mm larger than the minimal vessel diameter; conically shaped vessels are more challenging to occlude with the GGVOD. Some conically shaped vessels may not be candidates for GGVOD implant. Make sure the sack is the appropriate size and in the optimal position before separating the pusher wire from the filler wire; the wire and sack are easily removable before the wires are separated. Once the wires are separated, the device is difficult to remove and may have to be taken out surgically. When separating the filler wire from the pusher wire, extend the handle (allowing the ends of the wires to exit the thin plastic catheter and separate); then rotate the handle 90 degrees to make sure the smooth, spherical balls on the end of the pusher and filler wires completely disengage from each other. Using fluoroscopy, observe very carefully to make sure the wires disengage. If they do not, just repeat the handle extension maneuver. If the sack embolizes after the wires are separated but before the sack is released from the catheter, the catheter and sack may be pulled back to the right atrium. (Use caution when going through the tricuspid valve in case the initial end-hole catheter has gone through the chordae tendineae.) From the right atrium, the sack may be brought out through the femoral vein or SVC. The sack may come off the catheter as it is pulled through the subcutaneous tissue; a cut-down in the femoral (or jugular vein) may be required. If the sack embolizes after it is released from the catheter, a bioptome could be used to "bite" a hole in the sack. This would allow the wire to come out of the sack and be retrieved, then the sack is removed later.

RESULTS

Initially, the GGVOD was evaluated in a canine animal model (5,6). An acute study was performed to assess efficacy of the device, and a long-term model was created to evaluate the biologic response to the device. In the acute study, the GGVOD was implanted in carotid, subclavian, and renal arteries. Each GGVOD remained in position, all vessels were occluded completely, and no device emboliza-

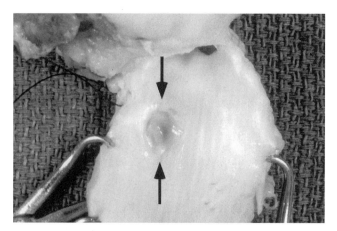

FIGURE 23.5. This specimen displays the aortic lumen from an animal model 4 months after occlusion of an aortopulmonary shunt placement with a GGVOD. The shunt lumen was completely occluded from the sack out to the aorta, where a layer of neointima has covered the shunt orifice *(arrows)*, providing a smooth aortic wall.

tions occurred. In the long-term study, a high-pressure, high-flow model (5- or 6-mm aortopulmonary shunt) was created, followed by transcatheter GGVOD occlusion. The GGVOD completely occluded every shunt by the initial formation of a thrombus plug. Over 2 to 6 months, the thrombus was replaced by collagen, and a smooth neointimal layer covered the vessel orifice (Figure 23.5). Microscopic studies revealed collagen had grown into the nylon sack fibers, fixing the sack in place, and there was no foreign-body reaction (Figure 23.6).

At Texas Children's Hospital, the GGVOD has been used to perform transcatheter occlusion of various vascular structures (9). The PDA has been the most common defect occluded using the GGVOD (Figures 23.7 and 23.8). Initially, we assumed that the GGVOD would be most useful for occluding vessels from 2 to 3.5 mm in diameter. Because

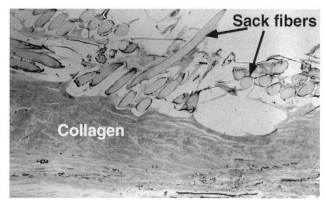

FIGURE 23.6. This cross-section microscopic slice of an occluded sack displays collagen interdigitating between the sack fibers *(arrows)*, ensuring a fixed sack position. No inflammatory reaction is present.

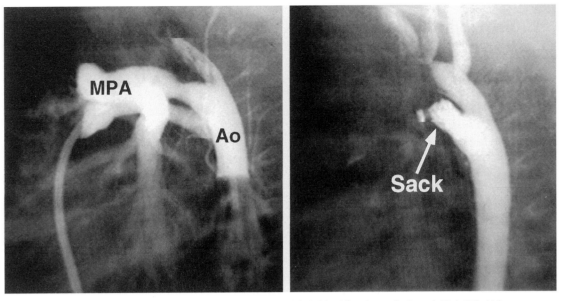

FIGURE 23.7. Lateral angiograms of a 2-month-old child with a large (4.4 mm) PDA **(A)**. Using the prograde (venous approach), a 5-mm GGVOD (*arrow*) was implanted in the mid-portion of the PDA, providing complete PDA occlusion and resolution of pulmonary overcirculation sequelae **(B)**. AO, aorta; MPA, main pulmonary artery.

of the excellent results using Gianturco embolization coils for PDAs of this diameter and the difficulty in occluding larger-diameter PDAs with coils, many of the vessels we have occluded using the GGVOD have been 3 to 8 mm in diameter (10,11).

To date, we have occluded 34 PDAs. The patients' weight ranged from 3.2 to 38 kg (median, 10 kg). The patients' ages ranged from 2 months to 13 years. The PDA minimal diameter ranged from 2.4 to 6.9 mm (median,

4.1 mm). The mean Qp:Qs ratio was 2.2:1. At follow-up evaluation, ranging from 9 to 54 months, complete PDA occlusion was obtained in 34 of 34 patients, determined by physical examination, color, and pulsed-wave Doppler evaluation. In 41% of patients (13 of 34), high-resolution angiography immediately after GGVOD implant displayed a miniscule jet of residual shunt through the neck of the sack. Complete PDA closure occurred in 91% of patients (31 of 34) within 24 hours, and in 97% of

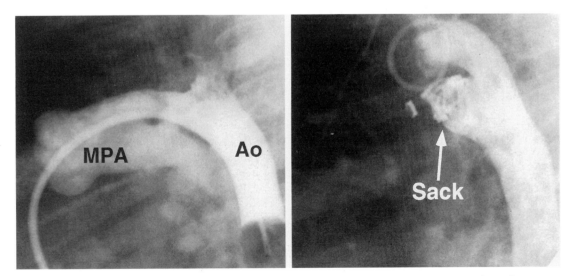

FIGURE 23.8. Lateral angiograms of a 10-month-old child who had a large PDA (6.9 mm), resulting in a large left-to-right shunt and elevated pulmonary artery pressure. A single 9-mm GGVOD was implanted in the mid-portion of the PDA, then released. Following implantation (right), the device (*arrow*) remains in the desired position, with immediate, complete PDA occlusion and no obstruction in the aorta (Ao) or pulmonary artery. MPA, main pulmonary artery.

patients (33 of 34) within 1 month after device implant. Only one patient had a (tiny) residual leak for more than 1 month after device implant; at evaluation 8 months after implant, the PDA was closed completely. This delayed closure was probably due to a short segment of filler wire (4 cm), which came out of the neck of the sack during release; the procedure was performed expeditiously in a 6-month-old infant who was hemodynamically unstable due a mitochondrial cardiomyopathy and large PDA. Thus for every PDA in which a GGVOD was implanted, we obtained complete PDA occlusion, without complication or embolization. The femoral vein was used for all PDA implants.

In one patient who had a large PDA (minimum diameter of 8.2 mm), a 9-mm GGVOD achieved complete occlusion. However, we pulled the device through the PDA (into the MPA) after the wires were separated but before the sack was released from the catheter. The sack was withdrawn into the right atrium, advanced up to the SVC, and removed through a small incision over the internal jugular vein.

APPLICABILITY IN ADULT PATIENTS

The GGVOD can be used in a wide range of patients, from small infants to adults. The only limitation is the ability to insert the 8F sheath into the vein or artery used for percutaneous entry. In adolescents and adults, their large size permits the sheath to be placed in either the femoral artery or the vein.

DISCUSSION

Transcatheter closure of the PDA, and other cardiovascular defects, has many advantages over surgical closure, including avoidance of general anesthesia and a thoracotomy procedure, less need for blood transfusions, decreased morbidity, less psychological trauma (especially in children), shorter length of hospitalization, and decreased total hospitalization cost. Many patients who would benefit from transcatheter device occlusion have other cardiovascular defects that require additional surgery. Transcatheter closure of a defect avoids the adhesions associated with surgical closure. These adhesions complicate subsequent surgeries and may preclude other procedures.

A number of transcatheter occlusion devices are available for the PDA and other vascular structures. Each device is effective for a limited number of defects. In an effort to develop an occlusion device that will add to the transcatheter armamentarium, we have developed the GGVOD. In comparison with other devices, the GGVOD has several advantages:

1. It is delivered through an 8F sheath, which can be placed in the femoral vein in all children 3 to 4 kg or larger, and in the femoral artery in older patients.
2. The flexible nylon sack will conform to the intravascular contour of any vessel.
3. If the wire-filled sack is not in the optimal position, the wire can be removed and the sack repositioned as many times as necessary.
4. If the wire-filled sack is too small (or too large), the wire and sack may be removed through the long sheath and replaced with a different-sized device.
5. Since the sack can be repositioned before device release, this should decrease the incidence of residual leaks and device embolizations.

Every transcatheter occlusion device has limitations, and the GGVOD is no exception. It is important to understand these limitations thoroughly. As with every device, the GGVOD cannot be used to occlude every PDA. Knowing when not to use a device can be as valuable as knowing when to use it. The limitations of the GGVOD include the following:

1. The PDA may be too short to implant the GGVOD. The exact site in the PDA where the sack is implanted should be 1.5 to 2.0 times the length of the sack size. If the PDA is too short, the sack has a higher possibility to embolize. The PDA cannot be too long to implant the GGVOD. Also, the PDA does *not* need to have a narrowing or stenosis to keep the GGVOD in position. As more experience is gained using the GGVOD, shorter-length PDA may be occluded.
2. For the sack to exert sufficient transmural pressure on the PDA wall, the sack diameter should be 1.0 to 1.5 mm larger than the PDA diameter at the exact site where the sack is implanted. If the sack size is too small, this could result in incomplete vessel occlusion or device embolization. Also, a large PDA (6 to 9 mm) may require a sack more than 1.0 to 1.5 mm larger to exert sufficient transmural pressure against the PDA wall to maintain the sack position.
3. To implant the GGVOD, a long delivery sheath must be positioned in the PDA. Sheath placement may be difficult if there is a tortuous course or the PDA makes an acute angle. The 8F sheath is a high-quality, kink-resistant Teflon material; a more flexible wire-braided sheath (Flexor sheath, Cook, Inc.) may be helpful for a tortuous path.
4. The 8F sheath may be too large if an arterial approach is required. This limits use of the GGVOD in infants.

CURRENT STATUS

The GGVOD has been approved by the FDA for transcatheter closure of unnecessary vascular structures, including the PDA. Transcatheter closure of the appropriate size and shape PDA is an excellent use of the GGVOD. The following defects have been occluded using the GGVOD: PDA, aortopulmonary collateral vessel, intrapulmonary arteriovenous fistula, left superior vena cava to left atrium, Glenn shunt, accessory pulmonary vein draining to the IVC (12–15).

CONCLUSION

The Gianturco-Grifka vascular occlusion device is safe and effective for transcatheter occlusion of tubular PDA and other vascular structures. To implant the GGVOD, the PDA (or other vessel) must have an appropriate length, and the 8F sheath must be placed into the PDA. In the future, minor modifications to the shape of the sack may result in additional transcatheter occlusion procedures.

REFERENCES

1. Rashkind WJ. Transcatheter treatment of congenital heart disease. *Circulation* 1983;67:711.
2. Rashkind WJ, Tait MA. Interventional cardiac catheterization in congenital heart disease. *Cardiovasc Clin* 1985;15:303.
3. Rashkind WJ, Cuaso CC. Transcatheter closure of a patent ductus arteriosus: successful use in a 3.5 kg infant. *Pediatr Cardiol* 1979;1:63.
4. Sato K, Fujino M, Kozuka T, et al. Transfemoral plug closure of patent ductus arteriosus: experiences with 61 consecutive patients treated without thoracotomy. *Circulation* 1975;51:337.
5. Grifka RG, Mullins CE, Gianturco C, et al. Initial studies using the Gianturco-Grifka vascular occlusion device in a canine model. *Circulation* 1995;91:1840–1846.
6. Grifka RG, Miller MW, Frischmeyer KJ, et al. Transcatheter occlusion of a patent ductus arteriosus in a Newfoundland puppy using the Gianturco-Grifka vascular occlusion device. *J Vet Intern Med* 1996;10:42–44.
7. Krichenko A, Benson LN, Burrows P, et al. Angiographic classification of the isolated persistently patent ductus arteriosus and implications for percutaneous transcatheter closure. *Am J Cardiol* 1989;63:877–880.
8. Forbess LW, O'Laughlin MP, Harrison JK. Partially anomalous pulmonary venous connection: demonstration of dual drainage allowing nonsurgical correction. *Catheter Cardiovasc Diagn* 1998; 44:330–335.
9. Grifka RG, Vincent JA, Nihill MR, et al. Initial clinical experience using the Gianturco-Grifka vascular occlusion device for congenital heart defects. *J Am Coll Cardiol* 1996;27(Suppl A): 119A.
10. Grifka RG, Vincent JA, Nihill MR, et al. Transcatheter patent ductus arteriosus closure in an infant using the Gianturco-Grifka device. *Am J Cardiol* 1996;78:721–723.
11. Ing FF, Mullins CE, Wolfe SB, et al. Relief of factitious coarctation following occlusion of large patent ductus arteriosus with Gianturco-Grifka vascular occluder. *Catheter Cardiovasc Diagn* 1998;45:409–412.
12. Jones TK, Garabedian H, Grifka RG. Right aortic arch with isolation of the left subclavian artery, moderate patent ductus steal syndrome: a rare aortic arch anomaly treated with the Gianturco-Grifka vascular occlusion device. *Catheter Cardiovasc Interv* 1999;47:320–322.
13. Geggel RL, Perry SB, Blume ED, et al. Left superior vena cava connection to unroofed coronary sinus associated with positional cyanosis: Successful transcatheter treatment using Gianturco-Grifka vascular occlusion device. *Catheter Cardiovasc Interv* 1999;48:369–373.
14. Gaskin P, O'Laughlin MP. Shunt closure with Gianturco-Grifka device [editorial; comment]. *Catheter Cardiovasc Interv* 1999;48: 368.
15. Hoyer MH, Leon RA, Fricker FJ. Transcatheter closure of modified Blalock-Taussig shunt with Gianturco-Grifka vascular occlusion device. *Catheter Cardiovasc Interv* 1999;48:365–367.

Catheter Based Devices: For the Treatment of Non-coronary Cardiovascular Diseases in Adults and Children. Edited by P. Syamasundar Rao and Morton J. Kern, Lippincott Williams & Wilkins, Philadelphia © 2003.

24

AMPLATZER DUCT OCCLUDER

SATINDER K. SANDHU
TERRY D. KING

Patent ductus arteriosus is present in 8% of the children born with congenital heart disease. It is twice as common in females as in males, and is more prevalent in preterm than in term infants. Gross and Hubbard (1) described the surgical ligation of the patent ductus arteriosus in 1939. Portsmann (2–4) and his colleagues were the first to describe the transcatheter closure of the patent ductus arteriosus with an Ivalon plug in 1966. Following the introduction of the Ivalon plug closure of the patent ductus arteriosus, the transcatheter techniques have continued to evolve, as reviewed elsewhere (5). The Gianturco coil (6,7) introduced in 1992 effectively closes the small patent ductus arteriosus with a residual shunt rate as high as 32% and an embolization rate of up to 8%. The Rashkind device (8,9) used to close the patent ductus arteriosus has a device embolization rate as high as 18% and a residual shunt rate of up to 22%. Other devices have similar limitations. The Amplatzer Duct Occluder (AGA Medical Corporation, Golden Valley, MN) described by Sharafuddin (10) and his colleagues was developed to address the problems of residual shunts and device embolizations related to transcatheter devices.

DEVICE

The Amplatzer Duct Occluder is a mushroom-shaped device with a low profile and is self-expanding and self-centering. The device frame is made from 0.0004 to 0.0005-inch Nitinol wire mesh. It is made up of a flat retention disk and a cylindrical main body into which are sewn polyester fibers to induce thrombosis. Nitinol and polyester both are biocompatible. There are platinum marker bands laser-welded to each end. The shape of the device is formed by heat treatment. After cooling, a stainless steel sleeve with a female thread is welded into the marker band. The screw is recessed inside the disk. The Nitinol frame of the device has

memory-retaining power and therefore does not elongate substantially on compression. The high hoop strength allows for positional stability in a stented ductus. The retention disk is thin and flat, and is 4 mm larger than the device to ensure secure positioning in the mouth of the PDA. The device ranges in size from 6–4 to 14–12 mm (Table 24.1). The 6-4-mm and 8-6-mm device are 7 mm in length; the remaining sizes are 8 mm in length. The device is delivered through a 5- to 7F sheath, depending upon the size of the device. The delivery system consists of a delivery cable, Mullins-type sheath, loader, and pin vise (Figure 24.1).

PATIENT SELECTION

The indications for transcatheter closure of the patent ductus arteriosus are no different from those for surgical ligation. Because of device size limitations, a ductus greater than 12 mm should not be closed with the Amplatzer Duct Occluder. The device should not be placed in patients <5 kg in weight, particularly if a larger device is needed because of the increased risk of acquired left pulmonary artery stenosis or coarctation. It is also contraindicated in patients with pulmonary vascular obstructive disease.

DEVICE IMPLANTATION TECHNIQUE

All patients should have a complete physical examination, including four extremity blood pressures. An echocardiogram

Satinder K. Sandhu: Associate Professor of Pediatrics, Louisiana State University Health Sciences Center; Director, Pediatric Cardiology, Children's Hospital, New Orleans, Louisiana

Terry D. King: Director, Pediatric Cardiology, Department of Pediatrics, St. Francis Medical Center, Monroe, Louisiana

TABLE 24.1. THE DEVICE SIZES AND DELIVERY SHEATHS

Device Diameter (mm)	Device Length (mm)	Delivery Sheath (F)
6–4	7	5
8–6	7	6
10–8	8	6
12–10	8	6
14–12	8	7

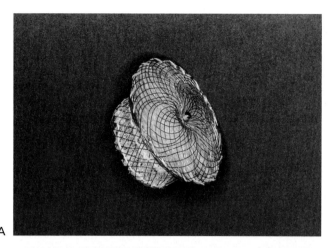

A

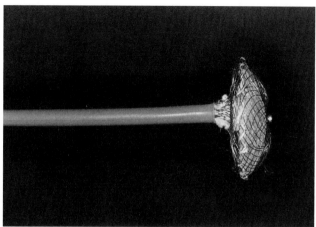

B

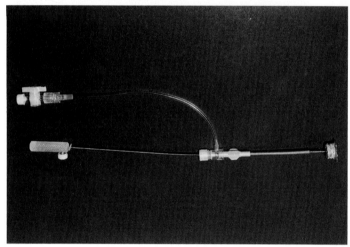

C

FIGURE 24.1. The device and the delivery system. **A:** The device with polyester fibers. **B:** The retention disc is extruded from the delivery sheath. **C:** The delivery system.

should be done to confirm the clinical diagnosis and to rule out the presence of associated lesions, with particular emphasis on the aortic arch and the branch pulmonary arteries.

The large majority of patients are discharged within 24 hours. At Children's Hospital, New Orleans, the procedure is done using light sedation. Both the femoral vein and the femoral artery are canulated percutaneously. A complete right and left heart catheterization is done with oximetry and pressure measurements obtained in room air. The ductal size and configuration are determined by an aortogram done in the anteroposterior and lateral projections. The minimum diameter, the diameter of the aortic ampulla, and the length of the patent ductus arteriosus are determined from the cineangiogram. The ductus arteriosus is then crossed from the pulmonary artery side using a 5F multipurpose catheter. The catheter tip is positioned in the descending aorta at the level of the diaphragm. The position of the catheter is then confirmed by fluoroscopy, oximetry, and pressure monitoring. The multipurpose catheter is exchanged over a 0.035-inch J-tipped exchange length wire for an appropriate (5 to 7F) delivery sheath and dilator. The dilator is removed and the sheath is flushed with heparinized normal saline. A device 1 to 2 mm larger than the smallest diameter of the PDA is selected and immersed in saline solution. The delivery cable

is passed through the loader and the occlusion device is screwed on clockwise to the tip of the delivery cable (Figure 24.2). The device and the loader are immersed in the saline solution and the device is pulled into the loader. The loader is introduced into the delivery sheath and the device is advanced without rotation into the descending aorta. The delivery technique is illustrated in Figure 24.3. The retention

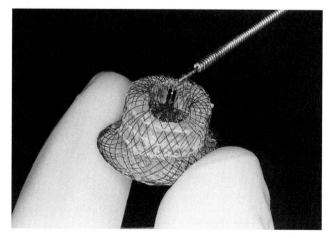

FIGURE 24.2. The recessed screw in the device where the delivery cable would attach.

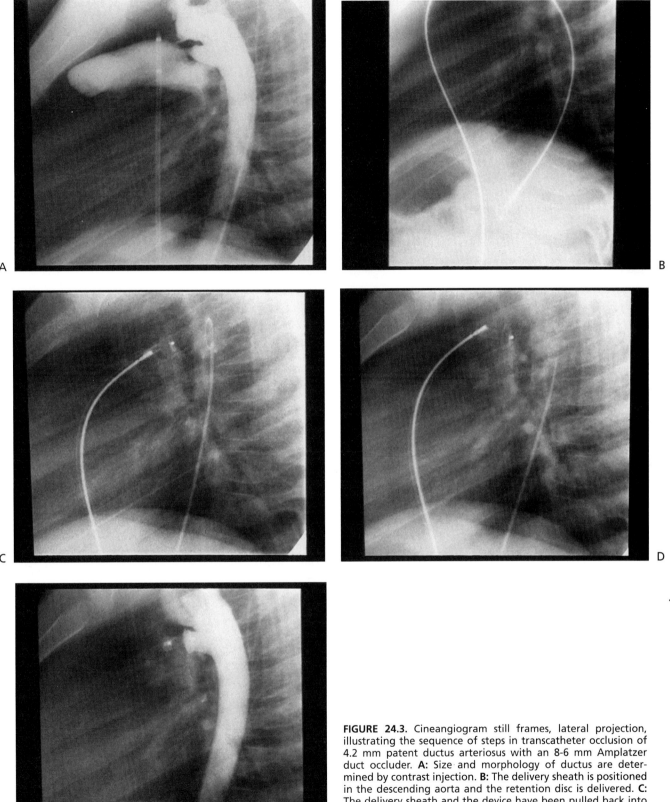

FIGURE 24.3. Cineangiogram still frames, lateral projection, illustrating the sequence of steps in transcatheter occlusion of 4.2 mm patent ductus arteriosus with an 8-6 mm Amplatzer duct occluder. **A:** Size and morphology of ductus are determined by contrast injection. **B:** The delivery sheath is positioned in the descending aorta and the retention disc is delivered. **C:** The delivery sheath and the device have been pulled back into the ductus. The retention disc is flushed against the ampulla. **D:** The cylindrical portion of the device is unsheathed with the device still attached to the delivery cable. **E:** Repeat aortogram confirms complete occlusion of the ductus arteriosus.

disk is deployed in the descending aorta. The device and the delivery sheath are pulled back as a single unit to the aortic ampulla. The device is pulled firmly against the ampulla and its position is confirmed by angiography. While applying gentle traction to the delivery cable the sheath is retracted and the cylindrical portion of the device is delivered. An aortogram is done to confirm the position of the device. A pulmonary artery hand injection is done through the side arm of the delivery sheath to delineate the length of the device in the pulmonary artery. Before releasing the device, if its position is questionable it can be retracted into the sheath and repositioned or removed from the patient. If the device is well positioned it is released by screwing the pin vise to the delivery cable and rotating the cable counterclockwise. A repeat aortogram is done 15 minutes later to evaluate the aortic arch and the residual shunt across the ductus. A pullback is done from the left pulmonary artery to the main pulmonary artery to look for acquired pulmonary artery stenosis. A pullback is also done from the ascending aorta to the descending aorta to exclude acquired coarctation. We administer heparin at 100 U/kg after femoral artery access has been obtained. Cefazolin is administered intravenously in all patients before placement of the Amplatzer Duct Occluder, and Caphalexin was administered orally for 24 hours. Patients who were allergic to cephalosporins received other antistaphylococcal antibiotics. Endocarditis prophylaxis is discontinued 6 months after successful duct occlusion. The patient is kept supine for 4 to 6 hours and then gradually ambulated. A chest x-ray, electrocardiogram (ECG), and echocardiogram are done at 24 hours to evaluate the position of the device, shunting across the ductus and the gradient across the aortic arch and the branch pulmonary arteries.

RESULTS

Immediate Results

Closure of the patent ductus arteriosus with the Amplatzer Duct Occluder has been associated with a 30% to 76%

immediate complete closure rate (11–15) and 100% complete closure rate at 6 months (12–15). The procedure is associated with minimal morbidity and mortality. Reports describing the results of ductus closure with the Amplatzer Duct Occluder are outlined in Table 24.2.

The first report of closure of the patent ductus arteriosus with the Amplatzer Duct Occluder was by Masura and his colleagues (11). They reported closure of the ductus in 24 patients (six male, 18 female) with the Amplatzer Duct Occluder. These patients ranged in age from 0.4 to 48 years (median, 3.8 years) and in weight from 6 to 70 kg (median, 5.5 kg). The mean minimal PDA diameter was 3.7 mm. According to the Krichenko (16) classification, 22 patients had a type A PDA and two had a type E PDA. The device was placed in 23 of the 24 patients. In 30% (7/23) there was immediate complete closure, 14 had a foaming shunt, and two had a jet. At 24 hours, there was complete closure in all patients by echocardiogram. The median fluoroscopy time was 13.5 minutes (range, 6.3 to 47 minutes). Twenty-one of the 23 patients were seen at 1 month and 18/23 were seen at 3 months with a 100% complete closure rate. The single patient in whom the device was not placed was a 9-kg patient with a 1.2-mm PDA in whom an attempt to place a 6/4-mm device resulted in obstruction of more than half the aorta. The device was retracted into the delivery sheath and the ductus was successfully closed with a coil.

Our experience is similar to that reported by other centers. We have attempted closure of the patent ductus arteriosus with the Amplatzer Duct Occluder in 23 patients. The patients ranged in age from 3 months to 12.5 years (median, 26 months) and in weight from 5 to 42.4 kg (median, 11.7). The diameter of the patent ductus arteriosus ranged from 1.6 to 7.2 mm (mean, 3.7) and the Qp/Qs was 1.2-4.7 (mean, 2.1). The PDA morphology as defined by the Krichenko classification was type A in 12, type C in three, type D in two, and type E in six. The fluoroscopy time was 5.2 to 46.4 minutes (median, 13.2). In 22 of 23 patients closure of the patent ductus arteriosus was successful.

TABLE 24.2. RESULTS OF PATENT DUCTUS ARTERIOSUS CLOSURE WITH THE AMPLATZER DUCT OCCLUDER

	Number	Age (yr)	Weight (kg)	Minimal PDA Dia (mm)	Imm	24 hrs	6 mo	12 mo	Complications
Masura et al. (4) (1998)	23	0.4–48 3.8 (median)	6–70 15.5 (median)	3.7 mean	30%	100%			None
Sandhu et al. (12) (1999)	25			1.2–4.8 3 (median)	76%	88%	100%	100%	Device displacement (n = 1) Decrease femoral pulse (n = 1)
Zellers et al. (13) (2000)	87	0.1–66 2.3 (median)	3.6–106 12.2 (median)	1.2–11.2 3 (median)	72%	85%	17/18	100%	Device displacement (n = 1) LPA obstruction mild (n = 1) Decrease femoral pulse (n = 2)
Leung et al. (14) (2000)	227	0.25–64 6.4 (mean)	5–56 19 (mean)	3.9 mean		91%	99.5%	99.5%	None
Bilkis et al. (15)	209	0.2–50 1.9 (median)	3.4–63.2 8.4 (median)	1.8–12.5 4.5 (median)		66%	97%	99%	Device embolization (n = 3)

Dia, diameter; Imm, immediate; LPA, left pulmonary artery; PDA, patent ductus arteriosus.

Immediately following placement of the device there was an 82% (18/22) complete closure rate. At 1 month there was complete closure of the ductus in 91% (20/22). Twelve patients seen at 6 months with a 100% complete closure of the ductus. Six patients were seen at 1 year and three patients were evaluated at 2 years with a 100% complete closure rate. All three patients with a residual shunt at 1 month had complete closure of the ductus by 6 months. There was one device embolization in a 3-month-old 5.4-kg infant. The patient had a type C PDA that measured 5.6 mm in diameter. An 8–6 Amplatzer was positioned and released with embolization of the device immediately into the left pulmonary artery. The device was removed surgically and the PDA was ligated. The embolization was related to placement of a device that was smaller than recommended. No patient had a residual shunt at 6 months. No patient had left pulmonary artery (LPA) stenosis or coarctation. There was no hemolysis.

Bilkis et al. (15) describe their results in 209 patients who underwent closure of the patent ductus arteriosus with the Amplatzer Duct Occluder. The patients ranged in age from 0.2 to 50 years (median, 1.9 years). They ranged in weight from 3.4 to 63.2 kg (median, 8.4 kg) with 27% of the patients being <5 kg. The smallest PDA diameter ranged from 1.8 to 12.5 mm (median, 4.5 mm). The fluoroscopy time ranged from 3.1 to 160 minutes, with a mean of 15.3 minutes. There was complete closure in 66% of the patients at 24 hours, 97% of the patients at 1 month, and 99% of the patients at 1 year. The single patient with a residual shunt at 1 year had complete closure at 15 months. There were three device embolizations, two immediate and one at 24 hours. One patient had a 15 mm Hg gradient across the aortic arch.

Complications

The complications reported (12,13,15) were device embolization ($N = 3$), aortic arch narrowing ($N = 3$), mild LPA stenosis ($N = 1$), and loss of femoral pulses ($N = 2$).

Device displacement resulting in aortic arch narrowing occurred in three patients. In a 1.3-year-old child with a 1.2- mm type A PDA after release of the 6–4 device the retention disk "tipped" back into the aorta, resulting in an 8 mm Hg gradient. This was felt to be hemodynamically insignificant and the device was left in place. In a 5-kg infant a 10–8 device was placed to close a 6.2-mm ductus, resulting in a 15 mm Hg gradient across the aortic arch. In another 5-kg infant with a 6.2-mm ductus, placement of a 10–8 device led to a 15 mm Hg gradient across the aortic arch (15). Patients less than 5 kg in weight appear to be at a greater risk of aortic arch narrowing following device closure.

Device embolization occurred in three patients (15). In one patient this was due to catheter manipulation, and in the other two it was spontaneous, occurring immediately in one and at 24 hours in another. All three patients had no hemodynamic compromise and underwent surgical ligation of the ductus and removal of the device. In most patients device embolization was related to implantation of a device smaller than recommended. Sharafuddin et al. (10) reported one device embolization in a canine model that was successfully retrieved with a gooseneck snare.

The device has a low profile; therefore acquired LPA stenosis is rarely seen. No patient with a residual shunt had hemolysis.

Follow-up

All patients had a chest x-ray, electrocardiogram, and echocardiogram at 6 and 12 months. Short- and mid- term follow-up studies (12–15) demonstrate a 99% to 100% closure rate of the patent ductus arteriosus at 6 and 12 months (13–15) (Table 24.2). No delayed device migrations or wire fractures were noted on chest x-ray. No recanalizations were noted on echocardiogram. No patient had endarteritis. Long-term follow-up is necessary to define the efficacy and safety of the device.

APPLICABILITY IN ADULT SUBJECTS

The patent ductus arteriosus in an adult may be calcified. Therefore transcatheter treatment of the ductus may be the preferred method of treatment. Adult patients up to 66 years of age (11–15) have undergone successful closure of the ductus with the Amplatzer Duct Occluder with no increased morbidity or mortality and a closure rate of 99.5% to 100% at 6 months.

DISCUSSION

Successful closure of the ductus (11–14) has been achieved in 99.5% to 100% of the patients at 1 year in a ductus measuring up to 11.2 mm in diameter. The Amplatzer Duct Occluder can be delivered through a small delivery system (5 to 7F) through the femoral vein, making it easy to use in infants and children. The mechanism by which the device works is by stenting the ductus and then inducing thrombosis. Therefore a device 1 to 2 mm larger than the smallest PDA diameter is used to close the ductus. The retention disk with its cylindrical body is extremely versatile, allowing closure of a variety of ductus, regardless of size and shape (Table 24.3). Although some oversizing of the device is necessary, care must be taken not to greatly exceed the PDA size in order not to compromise the left pulmonary artery or the aorta. Since the device is only 7 or 8 mm long and the average ductus is 5 mm in length, an extrusion of 2 or 3 mm can be expected into the pulmonary artery lumen, which should not compromise pulmonary flow or cause pulmonary stenosis. Although the follow-up of this device is limited, the residual shunt rate at 1 year is 0 to 0.5%,

TABLE 24.3. TYPE OF PATENT DUCTUS ARTERIOSUS UNDERGOING CLOSURE WITH THE AMPLATZER DUCT OCCLUDER

	A	B	C	D	E
Masura et al. (11)	22				2
Sandhu et al. (12)	15		1	2	7
Zellers et al. (13)	57	1	10		12
Bilkis et al. (15)	146		49		10

compared with the Rashkind device, which has a residual shunt rate of up to 38% (9) at 1 year. The flat aortic retention disk secures the device firmly against the aortic orifice, preventing dislodgment toward the pulmonary artery. Early device embolizations (15) were reported in three patients related to implantation of a smaller than recommended device. No late device embolizations have been reported. In infants less than 5 kg care should be taken to ensure that there is no acquired coarctation with the device. If there is acquired coarctation then the device can be removed before its release. Technically, the device is easy to use and does not have a steep learning curve.

CURRENT STATUS

The device is currently undergoing clinical trials in the United States. Phase I clinical trials were completed that have demonstrated that the device is safe and effective. Phase II clinical trials are ongoing.

CONCLUSION

The Amplatzer Duct Occluder is a safe and effective device to close a small to large patent ductus arteriosus. Closure with the Amplatzer Duct Occluder results in a 100% occlusion rate at 6 months. Larger numbers of treated patients and longer follow-up will be necessary to more precisely define the efficacy, safety, and most appropriate indications for this procedure.

REFERENCES

1. Gross RE, Hubbard JP. Surgical ligation of a patent ductus arteriosus: report of first successful case. *JAMA* 1939;112:729–731.
2. Porstmann W, Wierny L, Warnke H. Der verscluss des ductus arteriosus in persistens ohne thorakotomie (1, Miffeilung). *Thoraxchirurgie* 1967;15:109–203.
3. Porstmann W, Wierny I, Warnke H, et al. Catheter closure of patent ductus arteriosus: 62 cases treated without thoracotomy. *Radiol Clin North Am* 1971;9:203–218.
4. Wierny L, Plass R, Porstmann W. Transluminal closure of patent ductus arteriosus: long term results of 208 cases treated without thoracotomy. *Cardiovasc Interv Radiol* 1986;9:279–285.
5. Sandhu SK, King TD. Historical aspects of transcatheter closure of the patent ductus arteriosus. *Curr Interv Cardiol Rep* 2000;2:361–366.
6. Cambier PA, Kirby WC, Wortham DC, et al. Percutaneous closure of the small patent ductus arteriosus using coil embolization. *Am J Cardiol* 1992;69:815–816.
7. Lloyd TR, Fedderly R, Mendelsohn AM, et al. Transcatheter occlusion of patent ductus arteriosus with Gianturco coils. *Circulation* 1993;88:1412–1420.
8. Report of European Registry. Transcatheter occlusion of persistent arterial duct. *Lancet* 1992;340:1062–1066.
9. Hosking MCK, Benson LN, Musewe N, et al. Transcatheter occlusion of the persistently patent ductus arteriosus: forty-month follow-up and prevalence of residual shunting. *Circulation* 1991;84:2313–2317.
10. Sharafuddin MJ, Gu X, Titus JL, et al. Experimental evaluation of a new self-expanding patent ductus arteriosus occluder in a canine model. *J Vasc Interv Radiol* 1996;7:877–887.
11. Masura J, Walsh KP, Thanopoulous B, et al. Catheter closure of moderate to large sized patent ductus arteriosus using the new Amplatzer Duct Occluder: immediate and short term results. *J Am Coll Cardiol* 1998;31:878–882.
12. Sandhu SK, Hijazi ZM, Amin Z, et al. Transcatheter closure of patent ductus arteriosus using the Amplatzer Duct Occluder: results of Phase I US multicenter clinical trial. *Circulation* 1999;100(Suppl I):804.
13. Zellers TM, Hijazi ZM, Sandhu S, et al. Catheter closure of patent ductus arteriosus using the Amplatzer Device: interim report on US Phase I & II clinical trial. *Circulation* 2000;102:II-587.
14. Leung MP, Chin M, Chau O, et al. Multicenter trial for the occlusion of patent arterial duct by the Amplatzer Duct Occluder in China. *Circulation* 2000;102:II-587.
15. Bilkis AA, Mazeni A, Hasri S, et al. The Amplatzer Duct Occluder: experience in 209 patients. *J Am Coll Cardiol* 2001;37:258–261.
16. Krichenko A, Benson L, Burrows P, et al. Angiographic classification of the isolated persistently patent ductus arteriosus and implications for percutaneous catheter occlusion. *Am J Cardiol* 1989;63:877–880.

25

SUMMARY AND COMPARISON OF PATENT DUCTUS ARTERIOSUS CLOSURE METHODS

P. SYAMASUNDAR RAO

Since the initial description in the late 1960s by Porstmann and his associates (1,2) of a patent ductus arteriosus (PDA) occluding device, a number of other devices have been studied and reviewed elsewhere (Chapter 17) (3). During the 1990s, a number of devices to occlude PDA have been developed and tested. Some of these are available for clinical use, but many are in FDA-supervised clinical trials. Therefore the interventional cardiologist has a number of devices to choose from. Selection of any method of treatment of any condition is usually made on the basis of results of prospective, randomized clinical trials. There are some comparative studies (4–7), but most of these investigations were undertaken in small cohorts with a limited number of devices. They were conducted in a sequential fashion as the new devices became available. But, more important, they are neither prospective nor randomized in their design. At the present time, it is unlikely that a prospective randomized clinical trial with all the "eligible" devices is feasible or practical. Because of this, the selection of a device by the interventional cardiologist may have to be based on evaluation of results of the device implantation in large cohorts of patients, generally sponsored by the device designer and/or manufacturer.

This chapter provides a comparison of the PDA closure devices and discusses the selection of devices and methods to occlude the ductus based on its size and shape.

THE DEVICES

The devices are classified into those that have been tried only in experimental models (Table 25.1), those that underwent clinical trials but have been discontinued (Table 25.2), and those that are either in general clinical use or available for use on an investigational basis (Table 25.3). The tables list a brief description of the devices and year of their initial published report. The devices listed in Tables 25.1 and 25.2 are not available for clinical use and therefore are not detailed in this chapter.

TABLE 25.1. EXPERIMENTALLY USED PDA CLOSURE DEVICES

Authors (References)	Year	Description of Device
Mills and King (8)	1976	Dumbbell-shaped plug
Leslie et al. (9)	1977	Cylindrical Ivalon sponge plug tied securely to a stainless steel umbrella
Warnecke et al. (10)	1986	Detachable silicone double balloon
Magal et al. (11)	1989	Conical nylon sack filled with segments of modified guide wire with a 1.5-cm-long flexible wire cross bar attached to the distal end of the sack*
Echigo et al. (12)	1990	Temperature–shape changeable, shape–memory polymer (polynorbornene)
Nazarian et al. (13)	1993	Butterfly vascular stent plug
Pozza et al. (14)	1995	Conical-shaped stainless steel wire mesh
Liu et al. (15,16)	1993, 1996	Thermal shape–memory nickel–titanium coil
Grabitz et al. (17)	1996	Miniaturized Duct-Occlud pfm

*This device appears to a precursor of Gianturco-Grifka sac (18).
PDA, patent ductus arteriosus.
From Rao PS. Summary and comparison of patent ductus arteriosus closure devices. *Curr Interv Cardiol Rep* 2001;3:268–274, with permission.

P. Syamasundar Rao: Professor of Pediatrics, Medicine, and Cardiology, Department of Pediatrics, University of Texas-Houston Medical School; Director, Division of Pediatric Cardiology, Memorial Hermann Children's Hospital, Houston, Texas

TABLE 25.2. PDA DEVICES THAT HAVE UNDERGONE CLINICAL TRIALS BUT ARE CURRENTLY UNAVAILABLE FOR CLINICAL USE

Authors (References)	Year	Description of the Device
Porstmann et al. (1,2)	1967	Conical-shaped Ivalon foam plug
Rashkind and Cuaso (19)	1979	Polyurethane foam–covered single umbrella with miniature hooks
Rashkind (20)	1983	Two opposing polyurethane-covered umbrellas
Saveliev et al. (21,22)	1984, 1988	Polyurethane foam plug, Botallo occluder
Sideris et al. (23)	1990	Square-shaped polyurethane occluder and a rhomboid-shaped counter occluder attached to each other with a latex string
Bridges et al. (24)	1991	Clamshell ASD device
Sideris et al. (25)	1996	Two rhomboid-shaped polyurethane foam pieces mounted on single wires attached to each other *in vivo* by buttoning (infant buttoned device)
Grabitz et al. (26)	1997	Polyvinyl alcohol foam plug mounted on a titanium core pin

ASD, atrial septal defect; PDA, patent ductus arteriosus.
From Rao PS. Summary and comparison of patent ductus arteriosus closure devices. *Curr Interv Cardiol Rep* 2001;3:268–274, with permission.

DEVICE COMPARISON

The major considerations in the selection of a device for closure of PDAs are feasibility, safety, and effectiveness of occlusion. Other considerations are the size of the delivery sheath, the ease with which the device is implanted, cost, and availability.

Feasibility

Implantation feasibility for a given device may be gauged by examining the ratio of a number of implantations to the number of subjects taken to the catheterization laboratory with intent to close. The ease with which a given device is implanted is variable. Most require some training under the tutelage of an experienced operator. The implantation feasibility data for PDA device closures are sparse (Table 25.4). Implantation feasibility appears high for most devices, varying between 91% and 100%.

Safety

The most serious adverse effects of any device are misplacement, dislodgment, and embolization. Such displaced devices can be safely retrieved by snares and other transcatheter retrieval instruments. But in some instances surgi-

TABLE 25.3. PDA DEVICE CURRENTLY AVAILABLE FOR CLINICAL USE

Authors (References)	Year	Description of the Device
Rao et al. (27,28)	1991	Square-shaped polyurethane occluder and a rhomboid-shaped occluder attached to each other *in vivo* by buttoning
Cambier et al. (29)	1992	Gianturco coil
Le et al. (30)	1993	Duct-Occlud pfm
Cambier et al. (31)	1993	Cook detachable coil
Ozun et al. (32)	1996	Flipper detachable coil
Grifka et al. (33)	1997	Gianturco-Grifka sac
Owada et al. (34)	1997	0.052-in Gianturco coil
Masura et al. (35)	1998	Amplatzer duct occluder
Rao et al. (35)	1999	Folding plug buttoned device
Sideris et al. (36)	2001	Wireless PDA devices

From Rao PS. Summary and comparison of patent ductus arteriosus closure devices. *Curr Interv Cardiol Rep* 2001;3:268–274, with permission.

TABLE 25.4. COMPARISON OF DEVICES CURRENTLY AVAILABLE FOR CLINICAL USE IN OCCLUSION OF PDA

Device	Number of Patients	Implantation Feasibility	Device Dislodgement	Residual Shunt	
				24 hours	Follow-up
Buttoned device					
Rao et al. (36)	284	280/284 (99%)	0	40%	2.5%
Free Gianturco coils (38)*	488	369/387 (95%)	48/488 (9%)	18%	9%(40-42)†
Duct-occlude pfm					
Tometzki et al. (42)	51	44/51 (86%)	3/44 (7%)	9%	—
Oho et al. (43)	35	32/35 (91%)	0	—	16%
Lê et al. (44)	514	466/514 (91%)	16/466 (4%)	42%	5.5%
Detachable coils					
Temetzki et al. (45)	70	69/70 (99%)	1/69 (1.5%)	7%	3%
Podnar and Masura (46)	30	29/30 (97%)	2/29 (7%)	17%	10%
Bermudez-Canete et al. (47)	193	181/193 (94%)	5/181 (3%)	9%	6%
Ozun et al. (48)	76	—	—	28%	12%
Gianturco-Grifka device					
Grifka (18)	32	—	1/32 (3%)	9%	0
Amplatzer					
Masura et al. (35)	24	23/24 (96%)	0	0	0
Bilkis et al. (49)	209	205/209 (98%)	3/205 (1.5%)	34%	3%
Sandhu et al. (50)	23	100%	1/23 (4%)	14%	0
Waight et al. (51)	83	100%	0	5%	0
Folding plug buttoned device					
Sideris et al. (37)	20	100%	0	15%	5%
Wireless PDA device					
Sideris et al. (37)	4	100%	0	0	0

PDA, patent ductus arteriosus. N, number of patients.
*Summary of published reports on coil occlusion from 1992 to 1997; reviewed elsewhere (38), but not published.
†Follow-up residual shunt are based on follow-up results reported in selected studies (39–41).
From Rao PS. Summary and comparison of patent ductus arteriosus closure devices. *Curr Interv Cardiol Rep* 2001;3:268–274, with permission.

cal retrieval of the device along with surgical closure of the PDA may have to be undertaken for various reasons, including difficulty in transcatheter retrieval, embolization into a peripheral segment of the lung, or bulkiness of the device, not permitting transcatheter retrieval. A surgical approach has also been used in early experience with a given device. The device dislodgment rates are also listed in Table 25.4 and vary from 0 to 7%. Careful evaluation of the morphology and size of the ductus and their relationship with the device used may help prevent or reduce embolization after deployment and release.

Effectiveness

The effectiveness of occlusion is evaluated by angiography immediately following implantation and two-dimensional Doppler echocardiographic studies within 24 hours of the procedure. Repeat Doppler studies during follow-up are usually undertaken to determine the residual shunts. The prevalence of residual shunts within 24 hours of implantation appears to vary widely from one device to another (0 to 42%) and to decrease during follow-up (Table 25.4). The

variable residual shunt rate with different devices should not be attributed solely to the device because the types and sizes of PDA entering each study protocol varied widely.

Other Considerations

The size of the catheter/sheath required to implant the PDA closure device is variable (Table 25.5). Free Gianturco coils require a small-caliber (4F) catheter, whereas most devices require larger delivery sheaths. Devices are most expensive; Gianturco coils cost the least (Table 25.5). The implantation technique can easily be mastered with coils, but device implantation requires more training than that required for coil delivery. The coils are available for routine clinical use, but most devices are available under a protocol for investigational use at the participating centers (Table 25.5).

DISCUSSION

This section provides a few comments on the potential utility of the devices along with their advantages and disadvan-

TABLE 25.5. SIZE OF DELIVERY CATHETER, COST OF THE AVAILABLE PDA OCCLUDING DEVICES

Device	Size of Delivery Catheter/ Sheath	Cost	Availability
Gianturco coils (free)	4F	$40–60	Available for general clinical use
Detachable coils	5F	$65*	Available for general clinical use
Duct occlud pfm	4 or 5F		Available for clinical trials at participating institutions only
Buttoned device**	7 to 8F	$1,500	Available for clinical trials at participating institutions only
Gianturco-Grifka sac	8F	$600	Available for general clinical use
Amplatzer duct occluder	6 to 8F	$1,200	Available for clinical trials at participating institutions only
Wireless devices	10F	‡	Available outside US at institution participating in clinical trials§

*Cost does not include delivery system.
**FDA approval with IDE.
‡Cost not determined as yet.
§IDE from FDA is pending.
F, French size; FDA, US Food and Drug Administration; IDE, investigational device exemption; PDA, patent ductus arteriosus.
From Rao PS. Summary and comparison of patent ductus arteriosus closure devices. *Curr Interv Cardiol Rep* 2001;3:268–274, with permission.

tages. The comments are limited to devices that are currently available for routine clinical use or for investigational use (Table 25.3).

Regular Buttoned Device

The role of the buttoned device in occluding PDA in both children and adults has been studied extensively (28,36,52), and feasibility, safety, and effectiveness have been demonstrated. Although it requires a moderate-sized delivery sheath, it is delivered transvenously. All types of PDA, irrespective of the size, shape, and length, could be effectively closed with this device. However, the residual shunt rate (approximately 40%) at implantation is high, although the shunts decrease and disappear with time. To increase complete occlusion rates at implantation, it was modified by introducing a polyurethane foam plug over the button loop (36); this modified device will be discussed later in this section.

Gianturco Coils

The coils, originally developed to occlude renal arteries (53), were adopted to occlude PDA (29). They are readily available (initially, for off-label use) and relatively inexpensive. Whereas arterial delivery is most commonly used, transvenous delivery is also possible. The delivery catheter is small; a 4F catheter is sufficient for most cases. The method of coil implantation can easily be mastered. Indeed, Gianturco coil occlusion is the preferred method of occlusion of very small to small PDA at most institutions around

the world (54). Moderate-to-large ducti are difficult to occlude with coils (55), although a multiple-coil technique (56,57) and thicker-diameter (0.052-inch) coils (34,55) may be utilized to occlude moderate-sized PDA. It appears that coil occlusion will remain the preferred method to close very small PDAs. Most moderate-to-large PDAs may require device closure.

Detachable Coils

Control delivery is not possible with free Gianturco coils, and once released, they cannot be repositioned. To gain greater control during delivery and to prevent embolization, detachable coils (31,32) were developed. A review of available data (45–48) suggests that there continued to be a significant prevalence of coil dislodgment/embolization after release (Table 25.4). Therefore the perceived benefit of controlled coil delivery offered by detachable coils did not seem to accrue. Furthermore, the currently available wire diameters are relatively small (0.035-inch) and therefore may not be as effective as thicker-diameter (0.038- and 0.052-inch) coils in producing complete occlusion. Finally, cost of implantation of detachable coils is greater than that of free Gianturco coils.start here

Duct-Occlud Pfm

Duct-Occlud Pfm is a new stainless steel coil without Dacron fibers but with a diabolo configuration (30). A thicker, reinforced version was made available more recently

(44). The system provides for controlled delivery via small delivery catheters (4 to 5F) and is generally implanted transvenously. Slightly lower implantation feasibility, low but significant device dislodgment rates, a high rate of residual shunts at implantation (Table 25.4), cost, and availability only at institutions participating in clinical trials are the disadvantages of this device. In addition, it may not be useful in occluding large PDAs.

Gianturco-Grifka Vascular Occlusion Device

The Gianturco-Grifka vascular occlusion device appears to be a modified version of the device described by Megal et al. (11,58). It is useful in occluding large tubular ducti and can be implanted transvenously. Although it is approved for general clinical use, its disadvantages are the relatively large delivery system, difficulties in transcatheter retrieval if it dislodges, complex device implantation procedure, and usefulness in only specific types of PDAs.

Amplatzer Duct Occluder

The Amplatzer Duct Occluder is a relatively new device with rapid accumulation of implantation data (35,49–51). It can be delivered transvenously via a small delivery sheath. Deployment is simple and is retrievable and repositionable before device release. Also, complete closure rates are high. However, device dislodgment, though rare, requires surgical intervention (49,50), and this is a concern. Recent reports of aortic coarctation when used in small infants and nickel toxicity are of concern. Finally, at the present time it is only available for investigational use on a protocol basis at the participating centers.

Folding-Plug Buttoned Device

Incorporation of a polyurethane folding plug over the button loop improved complete and effective occlusion rates of the buttoned device (36,37). It can be implanted transvenously and can be used irrespective of the size (diameter), shape, and length of the ductus. It is particularly useful in large PDAs. However, it requires a large delivery sheath and is available only on protocol basis for investigational use at the participating centers. Thus far there is only a limited experience with this device. Recent FDA approval for clinical trials with IDE may provide additional data soon.

Wireless Devices

Lack of wires and utility in very large PDAs are attractive features. But, the clinical experience with this device is extremely limited. Experience in larger patient populations is needed before drawing any conclusion on their utility in occluding PDAs.

TABLE 25.6. CLASSIFICATION OF PDAS BASED ON SIZE

Type	Description
Silent PDA	Usually less than 1.0 mm*
	Without audible murmur of PDA
Very small PDA	≤1.5*
	Murmur of PDA present
Small PDA	1.5 to 3.0 mm*
	Murmur of PDA present
Moderate PDA	3 to 5 mm*
	Murmur of PDA present
Large PDA	>5 mm*
	Murmur of PDA present

*Minimal ductal diameters on lateral cineangiographic view. PDA, patent ductus arteriosus.
From Rao PS. Transcatheter closure of moderate-to-large patent ductus arteriosus. *J Invasive Cardiol* 2001;13:303–306, with permission.

APPROACHES TO PDA CLOSURE

Based on personal experience with PDA closure with a number of methods and review of the experience of others (54,55,59,60), it appears that the choice of the method of closure should be based on the size (minimal ductal diameter) and the shape (61) of the PDA (Tables 25.6 and 25.7).

SIZE OF THE PDA

Silent PDA

A new subset of patients, referred to as "silent ductus," has emerged because of widespread use of color Doppler echocardiography. Almost 1% of children undergoing such studies were found to have a PDA (62). These patients do not have a continuous murmur of PDA on auscultation, but PDAs are visualized by color Doppler. Some investiga-

TABLE 25.7. DEVICE SELECTION BASED ON DUCTAL SHAPE/MORPHOLOGY

Conventional Shape Description	Krichenko's Type	Devices Suitable for Closure
Conical	A1, A2, A3, D	Coils
		Amplatzer
		Buttoned device
Short	B	Buttoned device
Tubular	C	Gianturco-Grifka sac
		Buttoned device
Long and Bizzarre	E	Coils
		Amplatzer
		Buttoned device

From Rao PS. Summary and comparison of patent ductus arteriosus closure devices. *Curr Interv Cardiol Rep* 2001;3:268–274, with permission.

tors (63,64) have suggested that such PDAs should be closed because of potential risk of endocarditis (63); others (65), including our group (54,59,60), are opposed to closing such ducti. As more data become available, the weight of evidence may eventually resolve this controversy.

Silent Ductus After Device/Coil Occlusion

Residual shunts after device/coil closure are not uncommon as reviewed in the preceding sections of the chapter. Most of these have no associated murmur and therefore may be called "silent PDAs." Can we extend the noninterventional strategy to such PDAs? Latson and his associates (66) examined this issue in a piglet model. Latson initially occluded PDAs with Rashkind devices. Piglets with completely closed PDAs and those with residual shunts were studied for their risk of developing endocarditis. The data indicate that the piglets with no and "trivial" residual shunts were not at a greater risk than controls, whereas piglets with significant residual shunts developed endocarditis. These results led Latson to conclude that patients with silent PDA after device occlusion are not at a higher risk for developing endocarditis. However, it is not clear how trivial versus significant residual shunts in piglets compare with residual shunts without murmurs after device/coil closure in human subjects. Furthermore, subacute bacterial endocarditis prophylaxis is currently recommended if residual shunt exists after device/coil occlusion. Thus it is appropriate to recommend occlusion (mostly coil occlusion) if residual shunt persist 6 to 12 months after device/coil closure of PDA.

Very Small PDA

The PDAs may be characterized as small if the minimal ductal diameter ≤1.5 to 2 mm but with a continuous murmur (Table 25.6). Very small PDAs are easily occluded with free Gianturco coils, initially described by Cambier et al. (29). We personally prefer coils with a wire diameter of 0.038 inch with four or five loops so as to produce complete occlusion (38,67). Transarterial coil delivery is most commonly used and can be undertaken via 4F catheters. The procedure is relatively simple and the coils are inexpensive. Employing snares (68), forceps (69), detachable coils (70), and balloon (71,72) and tapered-tip (73) catheters during coil delivery is not necessary in all cases. Such procedures may increase fluoroscopic time and expense.

Small PDA

Small PDAs may be defined as minimal ductal diameters of 1.5 to 3 mm with a continuous murmur (Table 25.6). Complete occlusion may not be achieved with a single 0.038-inch Gianturco coil; therefore multiple coils (56,57) may be necessary to effect complete closure. Multicoil

deployment is a reasonable approach, but the potential for coil dislodgment and left-pulmonary artery stenosis exists. Because of this, 0.052-inch coils (34,74) are best. Such coils can be delivered via long 4F Blue Cook sheaths (Cook, Bloomington, IN) with the assistance of a biopsy forceps, in a manner similar to that described by Hays (69) and Grifka (58) and their associates.

While devices have been used (Table 25.3) to occlude very small and small PDAs, this is neither advisable nor necessary. Such devices increase the cost of the procedure.

Moderate-Sized to Large PDAs

Ducti with minimal diameter >3 mm may be closed by conventional surgical closure (75), video-assisted thoracoscopic interruption (76), and devices (Table 25.8). The relative advantages and disadvantages of the devices are listed in Table 25.8. The Rashkind PDA occluder (77), Botallo occluder (78), Clamshell device (24), and polyvinyl alcohol foam plug (79) have been discontinued and are unavailable for clinical use. The utility of Duct-Occlud Pfm (42) for closing moderate-to-large ducti has not been thoroughly investigated. The Gianturco-Grifka vascular occlusion device (33) is particularly useful in occluding tubular PDAs and is available for general clinical use. However, a large delivery sheath is required to deploy the device. In addition, retrieval of the dislodged devices is fraught with problems. The Amplatzer Duct Occluder (35,49–51) has been in extensive clinical trials. It has several favorable features, including relatively small delivery sheath (5 to 7F), ease with which it can be retrieved and repositioned before final detachment, and high closure rates. But device dislodgment requiring surgery (49,50) is of some concern. However, the device dislodgment rate (three of 209, or 1.4%) in a large series (49) is low. More recently, use of this device in infants has been reported to produce obstruction in the descending aorta, related to tilting of the device. A modified version of a buttoned device, the folding-plug modification (36), appears to have good occlusion rates. It requires 7- to 8F sheaths for device deployment. Both the Amplatzer and folding buttoned device are available only at institutions participating in FDA-approved clinical trials.

Finally, the transcatheter patch device may be useful in occluding large PDAs (37). International clinical trials are under way. A number of devices (Table 25.8) have been employed to occlude moderate-to-large PDAs. Some of the devices have been discontinued and others were modified. A few are available for general clinical use (33), and others are available under a clinical trial protocol (35,36). At the present time, the Gianturco-Grifka vascular occlusion device (33), the Amplatzer Duct Occluder (35), and the folding-plug buttoned device (36) are alternatives to conventional surgical closure (75) and videothoracoscopic closure (76). Given the current stage of device development

TABLE 25.8. DEVICES FOR MODERATE TO LARGE PDA

Device	Advantages/disadvantages
Rashkind PDA occluder	High residual shunt rate Device discontinued
Botalloccluder	Large delivery sheath Device discontinued
Clamshell occluder	Large delivery sheath Device discontinued
Duct occlude pfm	May not be useful in large PDA Availability only in clinical trials at participating institutions
Gianturco-Grifka sac	Relatively large delivery sheath Useful in tubular PDA Available for general clinical use
Polyvinyl alcohol foam plug	Large delivery sheath Not available for clinical use
Amplatzer duct occluder	Relatively small delivery sheaths Retrievable, repositionable Available only at institutions participating in clinical trials
Folding plug buttoned device	Small to moderate-sized delivery sheath Limited experience Available only at institutions participating in clinical trials
Wireless PDA devices	Large delivery sheath Limited experience Available only outside US at institutions participating in clinical trials*

*(IDE) from FDA is pending.
FDA, US Food and Drug Administration; IDE, investigational device exemption; PDA, patent ductus arteriosus.
From Rao PS. Transcatheter closure of moderate-to-large patent ductus arteriosus. *J Invasive Cardiol* 2001;13:303–306, with permission.

technology, the method for occlusion of moderate-to-large PDA is largely dependent upon the availability of expertise with a particular device or method at a given institution at a given time. Opportunity to perform randomized clinical trials may not arise until several devices become available for general clinical use. When available, such data may help to select the best method of PDA closure.

DUCTAL SHAPE

The classification described by Kriechenko (61) has largely replaced the earlier descriptions, such as *conical, tubular, short,* and *long.* If the PDA is very small or small, the shape may not play an independent role in determining the feasibility or effectiveness of closure of a given device. But if the ductus is moderate to large, the shape may play a significant role in determining the feasibility and effectiveness of device closure. Table 25.6 lists various shapes and the devices that are likely to be useful in closing moderate-to-large PDAs.

SUMMARY AND CONCLUSION

A number of transcatheter PDA closure devices have been designed and tested following the reports by Porstmann of

such a device. Some devices have been tested only in animal models, and others were used both in experimental models and in human subjects. Although the results appeared good, some devices were discontinued either because of lack of approval by appropriate regulatory authorities, bulkiness of the device, or excessive residual shunts. Some devices were further modified to improve their performance. Most of the devices were discussed separately in the preceding chapters of this book.

Whereas a number of these devices are available to the interventional cardiologist either for general clinical use or for investigational use, there are no prospective, randomized clinical trials to determine which is the best device or method for a given type of PDA. Therefore data of separate clinical trials with the devices supported by the device manufacturer are generally used to determine relative efficacy and safety of the devices.

The utility of free Gianturco coils for occlusion of very small and small PDAs is well established in current clinical practice. Options for closure of moderate-to-large PDAs are devices, videothoracoscopic interruption, and conventional surgical closure. Among the devices, the Gianturco-Grifka vascular occlusion device appears to be the only one that is approved for general clinical use. Other devices are currently undergoing FDA-approved clinical trials and are available for investigational use at the participating hospitals. These include the buttoned device, Duct-Occlud Pfm, the Amplatzer Duct Occluder, and the folding-plug buttoned device. Wireless PDA devices may be used for very large PDA and are undergoing clinical trials outside the United States.

Selection of the method of closure of PDA is generally determined by its size (minimal ductal diameter) and shape. Silent PDAs need not be closed. Very small PDAs can be successfully closed with the free or detachable Gianturco coils. Small PDAs may need multiple coils or a larger wire diameter (0.52-inch) coil. Devices or surgical methods are necessary for moderate to large PDAs. In the latter group, availability of the method or device plus expertise at a given institution at a given time largely determine the method selected.

REFERENCES

1. Porstmann W, Wierny L, Warnke H. Der Verschluß des Ductus arteriosus persistens ohne Thorakotomie (Vorläufige, Mitteilung). *Thoraxchirurgie* 1967;15:109–203.
2. Porstmann W, Wierny L, Warnke H, et al. Catheter closure of patent ductus arteriosus: 62 cases treated without thoracotomy. *Radiol Clin North Am* 1971;9:203–218.
3. Sandhu SK, King TD. Historical aspects of transcatheter closure of the patent ductus arteriosus. *Curr Interv Cardiol Rep* 2000;2: 361–366.
4. Galal O, de Moor M, Al-Fadley F, et al. Transcatheter closure of the patent ductus arteriosus: comparison between the Rashkind occluder device and the anterograde Gianturco coils technique. *Am Heart J* 1996;131:368–373.
5. Zeevi B, Berant M, Bar-Mor G, et al. Percutaneous closure of small patent ductus arteriosus: comparison of Rashkind double-umbrella device and occluding spring coils. *Catheter Cardiovasc Diagn* 1996;39:44–48.
6. Bulbul ZR, Fahey JT, Doyle TP, et al. Transcatheter closure of patent ductus arteriosus: a comparative study between occluding coils and the Rashkind umbrella device. *Catheter Cardiovasc Diagn* 1996;39:355–363.
7. Janorkar S, Goh T, Wilkinson J. Transcatheter closure of patent ductus arteriosus with the use of Rashkind occluder and/or Gianturco coils: long-term follow-up in 123 patients and special reference to comparison, residual shunts, complications and technique. *Am Heart J* 1999;138:1176–1183.
8. Mills NL, King TD. Non-operative closure of left-to-right shunts. *J Thorac Cardiovasc Surg* 1976;72:371–378.
9. Leslie J, Lindsay W, Amplatz K. Nonsurgical closure of patent ductus arteriosus: an experimental study. *Invest Radiol* 1977;12: 142–145.
10. Warnecke I, Frank J, Hohle R, et al. Transvenous double-balloon occlusion of the persistent ductus arteriosus: an experimental study. *Pediatr Cardiol* 1986;5:79–84.
11. Magal C, Wright KC, Duprat G, et al. A new device for transcatheter closure of patent ductus arteriosus: a feasibility study in dogs. *Invest Radiol* 1989;24:272–276.
12. Echigo S, Matsuda T, Kamiya T, et al. Development of a new transvenous patent ductus arteriosus occlusion technique using a shape memory polymer. *ASAIO Trans* 1990;36: M195–M222.
13. Nazarian GK, Qian Z, Vladaver Z, et al. Evaluation of a new vascular occlusion device. *Invest Radiol* 1993;28:1165–1169.
14. Pozza CH, Gomes MR, Qian Z, et al. Transcatheter occlusion of patent ductus arteriosus using a newly developed self-expanding device. *Invest Radiol* 1995;30:104–109.
15. Liu C, Shiraishi H, Yanagisawar M. Effectiveness of patent ductus arteriosus occlusion coil: *in vitro* study. *Jichi Med Schl J* 1993; 16:57–65.
16. Liu C, Shiraishi H, Kikuchi Y, et al. Effectiveness of a thermal shape-memory patent ductus arteriosus occlusion coil. *Am Heart J* 1996;131:1018–1023.
17. Grabitz RG, Neuss MB, Coe JY, et al. A small interventional device to occlude persistently patent ductus arteriosus in neonates: evaluation in piglets. *J Am Coll Cardiol* 1996;28: 1024–1030.
18. Grifka RG. Transcatheter PDA closure using the Gianturco-Grifka vascular occlusion device. *Curr Interv Cardiol Rep* 2001;3: 174–182.
19. Rashkind WJ, Cuaso CC. Transcatheter closure of a patent ductus arteriosus: successful use in a 3.5 kg infant. *Pediatr Cardiol* 1979;1:3–7.
20. Rashkind WJ. Transcatheter treatment of congenital heart disease. *Circulation* 1983;67:711–716.
21. Saveliev VS, Prokubovski VI, Kolody SM, et al. Interventional radiology: new directions in prophylaxis and treatment of surgical disease. *Khirurgiia (Mosk)* 1984;8:113–117.
22. Prokubovski, Kolody SM, Saveliev SV, et al. Transluminal closure of the patent ductus arteriosus with transvenous approach: alternative to surgery. *Grad Khirurgiia* 1988;1:42–47.
23. Sideris EB, Sideris SE, Ehly RL. Occlusion of patent ductus arteriosus in piglets by a double disk self-adjustable device (Abstract). *J Am Coll Cardiol* 1990;15:240A.
24. Bridges ND, Perry SB, Parness I, et al. Transcatheter closure of a large patent ductus arteriosus with the clamshell septal umbrella. *J Am Coll Cardiol* 1991;18:1297–1302.
25. Sideris EB, Rey C, DeLezo JS, et al. Infant buttoned device for occlusion of patent ductus arteriosus, early clinical experience (Abstract). *Cardiol Young* 1996;(Suppl 1):S32.
26. Grabitz RG, Schräder R, Sigler M, et al. Retrievable patent ductus arteriosus plug for interventional transvenous occlusion of the patent ductus arteriosus: evaluation in lambs and preliminary clinical results. *Invest Radiol* 1997;32:523–528.
27. Rao PS, Wilson AD, Sideris EB, et al. Transcatheter closure of patent ductus arteriosus with buttoned device: first successful clinical application in a child. *Am Heart J* 1991;121: 1799–1802.
28. Rao PS, Sideris EB, Haddad J, et al. Transcatheter occlusion of patent ductus arteriosus with adjustable buttoned device: initial clinical experience. *Circulation* 1993;88:1119–1126.
29. Cambier PA, Kirby WC, Wortham DC, et al. Percutaneous closure of small (<2.5 mm) patent ductus arteriosus using coil embolization. *Am J Cardiol* 1992;69:815–816.
30. Lê TP, Neuss MB, Redel DA, et al. A new transcatheter occlusion technique with retrievable double disk shaped coils: first clinical results in occlusion of patent ductus arteriosus. *Cardiol Young* 1993;3:I-38.
31. Cambier PA, Stajduhar KC, Powell D, et al. Improved safety of transcatheter vascular occlusion utilizing a new retrievable coil device. *J Am Coll Cardiol* 1994;23:359A.
32. Ozun O, Hancock S, Parsons JM, et al. Transcatheter occlusion of the arterial duct with Cook detachable coils: early experience. *Heart* 1996;176:269–273.
33. Grifka RG, Vincent JA, Nihill MR, et al. Transcatheter patent ductus arteriosus closure in an infant using Gianturco-Grifka device. *Am J Cardiol* 1996;15:78:721–723.

34. Owada CY, Teitel DF, Moore P. Evaluation of Gianturco coils for closure of large (>3.5 mm) patent ductus arteriosus. *J Am Coll Cardiol* 1997;30:1859–1862.

35. Masura J, Walsh KP, Thanopoulos B, et al. Catheter closure of moderate-to-large-sized patent ductus arteriosus using new Amplatzer Duct Occluder; immediate and short-term results. *J Am Coll Cardiol* 1998;31:1878–1882.

36. Rao PS, Kim SH, Choi J, et al. Follow-up results of transvenous occlusion of patent ductus arteriosus with the buttoned device. *J Am Coll Cardiol* 1999;33:820–826.

37. Sideris EB, Rao PS, Zamora R. The Sideris' buttoned devices for transcatheter closure of patent ductus arteriosus. *J Interv Cardiol* 2001;14:239–246.

38. Rao PS, Balfour IC, Chen S. Effectiveness of 5-loop coils to occlude patent ductus arteriosus. *Am J Cardiol* 1997;80:1498–1501.

39. Shim D, Fedderly RT, Beekman RH, III, et al. Follow-up of coil occlusion of patent ductus arteriosus. *J Am Coll Cardiol* 1996;28:207–211.

40. Goyal VS, Fullwani MC, Ramakantan R, et al. Follow-up after coil closure of patent ductus arteriosus. *Am J Cardiol* 1999;83:463–466.

41. Patel HT, Cao Q, Rhodes J, et al. Long-term outcome of transcatheter coil closure of small to large patent ductus arteriosus. *Catheter Cardiovasc Interv* 1999;47:457–461.

42. Tometzki A, Chan K, Giovanni JD, et al. Total UK multi-center experience with a novel arterial occlusion device (Duct Occlud pfm). *Heart* 1996;76:520–524.

43. Oho S, Ishizawa A, Koike K, et al. Transcatheter occlusion of patent ductus arteriosus with a new detachable coil system (Duct Occlud): a multicenter clinical trial. *Japn Circ J* 1998;62:489–493.

44. Le TD, Moore JW, Neuss MB, et al. Duct-Occlud for occlusion of patent ductus arteriosus. *Curr Interv Cardiol Rep* 2001;3:165–173.

45. Tometzki AJ, Arnold R, Peart I, et al. Transcatheter occlusion of patent ductus arteriosus with Cook detachable coils. *Heart* 1996;76:531–535.

46. Podnar T, Masura J. Percutaneous closure of patent ductus arteriosus using special screwing detachable coils. *Catheter Cardiovasc Diagn* 1997;41:386–391.

47. Bermudez-Canete R, Santoro G, Bialkowsky, et al. Patent ductus arteriosus occlusion using detachable coils. *Am J Cardiol* 1998;82:1547–1549.

48. Ozun O, Dickenson D, Parsons J, et al. Residual and recurrent shunts after implantation of Cook detachable coil. *Heart* 1998;79:220–222.

49. Bilkis AA, Alwi M, Hasri S, et al. The Amplatzer Duct Occluder: experience in 209 patients. *J Am Coll Cardiol* 2001;37:258–261.

50. Sandhu SK, King TD, Troutman WB, et al. Transcatheter closure of patent ductus arteriosus with the Amplatzer Duct Occluder: short-term follow-up. *J Invasive Cardiol* 2001;13:298–302.

51. Waight DJ, Cao Q, Hijazi ZM. Transcatheter closure of patent ductus arteriosus using the Amplatzer Duct Occluder. *Curr Interv Cardiol Rep* 2001;3:263–267.

52. Rao PS, Kim SH, Rey C, et al. Results of transvenous buttoned device occlusion of patent ductus arteriosus in adults. *Am J Cardiol* 1998;15:827–829.

53. Gianturco C, Anderson JH, Wallace S. Mechanical device for arterial occlusion. *Am J Roentgenol* 1975;124:428–435.

54. Rao PS. Coil occlusion of patent ductus arteriosus (editorial). *J Invasive Cardiol* 2001;13:36–38.

55. Rao PS. Transcatheter closure of moderate-to-large patent ductus arteriosus. *J Invasive Cardiol* 2001;13:303–306.

56. Hijazi ZM, Geggel RL. Results of antegrade transcatheter closure of patent ductus arteriosus using single or multiple Gianturco coils. *Am J Cardiol* 1994;74:925–929.

57. Hijazi AM, Lloyd TR, Beekman RH, Geggel RL. Transcatheter closure with single or multiple Gianturco coils of patent ductus arteriosus in infants weighing ≤8 kg: retrograde versus anterograde approach. *Am Heart J* 1996;132:828–835.

58. Grifka RG, Jones TK. Transcatheter closure of large PDA using 0.052-inch Gianturco coils: controlled delivery using a bioptome catheter through a 4 French sheath. *Catheter Cardiovasc Interv* 2000;49:301–306.

59. Rao PS, Sideris EB. Transcatheter closure of patent ductus arteriosus: state of the art. *J Invasive Cardiol* 1996;8:278–288.

60. Rao PS. Transcatheter occlusion of patent ductus arteriosus: which method to use and which ductus to close? (Editorial). *Am Heart J* 1996;132:905–909.

61. Krichenko A, Benson LN, Burrows P, et al. Angiographic classification of the isolated persistently patent ductus arteriosus and implications for percutaneous transcatheter closure. *Am J Cardiol* 1989;63:877–880.

62. Huston AB, Gnanapraksam JD, Lim MK, et al. Doppler ultrasound and the silent ductus. *Br Heart J* 1991;65:97–99.

63. Balzer DT, Spray TL, McMullin D, et al. Endocarditis associated with a clinically silent patent ductus arteriosus. *Am Heart J* 1993;125:1192–1193.

64. Moore JW, George L, Kirkpatrick SE, et al. Percutaneous closure of the small patent ductus arteriosus using occluding spring coils. *J Am Coll Cardiol* 1994;23:759–765.

65. Lloyd TR, Beekman RH, III. Clinically silent patent ductus arteriosus (Letter). *Am Heart J* 1994;127:1664.

66. Latson LA, McManus BM, Doer C, et al. Endocarditis risk of the USCI PDA umbrella for transcatheter closure of patent ductus arteriosus. *Circulation* 1994;90:2525–2528.

67. Rao PS, Balfour IC, Jureidini SG, et al. Five-loop coil occlusion of patent ductus arteriosus produces no recurrent of shunt at follow-up. *Catheter Cardiovasc Interv* 2000;50:202–206.

68. Sommer RJ, Gutierrez A, Lai WW, et al. Use of preformed Nitinol snare to improve transcatheter coil delivery in occlusion of patent ductus arteriosus. *Am J Cardiol* 1994;74:836–839.

69. Hayes MD, Hoyer NH, Glasgow PF. New forceps delivery technique for coil occlusion of patent ductus arteriosus. *Am J Cardiol* 1997;209–211.

70. Ozun O, Hancock S, Parsons JM, et al. Transcatheter occlusion of the arterial duct with Cook detachable coils: early experience. *Heart* 1996;176:269–273.

71. Berdjis F, Moore JW. Balloon occlusion delivery technique for closure of patent ductus arteriosus. *Am Heart J* 1997;133:601–604.

72. Dalvi B, Goyal V, Narula D, et al. A new technique using temporary balloon occlusion for transcatheter closure of patent ductus arteriosus with Gianturco coils. *Catheter Cardiovasc Diagn* 1997;41:51–62.

73. Prieto LR, Latson LA, Dalvi B, et al. Transcatheter coil embolization of abnormal vascular connections using a new type of delivery catheter for enhanced control. *Am J Cardiol* 1999;83:981–983.

74. Rao PS. Summary and comparison of patent ductus arteriosus closure devices. *Curr Interv Cardiol Rep* 2001;3:268–274.

75. Mavroudis C, Becker CL, Gewitz M. Forty-six years of patent ductus arteriosus division at Children's Memorial Hospital of Chicago: standards for comparison. *Ann Surg* 1994;220:402–410.

76. Laborde F, Noihomme P, Karam J, et al. A new video-assisted thoracoscopic surgical technique for interruption of patent duc-

tus arteriosus in infants and children. *J Thorac Cardiovasc Surg* 1993;105:278–280.

77. Gray DT, Walker AM, Fyler DC, et al. Examination of the early "learning curve" for transcatheter closure of patent ductus arteriosus using Rashkind occluder. *Circulation* 1994;90:11-36–II-42.

78. Verin VE, Saveliev SV, Kolody SM, et al. Results of transcatheter closure of patent ductus arteriosus with the Botallooccluder. *J Am Coll Cardiol* 1993;22:1509–1514.

79. Schräder R, Hofstetter R, Fabbender D, et al. Transvenous closure of patent ductus arteriosus with Ivalon plugs: multicenter experience with a new technique. *Invest Radiol* 1999;34:65–70.

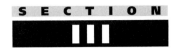

SECTION

III

DEVICE OCCLUSION OF VENTRICULAR SEPTAL DEFECTS AND PARAVALVAR REGURGITATION

26

RASHKIND AND CLAMSHELL DEVICES

T. H. GOH

The double-umbrella device invented by Rashkind (father of pediatric interventional cardiology) in its various sizes and modifications has proven to be the first interventional device versatile enough for closing intracardiac and extracardiac defects. The original 12- and 17-mm devices were initially used by Rashkind and his colleagues (1) to close patent ductus arteriosus (PDA). This heralded the era of pediatric transcatheter device closures, which was further expanded upon by Lock, who used the device for closing various extracardiac lesions (2). Lock modified Rashkind's atrial septal device, forming the clamshell device to close atrial and ventricular septal defects (VSD) (3,4). Lock and his associates then went on to amass the largest experience on transcatheter VSD closures worldwide. Redington, Rigby, and their colleagues confirmed the usefulness of the Rashkind device for closing various extracardiac lesions and perimembranous ventricular septal defects (5,6). We adopted these techniques to occlude PDAs and VSDs. We and others were eagerly awaiting the commercial availability of the clamshell device and were disappointed when it was withdrawn from clinical use because of the reported high frequency of device arm fractures after ASD closures (7). The clamshell device therefore did not leave the shores of the United States. Hence the international community only had the Rashkind device for use. This review will focus on the use of the Rashkind device for VSD closures worldwide and the experience of Rashkind and clamshell device closures in the United States.

Centers involved were Boston (United States), London (UK), New Delhi (India), and Melbourne (Australia). Data available were those published in the literature and, wherever possible, through personal communications.

RASHKIND DEVICE

The Rashkind double-umbrella device consists of two circular polyurethane foam umbrellas. The 12-mm device has

a three-arm spring assembly in each umbrella, and the 17-mm device has four supporting arms. Each device has a prosthetic ring for attachment to the delivery system (Figures 26.1 and 26.2). The 12-mm device requires an 8F delivery sheath, and the 17-mm device requires an 11F sheath, noting that sheath sizes could be reduced to 6, 8, and 9F using the front-loading strip-down technique (8).

LOCK CLAMSHELL DEVICE

The Lock clamshell device consists of two square Dacron-covered umbrellas, each with four steel arms, hinged at the center and with springs in the mid-portion. This allows bet-

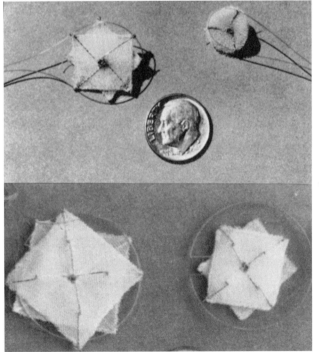

FIGURE 26.1. A: Photograph of Rashkind Device, 12 mm and 17 mm. **B:** Photograph of clamshell device, 28 mm and 40 mm.

T. H. Goh: Deputy Director of Cardiology, Royal Children's Hospital, Melbourne, Victoria, Australia

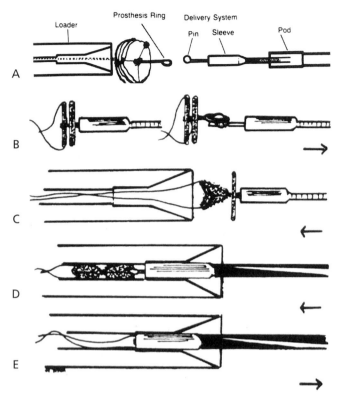

FIGURE 26.2. Attachment and loading sequence for Rashkind/clamshell device. **A:** Prosthetic ring is placed over pin knuckle and withdrawn and locked inside the sleeve. **B:** Traction by Prolene suture on distal umbrella collapses the arms forward into the loader. **C:** Further traction collapses the proximal umbrella arms backward over the sleeve in the loader. **D:** The pod is gently directed into the loader and the collapsed device pulled into the pod. **E:** After removal of Prolene suture, the device is now ready for delivery into the long sheath.

ter opposition of the open umbrellas to one another. The device comes in sizes of 17, 23, 28, 33, and 40 mm and requires 11F long sheath for delivery (Figures 26.1 and 26.2).

DEVICE SIZE SELECTION

The device size selected for use should be at least two times the measured VSD size, by angiography. Balloon sizing may not be necessary because of muscular reins of the defect.

CATHETER DELIVERY SYSTEM

The delivery catheter system has a central pin knuckle wire, which secures the prosthetic ring by drawing it into a small sleeve. This is attached to a second, larger "advance" wire and the delivery pod, inside which the collapsed device sits (Figure 26.2).

TECHNIQUE OF IMPLANTATION

The precise site, size, and location of each VSD are documented on transthoracic echocardiography and confirmed on transesophageal echocardiography and cineangiography. All patients undergo general anesthesia and full heparinization with antibiotic cover. The techniques for transcatheter closure of VSDs and transesophageal echocardiographic guidance have been well described (3,5,6). This article will describe certain modifications and innovations of the original techniques.

Technique 1

The right Judkins coronary catheter, cobra catheter, or balloon wedge catheter is advanced from the femoral vein into the right atrium across the atrial septum [through either a patent foramen ovale (PFO) or atrial septal puncture] into the left atrium, passing through the mitral valve and into the left ventricle. The "Glide" flow-directed double-length soft guide wire is then negotiated through the VSD, and wire and catheter are advanced into the right ventricle, right atrium, or pulmonary artery. The wire is then captured with a snare wire passed from the right internal jugular vein or from the opposite femoral vein and drawn out externally. The guide wire is thus positioned across the defect with either end of the guide wire outside the body. One end of this guide wire will contain the original catheter passed through the VSD to the right ventricle. Balloon sizing of the VSD is then undertaken. The appropriate-sized long sheath (made of nonkinkable material) is shaped in proportion to the size of the heart and the position of the VSD. The long sheath is then introduced either from the internal jugular for mid-muscular and apical VSDs or from the femoral vein for anterior muscular and high muscular VSDs. It is then advanced via the wire into the right ventricle, through the VSD, and into the left ventricle against the retreating opposing catheter from the other wire end. The procedure is usually a painstakingly slow and time-consuming process. Particular attention must be given to ensure that hemodynamic stability is maintained.

Technique 2

Technique 2 is similar to Technique 1 except that the catheter is passed retrogradely from the aorta into the left ventricle and manipulated with the help of the "Glide" wire across the VSD and subsequently snared.

Technique 3

For perimembranous VSDs, the venous catheter is introduced from the right ventricle through the VSD into the left ventricle or ascending aorta. The long sheath is also advanced through the VSD into the left ventricle or into the ascending aorta. For difficult anterior muscular VSDs, this technique is useful when the VSD is approached from the right outflow tract (3).

Technique 4

With Technique 4 the catheter is passed into the pulmonary artery as in Technique 1 but it is not snared. The catheter is then replaced by a long sheath through which a balloon wedge catheter is floated on the guide wire into the main pulmonary artery and subsequently wedged. The long sheath is then advanced on the balloon wedge catheter, which acts as a flexible introducer catheter, into the right ventricle, and, if necessary, the main pulmonary artery. This is the only technique where the device is deployed from the right ventricle.

General Comments on Transcatheter Crossing of the VSD

At all times, the soft guide wire should be covered by a catheter when across the VSD (Chuck Mullin's personal communication). This minimizes wire traction injury on the heart during catheter and wire manipulation.

During the advancing of the sheath into the heart (and including subsequent device advancing in the sheath), it is vital to prevent kinking of the sheath, as this halts further progress and necessitates backtracking to the start of catheter technique again. Prior balloon dilation of the VSD with a 4- or 5-mm balloon is one method to ease sheath passage through the VSD. Another tip is to float a second, smaller long guide wire through the VSD with either end outside the body. This is alongside the existing sheath so that if sheath kinking does occur, it is easy to retrieve the situation with the second wire. Close echocardiographic and fluoroscopic monitoring is essential throughout the whole procedure.

Device Deployment

After appropriate positioning of the sheath, the wire and introducer catheter are removed. The delivery catheter containing the collapsed device in the pod is positioned in the proximal end of the long sheath. The device is then pushed out of the pod into the long sheath by the sleeve advance wire. The advance to the distal end of the sheath can be a difficult and prolonged procedure because of the tight fit. Arrested advance is usually due to a kinked sheath necessitating the replacement of the sheath (i.e., repeating the procedure again).

Once the device is positioned at the distal end of the sheath, the sheath is retracted until the distal umbrellas open, with care being taken to ensure that the surrounding myocardium and AV valve apparatus are not interfered with. The whole system (i.e., delivery catheter, umbrella, and sheath) is then pulled back against the septum as one unit until the distal umbrella arms evert against the distal side of the VSD. Then, without moving the device, the sheath is retracted further until the proximal umbrella legs spring open on the proximal side of the defect. Again close scrutiny with fluoroscopy and echocardiography is maintained to ensure there is no interference with the tricuspid valve apparatus (9–11). At this point, angiography may be performed; however, more reliance is placed on echocardiography. The device can still be retrieved if the position is suboptimal, but once it is suitably placed, it is released by pushing the pin wire knuckle out of the sleeve, freeing the prosthesis ring from the pin wire.

For perimembranous VSD deployment (6) (i.e., Technique 3), the distal umbrella arms are initially deployed either in the left ventricle or in the ascending aorta and then pulled back into the VSD, followed by deployment of the proximal umbrella. Monitoring for aortic or tricuspid incompetence is essential.

RESULTS

Boston Pace-Setter Experience

Lock pioneered the technique for the Rashkind device closure of ventricular septal defects (3). From January 1987 to October 1987, he and his colleagues implanted Rashkind devices in six patients successfully. Three patients were adults post infarction VSD who died despite successful implants. A residual postsurgical iatrogenic VSD in an infant, an adult with a perimembranous VSD, and a 7-year-old with a mid-muscular VSD had successful Rashkind implants. They were subsequently spurred to the challenge of muscular VSD closures, given the technically difficult surgery.

From July 1989 to July 1990, Bridges et al. (9) reported the successful use of the clamshell device for 21 patients with complicated muscular VSDs. In all, 21 defects were closed. Fluoroscopy time was quoted at a range of 38 to 153 minutes, with a median of 104 minutes. Blood transfusion was required in 11 out of 21 patients.

The momentum continued to build, and from July 1987 to April 1993, Nykanen et al. (12) reported the implantation of 134 devices in 80 patients aged 1 month to 45 years with a median of 5.2 years and a weight range of 3.8 to 89 kg. One hundred and seventeen clamshell and 17 Rashkind devices were used on three groups: patients with single or multiple VSDs closed as a primary or preoperative procedure, patients with Swiss cheese VSDs closed with multiple devices, and patients with postoperative single or multiple residual defects. No mortality, emergent surgery, or serious permanent arrhythmias were reported. His results showed that patients are likely to have a successful outcome with preoperative closures. It was possible to close Swiss cheese VSDs with this technique. Postoperative residual defects may benefit from device implantation but usually with higher morbidity and mortality.

Laussen et al. (13) reported on the hemodynamic instability and anesthetic management of transcatheter closure of VSDs in the same institution. From February 1989 to September 1992, 70 VSD procedures were performed on 55 patients with insertion of 86 devices. He reported a total procedure time averaging 305 minutes, ranging from 127 to 580 minutes. Blood transfusion was necessary in 54% of patients. This was size related, with patients who weighed less than 10 kg requiring significantly larger transfusion volume. Hypotension was a complication in 40% of cases, arrhythmias occurred in 26%, and intensive care facilities were needed in more than 50% of cases after the procedure because of hemodynamic instability, procedure duration, or concerns about stability of device position. He concluded that hemodynamic instability is common during device closures and is likely to be an inescapable feature of this procedure in many patients because of the technique necessary for device placement.

In a later report Rocchini and Lock (14) reported on 148 VSD catheter closures from February 1989 to July 1998 with no deaths or late morbidity. This report likely includes the accumulated experience in the institution. Of the VSDs, 83% were deemed closed by echocardiographic evaluation with only minor leakage. The devices used were presumably a mixture of Rashkind, clamshell, and CardioSEAL.

Landzberg (15) reported on postinfarction VSDs in adults with better outcomes in the group that survived surgery and subsequently had device implantation (nine out of 11) than in those who had primary device implantation (three out of seven) with either clamshell or CardioSEAL devices.

Thus far, there have been no reports of clamshell arm fractures in the VSD closure group.

London Experience

Across the Atlantic, Redington and Rigby at Brompton Hospital, London, used the modified Rashkind PDA device by placing a gentle bend on each arm of the devices and used these for closure of ASDs, fenestrated Fontans and aortopulmonary collaterals (5,6,16). In a 3-year-old with "corrected TGA" with a residual VSD, they were able to implant three 17-mm devices on separate occasions to occlude the residual defect. An adult with perimembranous VSD and an infant with residual perimembranous VSD had successful device implantation.

After these successes, they proceeded to do a prospective trial of primary device closure in patients with large symp-

tomatic perimembranous VSD with QP:QS ratio in excess of 3:1, right ventricular pressure greater than 45% of the left ventricle, and VSD size less than 8.5 mm. Commencing in October 1990 (17), 13 patients entered this trial: six infants, five patients 1 to 5 years old, and the remaining two beyond 10 years old. Weight ranged from 1.8 to 46 kg and procedure time ranged from 75 to 220 minutes, with a mean of 122 minutes. Fluoroscopy time ranged from 15 to 46 minutes, with a mean of 32 minutes. Three patients were excluded with VSDs that were too large. The technique was especially difficult in infants. Complications encountered were device embolization to the pulmonary artery and to the aorta in two patients, hemolysis in two patients, and faulty placement requiring surgery in one patient. Of the ten successful implants, there was hemodynamic improvement with a residual shunt in five patients.

An infant with significant residual shunt developed aortic regurgitation 6 months later, and a number of smaller infants had complete heart block, one dying from asystole after surgical repair of VSD. Further follow-up was undertaken from September 1991 to 1994 of 17 patients from the same institution (18). Two patients required surgery, one for malposition of the device and the other for severe aortic regurgitation secondary to aortic valve perforation by the device arm (18). Six patients developed right bundle branch block with small residual shunts. This group recommended that Rashkind devices not be used for routine closure of large symptomatic perimembranous VSDs in infancy and early childhood.

Indian Experience

Karla et al. in New Delhi from April 1995 to April 1998 (19) used the Rashkind device for closure of VSDs in 30 patients, 28 being perimembranous VSDs and two muscular VSDs. Age ranged from 5.5 to 33 years, with a mean of 12.9 years, and VSDs measured between 3 and 8 mm. QP:QS ratio was from 2 to 2.6:1, and VSDs were separated from the aortic valve by at least 6 to 8 mm of septal tissue. Two patients had left-ventricle-to-right-atrial communication, and all patients were in no cardiac failure. Twenty-six patients (87%) had successful implantation of the Rashkind device, with three patients requiring a repeat procedure with the larger device. Small residual leaks were present in eight patients (30%). No residual aortic regurgitation or tricuspid regurgitation was noted, and the two patients with left-ventricular-to-right-atrial shunts had good outcomes. Procedure time was not mentioned. In this older age group with smaller perimembranous VSD, Rashkind device closure was successful in the vast majority with no untoward complications. Their conclusion was that the Rashkind device closure is an effective and safe procedure in selective cases of perimembranous VSDs, especially in the older patients.

Australian Experience

We at The Royal Children's Hospital in Melbourne implanted Rashkind devices for closure of PDA (20). Subsequently, between May 1995 and February 1997 (21), 16 children were enrolled for attempted transcatheter umbrella closure of muscular VSDs. Ages ranged from 0.1 to 4 years, with a median of 2 years, and weight ranged from 4.1 to 19 kg, with a median of 11 kg. Procedure time ranged from 120 to 300 minutes, with a mean of 200 minutes. Fluoroscopy time ranged from 51 to 205 minutes, with a median time of 110 minutes. Patients were divided into three groups.

The first group consisted of two patients who had primary transcatheter closure of VSDs; a 5-year-old girl with a mid-muscular and apical VSD (Figure 26.3), and a 4-month-old infant post coarctation repair with a single mid-muscular defect closed using Technique 4.

The second group consisted of nine preoperative patients where the muscular VSDs were closed to assist subsequent surgery. The majority had previous pulmonary artery (PA) banding; others had muscular VSDs associated with tetralogy of Fallot and perimembranous VSD requiring surgery.

The third group consisted of five postoperative patients with residual defects. One had a Swiss cheese septum. She had a preoperative apical device implant and remained symptomatic after subsequent cardiac surgery including left ventriculotomy. She underwent two further procedures in which a total of five devices were implanted with resolution of heart failure (Figure 26.4). A Down's infant with multiple VSDs and previous PA band had an apical VSD device and then went to surgery for closure of a perimembranous

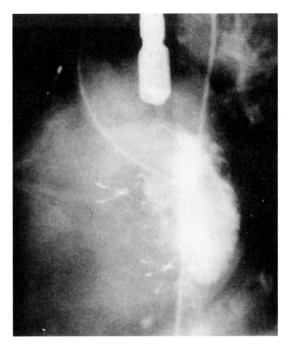

FIGURE 26.4. Selected frame of a left ventricular cineangiogram and left anterior oblique projection showing the apical and mid-muscular devices (splayed).

VSD and debanding. This unmasked a previously insignificant mid-muscular VSD. The child remained ventilator dependent. He was extubated after device closure of the mid-muscular VSD (Figure 26.5). The third patient was post arterial switch with multiple VSDs and heart failure. An apical device was implanted with good outcome. The fourth patient was a 4.5-kg infant (in our initial early experience) who had undergone recent repair of cor triatriatum,

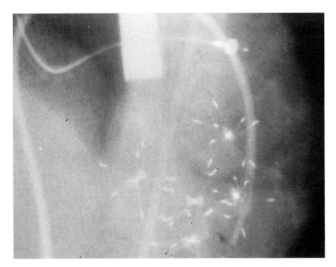

FIGURE 26.3. Selected frame of left ventricular cineangiogram in left anterior oblique projection demonstrating five devices in the anterior, apical, and mid-muscular septum.

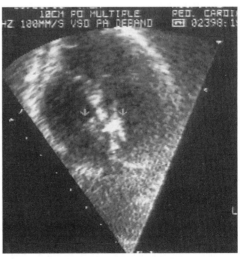

FIGURE 26.5. Subcostal transthoracic echocardiographic view demonstrating appropriate position of the Rashkind device across a mid-muscular ventricular septal defect.

and pulmonary artery banding with a mid-muscular VSD. A decision was made to close the VSD because of persisting symptoms. During the procedure, hemodynamic instability was noted by the splinting of the heart by the inadvertent use of the stiff guide wire. This resulted in cardiac arrest, and although successfully resuscitated, brain damage was evident. Elective termination of therapy occurred a few days later. The last patient had tetralogy of Fallot with criss-cross, Swiss cheese septum having undergone two open-heart procedures. He was hemodynamically unstable and brittle. During catheter intervention he suffered a cardiac arrest and was successfully resuscitated but developed brain damage and subsequently succumbed from pneumonia 4 months later.

VSD location was apical in 14 patients, mid-muscular in eight patients, and anterior muscular in three patients. Of the 25 attempted closures, 22 devices were placed successfully, nine patients received a single device, four received two devices, and one received five devices. The Melbourne experience agrees with the larger Boston experience that transcatheter closure of muscular VSDs is a technically demanding lengthy procedure with significant hemodynamic instability during catheter and device deployment.

Other Experience

In 1989 O'Laughlin and Mullins in Houston (22) implanted a Rashkind 17-mm device to close a residual VSD in a post Fontan patient. They have had other experiences with muscular VSDs, but the information is currently not available (personal communication).

INTRAOPERATIVE DEVICE CLOSURE OF MUSCULAR VSDS

The cardiac surgeons in Boston together with the cardiologists took the lead in using the Rashkind and clamshell devices intraoperatively, having seen the good results from transcatheter VSD closure in the laboratory (23). Ten patients with multiple complex abnormalities, including Swiss cheese defects, were chosen. Nine umbrella devices were implanted in nine patients, and there were five survivors in this technically difficult group.

Across the Atlantic at the Brompton Hospital (24), from January 1993 to May 1995, intraoperative apical ventricular septal defect closure was done in four patients successfully, one device per patient. There was one early death unrelated to VSD closure. Then in Italy, Murzi and colleagues (25) performed intraoperative closure of mid-muscular VSDs in three patients and apical VSDs in two patients. One patient required two devices, and there was one late death from intractable right heart failure. Four patients survived, most with a small residual leak. The sur-

geons have therefore demonstrated the feasibility of intraoperative device implantation with a reasonably good outcome.

DISCUSSION

VSD closure with the umbrella devices is the most demanding of all intracardiac interventions. The procedure is time-consuming, with high instances of hemodynamic instability due to catheter, long sheath, and wire manipulation. The Boston team has spearheaded the development of the techniques and has shown the feasibility of closure of muscular VSDs, postoperative residual VSDs, postinfarction VSDs, and perimembranous VSDs. The London experience centered on symptomatic perimembranous VSDs in infants and young children and these showed a high incidence of residual shunts, embolization, intravascular hemolysis, aortic and tricuspid valve regurgitation, complete heart block, and cardiac arrhythmias, especially in the infant group. The Indian experience showed better results in older patients with smaller perimembranous VSDs. The Australian experience agrees with the larger Boston experience regarding the complexity of the procedure (in the muscular VSDs) with long catheter time together with a high incidence of hemodynamic instability. The procedure can be therapeutic and aid in the overall surgical management of complicated VSDs. The combined worldwide experience has consolidated and fine-tuned the techniques for VSD crossing, long sheath placement, and device deployment. A dedicated interventional VSD team has grown together with experience gained.

CURRENT STATUS

The Rashkind device, although not ideal, has stood the test of time and is the forerunner for the "ideal" VSD device to come. Currently, the Rashkind and clamshell devices are no longer available for clinical use.

CONCLUSION

The late Dr. William Rashkind demonstrated a visionary approach to interventional cardiology when he invented the device that bears his name. The introduction of the Rashkind device for clinical use has been foundational for interventional device closure of intracardiac and extracardiac defects. The experience gained has provided the first crucial steps for further innovations. Lock and his Boston team have extended the frontiers into the "innermost sanctum" of the heart. Lock and his team are to be congratulated for setting the pace for transcatheter VSD closure and for passing the baton to the rest of the pediatric cardiology fraternity.

REFERENCES

1. Rashkind WJ, Mullins CE, Hellenbrand HE, et al. Nonsurgical closure of patent ductus arteriosus: clinical application of the Rashkind PDA occluder system. *Circulation* 1987;75: 583–592.
2. Lock JE, Cockerham JT, Keane JF, et al. Transcatheter umbrella closure of congenital heart defects. *Circulation* 1987;75:593–599.
3. Lock JE, Block PC, McKay RG, et al. Transcatheter closure of ventricular septal defects. *Circulation* 1988;78:361–368.
4. Rome JJ, Keane JF, Perry SB, et al. Double-umbrella closure of atrial septal defects, initial clinical applications. *Circulation* 1990; 82:751–758.
5. Redington AN, Rigby ML. Novel uses of the Rashkind ductal umbrella in adults and children with congenital heart disease. *Br Heart J* 1993;69:47–51.
6. Rigby ML, Redington AN. Primary transcatheter umbrella closure of perimembranous ventricular septal defect. *Br Heart J* 1994;72:368–371.
7. Prieto LR, Foreman CK, Cheatham JP, et al. Intermediate-term outcome of transcatheter secundum atrial septal defect closure using the bard clamshell septal umbrella. *Am J Cardiol* 1996;78: 1310–1312.
8. Perry SB, Lock JE. Front-loading of double-umbrella devices, a new technique for umbrella delivery for closing cardiovascular defects. *Am J Cardiol* 1992;70:917–920.
9. Bridges ND, Perry SB, Keane JE, et al. Preoperative transcatheter closure of congenital muscular ventricular septal defects. *N Engl J Med* 1991;324:1312–1317.
10. Vandervelde ME, Sanders S, Keane JF, et al. Transesophageal echocardiography guidance of transcatheter VSD closure. *J Am Coll Cardiol* 1994;8:721–730.
11. Rocchini A, Lock JE. Defect closure: umbrella devices. In: Lock JE, Keane JF, Perry SB, eds. *Diagnostic and interventional catheterization in congenital heart disease,* 2nd ed. Kluwer Academic Publishers 2000: Boston, Massachusetts, 192–193.
12. Nykanen DG, Perry SB, Keane JF, et al. Transcatheter occlusion of ventricular septal defects: experience in 80 patients with congenital heart disease. *Circulation* 1993;88:I-532.
13. Laussen PC, Hansen DD, Perry SP, et al. Transcatheter closure of ventricular septal defects: hemodynamic instability and anesthetic management (cardiovascular anesthesia). *Anesth Analg* 1995;80:1076–1082.
14. Rocchini A, Lock JE. Defect closure: umbrella devices. In: Lock JE, Keane JF, Perry SB, eds. *Diagnostic and interventional catheterization in congenital heart disease,* 2nd ed. Kluwer Academic Publishers 2000:194.
15. Landzberg M. Catheterization of the adult patient with congenital heart disease. In: Lock JE, Keane JF, Perry SB, eds. *Diagnostic and interventional catheterization in congenital heart disease,* 2nd ed. Kluwer Academic Publishers 2000:276–278.
16. Redington A, Rigby ML. Transcatheter closure of inter-atrial communications with a modified umbrella device. *Br Heart J* 1994;72:372–377.
17. Rigby ML, Heinsdijk M, Redington AN, et al. Medium term follow-up after transcatheter umbrella closure of perimembranous ventricular septal defect (VSD). *J Am Coll Cardiol* 1996; 119A.
18. Vogel M, Rigby ML, Shore D. Perforation of the right aortic valve cusp: complication of ventricular septal defect closure with a modified Rashkind umbrella. *Pediatr Cardiol* 1996;17:416–418.
19. Kalra GS, Verma PK, Dhall A, et al. transcatheter device closure of ventricular septal defects: immediate results and intermediate-term follow-up. *Am Heart J* 1999;138:339–344.
20. Janorkar S, Goh T, Wilkinson J. Transcatheter closure of patent ductus arteriosus with the use of Rashkind occluders and/or Gianturco coils: long-term follow-up in 123 patients and special reference to comparison, residual shunts, complications and techniques. *Am Heart J* 1999;138:1176–1183.
21. Janorkar S, Goh T, Wilkinson J. Transcatheter closure of ventricular septal defects using the Rashkind device: initial experience. *Catheter Cardiovasc Interv* 1999;46:43–48.
22. O'Laughlin MP, Mullins CE. Transcatheter occlusion of ventricular septal defect. *Catheter Cardiovasc Diagn* 1989;17:175–179.
23. Fishberger SB, Bridges ND, Keane JF, et al. Intraoperative device closure of ventricular septal defects. *Circulation* 1993;88: 205–209.
24. Chaturvedi RR, Shore DF, Yacoub M, et al. Intraoperative apical ventricular septal defect closure using a modified Rashkind double umbrella. *Heart* 1996;76:367–369.
25. Murzi B, Bonanomi GL, Giusti S, et al. Surgical closure of muscular ventricular septal defects using double umbrella devices (intraoperative VSD device closure). *Eur J Cardiothorac Surg* 1997;12:450–454.

Catheter Based Devices: For the Treatment of Non-coronary Cardiovascular Diseases in Adults and Children. Edited by P. Syamasundar Rao and Morton J. Kern, Lippincott Williams & Wilkins, Philadelphia © 2003.

27

BUTTONED AND OTHER DEVICES

ELEFTHERIOS B. SIDERIS

Transcatheter ventricular septal defect (VSD) occlusion is by far the most challenging heart defect occlusion. The reasons are both anatomic and technical. Most ventricular septal defects are perimembranous, in close proximity to critical structures such as the aortic valve and the tricuspid valve (1); most of these defects have deficient rim for disk device placement. Muscular VSDs are the ones traditionally considered to be good candidates for transcatheter occlusion (2). They usually have enough supportive tissue (rim) for disk device placement. They are also considered high risk for surgery, since they cannot always be approached from the tricuspid valve and require ventriculotomy (3).

There are also significant technical limitations, which include the following:

1. *Crossing the defect.* The easiest approach to cross a VSD is the transarterial approach. The size and location of the defect are the most important factors. Defects smaller than 3 mm and supracristal defects are the most difficult to cross. Large mid-muscular defects can be frequently crossed directly transvenously, from the right jugular vein.
2. *Establish an arteriovenous wire connection.* After crossing the defect a soft wire is be advanced into the pulmonary artery and snared to the most appropriate vein (femoral for outflow defects, right jugular for mid-muscular ones).
3. *Selection of the proper device.* Disk devices (4,5) are appropriate for most muscular VSDs; they certainly have an advantage with multiple defects, because of significant overlapping. In contrast, disk devices are applicable in only a small percentage of membranous VSDs (5) because of the close proximity to critical structures. Careful measurements are required to select the appropriate disk device size. The development of wireless devices (transcatheter patch and detachable balloon) that require minimal rim and do not interfere with crit-

ical structures (6,7) may revolutionize the transcatheter treatment of perimembranous VSDs.

4. *Difficulty delivering the device.* Most devices are delivered through long delivery sheaths. A straight rather an angulated route is preferable to avoid kinking of the sheath. Apical muscular VSDs are rather notorious in this aspect. Over-the-wire placement of the device and kink-resistant sheaths may be helpful in difficult VSD locations.

THE DEVICES

Since 1994 we have used the following devices for the occlusion of VSDs:

1. The buttoned device
2. The self-adjustable device
3. Wireless devices (detachable balloons and transcatheter patches)

Buttoned Device

The buttoned device is the same device as that was initially used for the occlusion of atrial septal defects (8). The current device is a fourth-generation device without centering, since VSDs are relatively small. The device has been described extensively elsewhere (9). In brief, it consists of an occluder with the button loop, a counteroccluder, and a loading or release wire. It can be placed directly through a long sheath or over a wire. Over-the-wire placement is quite attractive since loss of the arteriovenous connection in case of device misplacement or retrieval is minimized. The occluder is placed on the left ventricular side. The button loop adjusts for the septal thickness, and the counteroccluder is buttoned with the occluder from the right ventricle.

The Self-Adjustable Device

The self-adjustable device consists of two disks (proximal and distal) connected by a latex thread (10). It can therefore self-adjust according to the septal thickness (Figure 27.1).

Eleftherios B. Sideris: Director, Athenian Institute of Pediatric Cardiology and Custom Medical Devices, Athens, Greece

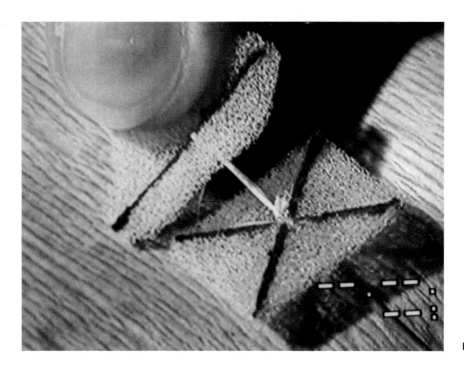

FIGURE 27.1. The self-adjustable device.

The disks are made by polyurethane foam and stainless steel skeleton wire. There are two-wire and one-wire disks in different combinations as follows:

1. Regular self-adjustable device, with a two-wire distal disk and a one-wire proximal disk.
2. Inverted self-adjustable device, with a single-wire distal disk and a two-wire proximal disk. This is the device most commonly used for transarterial VSD occlusion.
3. Two-disk device; both the proximal and the distal disks are made with two wires.
4. One-wire device; both the proximal and the distal disks are made with a single wire.

Wireless Devices

Two types of wireless occluders have been used in the occlusion of VSDs: detachable balloons and transcatheter patches (6,7). These devices have been described extensively in chapter 9.

In brief, the detachable balloon device consists of a detachable balloon occluder connected with a floppy disk. The detachable balloon occludes the defect from the left ventricle, and the floppy disk(s) supports the balloon from the right ventricle. The transcatheter patch is made with polyurethane foam in the form of a sleeve over a balloon. It is retrievable, retractable, and radiopaque. It is delivered and supported by a double balloon for 48 hours. It is totally wireless.

Both detachable balloons and transcatheter patches require minimal rim and are always centered. However, the detachable balloon method is an outpatient procedure, whereas the transcatheter patch application requires 48 hours of hospitalization.

PATIENT SELECTION

Indication for VSD occlusion is the presence of a significant shunt with or without evidence of pulmonary hypertension. Exceptions for occlusion include irreversible pulmonary hypertension with right-to left-shunt (pulmonary vasclar resistance [PVR] > 10 units) and anatomy preventing the application of the device (lack of sufficient rim).

Calculation of adequate rim and examples are given in the included diagram. The same rim requirements exist for both disk devices. The wireless devices require a minimal rim. Balloon test occlusion should be performed before a wireless device application (transcatheter patch). Providing that it results in full occlusion without impairment of critical structures, patch deployment should follow.

Ventricular septal defects of all types can be occluded, provided there is adequate rim for the deployment of the device. Baseline history, physical examination, electrocardiogram, echocardiogram, and chest x-ray should be obtained for screening purposes.

Exclusion Criteria

The following are reasons for excluding a patient:

1. Defects with severe pulmonary hypertension associated with significant right-to-left shunts (PVR > 10 units).
2. Defects without adequate rim for device deployment.

3. Patients too small for a possible retrieval of the device into an 11F sheath (10 kg) for disk devices or 9 to 10F for the transcatheter patch. Surgical retrieval should be performed in patients where the appropriate sheath for the retrieval cannot be introduced.

METHOD OF IMPLANTATION

Device Selection

The disk devices selected should have at least twice the size of the diameter of the VSD [similar to atrial septal defect (ASD) selection]. Caution should be used in selecting the proper device to avoid encroachment on the aortic valve leaflet. A long axial angiographic view should be obtained, and the distance between the center of the defect and the right aortic cusp (DA distance) should be measured as well as the diameter of the defect. The diameter of the required device should be less than double that of the DA distance and should be at least 2 mm away from the right aortic cusp. The minimal subaortic rim for the smaller available device (15 mm) is calculated therefore at 9.5 mm.

The transcatheter balloon/patch diameter should be selected as 2 mm larger than the test-occluding diameter (Figures 27.2 and 27.3).

The Procedure

The device implantation is performed in the cardiac catheterization laboratory. The patient is premedicated with a sedative mixture. Sedation is supplemented by Ketamine infusion. General anesthesia is reserved for the cases requir-

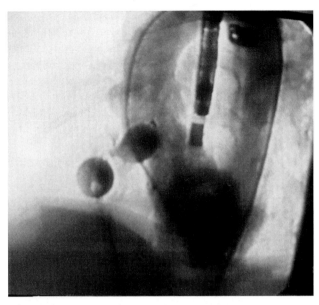

FIGURE 27.3. Transcatheter patch occlusion supported by a double balloon 14 mm in diameter.

ing transesophageal echocardiography or where simple sedation is considered inadequate. The procedure should be performed using sterile technique. After obtaining routine pressure and oxygen saturation data to confirm the diagnosis of VSD, angiography is performed, including long axial left ventricular angiogram. The location of the defect is noted and the size is measured digitally.

In addition to the size, the DA distance is measured and the appropriate disk device is selected. If the distance is too small for a disk device, use of a wireless device is entertained. Heparinization is started (100 U/kg).

The next step is crossing the VSD by a catheter. Crossing from the right side is preferable but not always possible. Therefore in most cases the defect is crossed from the left ventricle, utilizing a right Judkins or a modified Amplatz catheter.

Transvenous Approach

A regular 0.025-inch-long (260-cm) wire is utilized and is advanced into the pulmonary artery, from where it is snared to the femoral vein (membranous defects) or the jugular vein (muscular defects), being careful not to cause bleeding from the arterial and the venous sites. A long sheath of a size appropriate to the device is advanced over the wire from the venous side and is positioned in the ascending aorta.

Buttoned-Device (Fourth-Generation) Placement

The occluder is introduced over the wire into the sheath and is advanced to the aortic valve level, where releasing is

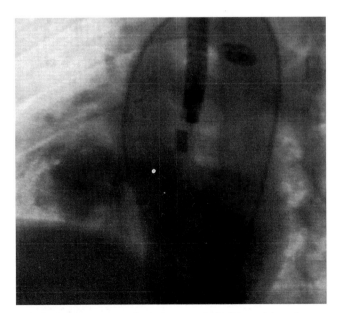

FIGURE 27.2. Large perimembranous VSD (12 mm) in a 4-year-old child, very close to the aortic valve (3 mm).

started. However, the sheath is slowly pulled back until the entire occluder is released into the left ventricle. The occluder is manipulated away from the aortic valve and is aligned with the ventricular septum. Echocardiography confirms the good position and the occlusion of the defect. The counteroccluder is buttoned as usual and a repeat left ventricular angiogram is performed. The wire is withdrawn through the device with the tip of the sheath placed against the device. The device is subsequently released.

Transvenous Approach Using the Transcatheter Patch

A long sheath in a size appropriate for the transcatheter patch used is advanced over the wire into the ascending aorta. The wire is taken out. Both the distal and the proximal balloons are initially positioned into the ascending aorta. The distal balloon/patch is inflated and is pulled until it obstructs the defect. Fluoroscopy, echocardiography, and pressure recording are utilized in guiding the procedure. After full occlusion is confirmed the proximal balloon in inflated. Subsequently, the balloon catheter and the long sheath are immobilized on the skin. A left ventricular angiogram and an aortogram confirm the result (Figures 27.3 and 27.4).

Transarterial Approach Using the Self-Adjustable Device

If the size and the location of the VSD are considered appropriate for disk device occlusion, a 0.025-inch stiff exchange wire is placed at the apex of the right ventricle. An

appropriate-sized sheath is placed over the wire in the right ventricle. An inverted self-adjustable device is loaded and is advanced until the distal (single-wire) disk is released in the right ventricle. Subsequently, the loading wire of the device is pulled until the distal disk becomes perpendicular to the tip of the sheath. The whole complex is pulled back until it stops at the ventricular septal level. The sheath is pulled back in the left ventricle and the proximal disk is released, occluding the VSD. The proximal disk could be manipulated away from the aortic valve. The distance between proximal and distal disk is self-adjusted according to septal thickness (Figure 27.1). The device is subsequently released in a similar fashion to the buttoned device.

Repeat oximetry will be reserved for patients with residual shunts, but it should be done carefully to avoid disturbing the device. ($Qp:Qs = 1$, no shunt; $Qp:Qs = 1$ to 1.2, trivial shunt; $Qp:Qs = 1.3$ to 1.5, small residual shunt; $Qp:Qs >1.5$, large shunt.)

Antibiotic prophylaxis should be started (preferably cephalosporins) with the first dose given intravenously in the catheterization laboratory and the subsequent ones given orally 6 and 12 hours later for the disk devices. Antibiotics are continued for 72 hours for the transcatheter patch. The patient should be discharged home within 24 hours from the release of the device. An echocardiogram, chest x-rays, and an electrocardiogram should be obtained before discharge. The patient should be discharged home with daily medication of aspirin (300 mg) for 6 weeks and endocarditis prophylaxis for 6 months for full occlusions. In patients with residual shunts, endocarditis prophylaxis will continue indefinitely.

RESULTS

Buttoned devices and their variants have been used to occlude 55 ventricular septal defects since 1994. Most of the defects (3,6) were occluded transvenously by the buttoned device. The transarterial approach with the self-adjustable device was used in 14 cases. Wireless devices were used in five cases.

Most occluded defects were perimembranous (4,5). Five congenital muscular and five postinfarction VSDs were occluded as well. One of the congenital muscular VSDs was of the Swiss cheese type.

The size of the VSDs varied from 3 to 12 mm (*median =* 5) for the congenital and from 12 to 25 mm for the post infarction. Patient ages varied from 1 to 45 years (*median =* 7) for the congenital VSDs and from 65 to 75 years (*median* = 70) for the post infarction. The average procedure time was 2.5 hours for transvenous procedures and 30 minutes for transarterial procedures utilizing the self-adjustable device. However, the transarterial procedure could not be performed in three attempted cases, which were performed transvenously instead. Wireless occlusions were performed

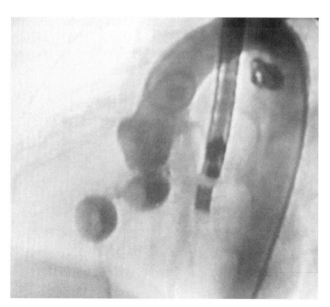

FIGURE 27.4. Aortogram shows no interference to the aortic valve.

in membranous VSDs inappropriate for disk device occlusion (three detachable balloons, two transcatheter patches).

Immediate effective occlusion occurred in all cases. Three early cases occluded transvenously with the buttoned device developed mild aortic insufficiency. In two the devices were extracted surgically in 48 hours. There was a transient third-degree A-V block in one case and transient PVCs in most cases during implantation.

Despite early symptomatic improvement only two of five cases after myocardial infarction are long-term survivors. No complications were seen with the self-adjustable device. One detachable balloon leaked in 24 hours and had to be extracted surgically.

Complications

Serious complications requiring reintervention occurred with the two early buttoned-device cases that developed aortic insufficiency and the case that involved early leakage of the detachable balloon, which required extraction. However, we are listing a series of potential complications. This list should be useful in obtaining informed consent from the patients.

Complications as seen in the ASD trials and the international VSD trials are defined as follows:

1. *Unbuttoning and embolization of the occluder on the left or on the right side of the heart* (self-explanatory).
2. *Cardiac perforation.* Perforation of a cardiac chamber by a catheter, a wire, or a device component during the procedure.
3. *Air embolism.* Introduction of air in the cardiac cavities from the introducing sheath, with findings of transient ST elevation, bradycardia, and transient drop of the systemic pressure. This is a self-limited phenomenon within 5 to 10 minutes, rarely seen during ASD occlusion. Such an episode is unlikely for VSD occlusion, since high-pressure bleeding prevents air entrapment.
4. *Excessive bleeding.* Small bleeding from the entry sites is not uncommon, especially if an arteriovenous connection is established. The investigator should be ready for the appropriate measures (sealing with pressure, new valve sheaths, etc.). Blood transfusions might be needed.
5. *Transient arrhythmia.* PVCs are common during catheter, wire, or device introduction in the ventricles. They are usually self-limited. Transient heart block has been seen as well.
6. *Mitral insufficiency.* This has been seen in ASD occlusion; highly unlikely with VSD occlusion.
7. *Tricuspid insufficiency.* Trivial tricuspid insufficiency has been seen without problems; in case of significant tricuspid insufficiency the device should be extracted.
8. *Aortic insufficiency.* This is the most common problem after membranous VSD occlusion, requiring extraction; it can be prevented by proper patient/device selection.
9. *Peripheral vascular problems.*

DISCUSSION

Concurrent use of three types of devices illustrates the inherent difficulties of VSD occlusion. The muscular VSDs were unquestionably the easiest to close by disk devices. Both the buttoned device and the self-adjustable device were used. The advantage of the significant overlapping of the disk devices could be best illustrated in the occlusion of a Swiss cheese type of VSD by the buttoned device.

The size of the self-adjustable device is restricted to 25 mm; therefore the use of the buttoned device was preferable for the large postinfarction muscular VSDs. Apical muscular VSDs are rather difficult for buttoned-device delivery, with the long sheath kinking in two occasions. Over-the-wire placement and kink-resistant sheaths may solve this problem. Despite the successful postinfarction VSD occlusion in five cases and their symptomatic improvement, only two of them are long-term survivors. The necessity of a stressful and high-risk procedure with questionable long-term outcome is raised.

The main procedural difficulty for transvenous VSD occlusion is crossing the VSD and establishing an arteriovenous connection. Over-the-wire placement with the buttoned device makes the procedure more secure. On the other hand, if the procedure can be done transarterially using the self-adjustable device, it is much faster. The average time for this procedure is only 30 minutes, in comparison to 2.5 hours for the transvenous procedure.

Most ventricular septal defects are perimembranous. This is why we focused our research effort in this category, and most of our occlusions were related to perimembranous defects (11). The first and the most commonly used device for perimembranous VSD occlusion was the buttoned device. The use of oversized devices early in the clinical trial was responsible for three instances of aortic insufficiency, two of which required surgical extraction of the device.

Careful measurements of the defect to right aortic cusp distance and selection of smaller devices positioned at least 2 mm away from the aortic cusp provided the solution to the problem. Indeed, no more cases of aortic insufficiency were noticed.

The presence of an aneurysm of the membranous septum was helpful in several cases, since the occluder could be pulled away from the aortic valve in the aneurysm.

The use of disk devices in the perimembranous VSD occlusion is limited, and most such VSDs are sent to surgery. The evolution of the wireless devices has the potential to change this practice. The five cases performed by us are in favor of this prediction. All were inappropriate for disk device occlusion and all were surgical candidates.

Both wireless devices used work on a balloon occluding principle. A balloon is a three-dimensional structure requiring a minimal rim for support. A subaortic rim as small as 1 mm is enough for the occlusion.

One detachable balloon device used leaked prematurely; it embolized in the pulmonary artery and had to be extracted surgically.

The transcatheter patch offers the efficacy of the detachable balloons but unparalleled safety with double cardiac and extracardiac immobilization and retractability in the introducing sheath. Despite the need for 48-hour balloon support, this wireless method has the potential to become the procedure of choice for most perimembranous VSDs.

CURRENT STATUS

The use of devices for the transcatheter occlusion of VSDs is investigational. All such devices are used under protocols and regulations acceptable in each center. In the United States, the FDA has approved clinical trials with the buttoned device in the occlusion of ventricular septal defects. Both perimembranous and muscular defects are occluded under the approved protocols.

An investigational device exception for the use of the transcatheter patch for occlusion of heart defects has been submitted to the FDA.

CONCLUSION

Transcatheter VSD occlusion using the different buttoned devices has been applied successfully since 1994. Three types of devices have been used to optimize the results. The buttoned device is the most common one used, over an arteriovenous wire, for transvenous occlusion. The self-adjustable device has the easiest application, since it can be applied transarterially. Wireless devices and especially the

transcatheter patch are the most promising methods for transvenous perimembranous VSD occlusion.

REFERENCES

1. Graham TP, Gutgesell HP. Ventricular septal defects. In: Emmanouilides GC, Riemenschneider T, Allen H, et al., eds. *Moss and Adams heart disease in infants, children, and adolescents*, 5th ed. Baltimore: Williams & Wilkins, 1995:724–746.
2. Lock JE, Block PC, McCay RG, et al. Transcatheter closure of ventricular septal defects. *Circulation* 1988:78:361–368.
3. Bridges ND, Perry SB, Keane JF, et al. Preoperative transcatheter closure of congenital muscular ventricular septal defects. *N Engl J Med* 1991;324:1312–1317.
4. Thanopoulos BD, Tsaousis GS, Konstantopoulou GL, et al. Transcatheter closure of muscular ventricular septal defects with the Amplatzer Ventricular Septal Defect Occluder: initial clinical application in children. *J Am Coll Cardiol* 1999;33:1395–1399.
5. Kalra GS, Verma PK, Dhall A, et al. Transcatheter device closure of ventricular septal defects: immediate results and intermediate term follow-up. *Am Heart J* 1999;138:339–344.
6. Sideris EB, Kaneva A, Sideris SE, et al. Transcatheter atrial septal defect occlusion in piglets, by balloon detachable devices. *Catheter Cardiovasc Interv* 2000;51:529–534.
7. Sideris E, Toumanides S, Alekyan B, et al. Transcatheter patch correction of atrial septal defects: experimental validation and early clinical experience. *Circulation* 2000;102(Suppl):II-588.
8. Sideris EB, Sideris SE, Thanopoulos BD, et al. Transvenous atrial septal defect occlusion by the buttoned device. *Am J Cardiol* 1990;66:1524–1526.
9. Rao PS, Berger F, Rey C, et al. Results of transvenous occlusion of secundum atrial septal defects with 4th generation buttoned device: comparison with 1st, 2nd and 3rd generation devices. *J Am Coll Cardiol* 2000;36:583–592.
10. Sideris EB, Zheng J, Wang Y, et al. Transarterial occlusion of membranous ventricular septal defects by a self-adjustable device. *Circulation* 1998;98:I-755.
11. Sideris EB, Walsh KP, Haddad JL, et al. Occlusion of congenital ventricular septal defects by the buttoned device. *Heart* 1997;77:276–279.

28

AMPLATZER MUSCULAR VENTRICULAR SEPTAL DEFECT OCCLUDER

DAVID J. WAIGHT
QI-LING CAO
ZIYAD M. HIJAZI

The Amplatzer Muscular Ventricular Septal Defect Occluder (MVSD) was designed to provide the most desirable characteristics for a percutaneous closure device that can be placed in the muscular ventricular septum. This device possesses some characteristics that render it ideal for catheter closure of muscular VSDs in children and adults. It has a simple, user-friendly delivery system and achieves high complete closure rates, limiting the need for repeat intervention. Furthermore, it requires small delivery sheaths, which permits its use in small infants. Therefore the device can be delivered from the traditional venous route or from the retrograde arterial route. The device is available in many different sizes that allow the operators to close a wide range of defects located in the apical, posterior, anterior, or mid-muscular portion of the ventricular septum. The device structure should have high fatigue resistance because of its position in the moving muscular septum until at least it is fully endothelialized. One of the most important features of this device and its delivery system, especially if misplacement occurs, is the ability to retrieve, reposition, or recapture the device before release. This feature results in low embolization rates.

The first use of the Amplatzer MVSD Occluder was reported in a study of closure of surgically created VSDs in dogs and naturally occurring VSDs in miniature pigs. The devices were placed through a catheter placed via right ventricular puncture with complete success and a 100% closure rate. The devices exhibited complete endothelialization at 3 months following occlusion autopsy examination (1). The

first human implantation of the device was included with a report on transcatheter use in canines. Complete occlusion was noted after the device was placed in an 8-month-old child with a residual VSD after attempted surgical closure (2). This device was placed intraoperatively through a right ventricular approach. Tofeig et al. reported a case of a 5-year-old child who underwent successful catheter closure of a MVSD (3).

The use of the Amplatzer MVSD device has continued to be explored with excellent results. Eight patients with MVSDs were all successfully occluded through a femoral arterial or jugular venous approach (4). Six patients were also reported with 100% complete occlusion (5). The device is currently being used in a Phase I trial in the United States.

THE DEVICE

The MVSD device is a self-expandable double-disk device made from a Nitinol wire mesh (Figure 28.1). Nitinol is an alloy of 55% nickel and 45% titanium with superelastic properties that provides shape memory (6,7). This allows the device to be stretched into an almost linear configuration and placed inside a small sheath for delivery and then to return to its original configuration within the VSD when not constrained by the sheath. Nitinol also has been proven to have excellent biocompatability (8,9). The device is constructed from Nitinol wires that are tightly woven into a thin retention disk that extends into the occluding waist and then into a second retention disk. The thickness of the wire is 0.004 inch for devices 10 mm and smaller and 0.005 inch for larger devices. The leading retention disk is 4 mm larger and the proximal disk is 3 mm larger than the diameter of the waist. To achieve immediate complete closure, three Dacron polyester patches are sewn securely with polyester thread into the two disks and the waist of the device. A stainless steel sleeve with a female thread is laser-welded

David J. Waight: Assistant Professor of Pediatrics, Department of Pediatrics, University of Chicago Pritzker School of Medicine; Cardiologist, Department of Pediatrics, University of Chicago Children's Hospital, Chicago, Illinois

Qi-Ling Cao: Assistant Professor, Department of Pediatric Cardiology, University of Chicago; Director, Pediatric Echocardiography Research Laboratory, University of Chicago Children's Hospital, Chicago, Illinois

Ziyad M. Hijazi: Professor of Pediatrics and Medicine, Department of Pediatrics and Medicine, University of Chicago; Director, Pediatric Cardiology, University of Chicago, Chicago, Illinois

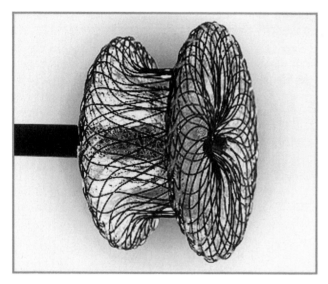

FIGURE 28.1. The Amplatzer muscular ventricular septal defect occluder device. The device consists of three components: a left ventricle disk, a connecting waist, and a right ventricle disk.

to the proximal end of the device. This sleeve is used to screw the delivery cable to the device. The device size corresponds to the diameter of the waist. The mechanism of closure involves stenting of the MVSD by the device and subsequent thrombus formation within the device with eventual complete neoendothelialization. The device is available in sizes from 6 to 24 mm that are delivered through 6- to 9F sheaths (Table 28.1). The delivery system is prepackaged with a long Mullins-type sheath, loader, diaphragm with side arm flush, delivery cable, and pin vise.

PATIENT SELECTION

Patients are selected for occlusion with the Amplatzer MVSD device based on the presence of a hemodynamically significant MVSD with left-to-right shunt. The patients are

evaluated with history, physical examination, electrocardiogram, and a transthoracic echocardiogram (TTE). All patients should have clinical and/or echocardiographic evidence consistent with a hemodynamically significant MVSD. Exclusion criteria include weight of less than 3.0 kg; distance of less than 4 mm between the VSD and the aortic, pulmonic, mitral, or tricuspid valves; pulmonary vascular resistance of greater than 7 Woods units; perimembranous VSD; sepsis; and conditions that might be exacerbated by the use of aspirin unless other antiplatelet agents could be used for 6 months. Informed consent is obtained from each patient or minor's parent.

DEVICE IMPLANTATION TECHNIQUE

The procedure is performed under general endotracheal anesthesia. Access is obtained in the femoral vein, the femoral artery, and the right internal jugular vein. The patients are fully heparinized with a target-activated clotting time (ACT) of greater then 200 seconds at the time of device placement. Routine right and left heart catheterization is performed to assess the degree of shunting and to evaluate the pulmonary vascular resistance. Axial angiography is performed to define the location, size, and number of VSDs. Transesophageal echocardiographic (TEE) monitoring is optional (4). However, for catheter closure of multiple MVSDs we strongly recommend the routine use of TEE guidance. On rare occasions, in very small children, TEE may not be well tolerated. Therefore transthoracic echocardiographic (TTE) monitoring may be used instead.

A complete TEE study is performed, including the standard imaging views: transgastric, frontal four-chamber, and basal short-axis views. Any associated abnormalities are noted and gross assessment of chamber size and function is made. Specific attention is then paid to the VSD and nearby structures, namely, the papillary muscles, moderator band, and chordae tendineae. The atrioventricular valves are interrogated as a baseline for any regurgitation. The

TABLE 28.1. AMPLATZER MUSCULAR VENTRICULAR SEPTAL OCCLUDER

Device Size (Waist Size, mm)	Device Length (mm)	Recommended Sheath Size (F)	Large Disc Diameter (mm)	Small Disc Diameter (mm)	Wire Diameter (inch)
6	7	6–7	14	12	0.004
8	7	6–7	16	14	0.004
10	7	6–7	18	16	0.004
12	7	7–8	20	18	0.005
14	7	7–8	22	20	0.005
16	10	7–8	24	22	0.005
18	10	7–8	26	24	0.005
20	10	8–9	28	26	0.005
22	10	8–9	30	28	0.005
24	10	8–9	32	30	0.005

VSD is measured in multiple views, including the frontal four-chamber and basal short-axis views. Tissue rims and distances from aortic and tricuspid valves are also measured in the preceding views.

The appropriate device size is chosen to be equal to or 1 to 2 mm larger than the VSD size as assessed by TEE and angiographic evaluation (maximal size at end-diastole). Some operators measure the balloon-stretched diameter of the MVSD by inflating a low-pressure balloon placed across the defect until no shunting is detected via color Doppler. We believe the stiffness of the muscular septum makes balloon sizing unnecessary. The waist of the device is designed to stent the VSD and produce closure by thrombosis. The Dacron patches within the device enhance thrombosis.

The next step in the closure sequence is placement of a long sheath (6 to 8F) across the VSD. Figure 28.2 demonstrates the steps of closure. This can be accomplished in a variety of ways. The most common approach used for mid-muscular VSDs is to advance a curved end-hole catheter (Judkins right, or Cobra) into the VSD from the left ventricular side. An exchange length 0.035-inch Amplatz wire is then advanced through the VSD and the right ventricle into the pulmonary artery. This wire is snared in the pulmonary artery or in the right atrium using the Amplatz gooseneck snare (Microvena Corporation, White Bear Lake, Minnesota) and is exteriorized out the right internal jugular sheath. This provides a stable rail to allow advancement of the 6- to 8F long sheath across the VSD. The sheath is preferentially advanced from the jugular approach to limit the sheath size in the artery. In some patients the catheter course is tortuous and this approach is impossible. The sheath can then be advanced from a retrograde approach through the femoral artery. On occasion, to eliminate kinking of the sheath in the aortic arch or VSD areas, a 0.018-inch glide wire is left inside the sheath while advancing the delivery cable and device. Once the device reaches the tip of the sheath, the wire is removed before deployment of the ventricular disk.

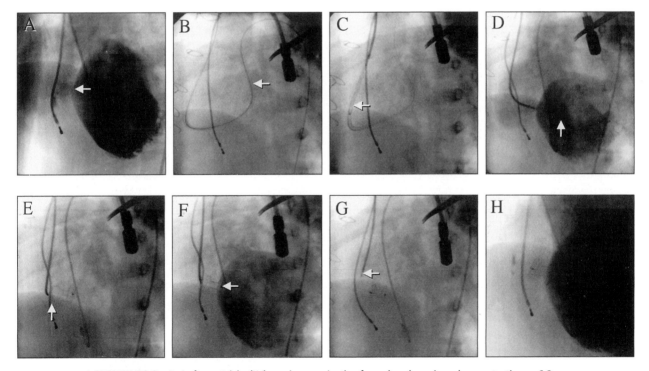

FIGURE 28.2. A: Left ventricle (LV) angiogram in the four-chamber view demonstrating a 6.3-mm mid-muscular VSD *(arrow)* in a 13-year-old, 40-kg child with acquired muscular VSD after surgical repair of hypertrophic cardiomyopathy, followed by Kono operation 5 years later. This operation was complicated by the development of muscular VSD and complete heart block requiring transvenous pacemaker. The Qp:Qs ratio was 2.3:1 and the systolic pulmonary artery pressure was 55 mm Hg. **B:** Cine image demonstrating arteriovenous wire loop from the femoral artery through the VSD and out the right internal jugular vein. **C:** Cine image of a 10-mm Amplatzer MVSD device passing through the sheath *(arrows)* while the guide wire is still positioned inside the sheath to prevent kinking. **D:** Angiogram in the LV after the LV disk has been deployed *(arrow)* in the LV. **E:** Cine image during deployment of the right ventricle disk *(arrow)*. **F:** Angiogram in the LV prior to release of device to assess position. **G:** Cine image immediately after the device has been released from the cable *(arrow)*. **H:** LV angiogram 10 minutes after the device has been released demonstrating good device position and minimal foaming through the device that disappeared the following day. The pulmonary artery pressure dropped to 38 mm Hg. MVSD, muscular ventricular septal defect; VSD, ventricular septal defect.

Patients with larger VSDs and some apical VSDs are easily crossed from the right ventricular side. If the VSD is crossed and a catheter can be placed in the body of the left ventricle, the stiff wire is advanced into the left ventricle (LV) and the sheath is advanced through the right internal jugular vein into the left ventricle.

The long sheath can also be advanced from the femoral vein. This approach produces a tortuous catheter course that makes advancement of the device more difficult. This approach should not be used unless access through the jugular vein is impossible.

Once the sheath is in proper position the appropriate-sized VSD device is screwed onto the delivery cable and pulled into the loader under water. The loader is then flushed with saline through the side arm of the valve supplied with the delivery system to prevent any air embolism. The loader is placed into the proximal end of the long sheath and the device is advanced with short pushes of the delivery cable to the distal tip of the sheath. The cable should be advanced without rotation to prevent premature unscrewing of the device. The device is then slowly advanced out the sheath to allow the distal disk to expand. Repeat small injections using the pigtail catheter positioned in the LV after each step are of paramount importance. These injections are used for optimal device positioning. The device and sheath are then retracted against the septum with gentle tension and the sheath is retracted to open the waist of the device in the VSD and open the proximal disk against the opposite side of the septum. The device position is then assessed with TEE in multiple views. Atrioventricular valves are assessed for any induced valvar regurgitation. Angiographic assessment of device position is performed using the pigtail catheter in the left ventricle or through the side arm of the delivery sheath if the arterial approach is used (or via a pigtail catheter from the contralateral femoral artery). If the device is not well positioned across the VSD or increased valvar regurgitation has been induced, the device can be easily recaptured into the long sheath. The preceding steps are then repeated and the device is repositioned.

If device position is satisfactory, the pin vise is fixed onto the delivery cable and the device is released with counter-clockwise rotation. A repeat angiogram is performed in the left ventricle 10 minutes after release to assess the closure. After device release a brief, complete TEE study is performed with additional imaging in multiple planes to confirm device placement and assess for residual shunting and any obstruction or regurgitation induced by the device. The device orientation commonly changes slightly as the device is released from the delivery cable and tension on the device is eliminated, which allows it to completely align with the septum.

The patients receive a dose of an appropriate antibiotic (commonly, cetazolin at 20 mg/kg) during the catheterization procedure and two further doses at 8-hour intervals. The patients are allowed to recover in an appropriate setting and are routinely discharged the following day. Observation of subacute bacterial endocarditis prophylaxis is recommended for 6 months or until complete closure is obtained. Patients are maintained on 3 to 5 mg/kg of aspirin per day for 6 months and are instructed to avoid contact sports for 1 month. Follow-up includes TTE, chest radiograph, and electrocardiogram (ECG) at 6 months after closure and yearly thereafter.

RESULTS

The results of our early clinical experience with eight patients have been previously reported and will be summarized (4). Patients' mean age was 5.4 ± 3.1 years (range, 2 to 10 years) and mean weight was 8.4 ± 6.5 kg (range, 11.5 to 29 kg). The mean VSD size by transthoracic echocardiographic measurement was 6.6 ± 1.3 mm (range, 5 to 9 mm). The mean VSD size by transthoracic echocardiographic measurement was 7.6 ± 2.4 mm (range, 4.5 to 12 mm). The mean Qp:Qs was 1.7 + 0.6 (range, 1.4 to 3). The mean device size was 9 ± 2.6 mm (range, 6 to 14 mm). The VSDs were mid-muscular in four patients, anterior in two, and apical and posterior in one each. The device was delivered through a transvenous sheath in five patients and through an arterial sheath in three patients (two with anterior and one with a posterior VSD). The mean fluoroscopy time was 37.1 + 13 minutes (range, 11.7 to 55 minutes). The mean procedural time was 165 + 65 minutes (range, 83 to 290 minutes). Complications were limited to a single transient episode of junctional rhythm. Transfusion was not required.

Complete closure was present in two patients in the catheterization suite. Complete closure was noted in seven patients at 24 hours after closure and in all patients by 1-year follow-up. No increased valvar regurgitation has been noted. No episodes of thromboembolism, hemolysis, device wire fracture, device disruption, or endocarditis were reported.

A summary of all the available published VSD occlusions with the Amplatzer VSD device includes 20 patients. The authors report complete occlusion of all these defects by 1-year follow-up. The reported complications include only transient changes in rhythm or ECG with complete resolution (2–5).

Since our report (4) we have done a few more patients with single or multiple "Swiss cheese" ventricular septal defects. The smallest patient we have attempted was a 4-month-old, 4.6-kg baby boy with very large mid-apical VSD measuring 12 to 13 mm with Qp:Qs of 5.9:1 and near systemic pulmonary artery pressure. This baby underwent closure from the right internal jugular vein using a 7F sheath and a 14-mm Amplatzer MVSD Occluder. Upon release of the device, the right ventricle disk migrated toward the LV. Twenty-four hours later, the device required surgical adjustment where, via a limited right ventriculotomy, the surgeon was able to pull the right ventricle disk through the VSD into the right ventricle. The device was sutured into the right ventricle to secure its position. This baby is being followed medically and is in good condition.

Another child (3 years of age, 11.4 kg) with multiple VSDs was referred for occlusion. She had undergone a pulmonary artery banding procedure early in her life. During the first intervention on this child, she received two Amplatzer MVSD devices of 8 mm each to close two large defects. The patient subsequently was transferred back to the referring institution, where she underwent debanding and attempted closure of additional VSDs. The patient had significant ventricular dysfunction postoperatively and a complicated hospitalization. Seven months after the initial procedure the patient returned to the catheterization suite and was noted to have a Qp:Qs of 3:1 through a large residual defect between the devices and a very small apical defect. A third Amplatzer VSD device of 6 mm size was placed in the larger VSD with effective occlusion. A minimal residual shunt was detected angiographically at the apical defect with the Qp:Qs ratio of 1:1 (Figure 28.3).

APPLICABILITY IN ADULT PATIENTS

The Amplatzer VSD device is easily used in adults with appropriate MVSDs. Our recent experience has included adults with congenital defects (Figure 28.4). The transcatheter closure of postinfarction MVSDs has been shown to be technically possible even in very ill patients (Mario Carminati, personal communication, 2000). The Amplatzer Septal Occluder has been used to close postinfarction VSDs with good initial results (10,11). One would expect the Amplatzer VSD device to be equally effective in the acute closure of these types of VSDs. However, the initial results using the MVSD device have not been encouraging (Mario Carminati, personal communication, 2000). It remains to be seen if long-term clinical improvement and improved outcome are achieved after closure in patients with immediate postinfarction VSDs (12).

DISCUSSION

VSD is the most common form of congenital heart disease. The management of hemodynamically significant VSDs has been medical and surgical. Most VSDs can be closed surgically with excellent results. There remains morbidity

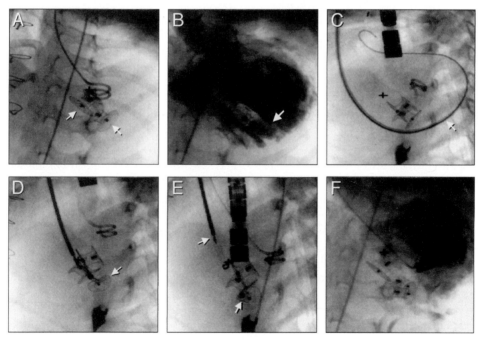

FIGURE 28.3. A: Cine image of the LV in a 3-year-old, 11.4-kg child who underwent placement of two 8-mm Amplatzer MVSD devices *(arrows)* for muscular VSDs. **B:** LV angiogram in the four-chamber view demonstrating large residual apical muscular VSD *(arrow)*. **C:** Cine image demonstrating the 7F sheath *(arrow)* with a guide wire through the VSD. **D:** Cine image of deployment of LV disk of a 6-mm Amplatzer device *(arrow)* in the LV. **E:** Cine image of device *(arrow)* released across the VSD from the cable *(arrow)*. **F:** LV angiogram 10-minutes after the device has been released demonstrating good device position with foaming through the device.

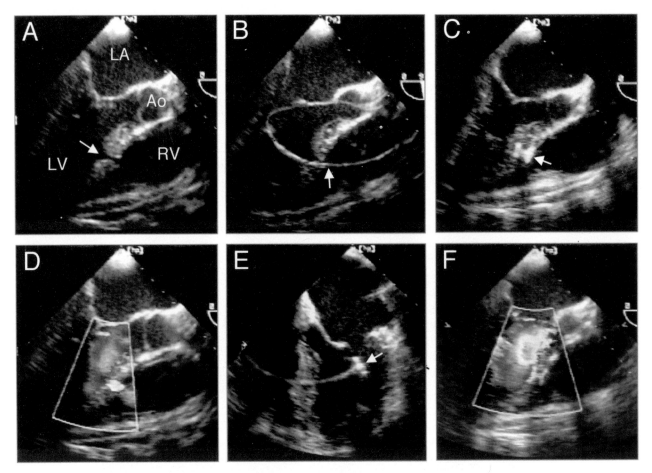

FIGURE 28.4. Transesophageal echocardiographic (TEE) images without (**A**) and with (**D**) color Doppler in a 31.5-year-old 123.5-kg male with a 4.5-mm mid-muscular VSD and a Qp:Qs ratio of 1.5:1. **B:** TEE image in the long-axis view demonstrating passage of the delivery sheath from the right to the left ventricle through the VSD. **E:** TEE image in the four-chamber view during deployment of the LV disk *(arrow).* TEE images without (**C**) and with (**F**) color Doppler after a 6-mm Amplatzer MVSD device *(arrow)* has been deployed demonstrating good device position and no residual shunt. (See Color Figures 28.4D and F.)

associated with the procedure and a very low mortality. The surgical results of the management of multiple VSDs demonstrate the increased morbidity and mortality associated with this complicated disease.

The success of device closure of atrial septal defects and patent ductus arteriosus has prompted the investigation of transcatheter closure of MVSDs. Many of the occlusion devices used for other shunts have also been used for VSD closure. Gianturco coils have been used to close small VSDs (13,14). The Grifka bag has been used to close both muscular and perimembranous defects. Perimembranous, muscular, and postinfarction VSDs have all been effectively treated using the Rashkind ASD and PDA devices (15–20). The buttoned device has also been used for VSD closure (21,22). However, the Amplatzer VSD Occluder device was designed specifically for MVSD closure and has been undergoing clinical trials since 1998. This device

is the only device designed for muscular VSD closure. This device has the characteristics necessary for effective use in VSD closure. It has a simple delivery system with simple mechanics, which shortens the fluoroscopy and procedure time. The device can be effectively repositioned or retrieved until it is released in an optimal position. The transvenous approach and a relatively small delivery system (6 to 8F) allow its use in smaller children with minimal vascular trauma.

The device has been used for anterior, posterior, mid-muscular, apical, postinfarction, and multiple Swiss cheese–type VSDs with excellent results. Patients with complex congenital heart disease requiring a staged approach may be treated with transcatheter repair of the VSD component of their disease. This can decrease the complexity of the subsequent surgical repair and eliminate the need for a ventricular incision.

CURRENT STATUS

The Amplatzer MVSD device is currently available at selected institutions as part of an investigational device exemption approved by the US Food and Drug Administration in May 2000. Also, the manufacturer of the device filed for Humanitarian Device Exemption status in the United States. The device is available internationally, depending on local regulations.

CONCLUSION

The initial experience with the Amplatzer MVSD occluder is very encouraging, with safe and effective results. The early results indicate a very high procedural success rate with excellent complete closure rates. All the common types of MVSDs can be effectively occluded with this device, including multiple VSDs. If further investigation and follow-up continue to produce similar results, this device may become an important component in the armamentarium of the interventional cardiologist caring for patients with congenital heart disease.

REFERENCES

1. Amin Z, Gu X, Berry JM, et al. Periventricular closure of ventricular septal defects without cardiopulmonary bypass. *Ann Thorac Surg* 1999;68:149–154.
2. Amin Z, Berry JM, Foker JE, et al. Intraoperative closure of muscular ventricular septal defect in a canine model and applicability of the technique in a baby. *J Thorac Cardiovasc Surg* 1998;115:1374–1376.
3. Tofeig M, Patel RG, Walsh KP. Transcatheter closure of a midmuscular ventricular septal defect with an Amplatzer VSD occlusion device. *Heart* 1999;81:438–440.
4. Hijazi ZM, Hakim F, Al-Fadley F, et al. Transcatheter closure of single muscular ventricular septal defects using the Amplatzer Muscular VSD Occluder: initial results and technical considerations. *Cathteter Cardiovasc Interv* 1900;49:167–172.
5. Thanopoulos BD, Tsaousis GS, Konstadopoulou GN, et al. Transcatheter closure of muscular ventricular septal defects with the Amplatzer Ventricular Septal Defect Occluder: initial clinical applications in children. *J Am Coll Cardiol* 1999;33:1395–1399.
6. Liu X, Stice JD. Shape-memory alloys and their applications. *J Appl Manufactur Syst* 1990;3:65–72.
7. Hebda DA, White SR. Hysteresis testing of Nitinol wires: adaptive structures and composite materials: analysis and application. New York: American Society of Mechanical Engineers, 1994:1–8.
8. Cragg AH, Jong SCD, Barnhart WH, et al. Nitinol intravascular stent: results of preclinical evaluation. *Radiology* 1993;189:775–778.
9. Putters JL, Kaulesar SDM, de Zeeuw GR, et al. Comparative cell culture effects of shape memory metal (Nitinol), nickel and titanium: a biocompatibility estimation. *Eur Surg Res* 1992;24:378–382.
10. Pesonen E, Thilen U, Sandstrom S, et al. Transcatheter closure of post-infarction ventricular septal defect with the Amplatzer Septal Occluder device. *Scand Cardiovasc J* 2000;34:446–448.
11. Lee EM, Roberts DH, Walsh. Transcatheter closure of a residual post-infarction ventricular septal defect with the Amplatzer Septal Occluder. *Heart* 1998;80:522–524.
12. Lock JE, Block PC, McKay RG, et al. Transcatheter closure of ventricular septal defects. *Circulation* 1988;78:361–368.
13. Latiff HA, Alwi M, Kandhavel G, et al. Transcatheter closure of multiple muscular ventricular septal defects using Gianturco coils. *Ann Thorac Surg* 1999;68:1400–1401.
14. Kalra GS, Verma PK, Dhall A, et al. Transcatheter device closure of ventricular septal defects: immediate results and intermediate-term follow-up. *Am Heart J* 1999;138:339–344.
15. O'Laughlin MP, Mullins CE. Transcatheter occlusion of ventricular septal defect. *Catheter Cardiovasc Diagn* 1989;17:175–179.
16. Rigby ML, Redington AN. Primary transcatheter umbrella closure of perimembranous ventricular septal defect. *Br Heart J* 1994;72:368–371.
17. Janorkar S, Goh T, Wilkinson J. Transcatheter closure of ventricular septal defects using the Rashkind device: initial experience. *Catheter Cardiovasc Interv* 1999;46:43–48.
18. Benton JP, Barker KS. Transcatheter closure of ventricular septal defect: a nonsurgical approach to the care of the patient with acute ventricular septal rupture. *Heart Lung* 1992;21:356–364.
19. Lock JE, Block PC, McKay RG, et al. Transcatheter closure of ventricular septal defects. *Circulation* 1988;78:361–368.
20. Bridges ND, Perry SB, Keane JF, et al. Preoperative transcatheter closure of congenital muscular ventricular septal defects. *N Engl J Med* 1991;324:1312–1317.
21. Sideris EB, Walsh KP, Haddad JL, et al. Occlusion of congenital ventricular septal defects by the buttoned device. *Heart* 1997;77:276–279.
22. Sideris EB, Haddad JL, Rao PS. The role of 'Sideris' devices in the occlusion of ventricular septal defects. *Current Intervent Cardiol Reports* 2001;3:349–353.

Catheter Based Devices: For the Treatment of Non-coronary Cardiovascular Diseases in Adults and Children. Edited by P. Syamasundar Rao and Morton J. Kern, Lippincott Williams & Wilkins, Philadelphia © 2003.

29

CARDIOSEAL/STARFLEX DEVICES

AUDREY C. MARSHALL
STANTON B. PERRY

Interventional cardiologists have accumulated more than a decade of experience using double-umbrella devices for transcatheter closure of intracardiac defects, including ventricular septal defect (VSD). Before 1996, VSDs were closed in 85 patients using the Bard Clamshell Septal Occluder at the Children's Hospital, Boston. In 1996, physicians at this hospital first used the CardioSEAL double-umbrella device to close a VSD. Since that time, the CardioSEAL and the STARFlex modification of this device, have been implanted in more than 75 additional patients with VSD. Transcatheter closure of VSD is an increasingly important therapy in the management of patients with multiple muscular VSDs, as well as those with hemodynamically significant postoperative residual defects.

DEVICE

The original Lock Clamshell Occluder (C.R. Bard, Boston, MA) consisted of two opposing, self-expanding Dacron umbrellas connected by a central post. Four metal arms supported each umbrella. Each of these arms, fabricated of 304v stainless steel, formed a single spring-loaded hinge. The original Clamshell was found to have a high rate of device arm fracture in intermediate-term follow-up (1). Concern about the potential for clinical sequelae of these fractures prompted the redesign of the device.

The addition of a second hinge along each arm of the Clamshell II device (C.R. Bard, Boston, MA) distinguished it from the original Clamshell. Furthermore, the metal framework of the Clamshell II consisted of MP35N, a nonferromagnetic alloy of cobalt, chromium, molybdenum, and nickel. This biocompatible alloy endowed the new device with improved resistance to metal fatigue and corrosion. In addition, the nonferrous nature of MP35N mini-

mized the risk for device dislodgment in patients undergoing subsequent magnetic resonance imaging.

The CardioSEAL, manufactured by NMT Medical, Inc. (Boston, MA), is equivalent to the Clamshell II in both materials and processes. The more recent STARFlex modification consists of the basic CardioSEAL device, with the addition of flexible Nitinol microsprings suspended between the arms of the opposing umbrellas. The intended function of these microsprings is to allow the device to center itself within a defect, both during delivery and after deployment (2). CardioSEAL and STARFlex are available in a range of sizes. Size designation is based on the distance along the diagonal of the Dacron umbrella. The CardioSEAL device is available in 17-, 23-, 28-, 33-, and 40-mm sizes; the STARFlex modification is not available in the 17-mm size.

PATIENT SELECTION

Candidates for transcatheter closure of VSD can be grouped into one of two broad classifications. Device closure should be considered in patients with hemodynamically significant, complex VSDs that, based on location, cannot be closed by standard transatrial or transarterial surgical approaches. In these patients, transcatheter therapy may obviate the need for a ventriculotomy. In addition, patients with underlying cardiac or medical disease putting them at high risk for surgical closure may be candidates for transcatheter closure. The hemodynamic impact of the defect may manifest as clinically evident heart failure, ventricular volume load, pulmonary hypertension, or, in the case of right-to-left shunting, cyanosis. Once potential candidates are identified, additional factors, such as VSD location and size, as well as patient size, must be considered.

Patients with multiple muscular VSDs were among the first treated with the Clamshell device (3). They continue to represent a large group of those undergoing transcatheter VSD occlusion at our institution. These patients, who are often initially palliated with a pulmonary arterial band, can subsequently be managed with a combination of transcatheter and surgical procedures to achieve a complete

Audrey C. Marshall: Instructor in Pediatrics, Department of Pediatrics, Harvard Medical School; Assistant in Cardiology, Department of Cardiology, Children's Hospital, Boston, Massachusetts

Stanton B. Perry: Associate Professor of Pediatrics, Stanford University Medical School; Director, Pediatric Cardiac, Catherization Laboratory, Lucile Packard Children's Hospital, Palo Alto, California

repair. Operative visualization of anterior and apical defects is often challenging and can be made more difficult by prior banding. In the catheterization laboratory, the defects can be visualized angiographically and crossed using a variety of techniques described later in this chapter.

In postoperative patients, VSDs may be located at the margin of, or within, a previously placed surgical patch. These defects are also amenable to device closure. Preminger et al. attempted umbrella closure of "intramural" VSD in seven patients who had previously undergone surgical repair of a conotruncal defect (4). This defect was located near the superior margin of the surgical patch, within the right ventricular free wall. Clamshell placement resulted in a decrease in the degree of residual shunting in all of these patients, as indicated by the pulmonary-to-systemic-flow ratio measured before and after device placement.

Love et al. recently presented a novel application of the CardioSEAL device, closure of fenestrated VSD patches in 24 patients with tetralogy of Fallot, and diminutive pulmonary arteries (5). At the time of surgery, partial VSD closure was accomplished by creating a fenestration within the patch material. The fenestration allowed decompression of potentially suprasystemic right ventricular (RV) pressures in the immediate postoperative period. Later, presumably after pulmonary arterial growth, some of these patients were able to tolerate complete closure of the VSD. A small group of four patients whose fenestration had failed to close spontaneously underwent device occlusion.

The framework of the CardioSEAL, consisting of eight independently sprung arms, lends itself to application in a variety of VSD configurations. The device can conform to the local anatomy, whether it is placed through RV muscle bundles (as reported by Kumar et al.), within a tunnel of thick ventricular septum, or bordering a patch of prosthetic material (6). The independent flexion of each arm also brings the periphery of the Dacron umbrella flush with surrounding structures, minimizing the profile of the device within the heart.

The CardioSEAL and STARFlex devices may be used to close intracardiac defects ranging in size from a few millimeters to 25 mm in stretch diameter. (Patients with intracardiac defects larger than 25 mm are currently excluded from clinical trials.) In practice, the typical stretch diameter of the VSD is 5 to 10 mm. In the case of two or more small defects close together, or one defect with multiple openings on the RV side, the body of the device can be delivered in any communication large enough to permit the delivery catheter. The coverage provided by the umbrellas will serve to occlude additional communications.

The size of the patient may limit consideration of transcatheter closure due to the size of the necessary delivery system. The CardioSEAL is delivered through an 11F sheath, while the STARFlex is delivered through a 10F sheath. In our experience, the average weight of patients receiving a CardioSEAL or STARFlex device for VSD has been approximately 20 kg. The device has been placed successfully in patients as small as 6 kg, although a weight of

10 to 12 kg is preferred to lessen the risk of damage to the vessel through which the device is introduced.

DEVICE IMPLANTATION TECHNIQUE

The catheter course is based on the location of the defect (7). Most often, the VSD is crossed from the left ventricular (LV) side. A venous end-hole catheter is passed through the atrial septum via an existing atrial septal defect or by transseptal puncture. The catheter is advanced to the LV. Using a flow-directed catheter in combination with either a tip-deflecting wire (Reuter tip deflector, Cook, Inc., Bloomington, IN) or a torque wire (Magic Torque, Boston Scientific, Watertown, MA), the catheter can usually be passed through the VSD and into the RV. Alternatively, a shaped catheter can be used to direct a torque wire through the defect. In the case of anterior muscular VSDs, the defect may be crossed from the RV side using a shaped catheter. The "intramural" VSD is crossed from the LV side using a retrograde arterial catheter.

After the defect is crossed from the LV side, the tip of the wire is advanced to the pulmonary artery and captured from a second venous site. When crossed from the RV side, the wire is snared in the descending aorta, using an arterial snare. The snared torque wire is then replaced by an exchange length wire. Most often, we use a 0.035-inch (210-cm) Rosen wire (Cook, Inc., Bloomington, IN) to guide the delivery system for the device. With this wire through the defect, both ends are secured outside of the body (Figure 29.1). Once this wire has been placed through the defect and is fixed at each end, the wire may prop open the atrioventricular and/or semilunar valve and severely compromise cardiac output. Excessive tension on the wire should be avoided for this reason.

Selective angiograms are performed using a cutoff pigtail catheter (Royal Flush II angiographic catheter, Cook, Inc., Bloomington, IN) over the wire. Camera angles must be tailored to the location and configuration of the VSD. The stretched diameter of the defect is determined using a pull-through technique. Filling the balloon of a 7F wedge catheter with dilute contrast and passing this balloon over the wire through the defect will sufficiently size most VSDs. The stretched diameter of the VSD is the major determinant of the size of device chosen. In general, we choose a device that measures twice the stretched diameter of the VSD when placing the CardioSEAL device. The self-centering properties of the new STARFlex may permit a slightly lower device-to-defect ratio.

Once the defect has been sized and the device size chosen, the device can be loaded into the delivery system. The CardioSEAL/STARFlex delivery system consists of three major components: a central rod, a coaxial pushing catheter, and a long sheath. The device is packaged separately and comes attached to a loading funnel. The device is first connected to the distal tip of the central rod using a locking pin/pin mechanism. Using the loading funnel in conjunction with the distal part of the pushing catheter, the

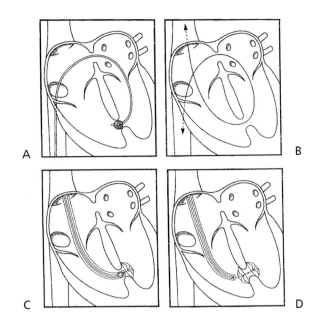

FIGURE 29.1. Steps in VSD closure using the CardioSEAL device. **A:** The VSD is first crossed with a catheter. **B:** An exchange length wire is positioned across the defect and secured at both ends. **C:** The delivery sheath is positioned over this wire and the device is loaded in the sheath. **D:** The distal and proximal arms of the device are deployed by withdrawal of the sheath.

device on the tip of the central rod is collapsed into the tubular configuration it will be maintained until delivered. Once the pushing catheter is locked into a fixed relation to the central rod, advancement of the pushing catheter will result in forward travel of the device. The device is now

ready to be introduced to the long sheath, which will deliver the device to the target lesion.

The device may be delivered from either the RV or the LV side, based on the location of the defect, the course of the wire, and the ability of the delivery system to track the wire course. Anterior VSDs are readily approached from the femoral vein via the RV. Apical defects may be closed from the RV side using the internal jugular vein, as depicted in Figure 29.1, or from the LV side using the femoral vein.

The long sheath and dilator are flushed on the table prior to advancing them over the guide wire across the defect. Next, the wire and dilator are removed as saline is continuously infused into the sheath. This prevents air from being drawn into the system and avoids a static column of blood within the large sheath. The device is then inserted into the long sheath and advanced until it reaches the distal end of the sheath. Withdrawal of the long sheath, while fixing the position of the device, deploys the distal arms. Retraction of the entire system allows the distal arms to engage the ventricular septum. If the distal arms are improperly positioned, they can be collapsed and repositioned by readvancing the long sheath. After the position of the distal arms is confirmed by fluoroscopy, angiography, or echocardiography, the proximal arms are deployed by further withdrawal of the long sheath.

Once fully deployed, the device remains connected to the central rod and the pushing catheter by the pin/pin mechanism (Figure 29.2). If the position of the device is incorrect or if the device interferes with intracardiac structures, the device can be removed and retrieved while still attached to the pusher catheter. Alternatively, the device can

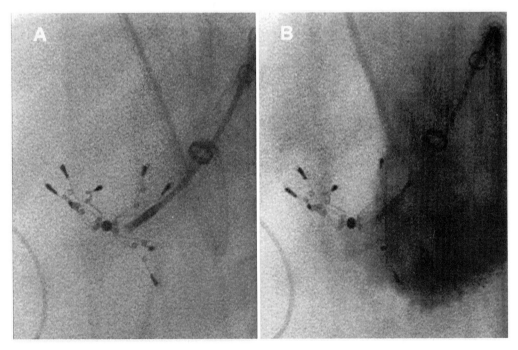

FIGURE 29.2. Long axial oblique angiogram during placement of a VSD device. **A:** The delivery system traverses the right atrium, left atrium, and left ventricle. Both the proximal and distal sets of arms have been deployed, though the device has not been released from the delivery system. **B:** Right ventricular arms are fixed between dense trabeculations, whereas left ventricular arms flex against the smooth septal surface.

be released and then retrieved from another site. The device is released by unlocking the pin/pin mechanism.

Full heparinization is maintained during the procedure. Antibiotics are given at the time of device implantation and for approximately 24 hours following the procedure. Patients are prescribed aspirin (approximately 1 mg/kg) for a period of at least 6 months.

Van der Velde et al. described the use of transesophageal echocardiographic (TEE) guidance of transcatheter VSD closure (8). Between January 1990 and November 1992, 31 of 83 (37%) catheterizations for transcatheter VSD closure were performed using TEE guidance. TEE during device deployment allows continuous visualization of device arms and their proximity to the septum and other cardiac structures. Arms that are positioned improperly or that interfere with valve function can be identified and repositioned before releasing the device.

RESULTS

Immediate Results

Between June 1989 and December 2000, a total of 160 patients received a double-umbrella device for closure of VSD at the Children's Hospital, Boston. Most of these patients (142, or 90%) had congenital heart disease. The remaining 18 patients had acquired VSDs. All patients catheterized before May 1996 received the original Clamshell device. Results of preoperative VSD closure using this device were reported by Bridges et al. (3). Subsequently, 75 patients with VSD have received a Clamshell II, CardioSEAL, or STARFlex device.

Sadr et al. reported results of VSD closure with the CardioSEAL device at the Scientific Sessions of the American Heart Association in September 1998 (9). At that time, the CardioSEAL had been implanted in 44 patients with VSD. The median age was 5.1 years (range, 0.5 to 76.5 years). Defects closed included congenital muscular VSDs (45%), postoperative residual defects (39%), fenestrated VSD patches (9%), and postmyocardial infarction defects (7%). A total of 88 devices were implanted during 52 procedures. Although most patients received a single device, 20 received more than one device, and one received seven devices. Small devices were used most frequently, with the 23-mm CardioSEAL accounting for half of the implanted devices and the 17-mm CardioSEAL accounting for another 29%.

Follow-up Results

Follow-up was available in all patients, with a median duration of 7.4 months (range, 0.3 to 21 months). Efficacy of defect closure using the CardioSEAL was assessed in two ways. The first method utilized a clinical outcome scale designed to quantify the degree of VSD flow in a clinically relevant manner. Patients were assigned to one of six categories on this scale, based on degree of shunt or heart fail-

TABLE 29.1. CLINICAL STATUS SCALE

0	Ventilator-dependent or intractable congestive heart failure (CHF)
1	Symptomatic CHF
2	Left ventricular volume overload, large shunt
3	Moderate shunt
4	Small shunt
5	No shunt

From Sadr IM, Jenkins KJ, Satou NL, et al. Transcatheter closure of complex ventricular septal defects using the CardioSEAL device (Abstract). *Circulation* 1998;98:I-755, with permission.

ure (Table 29.1). Patients were assigned a category prior to device placement, and again at each point of follow-up. A successful procedure was defined as one in which the patient experienced improvement by one or more steps on the clinical status scale following device placement. Based on this definition, 88% of patients had a successful procedure. This group of patients, who were described as having at least a moderate shunt prior to device placement, had either a small shunt or no shunt at follow-up.

A second method employed a quantitative assessment of residual flow by echocardiography. Residual flow was graded as trivial/absent, small, or more than small. Using these echocardiographic criteria, the patient group demonstrated a significant decrease in residual flow, with only 10% of patients having more than a small amount of residual flow visible at most recent follow-up.

Complications

Given the technical demands of this procedure, as well as the nature of the patient population, complications must be expected and managed in an anticipatory manner. Laussen et al. reviewed the adverse events encountered in a series of patients undergoing transcatheter closure of VSD with double-umbrella devices at our institution (10). Adverse events were identified retrospectively and classified as procedure related or device related. Of 70 consecutive transcatheter VSD closures with 86 devices, 38 (54%) resulted in blood loss requiring transfusion, 28 (40%) produced significant hypotension (defined as 20% reduction in systolic pressure from baseline), and 20 (26%) provoked an arrhythmia. After catheterization, 50% of the patients were admitted directly to the intensive care unit. There was no procedure- or device-related mortality.

Sadr et al. also found that procedure-related adverse events were frequent (70%), whereas device-related events were less common (2%) using the CardioSEAL device for VSD closure (9). Blood loss requiring transfusion occurred in 23% of this group. Hypotension was the next most common adverse event, and occurred in 16%. Arrhythmia occurred in 9%. Two mortalities were reported in follow-up, neither of which was specifically attributed to the procedure or the device. In univariate analysis, no predictors of adverse events could be identified. During follow-up, two patients experienced serious adverse events that may have been related to the procedure, ventricular tachycardia and aortic regurgitation. Device arm fractures were detected in 14% of patients, with no apparent clinical sequelae.

APPLICABILITY IN ADULT SUBJECTS

Use of the CardioSEAL and STARFlex devices in adult patients has been limited. At the Children's Hospital, Boston, double-umbrella devices have been placed in 18 patients with septal defects resulting from myocardial infarction or trauma. More than half ($N = 10$) of these patients had previously undergone an attempt at surgical closure of the VSD. All had large residual shunts, and all were felt to be at high risk for surgery. Among these 18 patients, 25 devices were placed during 22 separate procedures. With a median follow-up of 11 months (range, 0 to 105 months), there have been seven deaths, none of which was specifically attributed to the device or procedure. The six patients catheterized most recently received either a CardioSEAL or STARFlex device. In 14 months of follow-up (range, 6 to 27 months), there has been no mortality. Echocardiographically, four of these patients have a small residual shunt; two have no detectable shunt. More extensive application of the devices in this adult population may be limited by the currently available sizes, as defects following myocardial infarction or trauma tend to be large and potentially progressive.

DISCUSSION

Current results of transcatheter closure of VSD using the CardioSEAL device are promising, though patient numbers are small. The available reports conclude that the CardioSEAL device can be implanted safely and effectively in patients with complex VSD at high risk for surgical closure. The nature of the VSD may be congenital muscular, residual after surgical VSD repair (including fenestrated patches), or acquired following myocardial infarction. The procedure is successful in 88% of patients. Most patients experience a significant improvement in clinical status. Although adverse events frequently occur at the time of implantation (in up to 70% of patients), late events related to the device or procedure are rare. Data regarding the use of the STARFlex have yet to be reported.

CURRENT STATUS

The CardioSEAL and STARFlex devices have not yet received approval for marketing in the United States. They have earned the CE Mark and are available for sale in Europe, Latin America, and Asia. The CardioSEAL has been awarded a humanitarian device exemption by the US Food and Drug Administration for indications that include VSD, patent foramen ovale, and fenestrated Fontan. A trained practitioner must implant the device, and the local institutional review board must be informed of its use. The STARFlex is currently implanted in high-risk patients with VSD under an investigational device exemption.

Investigators at the Children's Hospital, Boston, are conducting a multicenter study of both the CardioSEAL and STARFlex in high-risk patients. Within the structure of this trial, patients with a VSD of sufficient size to require closure are eligible for entry if they are considered to be at high risk for surgery due to complex medical or cardiac disease. Patients who have an excessively large defect, a defect in close proximity to valves, or vasculature insufficient to accommodate the delivery system are excluded from this trial. An interventional cardiologist assesses technical feasibility of the procedure. If closure is feasible, an independent team, consisting of a cardiologist and a cardiovascular surgeon, reviews the case to determine whether the patient meets the high-risk admission criteria. Patients must agree to participate in follow-up and must provide informed consent.

CONCLUSION

The currently available closure devices and the cumulative experience in their use have brought to light the necessary characteristics of a successful VSD device. Because of the complex morphology of the interventricular septum, the device must be able to assume a stable position and conform to the local anatomy in a variety of defect configurations. It should be able to close a defect effectively without excessive projection into the cardiac chambers or impairment of valve function. The CardioSEAL and STARFlex devices have been designed and engineered to close even the most complex VSDs. These devices have been implanted in 75 patients to close defects ranging from tunnel-like muscular VSDs to fenestrations in surgical VSD patches. Additional prospective evaluation of these devices, as well as close review of the experience to date, will enlighten the ongoing practice of transcatheter VSD closure.

REFERENCES

1. Prieto LR, Foreman CK, Cheatham JP, et al. Intermediate-term outcome of transcatheter secundum atrial septal defect closure using the Bard Clamshell Septal Umbrella. *Am J Cardiol* 1996;78:1310–1312.
2. Kreutzer J, Ryan CA, Wright JA, et al. Acute animal studies of the STARFlex system: a new self-centering CardioSEAL septal occluder. *Catheter Cardiovasc Interv* 2000;49:225–233.
3. Bridges ND, Perry SB, Keane JF, et al. Preoperative transcatheter closure of congenital muscular ventricular septal defects. *N Engl J Med* 1991;324:1312–1317.

4. Preminger TJ, Sanders SP, van der Velde ME, et al. "Intramural" residual interventricular defects after repair of conotruncal malformations. *Circulation* 1994;89:236–242.

5. Love BA, Lang P, Jonas RA, et al. Ventricular septal defect patch fenestration in repair of tetralogy of Fallot with diminutive pulmonary arteries. *J Am Coll Cardiol* 1998;31:190A(Abstract).

6. Kumar K, Lock jE, Geva T. Apical muscular ventricular septal defects between the left ventricle and the right ventricular infundibulum: diagnostic and interventional considerations. *Circulation* 1997;95:1207–1213.

7. Rocchini A, Lock JE. Defect closure: umbrella devices. In: Lock JE, Keane JF, Perry SB, eds. *Diagnostic and interventional catheterization in congenital heart disease.* Norwell, MA: Kluwer Academic Publishers, 2000:179–198.

8. Van der Velde ME, Sanders SP, Keane JF, et al. Transesophageal echocardiographic guidance of transcatheter ventricular septal defect closure. *J Am Coll Cardiol* 1994;23:1660–1665.

9. Sadr IM, Jenkins KJ, Satou NL, et al. Transcatheter closure of complex ventricular septal defects using the CardioSEAL device (Abstract). *Circulation* 1998;98:I-755.

10. Laussen PC, Hansen DD, Perry SB, et al. Transcatheter closure of ventricular septal defects: hemodynamic instability and anesthetic management. *Anesth Analg* 1995;80:1076–1082.

30

NIT-OCCLUD
(NICKEL-TITANIUM SPIRAL COIL)

TRONG-PHI LÊ
PETER VAESSEN
FRANZ FREUDENTHAL
RALPH G. GRABITZ
HORST SIEVERT

Transcatheter occlusion of ventricular septal defects (VSDs) is considered to be one of the most sophisticated and complex interventional procedures. Most current transcatheter closure devices, however, target the muscular VSD. Some devices, mainly umbrella-shaped systems with radial arms, have been used to close subaortic VSD with relatively poor results. No device is yet considered established for the occlusion of subaortic VSD. Coils are proved to be flexible and therefore better adaptable to cardiac structures. Because of the superelastic properties, coils made of Nitinol have an excellent shape memory. In this chapter we will describe a new technique using a reinforced double-disk Nitinol coil to close subaortic VSD in an animal study. The same technique has been successfully used in the first four human subjects. Those data will also be presented.

DEVICE

Nitinol is biocompatible and has superelastic properties and excellent shape memory. The Nit-Occlud device (Pfm, Cologne, Germany) is constructed from 0.25-mm Nitinol wire and has primary windings and secondary coil loops. Primary windings are made around a straight core wire, producing a highly flexible, straight tension spring with an internal diameter of 0.25 mm and an outer diameter of 0.96 mm. A 0.04-mm flat wire is inserted into the lumen of the primary windings to enhance their stiffness. The thickness of the inserted flat wire becomes reduced toward the proximal part of the device. This spring is wound around a fixture with an hourglass shape and shock-heated. This process forms permanent secondary coil loops resulting in two disks with a 2-mm small central part. The distal (left ventricular) disk is larger and much stiffer than the proximal (right ventricular) disk. Devices with a distal loop diameter of 9 to 15 mm were available for study. The corresponding proximal loop diameters were 7 to 10 mm respectively. The proximal disk is reversed so that the device has a cone-in-cone shape. Once the device is placed the two disks are closely apposed to the septum. The device is shown in Figure 30.1. The proximal end of the device has a microscrew for attachment to the core wire of the delivery system. The detachment force is 12 to 15 N. Detachment of the Nit-Occlud is accomplished by forcefully pushing the pusher over the core wire, similar to the Duct-Occlud device (1). The Nit-Occlud device is mounted in a straightened fashion on a flexible delivery system connected to a disposable deployment handle (Figure 30.2).

With the device properly positioned, the safety clip is removed from the handle and the rotation screw is turned clockwise until the coil is released under fluoroscopic control.

Trong-Phi Lê: Consultant, Department of Pediatric Cardiology, University of Hamburg, Hamburg, Germany; Chief, Department of Pediatric Cardiology, Central Hospital lindes der Weser, Brennen, Germany

Peter Vaessen: Fellow, Department of Pediatric Cardiology, University of Achen, Achen, Germany

Franz Freudenthal: Fellow, Department of Radiology, Technical University of Achen, Achen, Germany

Ralph G. Grabitz: Associate Professor, Department of Pediatric Cardiology, University of Kiel, Kiel, Germany

Horst Sievert: Professor of Internal Medicine and Cardiology, Cardiovascular Center Bethanien, Frankfurt, Germany

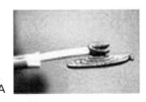
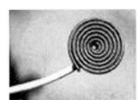

FIGURE 30.1. The Nit-Occlud device. The distal disk is configured outside the implantation catheter (**A**) that was introduced in the 8F long sheath (**B**).

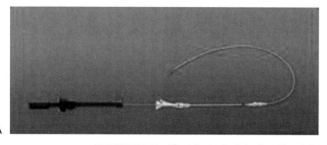
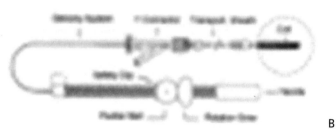

A   B

FIGURE 30.2. The Nit-Occlud device. The delivery system of the deployment handle is connected to a 5F implantation catheter through a Y-connector. The safety clip has to be loosened before moving the pusher ball forward for device detachment.

EXPERIMENTAL STUDIES

Hemodynamic and Angiographic Evaluation

A special breed of Yucatan micropigs with congenital subaortic VSD (Figure 30.3) was selected for the experimental studies. The approximate size of each defect was assessed with cross-sectional transthoracic echocardiography, which was performed in the catheter laboratory using a Kontron ultrasound scanner (Sigma 44 HVCD) with a 5-MHz transducer. Before the interventional procedure the micropigs underwent right and left cardiac catheterization. After obtaining vascular access percutaneously from the right femoral vein and artery, oxygen saturations and pressures were measured in left and right heart chambers. The location and size of the VSD were determined by angiography using 30- to 40-degree left anterior oblique view with cranial angulation. Measurements were corrected for magnification based on known spacing of radiopaque markers

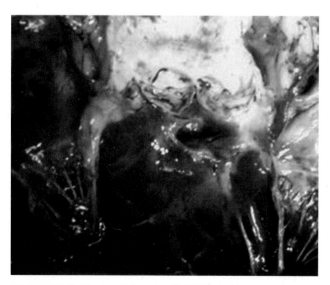

FIGURE 30.3. Congenital subaortic VSD in a Yucatan micropig. Left ventricular view. Note the close proximity to the aortic valve.

on the catheter (OccluMarker, Pfm, Cologne, Germany). The location of the VSD was correctly predicted from echocardiography in five of 12 micropigs. Based on the information available in each angiogram, we measured the distance between the septal rim and the aortic annulus. The distance from the VSD to the aortic valve was also measured to ensure that device placement would not compromise the aortic valve function. We did not measure the defect diameter using the balloon occlusion technique.

Occlusion Technique

After confirming the location, the VSD was crossed from the left ventricle with a coronary catheter or an end-hole balloon catheter. To create an arteriovenous loop a guide wire (Terumo) was advanced through the end-hole catheter into the pulmonary artery or the vena cava. The tip of the Teruno wire was captured with a snare (Microvena Corporation, White Bear Lake, MN). Thus at this stage the one end of the loop wire remained outside the body at the femoral artery and the other end was retrieved and brought outside the body through the femoral vein. A venous 8- or 9F long sheath was then introduced over the wire loop and was advanced into the ascending aorta. Before introducing the long venous sheath a 5F end-hole catheter was advanced arterially over the wire loop to prevent injury of the aortic valve due to the traction force on the wire loop. After confirming the correct position of the long sheath with its tip placed in the left ventricular outflow tract or in the ascending aorta, the wire loop was removed. Cartoon representation of these steps is shown in Figure 30.4.

The sizes of the left ventricular disk were selected to achieve a device-to-defect diameter ratio of approximately 2:1. The 5F delivery catheter with the premounted coil was introduced into the long sheath. The coil was then advanced and configured in the ascending aorta in such a way that only two or three proximal coil loops remained inside the implantation catheter. Then the whole delivery system (i.e., long sheath and delivery catheter) was carefully withdrawn into the left ventricle. By doing this the coil moves toward the septum and rotates when it adapts to the

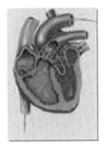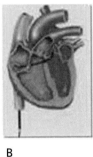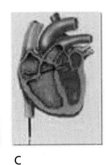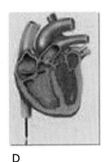

A   B   C   D

FIGURE 30.4. Key steps of the coil implantation procedure. **A:** After crossing the VSD by a guide wire an arteriovenous loop is created. **B:** The distal disk of the Nit-Occlud is constituted in the ascending aorta. **C:** The configured coil is pulled back into the left ventricular outflow tract. **D:** The Nit-Occlud coil is placed in the VSD.

defect. At this point the long sheath was moved very carefully back into the right ventricle with its tip kept close to the septum. The implantation catheter was then pulled into the right ventricle. At the same time the proximal two or three loops of the coil were pushed out of the implantation catheter to be positioned on the right side of the defect. Repeated hand injections of contrast medium were performed through a pig-tail catheter that was kept close to the coil during the implantation procedure to document the position of the device (Figure 30.5). After confirming the correct and safe configuration of the coil in the defect, the pusher was forcefully moved forward to free the coil from the attaching mechanism at the tip of the core wire. Left ventricular and the aortic angiograms were performed after device detachment to assess its position and the efficacy of closure (Figure 30.6). Follow-up studies with clinical examination and angiogram were undertaken at various times after coil implantation.

Follow-up Evaluation

The follow-up studies with angiograms of both ventricles and the aorta were performed at variable intervals. To investigate the effects of long-term implantation, the animals were restudied at 3, 6, and 11 months after defect closure. After angiography was performed, the animals were eutha-

nized. Both ventricles along with the aortic and the tricuspid valve were opened for gross examination. The device and surrounding ventricular septum were subjected for histopathologic examination.

Results

Twelve Yucatan micropigs with the clinical evidence of a VSD entered the study. The body weight of the micropigs ranged from 25 to 65 kg. In all animals the VSD was subaortic. The sizes of the defect ranged from 4 to 12 mm, measured by means of transthoracic echocardiography and/or left ventricular angiography. In all cases the distance between the defect rim and the aortic annulus was less than 10 mm. The pulmonary/systemic flow ratio (Qp:Qs) varied from 2.0 to 3.8 (mean, 2.7). Systolic pulmonary artery pressure was normal in all cases. Two animals had moderate mitral regurgitation. No incompetence of the aortic and atrioventricular valves was observed.

No implantation could be performed in three cases. Two animals died of complete heart block during creation of the arteriovenous loop before the device implantation procedure. In one animal the defect size was too large to close with the available devices at that time; therefore we abandoned the procedure. Additional procedural problems occurred in our study. The device embolized into the pul-

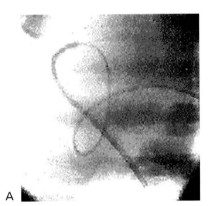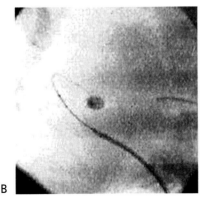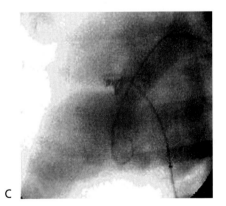

A   B   C

FIGURE 30.5. Implantation procedure in Yucatan micropigs. **A:** Long sheath advanced transvenously over the arteriovenous loop. **B:** Coil positioned in VSD. **C:** Control left ventricular angiogram before coil detachment.

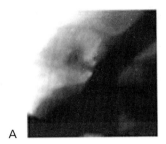
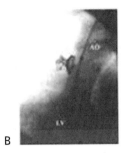
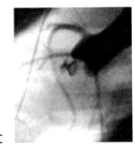

FIGURE 30.6. VSD occlusion in a Yucatan micropig. **A:** Angiogram of the LV. **B:** The Nit-Occlud coil is well positioned in the VSD. **C:** The aortic valve remained competent despite the close proximity to the device.

monary artery immediately after detachment in two cases. These were left in place and another larger device was implanted. In two cases the coil got entangled in the mitral valve. However, this occurred in the early phases of the study, when we were exposing the coil in the left ventricle and not in the ascending aorta.

We have successfully implanted the Nitinol coil in nine animals. The defect diameters ranged from 4 to 10 mm, with an average of 7 mm. In five cases the procedure was successful at first attempt. In the remaining four cases a second procedure was necessary that was carried out a few weeks after the first attempt. At the time of the last follow-up angiogram before the sacrifice, complete occlusion was observed in five cases, in which the coil had been implanted, respectively, 11 months ($N = 3$) and 6 months ($N = 2$) before. In four cases in which the coil implantation procedure had been performed 3 months ($N = 3$) and 6 months ($N = 1$) previously, a residual leak remained. Of the residual shunts two were small and two were moderate.

Neither insufficiency of the aortic and tricuspid valve nor arrhythmias were noted during follow-up. In one of the two cases with moderate residual leak, the coil was found embolized into the pulmonary artery at the followup angiogram 3 months after implantation. One coil fracture was detected at control angiogram 6 months after implantation. However, the device remained in a stable position without impairment of the aortic and tricuspid valve and the defect was completely closed.

Anatomic and Histopathologic Study

Three months after implantation, the device was partially covered by a tissue layer. The device was subtotally embedded into the tissue after 6 months of implantation. At 11 months after implantation the device was totally covered by a smooth tissue layer. In all cases histopathologic examinations revealed the existence of endothelium with some signs of nonspecific local inflammation and partial calcification. These findings are very similar to the results of studies of other implants performed previously (2).

CLINICAL STUDIES

Patients and Methods

Thus far the Nit-Occlud device has been implanted in five adult patients (aged 36 to 60 years; mean, 46) following successful device implantation in animal models. Patients were selected based on prior echocardiographic examination that demonstrated a defect size of less than 5 mm. Three patients had a subaortic VSD and two patients had a high muscular VSD. The pulmonary vascular resistance was normal in all patients. Unlike the animal study described earlier, the VSD in the human was also measured using the balloon-stretching technique to prevent underestimation of the defect size. For this purpose a 7F end-hole balloon catheter was advanced over the loop wire into the left ventricle. The angiographically measured diameter of the VSD was 4 or 5 mm; the corresponding balloon sizing diameter was 7 or 8 mm. In all cases the distance between the defect and the aortic annulus was more than 10 mm. In patients with subaortic perimembranous VSD a 15-mm device was used. In patients with high muscular VSD the selected device had a distal diameter of 11 mm.

Results

The Nit-Occlud device has been safely implanted in four cases: two subaortic and two high muscular VSD. The implantation procedure was abandoned in one patient with subaortic VSD as a result of unsatisfactory device configuration. Neither procedure-related problems nor other complications occurred. Neither impairment of the tricuspid and aortic valve nor arrhythmia was observed. A trace of residual shunt was demonstrated in the angiogram immediately after device detachment (Figure 30.7). Complete occlusion was proved using color flow mapping in two patients with perimembranous VSD in one patient with high muscular VSD. Further follow-up data are not available at this time.

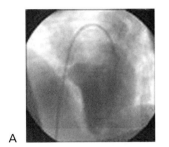 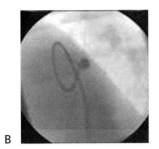 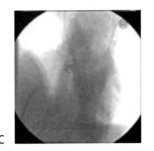 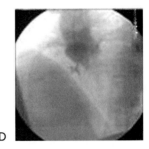

A   B   C   D

FIGURE 30.7. VSD occlusion in human. **A:** Angiogram of the left ventricular (LV). **B:** Balloon sizing of the VSD using a 7F end-hole balloon catheter. **C:** Angiogram of the LV after coil implantation. **D:** Angiogram of the aorta.

DISCUSSION

Umbrella-shaped devices have been shown to be suitable and effective in occlusion of muscular VSDs (3–7). In subaortic VSDs with close proximity of the aortic and the tricuspid valve there is a great potential of valve impairment. Occlusion devices with metallic struts radiating from the center for support of the fabric patches or with sharp edges are likely to cause perforation or laceration of the aortic valve (4,8). If the metal frame of the device is rigid, the cardiac structures around the VSD and even the ventricular geometry may be compromised (5).

The Gianturco coil was occasionally used for occlusion of very small muscular or membranous VSD with aneurysm (9,10). The Nit-Occlud device with its disklike circular geometry and rounded edges is less rigid. The central portion of the Nit-Occlud system is much more flexible than other currently available devices. The spiral loops of the disk are close but not adhesive to each other, so they could easily get into contact with the ventricular wall. This elastic property enables better adaptation of the device to the anatomy of the respective VSD. Distortion of the adjacent cardiac structure is avoided. Also, the circular geometry of the spiral loops seems to cause less diastolic disturbance of the ventricle.

The formation of the distal disk of the Nit-Occlud device in the left ventricular outflow tract was proved undesirable because of the risk of involvement of the mitral valve apparatus. Because of the flexible central portion of the device, withdrawal of the configured distal disk from the ascending aorta into the left ventricle was not injurious to the aortic valve.

For the choice of a proper size of the device to be used, it is very important to measure the stretched diameter of subaortic VSD, which is probably more elastic than the muscular defect. The subaortic and muscular VSD are frequently oval rather than round. Using an echocardiogram or angiogram of the left ventricle, only the smaller diameter of the oval VSD can be measured.

We advocate the use of an 8F long sheath for the implantation procedure because it is useful to stabilize the 5F implantation catheter. The long sheath appears to avoid engagement of coil loops with the adjacent valve apparatus. If necessary, the configured coil could be pulled back into the sufficiently large lumen of the long sheath to be safely removed.

Because the Nit-Occlud device does not bear thrombogenic fibers, complete occlusion of the defect is usually delayed. This phenomenon is comparable to the data of occlusion of patent ductus arteriosus using the stainless steel Duct-Occlud device, which is also free of thrombogenic fibers (1). The overall occlusion rate in PDA was reported to be 95% after 6 months of implantation. A similar occlusion rate could probably be expected in VSD using the Nit-Occlud device. The Nit-Occlud device with a maximum distal disk diameter of 16 mm is suitable for subaortic VSD with a stretched diameter of up to 8 mm. The Nit-Occlud device seems to be well suited for avoiding the risk of impairment of the aortic and tricuspid valves. Further data are necessary to judge the efficacy and safety of this new occlusion technique.

ACKNOWLEDGMENTS

We thank our friend and colleague Dr. Malte Neuss for his artwork and the Pfm Company (Cologne, Germany) for technical support.

REFERENCES

1. Lê TP, Moore JW, Neuss MB, et al. Duct-Occlud for occlusion of patent ductus arteriosus. *Curr Interv Cardiol Rep* 2001;3:165–173.
2. Sigler M, Handt S, Seghaye MC, et al. Evaluation of *in vivo* biocompatibility of different devices for interventional closure of the patent ductus arteriosus in an animal model. *Heart* 2000;83: 570–573.
3. Lock JE, Block PC, McKay RG, et al. Transcatheter closure of ventricular septal defects. *Circulation* 1988;78:361–368.
4. Sideris EB, Walsh KP, Haddad JL et al. Occlusion of congenital ventricular septal defects by the buttoned device. *Heart* 1997;77: 276–279.
5. Janorkar S, Goh T, Wilkinson J. Transcatheter closure of ventric-

ular septal defects using the Rashkind device: initial experience. *Catheter Cardiovasc Interv* 1999;46:43–48.

6. Thanopoulos BD, Tsaousis GS, Konstadopoulou GN, et al. Transcatheter closure of muscular ventricular septal defects with the Amplatzer ventricular septal defect occluder: initial clinical applications in children. *J Am Coll Cardiol* 1999;33:1395–1399.

7. Hijazi ZM, Hakim F, Al-Fadley F, et al. Transcatheter closure of single muscular ventricular septal defects using the Amplatzer muscular VSD occluder: initial results and technical considerations. *Catheter Cardiovasc Interv* 2000;49:167–172.

8. Vogel M, Rigby ML, Shore D. Perforation of the right aortic valve cusp: complication of ventricular septal defect closure with a modified Rashkind umbrella. *Pediatr Cardiol* 1996;17:416–418.

9. Latiff HA, Alwi M, Kandhavel G, et al. Transcatheter closure of multiple muscular ventricular septal defects using Gianturco coils. *Ann Thorac Surg* 1999;68:1400–1401.

10. Kalra GS, Verma PK, Singh S, et al. Transcatheter closure of ventricular septal defect using detachable steel coil. *Heart* 1999;82: 395–396.

31

TRANSCATHETER APPROACH TO POSTMYOCARDIAL INFARCTION VENTRICULAR SEPTAL RUPTURE AND PARAVALVAR REGURGITATION

MICHAEL J. LANDZBERG

The modern translational approach to medical research utilizes concepts recognized by one scientific discipline and adapts and applies them to a second, related field. By these means, previously held beliefs regarding restrictions to understanding or care can occasionally be torn down, new paradigms can be fashioned, and improved solutions to "unsolvable problems" may be formulated.

This chapter focuses on adaptations of accepted transcatheter approaches to congenital cardiac disease applied to two threatening causes of cardiac failure encountered primarily in the world of acquired adult cardiovascular disease. These include management of (a) patients with postmyocardial infarction (MI) ventricular septal rupture (VSR) and (b) patients with symptomatic paravalvar regurgitation. To date, although anecdotal use of various occlusion devices for such purposes has been noted (Amplatzer, AGA Medical, Golden Valley, MN), the greatest reported experience remains with double-umbrella device strategies, utilizing the Rashkind PDA Occluder (USCI, Billerica, MA), Bard Clamshell Septal Occluder (USCI, Billerica, MA), CardioSEAL (Nitinol Medical Technologies, Boston, MA), and STARFlex (Nitinol Medical Technologies, Boston, MA) devices, as well as transcatheter-delivered coils (Embolization coils, Cook Incorporated, Bloomington, IN). These experiences will be highlighted.

POSTMYOCARDIAL VENTRICULAR SEPTAL RUPTURE

Despite advances in the management of acute coronary syndromes, rupture of the interventricular septum remains

Michael J. Landzberg: Assistant Professor, Department of Medicine, Harvard University; Director, Boston Adult Congenital Heart (BACH) Service, Department of Cardiology, Brigham and Women's Hospital and Children's Hospital, Boston, Massachusetts

one of the most threatening complications of MI. With the more widespread utilization of acute reperfusion strategies, the incidence of post-MI VSR has been reduced to under 0.5% of all persons with MI, yet its occurrence carries highest risk of mortality (1). Surgical strategies emphasizing total exclusion of infarcted regions of the ventricular septum (typically from left ventricular apex to base, and free wall to mitral valve annulus) have markedly improved outcomes, but, to date, they have not been universally applied, and described success has not been generally reproduced (2).

In the late 1980s and early 1990s, Bridges and colleagues proposed the sentinel use of transcatheter occlusion of congenital muscular ventricular septal defects, a strategy aimed at supporting available surgical repair (3). They emphasized (a) use of the left ventricular approach to intubate the defect (to ensure positioning through the widest aspect of the passage); (b) a transseptal approach, as feasible, to the left ventricle (decreasing intraprocedural, catheter-induced aortic regurgitation, and allowing for potential for either transvenous or transarterial device delivery, as appropriate by defect location); (c) finessed angiography performed by injection of contrast within the defect using biplane imaging (to best understand anatomically the defect and its relationship to surrounding structures); and (d) maintenance of position with secure extra-long stiff wires (to best enable delivery system and device passage to, and within, the defect). Double-umbrella devices appeared sufficiently suited to the application of transcatheter VSD closure given their ability to (a) have differing conformations (flattening against the interventricular septum, or, remaining partially expanded, to provide for best defect occlusion); (b) be applied from either an RV or LV approach, to allow for safest and most secure device deployment; and (c) be retrieved, or repositioned, from a transcatheter approach, with relative ease and safety. The success of transcatheter closure techniques for management of congenital muscular VSDs, combined with both the presence of a joint pediatric and adult cardiovascular team and program (intimately familiar with anatomic and physiologic principles of acquired and congenital disease) and the lack of sufficient success with existing surgical therapies, led to our consideration of transcatheter device closure techniques for the management of patients with post-MI VSR.

Success of surgical repair of post-MI VSR appeared to be limited by (a) patch dehiscence (due either to lack of sufficient "healthy" tissue to anchor sutures or to continued necrosis at suture sites), (b) "acute or chronic" cardiac pump failure, worsened by the combination of MI, increasing intracardiac shunting, and cardiopulmonary bypass; and (c) development of multisystem organ failure, related to worsening systemic cardiac output. Transcatheter techniques offered potential relief from these restrictions due to device ability to fill a defect rather than to suture to its margins, as well as to provide patients with extremely rapid, if not immediate, access to "cardiopulmonary-bypass-free" therapy, in the catheterization laboratory.

Knowledge of the anatomy and physiology of post-MI VSR suggested particular challenges for transcatheter closure. Infarction led to necrosis along atypical planes, with

formation of rents within the ventricular septum that did not conform to similar locations on both ventricular surfaces. Necrotic holes within these serpiginous tracts were apparent, adding to potential spaces that might lead to multiple burrowing exits to the right ventricle. Conformational flexibility of double-umbrella devices appeared to allow adjustment for these anatomic variations. Ischemic injury raised the risk of development of intraprocedural heart block or ventricular tachycardia. Cardiology and anesthesia staff who are experienced managing congenital and ischemic cardiopulmonary disease and failure in both children and adults were essential to reduce the potential for such intraprocedural hemodynamic and electrical compromise.

From December 1989 until February 2001, 21 patients (median age 70 years) with post-MI VSR who were considered to have severe or prohibitive risk for surgical defect closure presented for consideration of transcatheter closure (4). Prior VSR surgical closure had been attempted in 14 of 21 patients. At catheterization, shunt was significant in all but one patient. One or more devices (Bard Septal Clamshell Occluder, CardioSEAL, or STARFlex: Nitinol Medical Technologies, Boston, MA) were successfully placed in either the primary interventricular necrotic lake or an operative patch margin, depending upon where the minimal

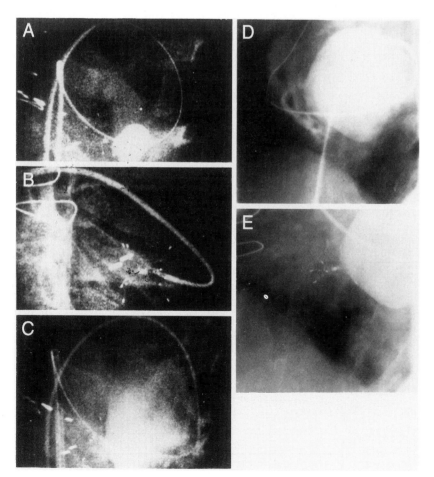

FIGURE 31.1. Balloon stretch sizing (**A**) of the central necrotic portion of a postoperative residual patch margin defect after primary suture repair of VSR following MI in a patient requiring mechanical inotropic support. Transseptal deployment of a Clamshell Occluder (**B**) led to moderate acute decrease in angiographic shunt (**C**), but patient markedly improved to NYHA II symptoms. Shunt flow (**D**) can be totally eliminated (**E**) in some patients with transcatheter closure of postoperative residual shunting of VSR post-MI.

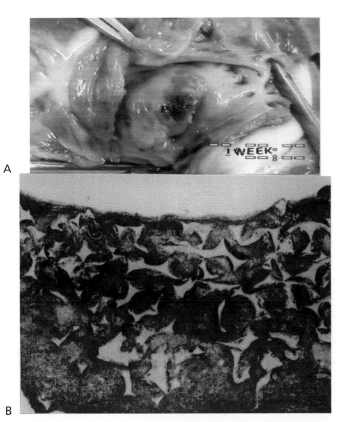

A

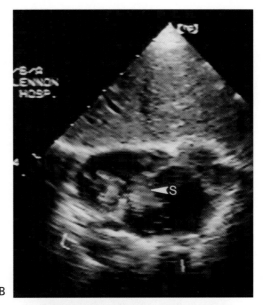

B

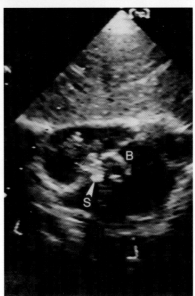

D

B

COLOR FIGURE 9.4. A: Patch pathology 10 days after implantation. The patch is fully covered by endothelium. **B:** Histology of transcatheter patch 48 hours after implantation. The patch is covered by fibrin and is attached to the endocardium.

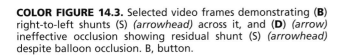

COLOR FIGURE 14.3. Selected video frames demonstrating **(B)** right-to-left shunts (S) *(arrowhead)* across it, and **(D)** *(arrow)* ineffective occlusion showing residual shunt (S) *(arrowhead)* despite balloon occlusion. B, button.

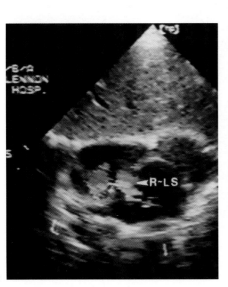

B

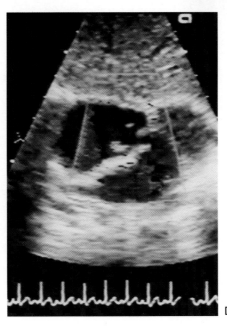

COLOR FIGURE 14.7. Selected frames from video recordings of two-dimensional echocardiographic studies from subcostal four chamber views demonstrating right-to-left shunt (R~LS) *(arrowhead)* in **(B)**. Following inverted button device, the shunt is no longer seen **(D)**.

D

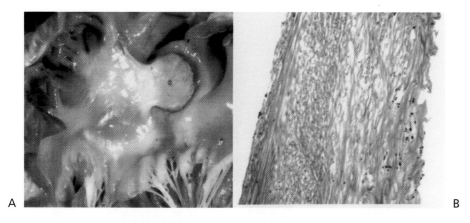

A

B

COLOR FIGURE 13.3. A: Postmortem cardiac specimen harvested from a minipig 3 months after implantation of an Amplatzer PFO Occluder revealing complete coverage of the device with neoendocardium. **B:** Microscopic view (original magnification, 160×) of specimen in (**A**) revealing coverage of both sides of the device with intact neoendocardium. (Both figures were obtained from Han YM, Gu X, Titus JL, et al. New self-expanding patent foramen ovale occlusion device. *Catheter Cardiovasc Interv* 1999;47:370–376, with permission of Wiley-Liss Publishing Company, New York.)

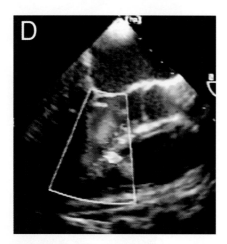

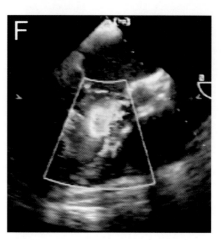

COLOR FIGURE 28.4. Transesophageal echocardiographic (TEE) images. **D:** TEE image with color Doppler in a 31.5-year-old 123.5-kg male with a 4.5-mm mid-muscular VSD and a Qp:Qs ratio of 1.5:1. **F:** TEE image with color Doppler after a 6-mm Amplatzer MVSD device *(arrow)* has been deployed demonstrating good device position and no residual shunt. MVSD, muscular ventricular septal defect; VSD, ventricular septal defect.

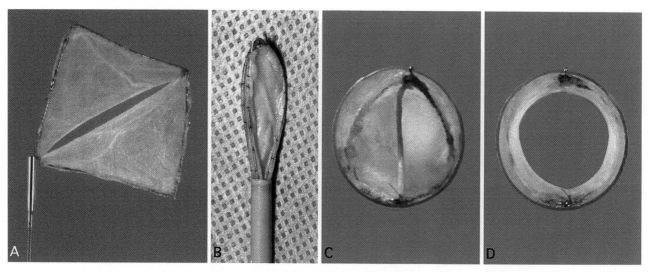

COLOR FIGURE 49.1. Small intestine submucose (SIS) aortic valve model. **A:** Unrestricted valve 30 mm long retained by a wire pusher connected to a barb. **B:** Valve partially front-loaded into a 10F sheath. **C:** Valve deployed in a plastic tube 20 mm in diameter, closed position. **D:** Open position.

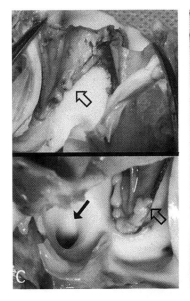
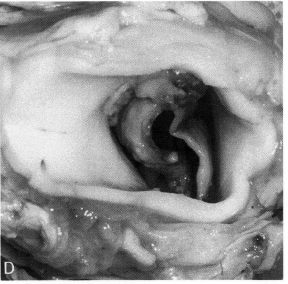

COLOR FIGURE 49.2. SIS aortic valve in supracoronary position in ascending aorta of a swine 2 weeks after placement. **C:** Side views of the specimen show incorporation of the bicuspid valve into aortic wall *(open arrows)* and patent coronary arteries *(arrow).* **D:** View from above shows bicuspid valve.

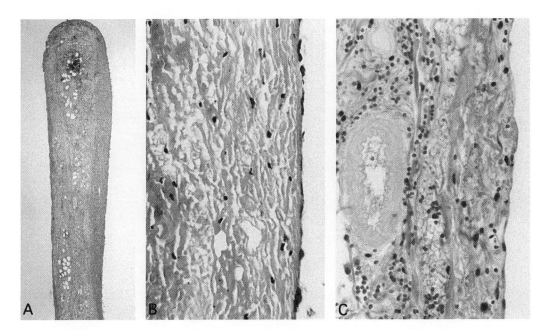

COLOR FIGURE 49.3. Photomicrographs of the SIS aortic valve 2 and 4 weeks after implantation into porcine aorta. **A:** A longitudinal cross section of aortic valve at 2 weeks shows early remodeling. **B:** Magnified view of the partially remodeled part of the SIS leaflet at 2 weeks shows collagenous tissue stroma with fibrocytes and endothelial cells covering valve leaflet (Hematoxylin and eosin stain, original magnification, 200×.) **C:** High magnification of the SIS leaflet with endothelial lining at 4 weeks shows remodeling of the SIS by collagenized fibrous tissue and numerous capillaries. (Hematoxylin and eosin stain; original magnification, 400×.)

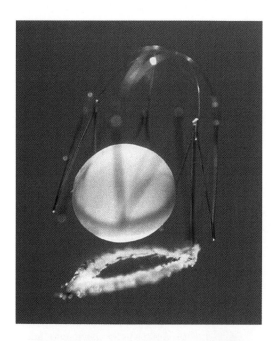

COLOR FIGURE 49.4. Caged-ball valve for percutaneous transcatheter placement. The three main components of the prosthesis (cage, ring, and ball) are depicted.

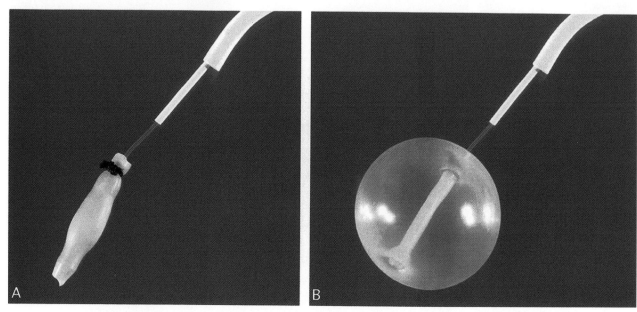

COLOR FIGURE 49.5. Detachable latex balloon used as the ball. The balloon is attached to a 5F catheter, which is passed coaxially through the Teflon introducer sheath. **A:** Noninflated latex balloon. **B:** Latex balloon filled with the air.

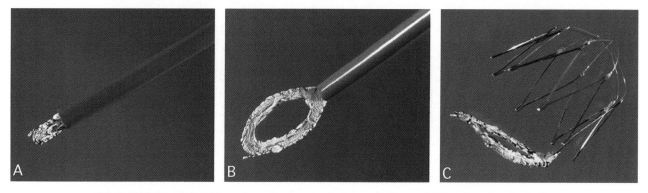

COLOR FIGURE 49.6. Collapsed prosthetic valve being pushed out of 12F Teflon sheath. **A:** The ring with anchoring barbs is just beginning to emerge from the sheath. **B:** Self-expanding ring is covered with nylon mesh. **C:** Self-expanding ring and the cage.

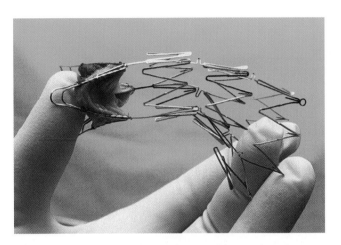

COLOR FIGURE 49.9. Nitinol stent aortic bioprosthetic valve. (Reproduced, courtesy of Dr. T Peschel.)

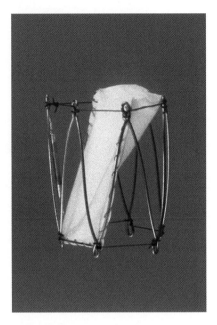

COLOR FIGURE 49.12. Monocusp Z-stent valve. (Reproduced, courtesy of Barry Uchida.)

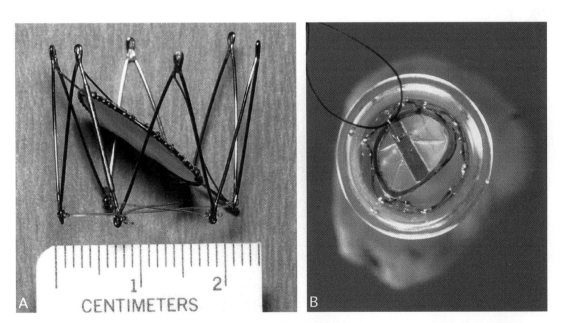

COLOR FIGURE 49.10. Expanded valve cage with anchored disk in a plastic tube. **A:** Side view. **B:** Axial view from above. (From Sochman J, Peregrin J, Pavčnik D, et al. Percutaneous transcatheter aortic disc valve prosthesis implantation: a feasibility study *Cardiovasc Intervent Radiol* 2000;23:384–388, with permission.)

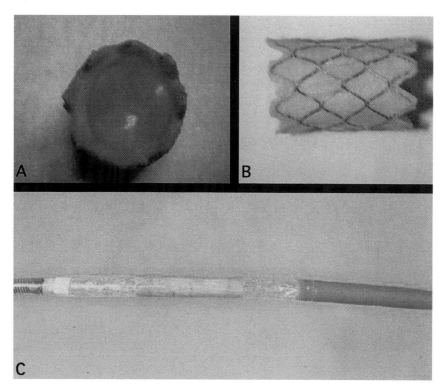

COLOR FIGURE 49.13. Valved stent. **A:** Closed jugular valve mounted in the stent. **B:** Profile of the valved stent before compression. **C:** Valved stent in the delivery system. (From Bonhoeffer P, Boudjemline Y, Saliba Z, et al. Percutaneous replacement of pulmonary valve in a right-ventricle to pulmonary-artery prosthetic conduit with valve dysfunction. *Lancet* 2000;356:1403–1405, with permission.)

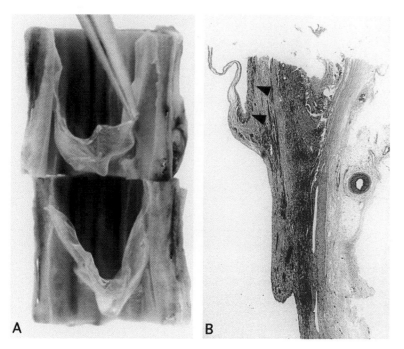

COLOR FIGURE 49.17. Histology of the bioprosthesis. **A:** Gross photograph of the venous valve leaflets (longitudinal bisection). **B:** Microscopic view of venous valve segment shows no thrombus in the lumen. More prominent endothelial cells noted at the base of the valve *(arrowheads).* (Reproduced, courtesy of Dr. Jackeline Gomez-Jorge.)

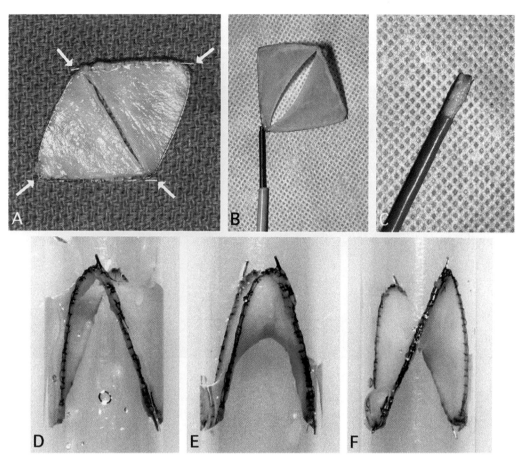

COLOR FIGURE 49.18. Venous valve model. A: Nonrestricted valve 20 mm long with four barbs *(arrows)*. B: Valve retained by a wire pusher connected to one barb. C: Valve front-loaded into a 9F guiding catheter. D: Deployed valve in a plastic tube, open position. E: Deployed valve in a plastic tube, closed position. F: Deployed valve in a plastic tube, oblique view, closed position.

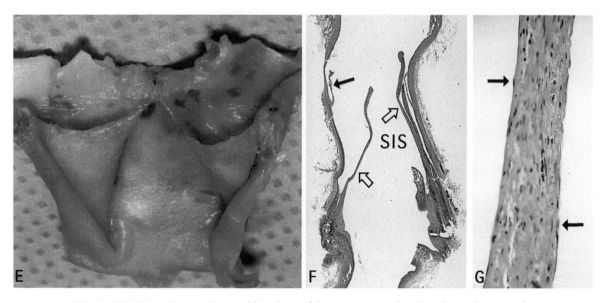

COLOR FIGURE 49.20. Function and histology of the SIS venous valve placed into sheep jugular vein 13 mm in diameter. E: One-month jugular vein specimen shows smooth incorporation of the valve into the vein wall. F: Longitudinal microscopic view of both SIS leaflets *(open arrows)* in original size. Native valve is visible *(arrow)*. G: Magnified view of the remodeled SIS leaflet reveals host tissue replacement and collagenous stroma remodeling with fibrocytes, plasma cells, and lymphocytes. Vascular endothelial cells *(arrows)* cover valve leaflet. (Hematoxylin and eosin stain; original magnification, 400×.)

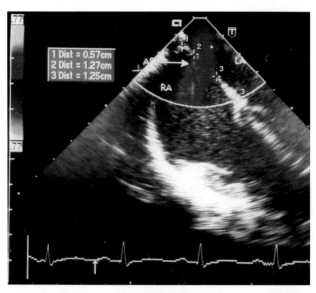

COLOR FIGURE 52.1. Transesophageal echocardiographic four-chamber view of the heart in transverse plane, showing the lengths of superior (1) and inferior (3) rims and the size of the atrial septal defect (2). The color flow through the defect *(arrow)* from the left atrium (LA) to the right atrium (RA) helps to delineate the size of the defect. ASD, atrial septal defect.

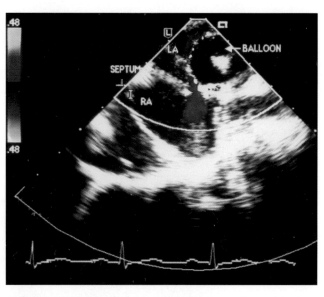

B

COLOR FIGURE 52.2. Transesophageal echocardiographic view. **B:** Residual leakage around the balloon, not apparent in two-dimensional echocardiography, became evident on color flow mapping indicated by *arrowheads.* LA, left atrium; RA, right atrium.

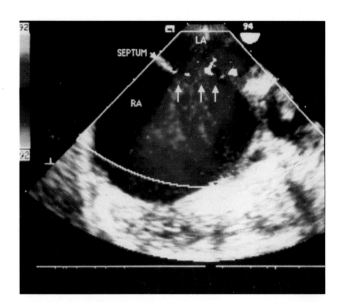

COLOR FIGURE 52.3. Basal four-chamber view in transverse plane showing fenestrated atrial septal defects with multiple holes indicated by *arrows.* The color flow through the three defects delineated the fenestrated defect. LA, left atrium; RA, right atrium.

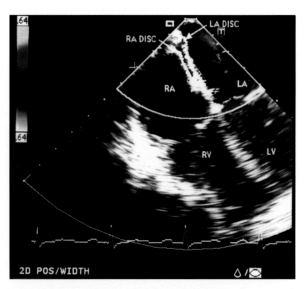

COLOR FIGURE 52.5. B: Color flow mapping in the same view shows no residual leakage across the defect and device, indicating the complete closure of the defect. LA, left atrium; LV, left ventricle; RA, right atrium; RV, right ventricle.

balloon stretch diameter of passage was found, in all remaining 20 patients. An initial transseptal approach to the ruptured septum was favored. Angiographic shunting improved in nearly all, with few patients having complete relief of intracardiac passage (Figure 31.1). When measured, oximetric shunt showed little immediate change. Success was similar, regardless of inferior or anterior VSR location. Procedural complications included blood loss eventuating in transfusion ($N = 8$), worsening of renal insufficiency ($N = 1$), device embolization ($N = 1$), transient catheterization-induced arrhythmia ($N = 3$), and ICD lead failure ($N = 1$). Clinical evidence of improved hemodynamics was evident in 20/20 patients undergoing transcatheter post-MI VSR closure. However, death within the first few postprocedural weeks ensued in five of seven surgically unoperated patients, and in three of 14 patients with prior surgical attempt at VSR closure. This occurrence of early, postprocedural death (associated with failure to maintain improved hemodynamics and shunt reduction) correlated with decreasing time between VSR occurrence and transcatheter device implantation (suggesting insufficient post-VSR tissue and scar maturation to support a mechanical device). Survival in the remaining 13 patients (median follow-up more than 5 years) has not been influenced by residual shunting.

Our experience with transcatheter VSR closure with double-umbrella devices highlights several issues. Although transcatheter VSR closure was technically feasible in nearly all patients, devices designed to close 8- to 15-mm defects early after MI generally proved clinically unsuccessful, with early shunt recurrence (suggesting need for a new transcatheter strategy for acute VSR closure). Device closure of "mature" VSR after MI (≥ 2 to 3 weeks after MI) was much more successful, with 12 of 14 such patients surviving. The impact of utilizing (a) newly designed, oversized, nonrigid devices with self-centering and self-adjusting potential (six-armed 38-mm and 43-mm STARFlex devices), potentially combined with (b) concomitant percutaneous coronary revascularization, as needed, remains to be evaluated.

PARAVALVAR LEAK CLOSURE

Clinically Significant Paravalvar Regurgitation

Clinically significant paravalvar regurgitation (causing heart failure, hemolysis, or both) complicates "routine" operative valve replacement in the adult, in large part because of the presence of heavy annular calcification associated with rheumatic and senile calcific degeneration, as well as the occurrence of bacterial endocarditis. With current surgical technique, freedom from paravalvar leakage at 15 years is 95%, though persistence of leakage and need for reoperation leads to decreasing 6-month freedom from significant leakage (approximating 85%, 78%, and 65% for first, second, and third reoperations, respectively) (5). The clinical burden of medical therapy for paravalvar leakage frequently necessitates either complex transfusion schemes or complicated heart failure programs for affected individuals and caregivers. Our experience, as outlined earlier, incorporating pediatric and adult caregivers at all facets of medical, surgical, anesthetic, intraprocedural, and nursing care, led to consideration of utilizing transcatheter techniques in an attempt to reduce the hemodynamic effects of paravalvar regurgitation.

We recognized several challenges involved with potential transcatheter closure of paravalvar leaks: (a) Three-dimensional reconstruction of such leaks in the operating amphitheater as well as by transesophageal echocardiography suggested that in an en face plane defects were crescentic, whereas in a side profile they appeared to have an hourglass shape. The optimal definition of defect anatomy (utilizing power injections of contrast through the side holes of a "cut-off" pigtail catheter positioned over a guide wire, locally within the defect) was necessary. Therefore both en face and side-profile views that would maximally separate the defect from the valve ring were essential (6). (b) Adequate closure of nonuniform defects would be suboptimal with rigidly defined devices that could not conform to defect anatomy. Within the recognized constraints of not having existing transcatheter devices suitable for closure of crescent-shaped defects, the ability of double-umbrella devices to "stuff" an hourglass space was felt to be superior to other investigational devices. (c) Valve leaflet mobility could not be compromised by the implanted closure device. We reasoned that the central portion of a paravalvar leak would need to be ≥ 6 to 8 mm from the coaptation point of the valve leaflet with the suture ring, to allow for device implantation with the smallest double-umbrella devices available at the time (12-mm Rashkind PDA Occluders or 17-mm CardioSEAL devices). (d) The coronary arterial ostium could be compromised by implanted devices (for paravalvar aortic valve regurgitation). In such circumstances, preimplantation aortography with potential for selective coronary angiography would be necessary to determine the potential for safe device deployment. (e) Typical 75-cm or 100-cm "long" guiding sheaths might not supply adequate access to paravalvar leaks in the aortic position from a femoral arterial approach in some larger adult patients. Special longer sheaths, or change in vascular access, would be required in such circumstances.

From May 1988 until January 2001, 31 patients (median age 55 years) with symptomatic paravalvar regurgitation (predominantly with associated heart failure), who were considered to have severe or prohibitive risk for surgical defect closure, presented for consideration of transcatheter closure. Affected valve location reflected incidence of rheumatic valve disease (mitral > aortic >> tricuspid). At catheterization, all patients were found to have significant paravalvar regurgitation. Devices were successfully implanted in all but two patients (in whom

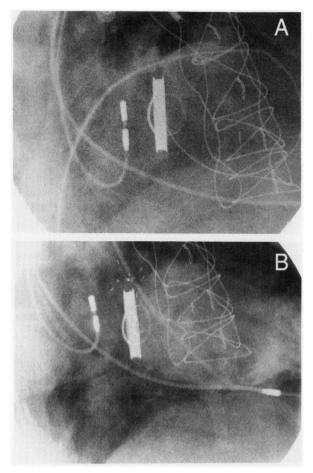

FIGURE 31.2. Paravalvar mitral regurgitation (**A**) resulting in left atrial hypertension and dyspnea is visualized with power injection through a "cut-off" pigtail catheter anchored over a stiff guide wire through the paravalvar leak. Shunt flow is eliminated after placement of a Bard Clamshell Septal Occluder (**B**), with resolution of symptoms.

regurgitant defects were considered excessive in size and in whom implantation strategy did not yet include deployment of more than one device/catheterization). Double-umbrella devices were predominantly employed (CardioSEAL devices > Rashkind PDA Occluders >> Bard Septal Clamshell Occluders), with lesser use of embolization coils (with use of an Amplatzer ASD occlusion device on one occasion). (Figure 31.2). Device encroachment on valve leaflet mobility was a rare occurrence and could always be corrected at the time of implantation. Residual leaks, both immediately at the time of implantation and in the longer term, were common but well tolerated hemodynamically, with the overwhelming majority of patients sustaining hemodynamic benefit over a 4- to 5-year fol-

low-up period. In patients with isolated hemolysis as a presenting symptom, improvement, without resolution, of transfusion requirement was common. Five-year freedom from cardiac-surgical reintervention due to paravalvar leakage approximated 70% to 80%. Late deaths occurred, but appeared to be due to underlying cardiac disease and not secondary to the hemodynamic effects of residual paravalvar leakage.

Our experience with transcatheter paravalvar leak closure (predominantly with double-umbrella devices) highlights several issues. While device implantation was technically feasible in nearly all cases, residual leakage was common, despite general substantial hemodynamic improvement. Current mechanical limitations suggest the need for construction of devices designed to better close crescent-shaped defects. The effects of such changes on short- and long-term closure rates, as well as on the need for surgical reoperation, remain to be evaluated.

CONCLUSION

Adaptations of accepted transcatheter occlusion approaches to congenital cardiac disease appear promising when applied, in translational fashion, to the management of high-risk adult patients with (a) post-MI VSR and (b) symptomatic paravalvar regurgitation. Modification of current device design may add substantial benefit for affected patients. Successful outcomes have required the presence of a combined pediatric/adult periprocedural care-giving team.

REFERENCES

1. Crenshaw BS, Granger CB, Birnbaum Y, et al. Risk factors, angiographic patterns, and outcomes in patients with ventricular septal defect complicating acute myocardial infarction. *Circulation* 2000; 101:27–32.
2. Komeda M, Fremes SE, David TE. Surgical repair of postinfarction ventricular septal defect. *Circulation* 1990;82(Supp I):IV-243–IV-247.
3. Bridges ND, Perry SB, Keane JF, et al. Preoperative transcatheter closure of congenital muscular ventricular septal defects. *N Engl J Med* 1991;324:1312–1317.
4. Landzberg MJ, Lock JE. Transcatheter management of ventricular septal rupture after myocardial infarction. *Semin Thorac Cardiovasc Surg* 1998;10:128–132.
5. Kirklin JW, Barratt-Boyes BG. *Cardiac surgery: morphology, diagnostic criteria, natural history, techniques, results and indications.* 2nd ed. New York: Churchill Livingstone, 1993.
6. Verma R, Keane JF. Use of cut-off pigtail catheters with intraluminal guidewires in interventional procedures in congenital heart disease. *Catheter Cardiovasc Diagn* 1994;33:85–88.

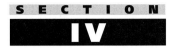

STENTS

32

MECHANICAL AND BIOPHYSICAL ASPECTS OF STENTS

GERD HAUSDORF

It was for some time suggested that the word *stent* was derived from Charles Stent, a British dentist of the nineteenth century (1807–1885). The *New England Journal of Medicine* refused in 1986 to print the word *stent,* arguing that it was not an English word (1). In 1996, two British surgeons (Morgan and Osborn) reported that the word had been known since the fourteenth century, suggesting that probably the English dictionaries from the "old world" got lost during the Boston Tea Party. In the meantime more than 74 different stent designs have been developed, and now implantation of stents is a generally accepted therapy. A stent prevents a vessel from collapsing after balloon dilatation because the recoil forces developed by the vessel are much smaller than the mechanical stability of the stent. When the stent is implanted into a vessel, it not only prevents recoil but applies force to the vessel wall either actively (self-expandable stent) or due to plastic deformation of the stent and the energy stored during balloon expansion (balloon-expandable stent). The force necessary to collapse the stent are generally higher than the recoil forces developed by the vessel.

Stents are used for several indications (2–19), the most important being the enlargement of stenotic vessels. In addition, stents are used to create a defined communication as the stent is expanded to a defined diameter and prevents recoil, which is unpredictable after balloon dilatation (e.g., in pulmonary atresia). Rare indications are for use as carrier for the implantation of conduits (covered stents) or valves, and as an occlusion device (Amplatzer devices). Endoluminal stents are used not only in the cardiovascular system (coronary arteries, pulmonary arteries, aorta, large systemic veins and arteries, etc.), but also in the tracheobronchial, biliary, and urogenital systems. The therapeutic efficacy of stents depends exclusively on their mechanical properties, like plumbing.

FUNDAMENTALS OF MATERIAL STRENGTH

Most stents are made from metals, as the mechanical properties of polymers are disappointing. Although the successful use of polylactides for coronary stents has been recently reported (20), most stents are still made from metallic alloys. Therefore this chapter will focus on the mechanic properties of metals, which are unique. The basic mechanical properties of metals can be defined as their strength. Stress and strain are, according to Hook's law, proportional when an isotropic material like a metal is deformed. Metals are polycrystalline materials, consisting of microscopically small crystals but behaving mechanically as isotropic material. The linear relation between stress and strain reflects the elastic behavior of metals, which is a temporary, reversible deformation (Figure 32.1A). When the stress is increased, plastic deformation occurs, which is a permanent deformation of the material. The stress where plastic (permanent) deformation occurs is called the yield stress and is constant for a specific material. Plastic deformation is irreversible and permanent. Plastic deformation can be a disadvantage (e.g., when a nail is deformed). On the other hand, plastic deformation can be advantageous (e.g., when a guide wire is preshaped to a particular curve or when a balloon-expandable stent is expanded). Expansion of a balloon-expandable stent results in plastic deformation, a permanent and (nearly) irreversible deformation of the stent. If the stress is increased beyond the point of plastic deformation, then fracture of the material occurs. The ability of a material to undergo plastic deformation is called its *ductility.* A ductile material shows a large range of plastic deformation, in contrast to a brittle material, which has low ductility and low fracture toughness beyond the yield stress; instead of permanent deformation, the material breaks (Figure 32.1B).

The mechanical properties of metals depend on the crystallographic structure (cubic, octahedron, hexagonal), pureness, environmental conditions (temperature), and manufacturing process (heat treatment, strain hardening). The

Gerd Hausdorf: *Deceased*

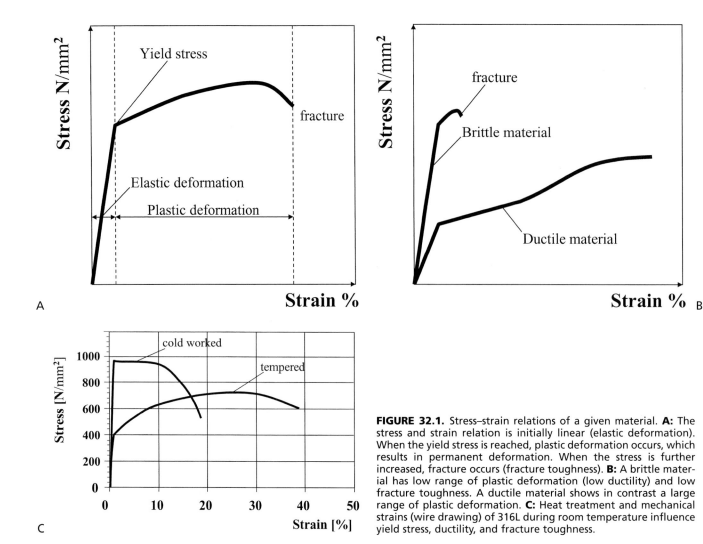

FIGURE 32.1. Stress–strain relations of a given material. **A:** The stress and strain relation is initially linear (elastic deformation). When the yield stress is reached, plastic deformation occurs, which results in permanent deformation. When the stress is further increased, fracture occurs (fracture toughness). **B:** A brittle material has low range of plastic deformation (low ductility) and low fracture toughness. A ductile material shows in contrast a large range of plastic deformation. **C:** Heat treatment and mechanical strains (wire drawing) of 316L during room temperature influence yield stress, ductility, and fracture toughness.

manufacturing process is of crucial importance for the mechanical properties of all alloys, being often more important than the composition. Heat treatment reduces the carbon content of steel and can influence their crystallographic structure (21), thereby increasing ductility and fracture toughness (Figure 32.1C). In contrast, mechanical strains (wire drawing) during room temperature affect the mechanical properties of alloys (steel). Yield strength is increased and therefore the range of elastic behavior, fracture toughness, is also increased, but ductility is reduced and strain hardening of the alloy occurs (Figure 32.2A). Strain hardening is of particular interest (21); it results in strengthening of the material and increasing stiffness. Strain hardening occurs during deformation at room temperature. It is used for the manufacturing of cold worked steels or while drawing a wire. Strain hardening is of interest for the mechanics of stents, as the expansion of a balloon-expandable stent occurs at room temperature and results in strengthening of the material. Thus during stent implantation the mechanical properties of the material change to a less ductile behavior.

STENT MATERIALS AND THEIR MECHANICAL PROPERTIES

A wide variety of alloys are currently used for stents. Their mechanical properties depend not only on their material composition, but also largely on grain size, soiling, and the manufacturing process, including forging, forming, heat treatment, rolling, drawing, and strain hardening (Figures 32.1C and 32.2A). Most of the alloys used as stent material have been developed for technical solutions but not for medical purposes.

Stainless Steel: 316L

Corrosion-resistant steel has been developed for technical purposes and is called *stainless steels*. To increase the corrosion resistance, chromium, nickel, and molybdenum are alloyed to iron. Corrosion is prevented by a Cr_2O_3 layer on the surface of the material. As long as this layer is intact and no galvanic corrosion occurs (breakthrough potential 0.2 to

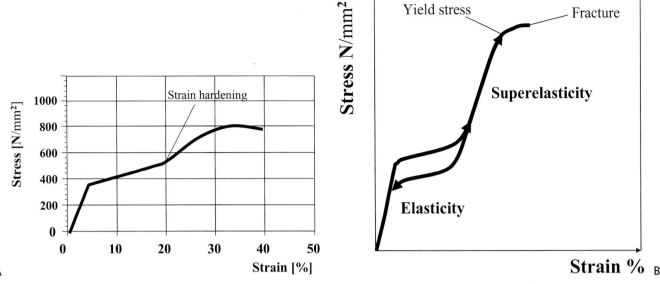

FIGURE 32.2. Strain hardening and superelasticity. **A:** Strain hardening occurs during deformation of the material at room temperature (cold worked steels or wire drawing). **B:** Superelasticity of NiTi results in a memory-effect and is due to a change from the austenitic to the martensitic phase. The stress–strain curve shows initially elastic deformation followed by a nonlinear "supereleastic" phase. If the stress is not increased beyond the yield point, the deformation is reversible.

0.3 V), the material is not corroding. Most stents are made from 316L stainless steel, an iron-based group of alloys containing chromium, nickel, and molybdenum that has the advantage of being inexpensive and being easy to manufacture. Therefore 316L is often used for balloon-expandable stents. Despite this, in a biologic medium minimal corrosion occurs, which results in ion leakage; however, biocompatibility is excellent.

Cobalt-Based Steels

Cobalt-based steel has been developed because of its superior corrosion resistance. The Wallstent is made from cobalt alloyed with chromium and molybdenum (CoCr30Mo5). Another cobalt-based alloy is MP35N (cobalt, chromium, nickel, molybdenum), which is used for orthopedic and cardiovascular implants because of its excellent corrosion resistance. Cobalt-based alloys have the advantage of high corrosion resistance, excellent biocompatibility, high yield stress, and thereby high elasticity and fracture toughness. The ductility of the material is low, so that the material is used only for self-expanding stents.

Tantalum

Tantalum has the advantage of high corrosion resistance and excellent radiopacity due to the high atomic number of tantalum. Several stents are made from tantalum, namely, the Strecker stent (one of the first available), Wiktor stent,

CrossFlex stent, and Tensum stent. The Tensum stent has been coated with amorphous silicium carbide (SiC) to reduce thrombogenicity.

Platinum

Platinum is alloyed either with iridium or with tungsten for use as a medical implant material. Because of the high thrombogenicity of precious metals, platinum-iridium and platinum-iridium alloys are used for micro coils. The corrosion resistance of these materials is extremely high, as is the radiopacity, because of the high atomic number. The Coronary Angiostent and the CP stent (Numed) are made from a platinum (90%) and iridium (10%) alloy.

Titanium

Titanium and titanium alloys are used for orthopedic implants. The corrosion resistance and biocompatibility are high, with excellent mechanical properties. The mechanical properties depend largely on the manufacturing process. The radiopacity is low because of the low atomic number. Titanium is an interesting material for stents but has been used until now only experimentally.

Nickel-Titanium Alloys

Nickel-titanium alloys with approximately equimolar nickel and titanium content have unique mechanical properties, called *superelasticity*. This superelasticity results in a memory effect: the alloy can be preshaped at a certain temperature (baking) and will regain this shape after deformation. The yield stress of Ni-Ti alloys is high, the stress–strain curve shows an initial elasticity followed by a nonlinear but reversible stress–strain relation. This "superelastic" phase is due to changing crystallographic characteristics of the alloy (from austenitic to martensitic phase) (Figure 32.2B) (22–24). If the stress is not increased beyond the yield point, the deformation is reversible and a hysteresis of the stress–strain curves between the loaded and unloaded material occurs. If the stress is increased beyond the yield point, only a small amount of plastic deformation is observed, and the material fractures just beyond the yield stress. Because of the elasticity and superelasticity of Ni-Ti alloys, the fracture toughness can be up to 60%.

TYPES OF STENTS AND BIOMECHANICS

There are two major types of stents. The most fundamental difference is that between balloon-expandable and self-

expandable stents. The balloon-expandable stents (Figure 32.3A) are expanded by inflating a balloon catheter within the stent. The balloon applies forces to the stent, which result in plastic (permanent) deformation of the stent (25–27). For balloon-expandable stents, high ductility of the material is crucial. Otherwise the material would fracture. In contrast to this, self-expandable stents are elastically deformed (compressed) before implantation within a delivery system (Figure 32.3B) (1,28). The energy stored in the compressed stent results in spontaneous expansion of the stent, when the stent is deployed. For self-expanding stents the elasticity (or superelasticity) of the material is crucial. The yield stress has to be high to prevent plastic deformation of the material.

Self-Expandable Stents

Self-expandable stents are deformed within a delivery system and the energy stored in the stent results in its spontaneous expansion (Figure 32.3B). The ability for spontaneous expansion depends on the elastic/superelastic properties of the material or on its specific design. While

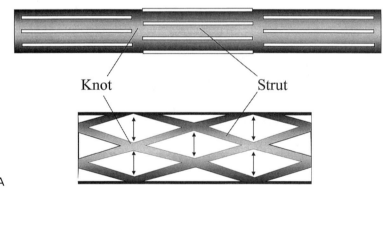

A

FIGURE 32.3. Types of stents. **A:** Balloon-expandable stents are expanded by inflating a balloon catheter within the stent, resulting in plastic (permanent) deformation of the stent. The cells of the stent open radially. **B:** Self-expandable stents (Wallstent) are elastically deformed (compressed) before implantation within a delivery system, spontaneous expansion of the stent occurs due to the energy stored in the compressed stent. **C:** Shortening of a stent can be prevented by use connecting elements between the cells, which elongate during expansion (top) or by longitudinally expanding elements within the radially expanding cells (bottom).

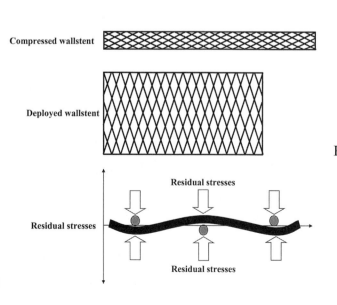

B

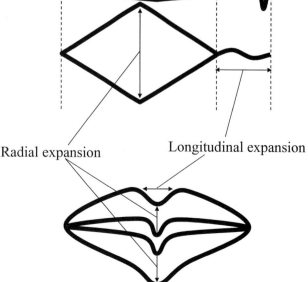

C

early attempts relied on the spring-back of spring-steel alloys, others used a zigzag design and stainless steel. It was Sigwart who invented the first self-expandable stent—the Wallstent. The Wallstent is self-expanding because of its design. It is made of weaved wires, and self-expansion depends on the forces and tensions between these woven wires. The wires need to have a high yield stress, high fracture toughness, and low ductility. Expansion of this stent occurs due to the residual stresses between the crossings of the woven wires. Although the elastic deformation between each crossing is small, because of the large number of crossings, these small elastic deformations result in an adequate recoil of the meshwork (Figure 32.3B). Expansion of the stent results in a reduction of residual stresses and thereby in a reduction of potential energy stored during compression. Because of the large number of small residual stresses, the stent has adequate radial forces and is not compressed by the surrounding tissue, but shows in practice some radial motion during the heart cycle.

In contrast to the Wallstent, Ni-Ti alloy–based stents rely on the material properties of the alloy alone (Figure 32.2B). The design is less important. The superelasticity of Ni-Ti alloys allows large strains without plastic deformation or fracture (Scimed RADIUS Stent, Aneurx stent).

Balloon-Expandable Stents

Balloon-expandable stents are expanded due to plastic deformation of radial expanding cells of the stent by a balloon catheter. Mechanically, plastic deformation depends on the ductility of the basic material. The most common type of stent is the "slotted-tube" stent, the prototype being the Palmaz stent (Figure 32.3A), which consists of a tube with longitudinal slits. When a slotted-tube is expanded with a balloon inside the slotted-tube, the slits open like a rhomb. The material between the slits is named a *strut*. The junction between struts is a *knot*. During expansion the struts deform at the knots, so that the cells form a rhomb. The highest amount of plastic deformation occurs certainly at the knots, which can result in roughening of the surface due to sliding bends within the material.

This simple design of the original Palmaz stent has two disadvantages: (a) the stent is rather stiff, particularly before expansion, because of its low longitudinal flexibility, and (b) the stent shortens significantly during expansion. To overcome these disadvantages modern stent designs use different cells for radial and longitudinal expansion. To prevent shortening of the stent during expansion a simple solution is to create longitudinal struts throughout the stent (Multilink stent), which act like a "spine" (GR II stent) that prevents shortening of the stent. Another design uses different cells for radial expansion and additional cells for longitudinal expansion. Alternatively, rounded connecting elements are used between the cells for longitudinal expansion or within these cells (Figure 32.3C), which prevents shortening as they elongate during expansion of the stent, neutralizing the shortening of the radially expanding cells.

The vast majority of currently available stents are balloon-expandable. According to the basic design of the stent, several types of balloon-expandable stents can be differentiated.

- *Slotted-tube stents.* These stents are laser-cut from a small tube with a diameter of 1.1 to 1.4 mm for coronary stents and 2.0 to 3.0 mm for peripheral (noncoronary) stents. The wall thickness ranges usually between 60 and 200 μm. After laser-cutting, the stents are electropolished. Most currently available stents are slotted-tube stents. To improve longitudinal flexibility and to prevent shortening of the stent during expansion modern stent designs use different cells or loops for radial and longitudinal expansion, which also improves the flexibility significantly.
- *Mesh stent.* These stents are made from a meshwork of wire. A typical mesh stent is the Strecker stent, which is made from knitted tantalum wire. Although no longer used for cardiovascular applications, it is still used for biliary stenting. Another mesh stent is the self-expanding Wallstent.
- *Coil stents.* Coil stents are made from wire as the mesh stents, but without creating a meshwork by weaving or knitting the wires. The wire is preshaped to coil-loops (usually in a zigzag pattern). These coil loops are stretched and straightened during balloon expansion and enlarge radially like the cells of slotted-tube stents. The major advantage of coil stents is their excellent flexibility. These stents can be advanced even around edges with steep angles and are flexible after implantation. A disadvantage of most coil stents is their low radial strength. Typical coil stents are the Wiktor stent, GR-I stent, CrossFlex stent, Freedom "fish scale" stent, and the Angiostent. Nowadays some stents with the basic design of a "coil stent" are laser-cut from a tube comparable to a slotted-tube stent. An example is the GR stent family: the GR I stent was made from wire, and the GR II stent has a similar design (with a spine that prevents shortening during expansion) but is laser-cut from a tube.
- *Ring stents.* This stent type is designed out of ring segments of wire folded in a zigzag pattern. The ring segments are connected by welding them together (Micro stent), by using sutures (Aneurx, self-expanding covered stent), or by interlocking the ring segments (Z stent). Ring stents have a high longitudinal flexibility and flexibility after implantation, and the radial strength is usually lower than in slotted-tube stents.
- *Covered stents.* Covered stents are a combination of a stent and a conduit. The conduit is either sutured to the framework of the stent (Aneurx) (19) or sandwiched between two stents (Jostent).
- *Degradable stents.* Several attempts have been made to design biodegradable stents. A promising approach seems to be the Igaki-Tamai stent, which is made from polylactic acid (PLLA) and is designed as a helical coil with a zigzag pattern. Other approaches are directed toward the use of corrosion for medical implants. Of interest are pure iron, iron-based alloys, or magnesium-lithium alloys.

Although there are several types of balloon-expandable stent designs and each type comprises several individual designs, all these stents have the expansion mechanism in common. Balloon-expandable stents are expanded by inflating a balloon within the stent. Either noncompliant balloons or semicompliant balloons are used. When a noncompliant balloon is inflated, the relation between pressure and diameter is constant, and pressure increases without any increase in diameter. In contrast to this, inflation of a semicompliant balloon occurs in several phases (Figure 32.4A). Opening of the balloon starts at a critical inflation pressure. Beyond this critical inflation pressure, a nearly linear increase of pressure without change of diameter (noncompliant behavior) is observed, which is followed by a phase of semicompliant behavior: With increasing inflation pressures a nearly linear increase of the balloon diameter occurs, until the burst pressure is reached. If the inflation pressure is kept below the burst pressure of the balloon, deflation of the balloon is characterized by hysteresis. When a semicompliant balloon is inflated several times, the pressure–diameter curves change during the first two inflations substantially; thereafter the pressure–diameter curve stabilizes at a lower level of inflation pressure. From this observation it would make sense to inflate a balloon several times before it is used in the patient. Another reason for preinflating the balloon is a hydrophilic layer on the balloon, which improves the pushability of the balloon and reduces friction but increases the risk of stent migration. Before a stent is crimped on a balloon, this gliding layer must be removed with a swab. However, when a balloon has been inflated, its profile will not come back to the initial profile. The profile of the balloon will increase after inflation, as the formation of wings will not occur with the same precision as before the first inflation. In coaxial balloon catheters the profile can be reduced and the surface of the balloon smoothened when the balloon is partially filled with fluid (outside the body) and deflated while the balloon is elongated by pulling on both ends of the balloon. (In coaxial balloons the distal balloon is connected to an inner shaft, the proximal end to an outer shaft. During inflation the inner shaft usually elongates slightly and thereby interferes with the folding of the balloon.)

Before a balloon-expandable stent is implanted it has to be premounted on a balloon, either by the manufacturer or by the operator. This procedure is called "crimping" and results in plastic deformation of the slotted-tube stent. The struts are pressed toward the balloon and are plastically deformed toward the center of the slotted tube. During this crimping the diameter of the slits is reduced, because the stent circumference is reduced. To improve the adhesion of the stent to the balloon, most operators crimp the stent on the balloon while applying a vacuum to the balloon and insert a guide wire into the lumen of the balloon catheter so as not to compress the lumen during crimping. When crimping has been completed, the pressure is neutralized, so that a minimal expansion of the balloon occurs due to capillary forces and adhesion of the stent is improved. To improve the adhesion of the stent to the balloon, the bal-

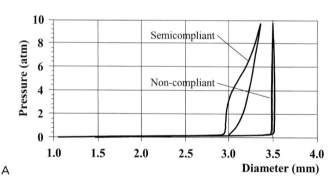

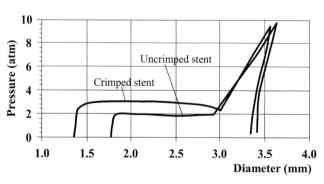

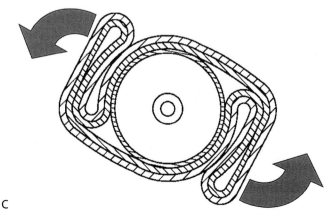

FIGURE 32.4. Balloon inflation. **A:** Inflation of a semicompliant balloon occurs in phases. Opening of the balloon at a critical inflation pressure, followed by a nearly linear increase of pressure without change of diameter (noncompliant behavior) and a phase of semicompliant behavior. With increasing inflation pressures a nearly linear increase of the balloon diameter occurs. **B:** Crimping of a stent results in strain hardening of the stent. **C:** The balloon is folded into two or four wings wrapped around the catheter shaft. Therefore inflation of a balloon results in a rotational movement of the balloon wings until they are completely inflated.

loon can be inflated slightly with an inflation pressure below the opening pressure (usually, <1 to 1.5 atm is safe, so that no stent expansion occurs). Theoretically and in practice, crimping results in strain hardening of the stent, with an increase of yield stress and the need of higher inflation pressures for stent expansion (Figure 32.4B).

To minimize the profile, the balloon is folded into two or four wings (depending on the manufacturer), which are wrapped around the catheter shaft (Figure 32.4C). Therefore inflation of a balloon results in a rotational movement of the balloon wings until they are completely inflated. The same rotational movement occurs during stent implantation, when the stent opens completely. When a balloon longer than the stent is used for inflation (Figure 32.4C) the rotational movement occurs when both ends are expanded ("flaring"), so that these ends will rotate around the axis of the balloon shaft during complete expansion of the stent and can act as a circular saw on the surrounding vessel. A small rotational movement of both balloon ends also occurs if they expand initially outside the stent, before the stent opens. This is one of the reasons for balloon perforation, particularly in large balloons, because the rotational movement of the balloon against the ends of the unexpanded stent will be more marked.

Implantation of balloon-expandable stents is a complex mechanical process. Crimping of the stent on the balloon reduces the stent diameter. Plastic deformation of the slotted-tube stent occurs and results in strain hardening of the stent. During insertion and positioning the adhesion of the stent to the balloon is the major problem, as is the longitudinal flexibility of the stent. When the stent is in an appropriate position, it is expanded by inflating the balloon. Expansion of balloon-expandable stents occurs in five phases (Figure 32.5) (21), as follows:

- *Phase 1.* The balloon is filled with fluid. Filling of the balloon occurs without any increase of pressure. As the balloon fills, the wings of the balloon inside the stent start to expand, and show some rotational movement. When the balloon is completely filled with fluid (without developing pressure within the balloon), the balloon fits inside the stent crimped on the balloon.

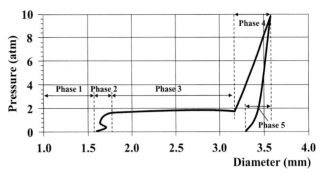

FIGURE 32.5. Stent expansion. Implantation of a balloon-expandable stent is a complex mechanical process. Expansion occurs in five phases.

- *Phase 2.* In phase 2 the inflation pressure starts to increase, but still the stent is not expanding. During this phase the inflation pressure stays constant, the ends of the stents start to expand, resulting in a "bone structure" of the balloon stent unity ("flaring") (Figure 32.4D). Concomitantly, the balloon applies radial stress to the stent, resulting in a small increase in stent diameter. This small increase of strain and reshaping of the stent results in storage of elastic energy within the stent.
- *Phase 3.* At an inflation pressure characteristic for the stent design and the material used, the stent suddenly opens: "burst-open pressure." The energy stored within the stent during elastic deformation suddenly results in plastic deformation due to sliding bends within the material. During this "burst-open" phase the stent expands without any increase in pressure. Actually, a reduction of the inflation pressure can occur. This occurs when the balloon cannot follow the plastic deformation of the stent. Because of this effect a slow inflation of the balloon can result in loss of adhesion between stent and balloon and in stent migration. The risk of stent migration is less when stent expansion occurs from both ends of the stent, because the "bone structure" of the balloon prevents stent migration by the expanded ends of the balloon (Figure 32.6).

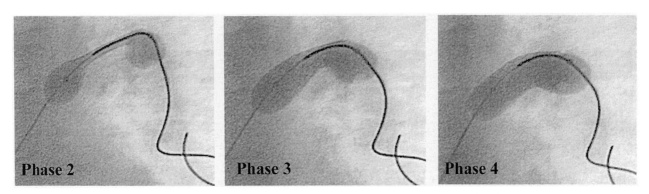

FIGURE 32.6. Self-centering due to flaring. The risk of stent migration is reduced when stent expansion occurs from both ends of the stent, resulting in flaring, as the middle of the stent is centering within the stenosis.

- *Phase 4.* After the abrupt transformation of elastically stored energy into plastic deformation during phase 3, the inflation pressure results in a slow plastic deformation of the stent, related to the inflation pressure. High pressures are needed to achieve further stent expansion. This is due to the balloon compliance and strain hardening of the stent beyond the yield stress (Figure 32.2A).
- *Phase 5.* Balloon inflation has been completed and the balloon is deflated. During this process a varying amount of recoil occurs. This depends on the elastic deformation of the stent that occurred during phase 2. The recoil results in complete relief of the elastic energy stored in the stent.

ENDOVASCULAR STENTING IN PRACTICE: MECHANICAL BASIS

At least two requirements must be met before stent implantation. The practitioner must have adequate knowledge about (a) the mechanical behavior of the stent itself and (b) the biomechanical properties of the vessel.

Although several types of interactions between stent, balloon, and vessel occur, the most important mechanical interaction is static friction between the stent and balloon, as well as that between the stent and vessel wall. Static friction prevents stent migration and is always higher than dynamic friction. Therefore the mechanical principles of static friction and adhesion should be discussed briefly (Figure 32.7). When a force F is applied with an angle α to a solid body which is in contact with a surface, forces parallel (F_τ) and perpendicular (F_n) to the contact surface are generated:

$$F_n = F \cos \alpha$$

$$F_\tau = F \sin \alpha$$

The stent remains immobile as long as $F_\tau < F_n \mu$ (μ is the constant for static friction). Within a critical angle ρ (Figure 32.7), the force F cannot result in migration because it cannot overcome static friction. The angle ρ depends on the material constant μ. As long as $F_\tau < F_n \tan \rho$ or, simpler, α is smaller than ρ, the stent remains immobile or static independent of the force F. When α becomes larger than the angle ρ, stent migration will occur. As dynamic friction is always smaller than static friction, the stent will migrate if the force F can overcome static friction. In a liquid environment μ and ρ are quite small, but as the forces applied by the expanding balloon to the stent during stent implantation are nearly perpendicular to its surface, the angle α is nearly zero. However, during insertion and advancing of the stent through a long sheath the angle α is nearly 90 degrees and thereby larger than ρ, so that the stent easily slips off the balloon. This risk can be reduced by the use of "Mullins glue" (radiopaque material). Contrast medium between stent and balloon increases μ and results in firm adhesion of the stent to the balloon as static friction is increased.

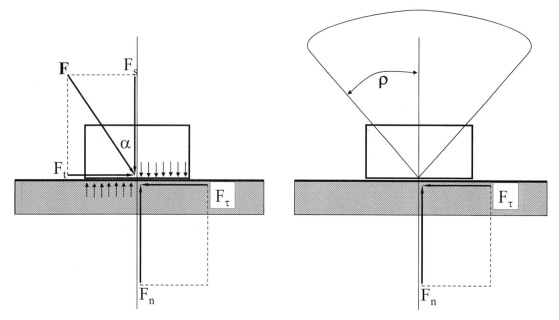

FIGURE 32.7. Static friction. The basic principles of static friction are shown. When a force *F* is applied with an angle α to a solid body that is in contact with a surface (hatched area), forces parallel (*F$_\tau$*) and perpendicular (*F$_n$*) to the contact surface are generated. The stent remains immobile as long as *F$_\tau$* < *F$_n$* μ (μ is a constant for static friction). Within a critical angle ρ the force *F* cannot result in migration as it cannot overcome static friction. When α becomes larger than the angle ρ, stent migration will occur.

Friction and adhesion to the vessel wall are of particular importance when a stent has to be implanted into a tapering vessel (Figure 32.8A). In a tapering vessel the distal diameter of the vessel is smaller than the proximal diameter. The force applied by the balloon to the stent is no longer perpendicular to the stent–vessel interface and α can become larger than ρ, so that the stent starts to migrate (29,30). A residual waist at the distal end of the stent substantially increases the risk of stent migration during implantation and during redilatation. In contrast, if a stent shows a residual waist in its middle, the dislocating forces on both ends neutralize each other and stent migration needs a force to overcome the noncompliant waist (Figure 32.8A). A stent with a (small) residual waist needs forces that result in elastic or plastic deformation of stent and vessel wall to overcome static friction. Thus a stent with a residual waist is a "safe stent" in respect to stent migration or dislocation. Because of these basic mechanical principles, assessment of the mechanical properties of the vessel at the site of stent implantation is indispensable. The purpose is to evaluate the regional compliance of the vessel wall. To assess the static compliance of a vessel, a balloon is slowly inflated to achieve distention of the vessel within the range of elastic deformation. In practice, inflation of the balloon is performed with inflation pressures of less than 1 to 2 atm. The waists within the balloon "point" to local areas of reduced compliance, which are often not suspected from the angiogram alone. In tubular stenosis circumscribed areas of reduced compliance are often observed, when regional compliance is assessed by inflating a balloon. "Balloon sizing" is of particular importance in "tubular" stenosis and in tapering vessels to localize the optimal position of the stent: the localized area of reduced compliance should be in the middle of the stent. In tapering vessels "balloon sizing" gives important additional information (31): Is the vessel compliance adequate to allow expansion of a given balloon selected for stent implantation, or does dislocation of the balloon occur during inflation, which would result in stent dislocation during stent implantation?

Before a balloon-expandable stent can be implanted it must be crimped on the balloon. Coronary stents are often crimped on the balloon by the manufacturer; peripheral stents are usually crimped by the operator. To place the stent on the balloon its inner diameter has to be larger than the balloon profile. Crimping results in deformation of the struts toward the balloon. This is performed until the stent adheres to the balloon. Crimping of the stent results in strain hardening of the stent and the need for higher inflation pressure to expand the stent (phase 3). In practice, it is of great importance that the difference between the luminal diameter of the stent and the profile of the balloon be small, in the range of 1 to 2F, depending on the unexpanded stent diameter. If a balloon with a particularly small profile is selected (more than 2F smaller than the stent lumen), the stent will be damaged during crimping. The circumference of the stent has to be reduced significantly to achieve adhesion between stent and balloon, so the struts are deformed strongly inward and start to bend. Moreover, the knots have to be deformed inward to reduce the stent circumference. "Overcrimping" occurs and results in failure to expand the stent. This failure to expand the stent occurs for several reasons: stress hardening of the stent material, interlocking of the neighbored struts, and strong strut deformation, resulting in an angle between expanding forces and struts that are no longer perpendicular, so that radial forces during expansion are reduced. "Overcrimping" of a stent occurs, for example, if a Palmaz series 6 ("renal stent") or Palmaz series 8 stent ("iliac stent") is crimped on a percutaneous transluminal balloon angioplasty (PTCA) balloon (3F diameter). This inevitable result is failure of the stent to expand, even when high-pressure PTCA balloons that can withstand more than 20 atm inflation pressure are used. If overcrimping occurs, virtually no inflation pressure will be able to expand the stent. The Palmaz-XL stent should be crimped at least on a 7F balloon to prevent

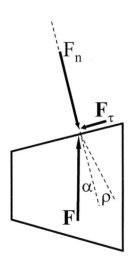
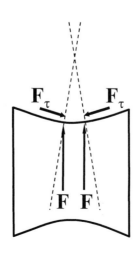

FIGURE 32.8. Static friction: clinical applications. When a stent is implanted into a tapering vessel, the force applied by the balloon to the stent is no longer perpendicular to the stent–vessel interface, α can become larger than ρ, so that the stent starts to migrate *(left)*. If a stent shows a residual waist in its middle, the dislocating forces on both ends neutralize each other and stent migration would need a force able to overcome the noncompliant waist *(right)*.

overcrimping. Overcrimping can be felt during manual crimping as a snapping sensation accompanied by a "clicking" sound, when the struts interlock. Although the smallest balloon profile should always be used to reduce vascular trauma, for endovascular stenting it is important not to select a balloon with too small a profile. Selection of a balloon with too large a profile virtually cannot occur because if the profile of the balloon is too large, it is impossible to slip the stent onto the balloon. However, if the stent is forced on the balloon it can damage the balloon and the stent will not expand. Perforation can also occur during phase 2 of stent implantation (as mentioned earlier). A solution (that honestly rarely works in practice) is to perform "power inflation" by performing balloon inflation with the injection pump used for angiography.

Finally, technical problems related to "inadequate" crimping must be mentioned. During crimping any twisting of the stent must be prevented: both hands should perform crimping in the same direction, either clockwise or counterclockwise. If the left hand is crimping the stent clockwise and the right hand is crimping it counterclockwise, the stent will be twisted in the middle. Because of the resulting plastic deformation, stress hardening and bending of the struts occur, which can result in failure to expand adequately during deployment:

■ If the middle of the balloon is occluded because of excessively intense compression of the stent or twisting, only the proximal part of the balloon can fill during balloon inflation but the distal balloon will remain unfilled because its lumen is completely occluded. The stent opens only proximal and is pushed distally by the proximal balloon inflating from the proximal to the distal end. This problem occurs particularly when a balloon coated with a hydrophilic gliding layer is used.

■ If the stent has been twisted in the middle of the balloon, both ends of the stent expand; while the middle of the stent is not expanding, the longitudinal forces can become larger than the radial forces, so that the middle of the stent is compressed by the inflating balloon toward the center of the stent.

To prevent asymmetric stent expansion the balloon-in-balloon (BIB) balloon (NuMed) is helpful for the expansion of stents with a large radial diameter. The BIB balloon consists of a smaller inner balloon and a larger outer balloon that are inflated sequentially. The inner balloon is used for "preexpansion" of the stent. As the angle between the balloon and the stent tips is smaller, when a smaller balloon is used, less flaring occurs than with a large balloon. Flaring of both ends of the stent ("bone-structure") is reduced, which could result in laceration of the vessel wall and perforation of the balloon. To prevent flaring of the stent some stent designs (coronary stents) use smaller cells at both ends of the stent than in the middle of the stents (NIR stent). Another simple technique to prevent flaring is to use a balloon with the same length as, or even slightly shorter than, the stent. Expansion will start in the middle of the stent ("short balloon technique" according to Mullins).

Although flaring is a disadvantage for several applications, it offers advantages. Flaring can result in self-centering of the stent, if the ends of the balloon stent unit expand on both sides of a severe and noncompliant stenosis. Stent expansion occurs from both ends of the stents toward the middle of the stent and will center the middle of the stent within the stenosis (Figure 32.6). The least distensible part of the vessel will always be localized in the middle of the stent.

In general, expansion of balloon-expandable stents occurs in several (five) phases, as described earlier (Figure 32.5). For the selection of the balloon, phase 3 is critical: the "burst-open pressure" resulting in stent expansion without any pressure increase. The balloon must be able to deliver an inflation pressure at least 2 atm higher than the "burst-open pressure." This can be critical when stents with a large diameter (Palmaz XL) are to be implanted: The larger the balloon diameter, the lower the burst pressure of the balloon. Therefore "overcrimping" is particularly critical with large stent diameters. For the "burst-open pressure" the stent design seems to be of superior importance, whereas the material of the stent is of lesser importance.

While self-expanding stents have a predefined diameter after expansion and will apply force to the vessel until they have expanded to this diameter, balloon-expandable stents can be expanded to varying diameters. The stent design limits the maximal expansion of balloon-expandable stents. Expansion of a slotted-tube stent like the Palmaz stent has to come to an end when the longitudinal struts achieve a radial orientation. The struts then form a ringlike structure Further expansion is impossible until stent fracture occurs. Such an overexpansion of a stent is associated with significant shortening of the stent and a plastic deformation near to the point where fracture of the stent occurs. Thus, although balloon-expandable stents can be redilated in the growing organism, redilatation is limited by the maximal stent diameter, which again depends on the stent design, not on the stent material. Significant shortening of the stent during overexpansion can be helpful before surgery, as the surgeon has to remove a shorter segment.

MATERIALS AND ENDOVASCULAR STENTING

Most stents are made from metallic alloys, because their ductility and mechanical strength are superior, and radial strength increases during expansion due to strain hardening. The only polymer stent currently under investigation is the Igaki-Tamai stent (polylactic acid). All materials are prone to fatigue, wear, and corrosion. The corrosion of alloys used for technical purposes is typically analyzed in

Hank's solution or other electrolyte solutions with a composition comparable to that of seawater. As seawater has nearly the same composition as the extracellular fluid of the human body, corrosion of permanent metallic implants is a matter of concern because of galvanic corrosion. Corrosion is in most instances due to oxidation of the metal and depends on the electronegativity of the metal. When a metallic surface is exposed to extracellular fluid, corrosion occurs on its surface immediately. This surface corrosion is surprisingly of outstanding importance to prevent corrosion, as further corrosion is prevented by a thin (10 nm), stable layer of Cr_2O_3, Fe_3O_4, and Ti_2O_5. This layer is also called the "passivation layer." The formation of a stable passivation layer can be inhibited by inclusion of MnS or other inclusions, which locally destabilize this passivation layer and result in pitting corrosion (32–34). The risk of corrosion can be increased by the manufacturing process. Intergranular (intercrystalline) corrosion occurs after welding of stainless steels: temperatures between 450°C and 850°C result in the formation of chromium carbides $Cr_{23}C_6$ and $Cr_{23}C_7$ that prevent the formation of a stable passivation layer. As these chromium carbides form between the crystals, corrosion occurs at the intergranular borders.

Corrosion also depends on the mechanical stress (stress corrosion, fatigue corrosion, crevit corrosion) and can be important if a stent is implanted in a region where it is exposed to continuous mechanical stresses, as in the right ventricular outflow tract or the pulmonary arteries. Stresses result in elastic deformation at the knots of the stent; fatigue results in small fractures where crevit corrosion can occur. When the metallic surface is exposed to an abrasive stress due to a fluid or another metallic surface that is "rubbing" on its surface (Figure 32.3B), this can result in abrasion of the passivation surface and erosion corrosion occurs. From these basic principles of corrosion, it is not surprising that in an aggressive medium like extracellular fluid, corrosion of metallic stents is unavoidable. Although the degree of corrosion is low, it results in a measurable ion leakage into the surrounding tissue and into the extracellular fluid. This ion leakage can be simulated in seawater, serum, or Hank's solution. For the ion leakage from a metallic surface the surface area in percentage of the stent surface is important, which varies according to the stent design. The long-term biologic relevance of ion leakage from stents or other cardiovascular implants is still unknown. The nickel released from stents and other permanent medical implants has been accused of causing restenosis after coronary stenting due to nickel allergy. Loosening of orthopedic implants due to nickel allergy is well known in orthopedics. The clinical symptoms are nonspecific and result in loosening of the implant. However, in orthopedics, wear causes microscopic particles that result in a large surface. Whether nickel allergy is relevant for cardiovascular metallic implants is still an unsolved question but could be of concern. Whether corrosion and thereby ion leakage can be prevented by sur-

face coatings like SiC (silicium carbide) (Tensum stent) or carbon coatings (Sorin stent) must yet be proven. Of interest is the observation that a surface coating of a 316L stent with gold resulted in a substantial acceleration of corrosion, as the gold granules act as local cathodes, which destabilize the passivation layer. This principle is of interest for developing biodegrading implants, which use biocorrosion as a degradation mechanism. Of particular interest are alloys from iron and magnesium, as both elements are essential for the human body.

Another concern with permanent medical implants is fractures of the implant with the potential risk of implant loosening and migration of fragments. Fractures of medical implants resulting in implant failure were initially observed in orthopedics. They occurred most frequently 8 to 15 years after implantation and were due to wear and fatigue. Fractures of pacemaker leads are well known in practice and can even occur within months when the leads are exposed to mechanical stresses and/or kinking. Incessant mechanical stresses can also result in fractures of a stent. This has been reported for certain locations as the right ventricular outflow tract and the ventricular septum in patients with a restrictive ventricular septal defect. Whereas mechanical stresses are high and can result in fatigue when a stent is implanted into the myocardium, they are much lower when stents are implanted into vessels. However, depending on the strut thickness, fractures can also occur after stent implantation into coronary arteries. For coronary stents a thickness below 60 to 80 μm can result in stent fracture during medium-term follow-up.

BIOLOGIC EFFECTS OF STENTING

A medical implant will inevitably interact with the biologic function of the surrounding tissue as a result of mechanical and chemical (toxic) interaction. Gross mechanical interactions between implant and organism are known from orthopedic implants. The mechanical properties of current implants and that of the surrounding tissue differ substantially. For orthopedic implants the Young's modulus and tensile strength of current implant materials (ceramics, alloys, and polymers) are significantly higher than those of human bone. Therefore mechanical stresses are diverted from the bone adjacent to the implant into the implant, resulting in "stress shielding" of the surrounding bone. Mechanical stresses that are normally directed into the bone are neutralized by the implant. As bone formation and degradation are dependent on the stresses within the osteons, bone formation ceases and the equilibrium between osteoblastic bone formation and osteoclastic breakdown is disturbed toward osteoclastic activity. This results in atrophy and thinning of the bone surrounding the implant. Loosening of the implant and fracture of the bone can occur, leading to implant failure. This "stress shielding" occurs due to the mechanical properties of the implant. If the Young's modulus and tensile strength of implant material and bone were comparable, stress shielding would not occur or would be very small.

The mechanical properties of stent materials and soft tissues differ significantly. Stents also result in "stress shielding" of the adjacent vessel, the Young's modulus and tensile strength of a stent are significantly larger than those of vessels, myocardium, or other soft tissues. In contrast to bone (which is anisotropic, stiff, and brittle), vessels show predominantly elastic and viscoelastic properties. The ductility of vessels is low, as is fracture toughness. It is difficult or even impossible to define Young's modulus, tensile strength, yield stress, ductility, and fracture toughness for vessels, because their mechanical properties vary with the anatomic site and functional status of the vessel. Furthermore, spasm of a vessel can reduce vessel compliance dramatically. Even with high-pressure balloons it can be impossible to relieve obstruction caused by a spastic vessel. In vessel spasm often 4 to 8 atm, and sometimes inflation pressures of up to 20 atm, are necessary to overcome the spasm. Normally, Young's modulus and tensile strength of current stents are much higher than those of any (nonspastic) vessel. Because of the cyclic, radial oscillations of the vessel and the longitudinal and radial stiffness of the stent, both ends of the stent will move against the vessel wall. Continuous stresses between stent and vessel occur particularly in curved vessels. This mechanical stimulus may be a reason for intimal proliferation at both ends of the stent and in in-stent stenosis. The motions of both ends of the stent are in part due to leverage and are therefore reduced with shorter stents.

Further mechanical interactions between stent and tissue can result from the rotational movement of the stent during expansion (phase 3) and from extensive flaring of both ends of the stent. Finally, longitudinally expanding elements engineered to prevent shortening of the stent can rotate during balloon inflation toward the vessel wall, resulting in additional laceration of the vessel. In contrast to these harmful mechanical effects, toxic effects due to ion leakage from the stent seem to be of less importance for the biocompatibility of the stent. If nickel allergy is a reason for early in-stent stenosis after coronary stenting, it has not been proven yet.

Stent implantation in the growing organism involves additional problems, as a stent cannot grow and therefore cannot adjust to growth-related changes of the organism. The same holds true for grown-ups with hypoplastic vessels with growth potential. Redilatation of the stent is the only way to adjust the stent diameter to the growth of the stented vessel. Redilation of balloon-expandable stents is easily performed and safe when the stent is covered by a neointima, so that stent dislocation during redilatation cannot occur (35). Redilatation of a stent is limited by the maximal stent diameter, which is dependent on the stent design (see earlier). In slotted-tube stents the maximal diameter of the stent is defined by the length (or circumference) of the cells for radial expansion. When a stent is expanded to its maximum diameter and the struts are forming ringlike structures, the radial stability of the stent is substantially reduced and substantial shortening of the stent occurs. To allow for later redilatation, stent selection should anticipate the final diameter of the stented vessel.

Some stent designs prevent shortening during expansion (Figure 32.3C). This is of particular interest for coronary stenting, as the combined effects of flaring and shortening during expansion can result in denudation of the endothelium during implantation. In the growing organism shortening of the stent during redilatation can be an advantage, particularly if surgery has to be performed, as the stented segment becomes short enough to be completely removed. Shortening of the stent has another advantage in the growing organism: the mechanical interactions between vessel and stent are reduced with a shorter stent. Self-expandable stents, such as the Wallstent, have certain disadvantages in the growing organism, because of their predefined radial diameter and as they apply stresses to the surrounding vessel until complete expansion has been achieved. Redilatation cannot be performed, and because of the cyclic, radial oscillations of the stent during the cardiac cycle most self-expandable stents result in continuous mechanical stimuli to the surrounding tissue, which can lead to intima proliferation. Thus in the growing organism self-expandable stents exhibit certain disadvantages and are of little value.

To overcome early redilatation of the stent, "overexpansion" of the stent to a diameter larger than the adjacent vessel (proximal and distal to the stent) seems to be an attractive approach. Overexpansion of a stent results in a reduced shear stress within the stent, leading to intimal proliferation, which in turn normalizes shear stresses. Thus overexpansion of a stent results almost always in substantial intimal proliferation, which continues until the vessel lumen within the stent is the same as that of the adjacent vessel. This intimal proliferation does not, unfortunately, regress when growth of the adjacent vessel occurs (36–39). Thus overexpansion of a stent should not be undertaken in the growing and grown-up organism. This can be achieved by graded expansion of the stent, a strong argument not to use oversized balloons for stent implantation. The problems associated with overexpansion are a particular disadvantage of self-expandable stents. The final stent diameter is predefined and allows no individual variability; the operator has no influence on the stent diameter (40,41).

Biocompatibility of current stent materials is excellent according to the current criteria. Endothelial cells are growing on the currently used alloys, as are fibroblasts. Even smooth muscle cells are not disturbed; however, their growth can be inhibited by certain ions, such as nickel, chromium, iron, and others, depending on their local concentration. In this context it has to be mentioned that the definition of medical biocompatibility is unclear: Is biocompatibility the same as biologic inertness of a material, or is it lack of interference between implant and organism (42,43)? The latter cannot be achieved by an inert material, as the mechanical interaction between implant and organism results in a biologic response by itself. Should a stent material therefore have some local toxicity to prevent intimal proliferation? Expanding the discussion of the "idea" or concept of biocompatibility is beyond the scope of this chapter, but inertness is definitely not the same as biocompatibility. Perhaps the definition of biocompatibility needs to include biodegradation: Is a medical implant only biocompatible when it disappears with time?

One component of biocompatibility for stents is thrombogenicity. A simple rule helps: The more precious a metal or alloy, the higher its thrombogenicity (44,45). Also the surface of the stent plays an important role: a smooth surface reduces the thrombogenicity of a stent but does not diminish it. Even more important is the surface of the vessel after stent implantation. Laceration of the endothelium and rupturing of unstable plaques enhance thrombus formation. Of particular interest is the observation that a stent diameter below 4 to 5 mm has an increased risk for thrombus formation.

CONCLUSION

Endovascular stent implantation is a simple and effective solution for the relief of stenotic lesions. However, it has something in common with ordinary plumbing. Despite this, stent implantation offers advantages to and does not interfere with surgery. Matters of concern are the long lifespan of these permanent implants, with continuous mechanical interference and ion leakage. This is certainly true for their use in children with a life expectancy of 70 years or more. This is a time period far beyond the scope of current investigators and engineers.

REFERENCES

1. Sigwart U, Puel J, Mirkovitch V, et al. Intravascular stents to prevent occlusion and restenosis after transluminal angioplasty. *N Engl J Med* 1987;316:701–706.
2. Hanley HG; Sheridan FM, Rivera E. Carotid stenting: a technology in evolution. *J La State Med Soc* 2000;152:235–238.
3. Isotola T, Alarakkola E, Talja M, et al. Biocompatibility testing of a new bioabsorbable X-ray positive SR-PLA 96/4 urethral stent. *J Urol* 1999;162:1764–1767.
4. Abou Zamzam AM Jr, Porter JM. Does endovascular grafting represent a giant step forward? *Semin Vasc Surg* 1999;12:235–241.
5. Bader R, Somerville J, Redington A. Use of self-expanding stents in stenotic aortopulmonary shunts in adults with complex cyanotic heart disease. *Heart* 1999;82:27–29.
6. Haage P, Vorwerk D, Piroth W, et al. Treatment of hemodialysis-related central venous stenosis or occlusion: results of primary Wallstent placement and follow-up in 50 patients. *Radiology* 1999;212:175–180.
7. Mehta AC, Dasgupta A. Airway stents. *Clin Chest Med* 1999;20:139–151.
8. Stockx L. Stent-grafts in the superficial femoral artery. *Eur J Radiol* 1998;28:182–188.
9. Palmaz JC. New advances in endovascular technology. *Tex Heart Inst J* 1997;24:156–159.
10. Schurmann K, Vorwerk D, Uppenkamp R, et al. Iliac arteries: plain and heparin-coated Dacron-covered stent-grafts compared with noncovered metal stents-an experimental study. *Radiology* 1997;203:55–63.
11. Kulkarni RP, Bellamy EA. A new thermo-expandable shape-memory nickel-titanium alloy stent for the management of ureteric strictures. *BJU Int* 1999;83:755–759.
12. Ing FF, Mullins CE, Grifka RG, et al. Stent dilation of superior vena cava and innominate vein obstructions permits transvenous pacing lead implantation. *Pacing Clin Electrophysiol* 1998;21:1517–1530.
13. Shaffer KM, Mullins CE, Grifka RG, et al. Intravascular stents in congenital heart disease: short- and long-term results from a large single-center experience. *J Am Coll Cardiol* 1998 1;31:661–667.
14. Marshall AC, Perry SB, Keane JF, et al. Early results and medium-term follow-up of stent implantation for mild residual or recurrent aortic coarctation. *Am Heart J* 2000;139:1054–1060.
15. Hijazi ZM, al Fadley F, Geggel RL, et al. Stent implantation for relief of pulmonary artery stenosis: immediate and short-term results. *Catheter Cardiovasc Diagn* 1996;38:16–23.
16. Ovaert C, Caldarone CA, McCrindle BW, et al. Endovascular stent implantation for the management of postoperative right ventricular outflow tract obstruction: clinical efficacy. *J Thorac Cardiovasc Surg* 1999, 118:886–893.
17. Magee AG, Brzezinska Rajszys G, Qureshi SA, et al. Stent implantation for aortic coarctation and recoarctation. *Heart* 1999;82:600–606.
18. Suarez de Lezo J, Pan M, Romero M, et al. Immediate and follow-up findings after stent treatment for severe coarctation of aorta. *Am J Cardiol* 1999 1;83:400–406.
19. Klima U, Peters T, Peuster M, et al. A novel technique for establishing total cavopulmonary connection: from surgical preconditioning to interventional completion. *J Thorac Cardiovasc Surg* 2000;120:1007–1009.
20. Tamai H, Igaki K, Kyo E, Kosuga K, et al. Initial and 6-month results of biodegradable poly-l-lactic acid coronary stents in humans. *Circulation* 2000 25;102:399–404.
21. Mahr R, Fischer A, Brauer H, et al. Biophysical study of coronary stents: which factors influence the dilatation and recoil behavior. *Z Kardiol* 2000;89:1–9.
22. Shih CC, Lin SJ, Chen YL, et al. The cytotoxicity of corrosion products of Nitinol stent wire on cultured smooth muscle cells. *J Biomed Mater Res* 2000; 52:395–403.
23. Trepanier C, Leung TK, Tabrizian M, et al. Preliminary investigation of the effects of surface treatments on biological response to shape memory NiTi stents. *J Biomed Mater Res* 1999;48:165–171.
24. Trepanier C, Tabrizian M, Yahia LH, et al. Effect of modification of oxide layer on NiTi stent corrosion resistance. *J Biomed Mater Res* 1998;43:433–440.
25. Skerven GJ, Spain Stewart B. The Z-stent. *Gastrointest Endosc Clin N Am* 1999;9:367–372.
26. Schurmann K, Vorwerk D, Uppenkamp R, et al. Determination of stent stenosis: an in vivo experimental comparison of intravascular ultrasound and angiography with histology. *Cardiovasc Intervent Radiol* 1998; 21:189–198.
27. Roguin A, Beyar R. beStent: the serpentine balloon expandable

stent: review of mechanical properties and clinical experience. *Artif Organs* 1998;22:243–249.

28. Schurmann K, Vorwerk D, Kulisch A, et al. Neointimal hyperplasia in low-profile Nitinol stents, Palmaz stents, and Wallstents: a comparative experimental study. *Cardiovasc Intervent Radiol* 1996;19:248–254.

29. Squire JC, Rogers C, Edelman ER. Measuring arterial strain induced by endovascular stents. *Med Biol Eng Comput* 1999;37: 692–698.

30. Schrader SC, Beyar R. Evaluation of the compressive mechanical properties of endoluminal metal stents. *Catheter Cardiovasc Diagn* 1998;44:179–187.

31. Recto MR, Ing FF, Grifka RG, et al. A technique to prevent newly implanted stent displacement during subsequent catheter and sheath manipulation. *Catheter Cardiovasc Interv* 2000;49: 297–300.

32. Shih CC, Lin SJ, Chung KH, et al. Increased corrosion resistance of stent materials by converting current surface film of polycrystalline oxide into amorphous oxide. *J Biomed Mater Res* 2000;52: 323–332.

33. Smith GK. Systemic transport and distribution of iron and chromium from 316L stainless steel implants. Dissertation Metallurgy and Materials Science, University of Pennsylvania, 1982.

34. Moller D, Reimers W, Pyzalla A, et al. Residual stresses in coronary artery stents. *J Biomed Mater Res* 2001;58:69–74.

35. Mendelsohn AM, Dorostkar PC, Moorehead CP, et al. Stent redilation in canine models of congenital heart disease: pulmonary artery stenosis and coarctation of the aorta. *Catheter Cardiovasc Diagn* 1996;38:430–440.

36. Yu SC, Zhao JB. A steady flow analysis on the stented and nonstented sidewall aneurysm models. *Med Eng Phys* 1999;21: 133–141.

37. Keelan PC, Miyauchi K, Caplice NM, et al. Modification of molecular events in coronary restenosis using coated stents: the Mayo Clinic approach. *Semin Interv Cardiol* 1998;3:211–215.

38. Meerkin D, Bonan R, Crocker IR, et al. Efficacy of beta radiation in prevention of post-angioplasty restenosis: an interim report from the beta energy restenosis trial. *Herz* 1998;23: 356–361.

39. Bertrand OF, Sipehia R, Mongrain R, et al. Biocompatibility aspects of new stent technology. *J Am Coll Cardiol* 1998;32: 562–571.

40. Edelman ER, Rogers C. Pathobiologic responses to stenting. *Am J Cardiol* 1998;9;81:4E–6E.

41. Eton D, Warner DL, Owens C, et al. Histological response to stent graft therapy. *Circulation* 1996 1;94(Suppl):II-182–II-187.

42. Palmaz JC, Benson A, Sprague EA. Influence of surface topography on endothelialization of intravascular metallic material. *J Vasc Interv Radiol* 1999;10:439–444.

43. Bertrand OF, Sipehia R, Mongrain R, et al. Biocompatibility aspects of new stent technology. *J Am Coll Cardiol* 1998;32: 562–571.

44. Herrmann R, Schmidmaier G, Markl B, et al. Antithrombogenic coating of stents using a biodegradable drug delivery technology. *Thromb Haemost* 1999;82:51–57.

45. Heublein B, Pethig K, Elsayed AM. Silicon carbide coating N: a semiconducting hybrid design of coronary stents—feasibility study. *J Invasive Cardiol* 1998;10:255–262.

33

RECENT TECHNICAL DEVELOPMENTS IN IMPLANTATION OF STENTS FOR CONGENITAL AND POSTSURGICAL CARDIOVASCULAR ANOMALIES

JOHN D. COULSON
ALLEN D. EVERETT
CARL Y. OWADA

Initial reports of endovascular stent implantation in experimental animals and then humans were published more than a decade ago (1–3). A broad spectrum of clinical indications for use of stents is now recognized, including a variety of congenital and postsurgical cardiovascular anomalies found in both children and adults. The general method used by interventional pediatric cardiologists to deliver stents to treat these anomalies has changed little during the past decade (4). Guide wires are used to direct long sheaths to vascular narrowings. The sheaths in turn are used to position stents mounted on angioplasty balloons in the narrowings. Finally, the stents are expanded by balloon inflation. Self-expanding stents have found only limited application in the treatment of congenital and postsurgical anomalies.

THE CHALLENGES

Although the concept of stent implantation to treat congenital and postsurgical cardiovascular anomalies is simple, these procedures are technically challenging for a number of reasons. First, infants and smaller children, whose cardiovascular structures are relatively small, can only accommodate small stent delivery systems. Even the stent delivery systems used in larger children and adults are relatively large, 8 to 14F in diameter.

John D. Coulson: Director, Bakersfield Pediatric Cardiology Clinic, Department of Cardiology and Cardiovascular Surgery, Children's Hospital Central California, Bakersfield, California

Allen D. Everett: Associate Professor, Department of Pediatrics, University of Virginia, Charlottesville, Virginia

Carl Y. Owada: Director, Cardiac Catheterization Laboratory, Department of Cardiology and Cardiothoracic Surgery, Children's Hospital of Central California, Madera, California

Second, lengthy and tortuous stent delivery routes are often encountered. For example, two cardiac chambers and valves must usually be traversed when delivering stents to main or branch pulmonary artery narrowings. Such routes can make guide wire placement and maintenance of guide wire position difficult. Furthermore, these routes can make long sheaths and their dilators difficult to advance over guide wires even when the wires are very strong and optimally positioned. After a long sheath is satisfactorily positioned over a tortuous course, removal of its dilator can permit the lumen of the sheath to assume an elliptical section or, worse, collapse and form a "kink." In either case the reduced diameter of the long sheath can impede an advancing angioplasty balloon with a stent mounted on it. Some stents are longitudinally rigid and comply poorly with curves in delivery sheaths, thus compounding the difficulty encountered in advancing a stent and angioplasty balloon through a tightly curved long sheath.

Third, stents adhere poorly to angioplasty balloons on which they are mounted or "crimped." A stent can be "stripped" off its angioplasty balloon as the balloon and stent are advanced through a distorted or kinked long sheath. A stent can be "milked" off its angioplasty balloon during balloon inflation, typically when one end of the angioplasty balloon inflates in advance of the opposite end and pushes the stent along the balloon.

Fourth, some stents have sharp ends. These can lacerate an angioplasty balloon and cause balloon failure, leading to nonexpansion or only partial expansion of a stent. Thus the interventionalist must judiciously limit the force used to crimp a stent on an angioplasty balloon. The same sharp stent ends can perforate a vascular wall during or after stent deployment and cause severe injury.

Finally, even when the preceding challenges are overcome, a number of factors can cause the ultimate position of a deployed stent to be suboptimal. Considerable judgment is required to accurately predict the final position of an expanding and often foreshortening stent with respect to the vascular narrowing being treated, particularly when no reliable fluoroscopic landmark is present to precisely define the relationship between the narrowing and the stent. Stents can slip out of position as they are being deployed. This problem is especially apparent in the aorta, where high-pressure systolic blood flow tends to push an expanding stent and its angioplasty balloon distally before the stent can engage the aortic wall. Stents also tend to slip out of position as they are being expanded in tapering vessels. A stent can migrate out of position after deployment even when the initial position of the stent appears satisfactory. Such migration can occur immediately after stent implantation or at a later time. Stent fracture is an uncommon problem usually caused by metal fatigue associated with crimping or cardiac motion. Stents placed in ventricular outflow tracts are particularly subject to such failure. Over time, stent recoil, intimal proliferation, and in-stent restenosis can cause an immediately favorable outcome to become suboptimal.

Fortunately, technical aspects of stent implantation by pediatric interventionalists have evolved greatly in response to these challenges. Stent implantation procedures have thus become simpler, safer, and more effective than they were originally. The purpose of this chapter is to describe several recent technical developments in the implantation of endovascular stents for the treatment of congenital and postsurgical cardiovascular anomalies.

NEW PRODUCTS THAT FACILITATE STENT IMPLANTATION

Manufacturers are continuously introducing new products that may facilitate stent implantation in congenital and postsurgical cardiovascular narrowings. Conversely, manufacturers have withdrawn or will soon withdraw some products that were originally adapted for use in these applications (e.g., Mansfield angioplasty balloons and Cordis Corinthian IQ stents). With few exceptions, the techniques used by pediatric interventionalists to implant stents in congenital and postsurgical cardiovascular narrowings have been developed by adapting products intended for other stent applications, particularly hepatobiliary and peripheral vascular stent implantations. Thus the disappearance of familiar products and the appearance of unfamiliar products represent additional challenges for pediatric interventionalists. The changing array of products available must be carefully evaluated so that only those combinations of products are used that are likely to improve or at least maintain the safety and effectiveness of stent implantation.

Products available in one region may not be available in another. As a consequence, the authors are familiar primarily with products available to them in North America and in this chapter present information only about such products. Product cost will drive decisions regarding which products to use. Products that work well in the hands of one interventionalist may work less well in the hands of another. Thus each pediatric interventionalist will have his or her own individual preference for certain products or certain techniques. Fortunately, there is usually more than one suitable way to safely and effectively implant a stent in any given congenital or postsurgical cardiovascular narrowing.

STENTS

Palmaz

The first stents available for treatment of congenital and postsurgical cardiovascular anomalies were the Palmaz stents manufactured originally by Johnson and Johnson Interventional Systems and now by Cordis Endovascular, both divisions of Johnson and Johnson. The Palmaz stents have been widely used to treat congenital anomalies, and by far the greatest experience for these applications has accumulated with them. The Palmaz stents typically used are available in three sizes: medium (10, 15, 20, 29, and 39 mm long), large (12, 18, and 30 mm long), and extra large (30, 40, and 50 mm long).

The Palmaz stent is a balloon-expandable, slotted-tube design cut from type 316L stainless steel tubing using a laser. These stents offer the advantages of sufficient radial strength for most applications and adequate radiopacity for satisfactory fluoroscopic visualization during implantation. However, the Palmaz stents are longitudinally rigid. Thus they can be difficult to deploy via tortuous catheter courses, and they may not conform well to curvilinear vessels. They shorten considerably as they are expanded to large diameters (4). These stents tend to slip on angioplasty balloons on which they are mounted. The ends of Palmaz stents are sharp and can lacerate angioplasty balloons or perforate vessel walls (5,6). These stents rarely fracture.

The medium and large Palmaz stents are clearly an established element of the pediatric interventionalist's armamentarium. The extra-large Palmaz stents have more recently been put to use by pediatric interventionalists (Table 33.1). Benson and colleagues at the Toronto General Hospital and the Hospital for Sick Children in Toronto, Canada, have successfully used the extra-large stents to treat adolescent and adult patients with coarctation of the aorta. The extra-large stents have also proven useful in palliating obstructed right ventricular outflow tract conduits (4). Nugent and associates in Boston and Quebec have recently reported use of Palmaz stents covered with expanded polytetrafluoroethylene to treat 12 patients with congenital heart disease and a variety of cardiovascular narrowings (7).

TABLE 33.1. CHARACTERISTICS OF PALMAZ XL (EXTRA-LARGE) TRANSHEPATIC BILIARY STENTS*

Expanded Diameter (mm)	Expanded Length (mm)		Shortening (%)	Fit[†] (F)
	P4010	P5010		
10	39.0	49.0	2.5	—
14	37.8	47.0	5.1	10
15	37.4	46.5	6.0	10
16	37.0	46.0	7.0	10
17	36.5	45.4	8.3	—
18	35.9	44.7	9.8	10
19	35.3	44.0	11.3	—
20	34.7	43.2	12.8	11
21	34.0	42.3	14.6	—
22	33.3	41.4	16.3	—
23	32.4	40.3	18.6	—
24	31.6	39.2	20.9	—
25	30.6	38.0	23.1	—

*Specifications taken from Cordis literature.
Nominal lengths (mm) = 39.8 for P4010, 49.5 for P5010. Nominal outer diameters (mm) 4.55 for P4010, 4.55 for P5010.
[†]4010 mounted on Maxi LD angioplasty balloon.
—, Not applicable or no data given.

Cordis introduced the Corinthian IQ stent as an alternative to the medium Palmaz stent (Figure 33.1 and Table 33.2). The Corinthian IQ stent is flexible and has rounded ends, which reduces risk of angioplasty balloon laceration or vascular injury. The Corinthian IQ stents are available premounted on angioplasty balloons, resulting in lower delivery system profile and improved stent/balloon adherence. In fact, some pediatric interventionalists have found long sheaths unnecessary when implanting the Corinthian IQ stents. Although anecdotal reports have been favorable, little has yet been published by pediatric interventionalists regarding use of these stents (8).

Cordis recently replaced the Corinthian IQ stents with its new line of Palmaz Genesis stents (Figure 33.2). The Genesis stents are based on the same technology as the Cordis Bx VELOCITY coronary stents, and they are simi-

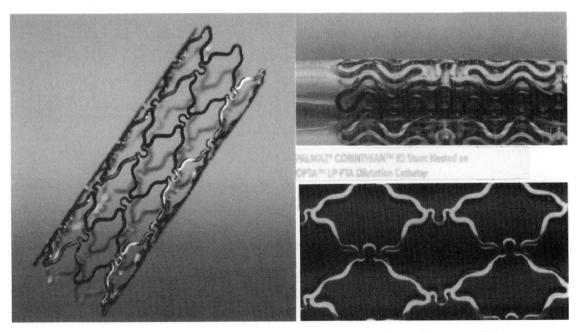

FIGURE 33.1. Cordis Corinthian IQ stent. (Courtesy, Cordis Endovascular, Warren, NJ.)

TABLE 33.2. CHARACTERISTICS OF CORDIS CORINTHIAN IQ STENTS*

Expanded Diameter (mm)	Expanded Length (mm)					Shortening (%)	Fit‡ (F)
	PQ124B	PQ154B	PQ184B	PQ294B	PQ394B†		
4	11	14	17	29	38	2.6–8.3	6
5	11	14	17	28	36	3.4–8.3	6
6	10	13	16	27	35	6.9–16.7	6
7	9	12	15	26	34	10.3–25	6/6.5
8	9	11	13	22	29	24.1–27.8	6/6.5
9	—	—	—	22	29	24.1–25.6	—

*Specifications taken from Cordis literature.
†Product codes. Nominal lengths (mm) = 12 for PQ124B, 15 for PQ154B, 18 for PQ184B, 29 for PQ294B, and 39 for PQ394B.
‡PQ124B, PQ154B, and PQ184B are compatible with 6 sheaths when expanded to 4–8 mm diameter. PQ294B and PQ394B are compatible with 6.5 sheaths when expanded to 7–8 mm diameter.
—, not applicable or no data available.

lar in appearance to the Bx VELOCITY stents. They have greater radial strength than the original Palmaz stents. They are also flexible, more so than the Corinthian IQ stents. They have rounded ends, thus reducing the risk of angioplasty balloon laceration or vessel wall perforation. They shorten during expansion, but shortening is less than 10% of nominal length at final diameters of 12 mm or less. These stents are available with nominal lengths of 12 to 79 mm. They are grouped into short (12, 15, 18, and 24 mm long), medium-long (19, 29, and 39 mm long), and very-long (59 and 79 mm long) categories. The medium-long and very-long Genesis stents are expandable to a diameter of 18 mm.

NuMED Cheatham Platinum Stent

The NuMED Cheatham Platinum (CP) stents are the product of collaboration between Dr. Cheatham and NuMED, Inc. (9–11). They were developed in conjunction with the balloon-in-balloon (BIB) catheters, also from NuMED, Inc. They are not yet FDA approved. The CP stent is a laser-welded assembly consisting of tandem rows of "zigs." Each row of zigs is formed from tempered, 0.013-inch, 90% platinum and 10% iridium wire. The stents are available in 6-, 8-, and 10-zig configurations, making them expandable to 25- to 30-mm diameters, and they are available in a variety of lengths, depending on the number of rows of zigs welded together. They are also available with a polytetrafluoroethylene (PTFE) cover. These stents have excellent radial strength and are somewhat flexible. Because of their high content of platinum, they are densely radiopaque and easily visualized fluoroscopically. The ends of these stents are rounded rather than sharp, making balloon laceration and vessel wall perforation unlikely. They adhere satisfactorily after crimping on BIB balloons. These stents are reputed to occasionally fracture during crimping,

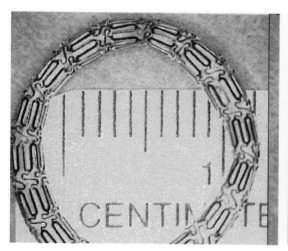
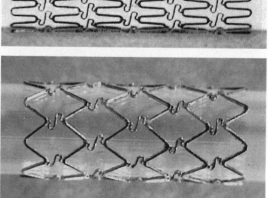

FIGURE 33.2. Flexible Cordis Genesis stent. (Courtesy, Cordis Endovascular, Warren, NJ.)

TABLE 33.3. SHORTENING OF 8-ZIG, 45-MM-LONG, COVERED NUMED CP STENT MEASURED ON BENCH TOP DURING EXPANSION WITH PROGRESSIVELY LARGER DIAMETER BALLOONS

Balloon Diameter at 6–7 Atmospheres	Minimum Length of Stent Itself	Minimum Length of PTFE* Cover	Stent Shortening (%)	Cover Shortening (%)
12	43	38–40	4.4	2.4–4.9
15	38–39	33–35	13.3–15.6	14.6–19.5
18	38	30–31	15.6	24.4–26.8
19	37–38	30–31	15.6–17.8	24.4–26.8
21–22	34	25	24.4	39

*Polytetrafluoroethylene. Estimated nominal length of cover 41 mm. No tears in the cover were discernible at the maximum expansion diameter of 21–22 mm.

although fracture has not been encountered in the authors' limited experience with them. The stents have a slightly higher profile after mounting on angioplasty balloons, although the increment in profile has not seemed objectionable. The stents do foreshorten as they are expanded.

The CP stents have been used in a variety of narrowings (9–11). Final stent diameters have ranged between 10 and 30 mm; final lengths, between 22 and 117 mm. Long introducer sheaths used to deploy these stents have ranged between 10 and 14F in diameter. The few covered CP stents known to have been implanted have been used to relieve severe coarctation of the aorta, to relieve coarctation with complete obstruction (atresia) of the aorta, to close multiple fenestrations in a Fontan lateral tunnel, and to relieve obstruction of a superior vena cava (SVC) compressed by a grossly dilated and severely hypertensive pulmonary artery. Shortening of the PTFE cover on the covered CP stent is relatively greater than shortening of the stent itself, as the covered stent is progressively expanded to increasing diameters (Table 33.3). Bonhoeffer, now working at the Great Ormand Street Hospital in London, has constructed valved stent grafts and implanted them in the right ventricular outflow tracts of several patients with outflow tract obstruction. These valved stent grafts are fabricated using CP stents and glutaraldehyde-treated, valved segments of bovine jugular veins.

Intrastent DoubleStrut LD

Intrastent DoubleStrut stents (Figure 33.3) have been introduced relatively recently by Intratherapeutics, a division of Sulzer Medica in Switzerland. Anecdotal reports of their use by interventional pediatric cardiologists have generally been favorable. More formal reports of such use are now beginning to appear (12–17). The Intrastent DoubleStrut LD stent is a balloon-expandable double-strut design cut from type 316L stainless steel tubing using a laser. The Intrastent DoubleStrut LD stents are available in a range of sizes suitable to treat many of the congenital and postsurgical cardiovascular anomalies requiring stent implantation (Table 33.4). However, they are not available

in sizes as large as the Palmaz XL and NuMED CP stents. The Intrastent DoubleStrut LD stents are sufficiently radiopaque for satisfactory fluoroscopic visualization. Their radiopacity is similar to that of the Palmaz stents but not as great as that of the NuMED CP stents. These stents are longitudinally flexible. Thus they are more readily advanced over tortuous catheter courses than the Palmaz or NuMED CP stents, and they better conform to curvilinear vessels in which they are implanted. The Intrastent DoubleStrut LD stents do *not* shorten as they are expanded to a 12-mm diameter. They do shorten as they are expanded to an 18-mm diameter (Table 33.4). The ends of these stents are less sharp than those of the Palmaz stents, although they are somewhat sharper than the ends of the NuMED CP stents. Furthermore, the ends of these stents are designed to be more flexible than their middle segments. Thus these stents have reduced tendency to lacerate angioplasty balloons or perforate vessel walls. These stents have a proprietary "Microgrip" internal finish claimed to reduce their ten-

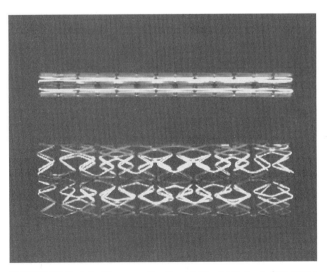

FIGURE 33.3. IntraTherapeutics DoubleStrut LD stent. (Courtesy, Sulzer IntraTherapeutics, Inc., St. Paul, MN.)

TABLE 33.4. INTRASTENT DOUBLESTRUT LD STENT SPECIFICATIONS*

Product Number	Nominal Dimensions	Dimensions Expanded	Dimensions Expanded > 12 mm Diameter
S15–16	3.8 mm diameter 16 mm long	9–12 mm diameter 16 mm long	
S15–26	3.8 mm diameter 26 mm long	9–12 mm diameter 26 mm long	18 mm diameter 17.4–19.2
S15–36	3.8 mm diameter 36 mm long	9–12 mm diameter 36 mm long	
S15–56	3.8 mm diameter 56 mm long	9–12 mm diameter 56 mm long	
S15–76	3.8 mm diameter 76 mm long	9–12 mm diameter 76 mm long	

*These stents do not shorten when expanded to 12-mm diameter. *In vitro* testing (9) showed 26% to 33% shortening of the 26-mm-long stent dilated directly to 18-mm diameter. However, stepwise dilation of the 26-mm-long stent to a final diameter of 18 mm using progressively larger-diameter angioplasty balloons produced no shortening because of a change in the stent cell geometry. Clinically, no shortening was discernible in stents expanded to 6 to 15, mean 8.9 mm, minimum final diameter (9).

dency to slip on angioplasty balloons on which they are mounted. However, some pediatric interventionalists believe that these stents are somewhat more difficult to crimp on angioplasty balloons and therefore are more prone to slipping, despite the proprietary internal finish. These stents have reduced radial strength when expanded to diameters greater than 12 mm, and stent recoil has been encountered after these stents have been expanded to large diameters (16). Intratherapeutics will soon introduce a new line of stents that have increased radial strength when expanded to large diameters. The tendency of the DoubleStrut LD stents to fracture is unknown.

Medtronic Bridge Stent

The Bridge stents from Medtronic AVE (Figure 33.4) are manufactured from 2-mm-long stainless steel, sinusoidal elements. These elements are fused with a laser to form eliptorectangular struts, which resist radial compression, and a dual-helical pattern, which promotes longitudinal flexibility. Heat and pressure are used to mount the stents on angioplasty balloons so that balloon material fills the space between the stent struts, creating "pillows," which promote stent retention. These stents are available premounted on angioplasty balloons with diameters of 6 to 10 mm. The stents are available in 28-, 40-, and 60-mm lengths. They have rounded ends and tend not to flare during expansion, reducing the risk of angioplasty balloon laceration and rupture or vascular injury. Rao and colleagues at Saint Louis University have successfully used these stents to treat vascular narrowings in a small number of children (18). One drawback of these stents is that they are not available in the larger diameters (12 to 18 mm) often required for treatment of congenital and postsurgical cardiovascular anomalies.

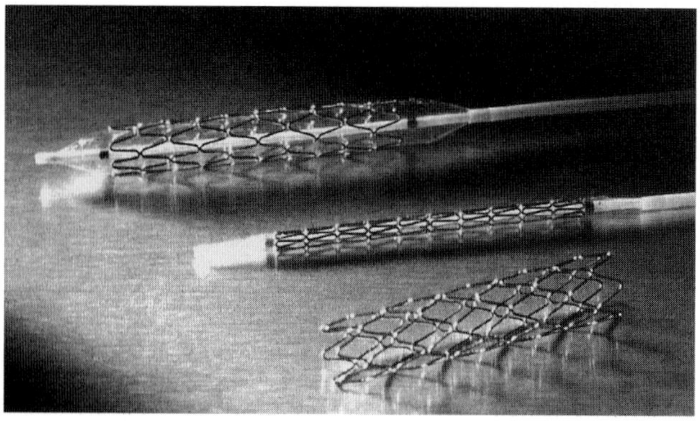

BALLOON ANGIOPLASTY CATHETERS

A variety of balloon angioplasty catheters are now available for implantation of endovascular stents. Although Cordis and NuMED recommend that their stents be deployed using balloon angioplasty catheters of their own manufacture, other companies' balloon angioplasty catheters can also be used effectively. Selection of a particular catheter for stent implantation in a specific narrowing depends on the size and location of the narrowing, the type of stent to be used, the technique to be used, and catheter cost and availability as well as the experience and personal preference of the interventionalist. Several of the balloon angioplasty catheters currently used to implant stents in congenital and postsurgical narrowings are briefly discussed next.

FIGURE 33.4. Medtronic AVE Bridge stent. (Courtesy, Medtronic AVE, Santa Rosa, CA.)

Slalom

The Slalom catheters from Cordis are recommended by the manufacturer for deployment of the Genesis stent when a 0.018-inch guide wire is to be used. The Slalom catheters have 3.7- or 4.2F shafts. Balloons are available in 3- to 8-mm diameters and 2- and 4-cm lengths. The balloons have rated burst pressures of 10 to 14 atm.

Opta Pro

The Opta Pro catheters from Cordis are recommended by the manufacturer for deployment of the Genesis stent when a 0.035-inch guide wire is to be used. The Opta Pro catheters have 5F shafts. Balloons are available in 3- to 12-mm diameters and 1- to 10-cm lengths. The balloons have rated burst pressures of 6 to 10 atm.

Marshal

The Marshal catheters from Medi-tech are recommended by the manufacturer for deployment of the Palmaz medium stents. These catheters accept 0.035-inch guide wires, and they have 5.0- to 5.8F shafts. Balloons 4 through 8 mm in diameter and 1.5, 2, 3, and 4 cm long on 90-cm shafts are intended for stent deployment. The balloons have a rated burst pressure of 12 atm.

Powerflex P3

The PowerFlex P3 catheters from Cordis have been used to deploy Palmaz large stents that are to be expanded to intermediate diameters. These catheters accept 0.035-inch guide wires and have 5F shafts. Balloons 7, 8, 9, 10, and 12 mm in diameter are available in 2-, 3-, and 4-cm lengths. Rated burst pressures range between 8 and 15 atm.

Maxi LD

The Maxi LD catheters from Cordis can be used to deploy Palmaz large and extra-large stents. These catheters accept 0.035-inch guide wires, and they have 7F shafts. Balloons are available in 14- to 20-mm diameters and 2- to 8-cm lengths. The balloons have a rated burst pressure of 6 atm. The manufacturer somewhat optimistically claims that 8F sheaths will accommodate P308 stents mounted on 14- to 18-mm-diameter Maxi LD balloons and that 10- to 11F sheaths will accommodate P4010 stents mounted on 14- to 20-mm-diameter Maxi LD balloons (Table 33.1). However, in practice, somewhat larger sheaths will usually prove necessary to accommodate these combinations of stents and balloons.

Z-Med II

The Z-Med II catheters manufactured by NuMED and distributed by Braun can be used to deploy Palmaz large stents. The Z-MED II catheters have 5- to 9F shafts and accept 0.025- to 0.035-inch guide wires. The catheters track well over guide wires. However, the shafts are thin-walled and can telescope if too much push is applied. The balloons are made of double extruded plastic that is resistant to puncture. The balloons are available up to 25 mm in diameter and 6 cm in length, and they have rated burst pressures of 4 to 15 atm. The balloons have an irregular surface, which may improve stent adhesion, and they are short-tapered, which assists maintenance of balloon position during stent expansion. Required introducer sizes range from 6 to 14F (7F for the 10-mm balloon, 10F for the 18-mm balloon).

Balloon-in-Balloon

The balloon-in-balloon (BIB) catheter from NuMED (Figure 33.5), is a novel design developed by John Cheatham in conjunction with the manufacturer. An inner balloon is centered inside an outer balloon. The inner and outer balloons have separate inflation ports. The inner balloon is half the diameter of the outer balloon and 1 cm shorter than the outer balloon. The inner balloon is inflated first to expand a stent to half its intended final diameter, thereby fixing the stent on the catheter without causing the ends of the stent to flare. With the inner balloon inflated, the position of the stent is adjusted if necessary. Then the outer balloon is inflated to expand the stent to its final diameter and fix it in the cardiovascular narrowing. Both Palmaz large stents

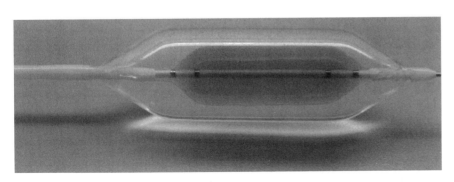

FIGURE 33.5. NuMED Balloon-in-Balloon (BIB) catheter. (Courtesy, NuMED, Inc., Hopkinton, NY.)

and NuMED CP stents can be deployed using the BIB catheters. All the catheters accept 0.035-inch guide wires. Outer balloons are 8 to 24 mm in diameter and 2.5 to 5.5 cm long. Inner balloons have rated burst pressures of 4.5 to 5 atm. Outer balloons are made of the same material as Z-MED II balloons and have rated burst pressures of 3 to 10 atm. Required introducer sizes are like those needed for Z-MED II balloons.

Accent

The Accent catheters from Cook have recently been used to implant large stents in pulmonary artery narrowings in infants and small children using a miniature stent delivery system developed by Ing and colleagues at the San Diego Children's Hospital in California. The Accent balloons have had dilator tips attached to them to facilitate passage of "front-loaded" stents tightly crimped onto the balloons. The Accent catheters have been used for this technique, because the geometry of the distal end of the balloons facilitates attaching the dilator tips. However, the balloon material has proven susceptible to damage during the tight crimping of the stents. Twenty-five percent to 35% of the balloons have developed pinpoint holes manifest during stent expansion. Ing's technique is described in greater detail later. Because of their susceptibility to balloon puncture, the Accent catheters have not otherwise been much used for stent implantation.

LONG SHEATHS

Long sheaths are commonly used to facilitate advancement of stents mounted on angioplasty balloons to distal vascular narrowings. A long sheath allows the interventionalist to retrieve a stent should it slip out of position on an angioplasty balloon as the stent and balloon are being advanced to the end of the sheath. A long sheath allows contrast material to be injected directly into the region of interest so that stent position can be adjusted prior to deployment and so that outcome can be evaluated immediately after deployment. A long sheath can also be used to control inflation of the proximal end of an angioplasty balloon or to stabilize the proximal end of a stent during stent expansion. The ideal long sheath should have a positive but compliant hemostasis valve and a sheath side arm, should be readily visualized by fluoroscopy, should be resistant to kinking, and should track readily over a guide wire.

The long sheaths originally used to implant Palmaz stents had no hemostasis valves. Hemostasis valves had to be fabricated for these long sheaths by mating modified introducer sheaths to them (4). Now, however, suitable long sheaths are available from Cook, Inc. and Arrow International, Inc. These long sheaths are manufactured with hemostasis valves and side arms. Stent implantation procedures are greatly simplified using these long sheaths. The

hemostasis valves manufactured by these vendors not only effectively prevent bleeding, most notably when only a guide wire is passed through them, but are large enough to readily accommodate angioplasty balloons with stents mounted on them. This characteristic allows stents to be "back-loaded" for delivery to the cardiovascular narrowings to be treated. The ease with which these long sheaths can be visualized fluoroscopically also significantly simplifies stent implantation. The long sheaths from Cook have a radiopaque marker band at the tip, whereas the long sheaths from Arrow are radiopaque throughout their lengths, with radiopaque marker bands at the tips. The newer Cook long sheaths are more resistant to kinking than the original Cook sheaths, although the newer sheaths will kink if sufficiently tightly curved. The Arrow long sheaths are extremely kink resistant. However, the Arrow sheath lumen will progressively distort from a circular to an oval cross section as the sheath is increasingly tightly curved. In addition, the Arrow sheath has an irregular or "ribbed" luminal surface due to its spiral design. These qualities can increase the resistance encountered when advancing a stent mounted on an angioplasty balloon through a tightly curved Arrow long sheath.

A large variety of long sheaths are available from Cook. The authors have found the "Large Check-Flo II Blue Introducer Sets with Radiopaque Band" to be particularly useful for stent implantation. These long sheaths are available in 9.0- to 14.0F diameters. Product numbers for these sheaths in 80 cm lengths are RCF-9.0-38-80-J-RB through RCF-14.0-38-80-J-RB, with the first set of numerals in the product number representing the sheath diameter in French units. Cook is introducing a new line of long sheaths. These "Flexor" sheaths, which will eventually be available in 5- to 16F diameters, have a spiral wound design similar to the Arrow long sheaths but with a smooth luminal surface.

A variety of long sheaths is also available from Arrow. The authors have used "Super Arrow-Flex Percutaneous Sheath Introducer Sets with Integral Hemostasis Valve Side Ports." These sheaths are available in diameters from 5 through 11F. Product numbers for these sheaths in 80-cm lengths are CL-07880, CL-07980, CL-07080, and CL-71180 for 8-, 9-, 10-, and 11F diameters, respectively.

GUIDE WIRES

Guide wires used for stent implantation must be sufficiently stiff to remain in position during stent delivery, must have a soft distal tip to minimize the risk of vascular injury, and must be long enough to perform catheter exchanges. The Amplatz Super Stiff guide wire available from Medi-tech remains the mainstay for stent implantation in many congenital and postsurgical cardiovascular narrowings. This wire is 0.035 inch in diameter and 260 cm long with a 7-cm soft tip. It is an extremely rigid wire except at its tip, which is highly flexible for a length of 7 cm. The wire's rigidity enables long sheaths, angioplasty balloons, and stents to be relatively easily advanced via the tortuous course through the right heart to narrowings in branch pulmonary arteries, main pulmonary arteries, and right ventricular outflow tract conduits. Thus the wire promotes pushability and trackability. The wire's rigidity also helps to stabilize the position of angioplasty balloons and stents as stents are being deployed. This feature is particularly helpful when deploying stents in coarctation of the aorta, where high-pressure systolic blood flow tends to push an expanding stent and its angioplasty balloon distally before the stent can engage the aortic wall. The soft tip of the wire protects the peripheral pulmonary arteries during stent implantation in pulmonary artery narrowings, and it protects the aortic root and aortic valve during stent implantation in coarctation of the aorta. A disadvantage of this wire is that the 7-cm soft tip may prove excessively long in infants and small children, whose pulmonary arteries are shorter and where wire rigidity closer to the end of the wire would be helpful. However, more recently 2 cm long soft tip wire are available and are useful in younger children. Another disadvantage of this wire is that it is poorly steerable. Because of its stiffness, the wire tends to distort cardiovascular structures such as the right atrial wall or tricuspid valve. Resulting bradycardia, heart block, tachyarrhythmias, or valve incompetence can lead to hemodynamic instability during stent implantation.

The Rosen guide wire available from Cook, Inc., is a utility wire that is not as stiff as the Amplatz Super Stiff guide wire. The Rosen wire is available in diameters of 0.025 and 0.035 inch and a length of 260 cm. It has a short floppy tip with a tight J-curve. The intermediate stiffness of the Rosen wire is often sufficient to position long sheaths for stent deployment with less distortion of cardiovascular structures and less attendant hemodynamic instability.

The Wholey Hi-Torque Floppy guide wire and its extension guide wire, the LOC wire, are available from Mallinckrodt. The Wholey wire is 0.035 inch in diameter and 145, 175, or 260 cm long. It is quite stiff throughout its length except at its end, which is progressively floppy over a distance of approximately 20 cm. The wire is highly steerable and therefore extremely useful when attempting to gain access to tortuous peripheral pulmonary artery branches. The LOC extension wire is a 0.035-inch wire that is 115 cm long. It can be threaded onto the proximal end of a 145-cm Wholey wire to create an exchange length wire. The extended Wholey wire can thus be used to introduce catheters to peripheral pulmonary artery branches and then exchanged for an Amplatz Super Stiff wire to be used for stent implantation.

The Magic Torque guide wire from Medi-tech is another highly steerable 0.035-inch wire. The wire features platinum radiopaque markers spaced at 10-mm intervals near the tip. The markers can be used as a reference to facilitate measurement of vascular narrowings during stent implantation procedures.

Nitinol guide wires available from both Microvena Corporation and AGA Medical deserve mention. Stiff versions of these wires that are 0.035 inch in diameter and 260 cm long with 14-cm soft tips are available. These wires, which will not kink, might, for example, prove quite useful during stent implantation in coarctation of the aorta.

RECENT PROCEDURAL INNOVATIONS THAT FACILITATE STENT IMPLANTATION

Procedural innovations that facilitate stent implantation in congenital and postsurgical cardiovascular narrowings are at least as important as the new products that facilitate these interventions. Several such innovations will be discussed in the following paragraphs. Again, techniques that work well in the hands of one interventionalist may work less well in the hands of another. Thus each pediatric interventionalist must decide whether these innovations will prove useful in his or her individual practice.

Over-the-Wire Angiography

Because guide wire position can be difficult to attain and then maintain during stent implantation procedures, over-the-wire technique can be used to measure pressures proximal and distal to a vascular narrowing and to image the narrowing without having to remove and then replace the guide wire traversing the narrowing. Two techniques are available. In the first, a high-flow angiographic catheter is advanced over the guide wire to the narrowing. The hub of the catheter is attached to a Y-adaptor. The Y-adaptor, in turn, is attached either to a pressure transducer to measure pressures or to a pressure injector to perform angiography. Some pediatric interventionalists prefer to use a shortened 7F pigtail catheter available from Merit Medical (South Jordan, Utah) (product number 1308-35-0007) and a Y-adaptor available from Braun (Bethlehem, PA) (product number AYC-013). This combination of catheter and Y-adaptor will permit contrast material to be injected via the catheter over a 0.035-inch guide wire at a flow rate of 15 mL/sec and a pressure of 600 lb/in.[2]. Y-adaptors available from other manufacturers tend not to accommodate such high flow rates and injection pressures, and they often fail during angiography. Some interventionalists prefer this technique, because the angiographic catheter traversing the wire is readily pushable. The disadvantages of this technique are that pressure tracings can be damped in the relatively narrow catheter lumen surrounding the guide wire and that flow rates and injection pressures for angiography are somewhat limited.

In the second, or monorail, technique, the tip of a monorail Multi-Track catheter available from Braun is advanced over the guide wire to the vascular narrowing, where pressure measurements and angiography can be performed. The Multi-Track catheter permits high-fidelity pressure recordings to be made, and the catheter accommodates higher flow rates and injection pressures than a modified angiographic catheter attached to a Y-adaptor. For example, the 6F Multi-Track catheter delivers contrast material at 25 mL/sec and 1,000 lb/in.[2] However, the disadvantage of this technique is that the monorail catheter is less pushable because only the catheter tip traverses the guide wire, and the remainder of the catheter shaft lies free in the vascular space parallel with the guide wire. This limitation can be overcome by advancing an appropriate-sized guide wire through the lumen of the Multi-Track catheter to stiffen the system and enhance pushability.

Miniaturization of Delivery Systems to Facilitate Implantation of Large Stents in Infants and Small Children

Ing and his colleagues have developed a novel method to deliver large stents via small-diameter long sheaths into stenotic branch pulmonary arteries in infants and small children (19,20). The large stents can later be dilated to adult pulmonary artery diameters as required. Ing's technique involves slightly enlarging the distal end of the long delivery sheath, mounting the stent using a novel crimping technique, fitting the angioplasty balloon with a dilator tip, and "front-loading" the assembly into the long sheath.

The diameter of a 7- or 8F long sheath is first slightly enlarged. It may occasionally be necessary to cut off the restrictive radiopaque marker band from the tip of the 7F long sheath before enlarging the tip of the sheath. The end of the sheath is heated with a hot air gun, and a dilator one French size larger than the sheath is inserted for a distance of 2 to 3 cm. The dilator is kept inside the sheath while it is cooled under water. Then the dilator is removed. The tip of the dilator supplied with the long sheath is cut off and twisted or glued using "superglue" (Surgical Simplex P) onto the end of the angioplasty balloon. Ing has used the Accent balloon angioplasty catheters available from Cook. This particular balloon has a slightly longer tip and larger profile than other balloons, and it accommodates the dilator tip particularly well. The angioplasty balloon with the dilator tip attached is advanced through the long sheath and out the distal end.

A large stent (Palmaz P188, Palmaz P308, or IntraStent DoubleStrut 16DS) is mounted on the angioplasty balloon. Crimping is accomplished by wrapping a single turn of suture or narrow cloth tape ("umbilical tape") around the stent and pulling firmly on the ends of the suture or tape. This method ensures that an even force is circumferentially applied to the stent during crimping. Using the same technique, the dilator tip is tightened onto the balloon tip. The assembly consisting of the dilator tip, the angioplasty balloon, and the tightly crimped stent is then withdrawn or front-loaded into the distal end of the long sheath. Only the dilator tip is left exposed beyond the end of the long sheath. The dilator tip on the angioplasty balloon allows the assembled dilator tip, angioplasty balloon, stent, and long sheath to pass smoothly as a unit through the skin to the narrowing where the stent is to be deployed.

Ing and his colleagues initially described this technique in ten infants and children (19). These patients weighed 6

to 38.7 kg. Twelve large stents (P188 and P308) were mounted on 8- to 14-mm-diameter angioplasty balloons and delivered using 7- or 8F long sheaths. Balloon perforation occurred during 25% of stent expansions. New balloons were used to complete implantation of partially expanded stents. Anatomic and hemodynamic results were excellent in all patients. No dilator tip separated from its angioplasty balloon. Ing and his colleagues have now extended this technique to 14 infants (20). These patients weighed 5.4 to 10, median 6.8 kg. Twenty large stents (10 Palmaz P188 stents and 10 IntraStent DoubleStrut 16DS stents) were mounted on 6- or 8-mm-diameter angioplasty balloons and delivered using 7F long sheaths. Pinpoint balloon rupture occurred during 35% of stent expansions. However, anatomic and hemodynamic results were excellent in all patients.

Ing's crimping technique can permit delivery of large stents via small-diameter long sheaths in small children without use of front loading or a dilator tip attached to the angioplasty balloon. For example, the authors used umbilical tape to crimp a Palmaz P188 stent onto a 10-mm-diameter Z-MED II angioplasty balloon. The balloon and stent were back-loaded into an 8F Arrowflex long sheath prepositioned in the left pulmonary artery of a 23.5-kg child. The balloon and stent were advanced to the left pulmonary artery via the usual somewhat tortuous course through the right heart without difficulty, and the stent was deployed with good result.

Protection of the Coronary Arterial Circulation

An expanded endovascular stent can compress or distort an adjacent coronary artery and interfere with coronary arterial flow. In fact, the authors know of two anecdotal reports of patient death attributed to coronary insufficiency following adjacent stent implantation. Thus stent implantation in a right ventricular outflow tract conduit, main pulmonary artery, ascending aorta, or right or left ventricular outflow tract should be approached with great caution to avoid causing myocardial ischemia (21,22). The potential effect of stent implantation in a narrowing lying near a coronary artery can be predicted by placing an appropriately sized angioplasty balloon in the narrowing and performing selective coronary angiography before and while the balloon is inflated. If balloon inflation is seen to cause no compression of the nearby coronary artery and if no electrocardiographic changes occur, then the interventionalist can generally conclude that stent implantation will cause no interference with coronary flow. Of course, the stent that is implanted must be expanded to no greater a diameter than that of the angioplasty balloon used during the test coronary angiography. In addition, the conclusion that stent implantation can safely proceed must be based on a decision that there are probably no dynamic factors that might affect the relationship between the stent and the adjacent coronary artery during increases in cardiac output. Great caution should be exercised when implanting a stent to treat right ventricular outflow tract obstruction associated with prior surgical manipulation of the coronary arteries.

Stent Implantation for Superior and Inferior Vena Cava Obstruction

It is often possible to patiently manipulate a guide wire through a totally obstructed superior or inferior vena cava, thereby establishing a track that can be serially dilated with angioplasty balloons and then kept open permanently by stent implantation. Pediatric interventionalists have also shown that total caval occlusions can be penetrated with modified transseptal needles, after which guide wires or dilators can be advanced to establish tracks for serial dilation and then stent implantation. These techniques have recently been extended for use in small infants (23–26).

MAGNETIC RESONANCE IMAGING FOLLOWING STENT IMPLANTATION

Until recently, there has been reluctance to perform magnetic resonance imaging for patients who have received metallic endovascular stents. There has been concern that exposure of stents to strong magnetic fields will cause stent dislodgment or vascular injury and that stents will introduce significant artifact into images obtained with this modality. Several pub-

lications appear to have allayed these concerns (27–31). Stents composed of several metals, including type 316L stainless steel and platinum, have been found to be nonferromagnetic and subject to minimal deflection forces in strong magnetic fields (27–29). Magnetic resonance imaging has usually been deferred during the first 6 weeks following stent implantation to allow time for tissue ingrowth to stabilize stent position. However, Rutledge and colleagues have reported that magnetic resonance imaging performed 2 to 13 days following implantation of Palmaz P188 and P308 stents (type 316L stainless steel) caused no adverse effect in a group of three patients (30). Imaging using spin-echo technique, as opposed to gradient echo technique, appears to adequately minimize introduction of artifact (30,31). Other imaging techniques, such as inversion recovery, may also satisfactorily minimize artifact.

CONCLUSION

An expanding range of products is becoming available to pediatric interventionalists using stents to treat congenital and postsurgical cardiovascular narrowings. Manufacturers are continuously introducing new products that may facilitate stent implantation in congenital and postsurgical cardiovascular narrowings (Table 33.5). Even though most of these products are intended for use in adults, they are also quite often suitable for use in children. Concurrently, imag-

TABLE 33.5. ADDRESSES AND TELEPHONE NUMBERS OF VENDORS MENTIONED IN THIS CHAPTER

AGA Medical Corporation
682 Mendelssohn Avenue
Golden Valley, Minnesota 55427
Phone: 763-513-9227
888-546-4407
FAX: 763-513-9296
www.amplatzer.com

Arrow International, Inc.
2400 Bernville Road
Reading, Pennsylvania 19605
Phone: 610-378-0131
800-523-8446
FAX: 610-478-3199
www.arrowintl.com

B. Braun Medical, Inc.
824 Twelfth Avenue
Bethlehem, Pennsylvania 18018
Phone: 800-523-9695
610-691-5400
FAX: 610-266-6122
www.bbraunusa.com

Cook, Inc.
Post Office Box 489
Bloomington, Indiana 47402-0489
Phone: 800-468-1379
FAX: 800-554-8335
www.cookgroup.com

Cordis Endovascular
7 Powder Horn Drive
Warren, New Jersey 07059
Phone: 908-755-830
FAX: 908-412-3060
www.cordis.com

IntraTherapeutics, Inc.
651 Campus Drive
Saint Paul, Minnesota 55112
Phone: 877-697-4840
FAX: 877-697-4841
www.IntraTherapeutics.com

Mallinckrodt Medical, Incorporated
900 Hornet Drive
Hazelwood, Missouri 63042
Phone: 800-635-5267
888-744-1414
FAX: 888-744-4646
www.mallinckrodt.com

Medi-tech
Boston Scientific
One Boston Scientific Place
Natick, Massachusetts 01760-1537
Phone: 508-650-8000
800-225-3238
FAX: 888-272-3767
www.bsci.com

Medtronic AVE
3576 Unocal Place
Santa Rosa, California 95403
Phone: 888-283-7868
FAX: 800-838-3103
www.medtronic.com

Merit Medical Systems, Inc.
1600 West Merit Parkway
South Jordan, Utah 84095
Phone: 801-253-1600
800-626-3748
FAX: 801-253-1681
www.merit.com

Microvena Corporation
1861 Buerkle Road
White Bear Lake
Minnesota 55110-5246 USA
Phone: 651-777-6700
800-716-6700
FAX: 651-777-4962
www.microvena.com

NuMED, Inc.
2880 Main Street
Hopkinton, New York 12965, USA
Phone: 315-328-4491
FAX: 315-328-4941
Email: numedorders@slic.com

inative pediatric interventionalists are refining established procedural techniques, inventing new techniques, and identifying new clinical indications for the use of stents. This convergence of new product availability and procedural innovation should make stent implantation by pediatric interventionalists simpler, quicker, safer, and more efficacious. The authors expect these welcome trends to continue indefinitely.

REFERENCES

1. Palmaz JC, Sibbitt RR, Reuter SR, et al. Expandable intraluminal graft: preliminary study. *Radiology* 1985;156:73–77.
2. Mullins CE, O'Laughlin MP, Vick GW III, et al. Implantation of balloon expandable intravascular grafts by catheterization in pulmonary arteries and systemic veins. *Circulation* 1988;77:188–199.
3. O'Laughlin MP, Perry SB, Lock JE, et al. Use of endovascular stents in congenital heart disease. *Circulation* 1991;83:1923–1939.
4. Coulson JD, Alekyan BG, Alia SJ, et al. Stents in the treatment of congenital heart disease: a five-year experience at two centers. In: Bockeria LA, Alekyan BG, Podzolkov, eds. *Endovascular and minimally invasive surgery of the heart and great vessels of children.* Moscow: Scientific Center of Cardiovascular Surgery, 1999:165–188.
5. Evans J, Saba Z, Rosenfeld H, et al. Aortic laceration secondary to Palmaz stent placement for treatment of superior vena cava syndrome. *Catheter Cardiovasc Interv* 2000;49:160–162.
6. Cheatham JP. A tragedy during Palmaz stent implant for SVC syndrome: Was it the stent or was it the balloon delivery system? *Catheter Cardiovasc Interv* 2000;49:163–166.
7. Nugent AW, Love B, Perry SB. Covered stents in congenital heart disease. *Cardiol Young* 2001;119(Suppl 1):62.
8. Turner DR, Rodriguez-Cruz E, Ross RD, et al. Initial experience using the Palmaz Corinthian stent for right ventricular outflow tract obstruction in infants and small children. *Catheter Cardiovasc Interv* 2000;51:444–449.
9. Cheatham J, Tower A, Ruiz C, et al. Initial experience using the NuMED Cheatham Platinum (CP) stent and a new balloon delivery catheter in children and adults with congenital heart disease. *Catheter Cardiovasc Interv* 1999;47:122.
10. Cheatham JP, Tower AJ, Ruiz CE, et al. Initial experience using the NuMED Cheatham Platinum stent and balloon in balloon delivery catheter in children and adults with congenital heart disease. *Circulation* 1999;100:I-30.
11. Kozlik-Feldmann R, Cheatham JP, Dabritz S, et al. Implantation of Cheatham Platinum (CP) stents for recoarctation in childhood. *Catheter Cardiovasc Interv* 2001;53:133.
12. Ing FF, Mathewson JW, Cocalis M, et al. The new DoubleStrut stent: *in vitro* evaluation of stent geometry following over dilation and initial clinical experience in congenital heart disease. *J Am Coll Cardiol* 2001;37:467A.
13. Rutledge JM, Grifka RG, Nihill MR, et al. Initial experience with IntraTherapeutics DoubleStrut LD stents in patients with congenital heart defects. *J Am Coll Cardiol* 2001;37:461A.
14. Kreutzer J, Rome JJ. Open cell design stents for vascular obstruction in congenital heart disease: a comparison of IntraStent versus Palmaz stents. *Catheter Cardiovasc Diagn* 2001;53:138.
15. Recto MR, Grifka RG. IntraStent DoubleStrut LD: collapse/recoil following use in post-operative stenoses. *Catheter Cardiovasc Diagn* 2001;53:146.
16. Recto MR, Elbl F, Austin E. Use of the new IntraStent for treatment of transverse arch hypoplasia/coarctation of the aorta. *Catheter Cardiovasc Diagn* 2001;53:499–503.
17. Cheatham JP. Initial use of the intratherapeutics, Inc. IntraStent Double Strut biliary endoprosthesis in the treatment of congenital heart disease. *Cardiol Young* 2001;11(Suppl 1):278.
18. Rao PS, Balfour IC, Singh GK, et al. Bridge stents in the management of obstructive vascular lesions in children. *Am J Cardiol* 2001;88:699–702.
19. Ing FF, Mathewson JW, Cocalis M, et al. A new technique for implantation of large stents through small sheaths in infants and children with branch pulmonary artery stenoses. *J Am Coll Cardiol* 2000;35:500A.
20. Ing FF, Perry JC, Mathewson JW, et al. Percutaneous implantation of large stents for the treatment of infants with severe postoperative branch pulmonary artery stenoses. *J Am Coll Cardiol* 2001;37:461A.
21. Maheshwari S, Bruckheimer E, Nehgme RA, et al. Single coronary artery complicating stent implantation for homograft stenosis in tetralogy of Fallot. *Catheter Cardiovasc Diagn* 1997;42:405–407.
22. Hijazi ZM. Interventionalists: watch out for coronary arterial anomalies in tetralogy of Fallot. *Catheter Cardiovasc Diagn* 1997;42:408.
23. Ing FF, Mullins CE, Grifka RG, et al. Stent dilation of superior vena cava/innominate vein obstructions permits transvenous pacing lead implantation. *Pacing Clin Electrophys* 1998;21:1517–1530.
24. Ing FF, Fagan TE, Grifka RG, et al. Reconstruction of stenotic or occluded ileofemoral veins and inferior vena cava using intravascular stents: reestablishing access for future cardiac catheterization and cardiac surgery. *J Am Coll Cardiol* 2001;37:251–257.
25. Mohsen AE, Rosenthal E, Qureshi SA, et al. Stent implantation for superior vena cava occlusion after the Mustard operation. *Catheter Cardiovasc Interv* 2001;52:351–354.
26. Frias PA, Johns JA, Drinkwater DC, et al. Percutaneous stent placement as treatment for an infant with superior vena cava syndrome. *Catheter Cardiovasc Interv* 2001;52:355–358.
27. Shellock FG, Morisoli S, Kanal E. MR procedures and biomedical implants, materials and devices. *Radiology* 1993;189:587–599.
28. Jost C, Kumar V. Are current cardiovascular stents MRI safe? *J Invasive Cardiol* 1998;10:477–479.
29. Strouse PF, Beekman RH III. Magnetic deflection forces from atrial septal defect and patent ductus arteriosus-occluding devices, stents, and coils used in pediatric-aged patients. *Am J Cardiol* 1996;78:490–491.
30. Rutledge JM, Vick W III, Mullins CE, et al. Safety of magnetic resonance imaging immediately following Palmaz stent implant: a report of three cases. *Catheter Cardiovasc Interv* 2001;53:519–523.
31. Fagan TE, Bolinger L, Scholz TD. Magnetic resonance imaging of the stented aorta: quantitative assessment. *Catheter Cardiovasc Interv* 2001;53:146.

Catheter Based Devices: For the Treatment of Non-coronary Cardiovascular Diseases in Adults and Children. Edited by P. Syamasundar Rao and Morton J. Kern, Lippincott Williams & Wilkins, Philadelphia © 2003.

34

STENT MANAGEMENT OF BRANCH PULMONARY ARTERY STENOSIS

COLIN J. MCMAHON
MICHAEL R. NIHILL

Management of branch pulmonary artery stenosis remains one of the most common procedures faced by the interventionalist, particularly given the prevalence of the postoperative tetralogy of Fallot patient. Several terms are used to describe pulmonary arterial obstruction distal to the pulmonary valve. These include *supravalvular pulmonary stenosis, peripheral pulmonary stenosis, hypoplasia of the pulmonary arteries,* and *coarctation of the pulmonary arteries.* Several classifications have been proposed, but those of French and Smith are the most widely used, describing the exact site of involvement: the proximal pulmonary arteries, branching pulmonary arteries, or distal pulmonary arteries (1,2). Rowe et al. proposed another classification: *simple* and *complicated,* based upon the presence of significant other congenital defects (3). Simple pulmonary stenosis is defined as affecting those patients with peripheral pulmonary arterial obstructions in association with simple underlying cardiac anomalies (e.g., ventricular or atrial septal defect). Complex pulmonary stenosis, on the other hand, is defined as occurring in association with transposition of great arteries or tetralogy of Fallot. In addition, stenoses are further classified based on location into *central, peripheral,* or *intermediate.* Perhaps the most practical classification, however, is *postoperative pulmonary arterial stenosis* (generally in the context of tetralogy of Fallot repair) or *native branch pulmonary artery stenosis.* Physiologic branch pulmonary stenosis should also be differentiated from peripheral branch stenosis. The former is a benign occurrence in neonates in which there is turbulence at the branching of the main pulmonary artery secondary to an acute take-off of the branch pulmonary arteries. This acute branching pattern generally resolves by 3 to 6 months and is without any clinical consequence.

Colin J. McMahon: Senior Fellow in Pediatric Cardiology, Texas Children's Hospital, Houston, Texas

Michael R. Nihill: Professor of Pediatrics, Department of Pediatrics, Baylor College of Medicine; Attending Cardiologist, Department of Cardiology, Texas Children's Hospital, Houston, Texas

PREVALENCE

Mangers reported the first case of peripheral pulmonary stenosis in 1802 (4). There is an estimated frequency of between 2% and 3% of all congenital heart defects (5). There is a strong association with tetralogy of Fallot and pulmonary atresia. Congenital rubella syndrome is much less frequent since the widespread introduction of immunization programs. Several genetic disorders are strongly associated with peripheral pulmonary stenosis. These include Williams syndrome, characterized by multiple pulmonary arterial obstructions, supravalvular aortic stenosis, mental handicap, hypercalcemia, and elfinlike dysmorphic facies. The occurrence of peripheral pulmonary stenosis is also associated with Alagille, Noonan, Ehlers-Danlos, Silver, and Leopard syndromes.

NATURAL HISTORY

The natural history of the condition is variable. Patients with Williams syndrome often have multiple severe stenoses of the branch pulmonary arteries, or in some cases even severe diffuse hypoplasia of the entire pulmonary arterial tree, which may be associated with systemic or even suprasystemic right ventricular pressure. Although these patients appear to have a terrible prognosis, they represent a distinct group in whom there often is a progressive improvement in the condition with time, and a reduction of the right ventricular pressure. Other non-Williams patients with multiple peripheral stenoses tend to carry a poor prognosis. These patients often show a progressive increase in severity of pulmonary obstruction with time and are predisposed to develop pulmonary arterial sclerosis, pulmonary arterial thrombosis, poststenotic aneurysmal dilation, and eventually severe right ventricular dilation and failure. The natural history may be rapid with severe right ventricular dysfunction, pulmonary thromboembolism, and hemoptysis occurring within the first 5 years of life. The distal nature of this disease process makes surgical intervention hazardous and in many cases nonviable because of the location of the disease process. There is another group of patients in whom there is mild to moderate peripheral pulmonary stenosis without a significant elevation in right heart pressures who do not develop any long-term sequelae.

NONINVASIVE ASSESSMENT OF PERIPHERAL PULMONARY STENOSIS

Cardiac catheterization is required to fully delineate the number and location of stenoses, in addition to measuring right ventricular pressures, and the gradient across any isolated branch stenosis. However, clinical examination, particularly paying attention to the degree of the right ventricular impulse, in accordance with the degree of right ventricular hypertrophy on electrocardiography, can aid the clinician in making an approximate assessment of the severity of stenosis and the presence or absence of right ventricular hypertension. A typical high-pitched murmur is heard over both lung fields posteriorly.

Transthoracic echocardiography, although extremely limited at assessing the distal pulmonary arterial vasculature because of the intrusion of the air-filled lung, is helpful in estimating right ventricular pressure (RVP) in the presence of a tricuspid regurgitation (TR) jet. Using the modified Bernoulli equation [RVP = $4TR^2$ + RA (right atrial) pressure], this gives an estimate of right ventricular pressure (6). A well-defined echocardiogram envelope is required for this to be valid. Likewise, the degree of right ventricular dilation and hypertrophy is an indication of the duration of elevated right heart pressure. However, it cannot be overemphasized that accurate delineation of the anatomic site of stenosis and the pressure gradient across a discrete stenosis requires the use of a catheter. Future developments in noninvasive imaging, including increasing use of MRI and gadolinium-enhanced MRA (magnetic resonance angiography), will see this technology applied to peripheral pulmonary stenosis. Again, estimation of pulmonary pressure or gradients across the area of stenosis is impossible using this modality and a limiting factor in complete assessment of patients.

CARDIAC CATHETERIZATION AND ANGIOGRAPHY

Catheterization allows precise anatomic and physiologic diagnosis. With the catheter positioned in the distal pulmonary vascular bed, slow pullbacks and simultaneous pressure transducing with an end-hole catheter should enable detection of the exact site of obstruction. A systolic pressure gradient greater than 10 mm Hg in the absence of

a significant left-to-right shunt is abnormal. In unilateral isolated pulmonary artery stenosis the pressure gradient is at the site of stenosis, with a normal pressure in the proximal pulmonary vasculature. In the absence of pulmonary valve stenosis the main pulmonary trunk pressure pulse can be used as an indicator of distal peripheral stenosis. Agustsson et al. first demonstrated that in peripheral pulmonary stenosis the main pulmonary artery diastolic pressure is normal but the dicrotic notch is markedly deeper, with a flattened diastolic descent after pulmonary valve closure (7). This characteristic pulse contour may relate to altered physiologic properties of the pulmonary trunk secondary to decreased distensibility of the relatively nonelastic pulmonary trunk. If the obstruction is more distal in the pulmonary arterial tree, this property becomes less marked. Angiography allows delineation of the site of obstruction, the number of stenoses, and poststenotic dilation, in addition to assessment of improvements in vessel diameter following stent implant. The proximal pulmonary artery branches are best assessed in the anteroposterior view or with a 40° cranial angulation with the posterior-anterior (PA) image intensifier with the origins of the right and left pulmonary arteries well seen with right anterior oblique (RAO) and left anterior oblique (LAO) with cranial angulation. The distal pulmonary vasculature can be better assessed by selective injection into each unilateral pulmonary artery viewing on straight lateral projection. Sufficient angiograms are required to ensure that the entire vasculature has been assessed. In those patients with suspected or confirmed Williams syndrome, additional angiography to assess the left ventricular outflow tract is warranted.

BALLOON ANGIOPLASTY: RESULTS AND LIMITATIONS

During the last two decades significant advances have been made in interventional treatment of peripheral pulmonary stenosis. This started with the first report of percutaneous transluminal angioplasty in the treatment of a postoperative peripheral pulmonary stenosis in 1980 in a patient following pulmonary atresia/ventricular septal defect repair (8). Subsequent to this, animal work resulted in the development of several protocols for balloon angioplasty of hypoplastic or stenotic peripheral pulmonary arteries (9,10). The introduction of high-pressure balloons for angioplasty by Gentles et al. resulted in a significant improvement in outcome (11). Several other authors reported their results with balloon dilation of peripheral pulmonary artery stenosis over the last decade. The initial techniques for balloon angioplasty using low-pressure balloon catheters required a diameter three to four times the stenosis segment. The initial results were certainly less than optimal. In a series reported by Lock et al. (12), five out of seven patients had a successful reduction with a significant drop in pressure gradient across the segment and an increase in vessel diameter, and Rocchini et al. reported an improvement in five of 13 patients (13). The early follow-up results from Boston Children's Hospital involving 218 angioplasty procedures in 135 patients reported a mean diameter increase from 3.8 ±1.7 mm to 5.5 ± 2.1 mm (14). However, only a 58% success rate was reported on the basis of an increase greater than or equal to 50% of the predilation diameter, an increase of more than 20% or more in flow to the involved lung, or a decrease in systolic RV:FA pressure ratio (right ventricle:femoral artery). Complications included death (four patients: vascular rupture in two patients with angioplasty), aneurysm, pulmonary edema, total occlusion of small adjacent vessels, hemoptysis, hypotension, and arrhythmia.

The VACA Registry reported 156 patients who underwent 182 procedures with a reduction of RV:FA ratio from 0.49 ± 0.25 to 0.37 ± 0.26 (15). There was an increase in vessel diameter from 4.5 ± 2.0 to 6.8 ± 3.0 mm. There were complications in 21 patients, with six deaths, including vessel rupture ($N = 2$), cardiac arrest ($N = 1$), paradoxical emboli ($N = 1$), and low cardiac output ($N = 1$). The low success rate (50% to 60%) associated with low-pressure balloons relates predominantly to an inability to eradicate balloon waists in those stenotic segments. Several other groups reported similar results with balloon angioplasty (16–18). These results prompted the use of high-pressure balloons by the Boston group using up to 17 to 20 atm (11). In this group, 63% of patients previously failing treatment with low-pressure balloons were successfully dilated with high-pressure balloon angioplasty, and 81% of patients not previously dilated were successfully treated. Criteria for successful treatment included a 50% or greater increase in vessel diameter, or a 20% or greater reduction in RV:FA pressure ratio. Those patients in whom there was disappearance of the waist on angioplasty had the most significant improvement. Although there was an 80% success rate using high-pressure balloons, up to 10% of patients developed restenosis, a similar outcome to the low-pressure angioplasty group.

HISTORY OF STENT DEVELOPMENT

Combined advances in technological development and increasing operator experience over the last decade have seen stent implant become the therapeutic modality of choice in the treatment of peripheral pulmonary stenosis. More than three decades ago, Dotter and Judkins foresaw the development of endovascular stents when they stated, "Once a pathway has been created through an occluded segment, repeated dilatation or temporary use of a Silastic endovascular (or in some cases, perivascular) splint could maintain an adequate false lumen until the natural processes of fibrosis and reintimalization have taken place" (19). It was 5 years later, in 1969, when Dotter first

reported the development of "tubular coil-spring endovascular prostheses," which were nonexpansible but enabled support of an already dilated vascular lumen (20). These were limited in lack of expansibility and lack of side branches. Julio Palmaz must be credited for his significant work in the development of intraluminal vascular grafts in the mid-1980s, which led to the application of this technology not only in pulmonary artery stenoses, but in all areas of congenital heart disease (21,22). He was the first to demonstrate the potential for these stainless steel intraluminal grafts in maintaining patency in surgically created arterial stenoses in 18 dogs. Initial results were encouraging, demonstrating 77% patency rate at 35 weeks, with complete endothelialization at 3 weeks. Sigwart et al. was one of the first to introduce balloon-expandable stents in treatment of peripheral vascular and coronary stenoses (23). Mullins et al. advanced this technology and demonstrated its efficacy in the management of stenoses in the pulmonary arteries and systemic venous obstruction (24).

STENT DESIGN

Several designs of stent are currently available. The Palmaz stent has become widely acceptable for treatment of peripheral pulmonary artery stenosis. This is a balloon-expandable stainless steel stent measuring 0.076 mm in thickness. It is available in several lengths. The large stents include 30, 18, and 12 mm (P-308, P-188, and P-128), which are capable of maximal dilation up to 18 mm in diameter. The medium-sized stents are 10, 15, and 20 mm (P-104, P-154, and P-204) in length, measure 2.5 mm in diameter, and can be dilated up to a maximum diameter of 10 mm. Each stent consists of several rows of slots, which form a diamond shape on complete expansion.

One of the limitations in design of the Palmaz stent is its relative inflexibility. Newer stent designs include the Intratherapeutics stent (St. Paul, MN.), which has increased flexibility, making traversing corners easier and giving the added advantage of increased space between the struts. This reduces the risk of occluding small branching vessels and the possibility of passing a balloon through the side of the stent in order to enable balloon dilation and implant of perpendicular placed stents. Self-expanding stents were initially used for adults with iliac and femoral arterial stenoses and malignant caval venous obstruction, and then applied to pediatric congenital heart disease, over the last 5 years. They were employed in treatment of peripheral pulmonary stenoses with the intended advantages of requiring a shorter sheath for deliverance, a longer length for placement across long stenotic segments, and decreased risk of embolization by premounting the stent onto the catheter. Benefits also included avoidance of risk of balloon rupture, with incomplete stent expansion seen occasionally with the Palmaz stents. (Other flexible stents became available subsequently (chapter 33).

TECHNIQUE FOR STENT IMPLANTATION

Before catheterization, fully informed consent must be obtained from the family or the patient, with the ever-increasing number of grown-up congenital heart patients coming to the fore. Most patients undergo cardiac catheterization under conscious sedation, with general anesthesia reserved for those children deemed too uncooperative to remain still during stent implant. Surgical back-up should be available with a type and cross-match of packed blood cells readily available if required. Routine arterial and venous access is obtained. Standard venous sheaths are then replaced with a larger-diameter long transseptal sheath over a stiff exchange-length wire previously anchored across the stenosis. It is important to obtain a stable stiff guide wire position with the short soft end as distal as possible in the lung. Anticoagulation is used (50 to 100 U/kg body weight) once initial activated clotting time (ACT) is measured. Reversal at the end of the procedure is required if the ACT exceeds 350 seconds. Prophylactic Ancef 25 mg/kg (1 g maximum) is administered before stent implant, with three doses of Keflex over the next 24 hours. Hemodynamic assessment and determination of pressure gradients on pull-back are essential before angiography. Angiography provides a roadmap before stent deployment. The vessel diameter at the site of stenosis and in the immediate adjacent areas to the stenosis must be measured. Certain catheterization laboratories have inherent calibration systems to enable measurement (e.g., Siemens catheterization laboratory) using a "cardiomarker" catheter as a calibration marker. Stents are mounted on low-pressure angioplasty balloons whose diameter should not exceed the diameter of the vessel adjacent to the stenosis.

The long sheath is advanced through the area of stenosis, and the balloon and stent apparatus are advanced within the sheath to the level of stenosis. Once the sheath is withdrawn to expose the balloon and stent, angiography is performed to confirm stent position. Following initial inflation and stent deployment, subsequent balloon dilation with both low- and high-pressure balloons optimizes results. Repeat hemodynamic and angiographic data should be obtained following stent implant. Specifically, the pressure gradient across stents, the RV:FA pressure ratio, and the luminal diameter should be determined for all patients. Mullins et al. developed a technique of bilateral simultaneous stent deployment in bifurcating branch pulmonary arteries to avoid compression of the smaller side branch. Generally, the most distal stent is implanted first and then, if required, additional proximal stents, with at least 2 to 3 mm of stent overlap. Occasionally, several interlocking series of stents are required to obtain maximal stent diameter, which have demonstrated excellent results. After all sheaths and catheters have been removed and hemostasis has been achieved, patients are returned to the high-dependency area. They are then monitored overnight and a chest x-ray is performed to assess the appropriate site of stents and rule out the presence of hemothorax. Patients are discharged on aspirin for 6 months following stent implant to prevent overabundant endothelialization. Follow-up catheterization is recommended at approximately 12 months to assess for restenosis, neointimal proliferation, or growth of vessel adjacent to the stent. Redilation may be required at this stage for restenosis, staged serial dilation, or neointimal proliferation.

RESULTS OF STENT IMPLANT FOR PERIPHERAL PULMONARY STENOSIS

The rationale for use of endovascular stents was to maintain vessel patency by preventing elastic recoil, external compression of the vessel, thrombosis, or intimal flap or tear obstructing the lumen.

Immediate Results

In one of the earliest combined studies from Houston and Boston, O'Laughlin et al. reported 58 patients who had 80 pulmonary artery stents implanted (25). The immediate results were encouraging, with a reduction in gradient from 55.2 ± 33.3 to 14.2 ± 13.5 mm Hg, with an increase in vessel diameter from 4.6 ± 2.3 to 11.3 ± 3.2 mm. There was a dramatic improvement in pulmonary perfusion with an increase in pulmonary blood flow to the stented lung from 29.4% ± 16.5% to 51.1% ± 13.1%. Repeat catheterization was performed at a mean of 8.6 months in 38 patients and demonstrated no significant change in luminal diameter. There was one mortality after initial stent implant in a Fontan patient who had a left pulmonary artery stent implanted and died from massive pulmonary embolism following dislodgment of atrial thrombus. Redilation was required of 17 stents in 14 patients at a mean of 10.2 months with a significant increase in stent diameter.

Long-Term Results

Shaffer et al. reported long-term results of 200 patients who had 357 stents implanted between September 1989 and June 1995 at Texas Children's Hospital (26). Of these patients, 48 had venous stenoses stented and the remaining 152 patients had either postoperative (136 patients) or congenital branch pulmonary stenosis (15 patients) stented. In both the postoperative and congenital PA stenoses groups, vessel diameters increased markedly, from 5.6 ± 2.1 mm to 12.1 ± 3.0 mm (p < .001) and 3.3 ± 1.2 mm to 8.9 ± 1.2 mm (p < .001), respectively. This represented a 100% increase in 65% of cases for the postoperative and 88% of cases for the congenital groups, respectively. The RV:FA systolic pressure ratio decreased from 0.63 ± 0.2 to 0.41 ± 0.02 (p < .001) in the postoperative group and from 0.71 ± 0.3

to 0.55 ± 0.35 (p = .04) in the congenital group. At follow-up catheterization, at a mean of 14 months the RV:FA ratio remained low at 0.45 ± 0.01 (p = .002) in the postoperative group, and the RV:FA ratio increased to 0.65 ± 0.3 (p = .8) in the native PA stenosis group. In those patients who required further dilation in the postoperative group there was a reduction in RV:FA ratio from 0.48 ± 0.14 to 0.38 ± 0.09 (p = .2), and in the congenital group in a limited number of patients from 0.74 ± 0.15 to 0.70 ± 0.14 (p = .2). Complications included stent migration in four cases, with surgical removal in two and expansion in a benign position other than the intended site. Three patients developed thrombosis of the PA within the stent. Self-limited hemoptysis developed in four patients. A pedunculated aneurysm with a stenotic mouth developed in one PA after a redilation procedure when the balloon "milked" distal to the stent. Follow-up MRI demonstrated no change after 6 months. Deaths occurred in two patients in this study cohort. One patient with familial congenital branch PA branch stenosis and suprasystemic RV pressure developed lethal ventilation–perfusion mismatch secondary to severe segmental pulmonary edema. The second death occurred in a 7-month-old child several weeks status post tetralogy repair who had systemic RV pressure with severe residual branch pulmonary stenosis. He sustained a main PA tear resulting in massive hemothorax and succumbed. No late deaths resulted from stent implant. Neointimal proliferation occurs to some degree in all patients, with a consistent 1- to 2-mm decrease in the lumen on both sides of the stent, which is secondary to "normal" or physiologic intimal lining of the stent. In the series reported by Shaffer et al. only three patients were identified who developed significant stenosis due to neointimal proliferation.

These aforementioned studies all reported on the use of balloon-expandable Palmaz stents. One recent study from Cheung et al. reported on 17 patients who had 20 Wallstents implanted for pulmonary arterial stenoses (27). Although there was impressive increase in vessel diameter from 4.1 ± 1.5 mm to 8 ± 2 mm and a decrease in systolic pressure gradient across the stent from 24.6 ± 15.8 mm to 12.1 ± 11.4 mm, at recatheterization at a mean of 14.8 months, 28% of the implanted stents demonstrated significant neointimal proliferation. This is extremely concerning, particularly in face of the low incidence in association with other stent designs. Further studies are required to compare the risk of neointimal proliferation, as this obviously varies significantly, depending on stent design.

Redilation of Stents

The potential for reexpansion of stents was first demonstrated by Morrow et al. (28). Reexpansion was performed at 11 and 18 weeks in thoracic aorta stents in 11 juvenile swine. Redilation resulted in a significant increase in mean

stent luminal diameter from 10.1 ± 1 mm to 12.3 ± 1.2 mm at 11 weeks and 11.2 ± 0.7 mm to 13.5 ± 1.1 mm at 18 weeks without significant injury to the neointima, media, or adventitia. Ing et al. reported early results of redilation of 30 pulmonary artery stents in 20 patients from Houston (29). Indications included initial limited dilation, restenosis due to neointimal proliferation or a residual waist within the stent. At recatheterization at a mean of 13 months all stents were patent, with a mean diameter decrease of 1.3 mm and a mean increase in gradient by 3 mm Hg. There was a 94% redilation success rate. The mean diameter increased from 9.5 to 12.2 mm and the mean gradient decreased from 14 to 8 mm Hg up to 3 years after dilation. Repeat dilation was possible in four cases using similar size and pressure balloons as on initial implant, demonstrating a "softening effect" of the stent on tissues with time. Redilation procedures were performed on 15 stents in 11 patients of 29 who underwent repeat catheterization from the Toronto group (30). Changes in pressure gradient and luminal vessel size were comparable to those reported from the Houston group.

APPLICABILITY IN ADULT SUBJECTS

With increasing numbers of pediatric congenital heart patients surviving into adulthood it goes without saying that this technology will be increasingly required in this subset of patients. This should be tolerated equally well by the adult population, with fewer complications (e.g., vessel trauma) related to sheath size. The maximal dilated stent diameter is 18 mm, which should accommodate growth within the largest pulmonary artery branches sufficient to reduce the RV:FA ratio and allow sufficient pulmonary blood flow in this group of patients.

DISCUSSION

Over the last decade, the application of endovascular stents in congenital heart disease has proven very successful. Stents have been particularly effective in the treatment of postoperative pulmonary artery branch stenoses, for which further surgical treatment is limited. Isolated balloon valvuloplasty of arterial and venous stenoses has been shown to be inadequate, with even early follow-up demonstrating restenosis rates as high as 40% (31). Redilation of endovascular stents may be required to accommodate the patient's somatic growth, for staged serial "further" dilation to avoid vessel overdilation during stent implant, for neointimal proliferation, or for the development of restenosis. Early follow-up studies demonstrated very low rates of significant stent neointimal proliferation and/or restenosis, occurring in only 3% of patients, with a mean duration of follow-up of 13 months (29).

We define *restenosis* as a reduction in the stent luminal diameter less than the nominal adjacent vessel diameter, and/or a development or increase in pressure gradient across the stent. This represents one of the primary reasons for performing repeat catheterization 1 to 3 years following initial stent implant, in order to assess vessel growth adjacent to the stent and the necessity for further stent dilation to accommodate somatic growth. Certain risk factors were determined to predispose to the development of restenosis. These include inadequate stent overlap of only 1 to 2 mm and the placement of stents with sharp angulation to the curvilinear pulmonary arterial wall, resulting in the development of restenosis at the distal end of the stent. This probably occurs as a reaction of the vessel wall to the stent struts. Patients with abnormal vasculature are also predisposed to develop restenosis. One patient in our group with Williams syndrome with severe diffuse pulmonary artery hypoplasia developed restenosis following redilation despite an increase in vessel diameter of 50% (32).

One recent study using self-expanding Wallstents (25 stents implanted in 22 procedures) in a small group of patients reported an incidence of neointimal proliferation of 28% at a mean follow-up of 8.1 months in 17 patients with pulmonary arterial stenoses and four patients with venous stenoses (27). These authors defined *neointimal proliferation* as "neointima growth greater than 30% of the vessel diameter," and reported its development in five of the pulmonary artery stents, one left superior vena cava stent, and one modified Blalock Taussig shunt; one of the pulmonary arterial stents was totally occluded. These results are markedly different from our experience using balloon-expandable (Palmaz) stents. We define *neointimal proliferation* with a more critical definition. Even using our stricter definition, our patients developed significantly less neointimal proliferation (33) in the early study by Ing et al. (29). One patient developed severe neointimal proliferation in a femoral vein stent following initial overdilation of the stented vessel, in comparison to the adjacent venous dimension. This resulted in an in-growth of neointima from the surrounding vessel into the stent with a significant reduction in stented vessel diameter. In the previously mentioned Wallstent study, excessive vessel wall dilation may have been responsible for the high incidence of neointimal proliferation, with a reported increase in vessel wall diameter of up to 95% for the pulmonary arterial stenosis group and up to 75% for the systemic venous group. Further studies comparing self-expanding stents (e.g., Wallstent) to balloon-expandable stents (Palmaz) may be warranted to address whether the self-expanding stents are inherently more prone to stenosis and pose a higher risk of neointimal proliferation. Avoidance of initial overdilation of the stent appears to result in a reduction of risk of neointimal proliferation and, it is hoped, avoidance of aneurysm formation and vessel perforation.

Initially, there were concerns regarding the potential for stent redilation to accommodate somatic growth. Published animal studies by Grifka (32) and Morrow (28) unequivocally demonstrated the potential to increase the diameter of previously implanted balloon-expandable stents using larger balloons to accommodate for somatic growth. When indicated, we advocate staged serial further dilation of arterial and venous stents, rather than attempting to gain maximal vessel diameter at initial stent implant, since this appears to predispose the patient to neointimal proliferation and restenosis, and may increase risk of complications. The aim of redilation should be to expand the stent diameter to equal that of the adjacent vessel wall. Our practice has been to restudy patients 1 to 3 years after stent implant, or when their weight has increased sufficiently to have hemodynamic implications. Repeat catheterization is indicated when their adult weight has been reached to achieve full dilation potential of the stented vessel.

CONCLUSION

Long-term follow-up studies continue to demonstrate the efficacy of endovascular stent implant for the treatment of peripheral pulmonary arterial stenoses and confirm this as the treatment of choice. Redilation is required in most patients for somatic growth, staged serial redilation, or restenosis secondary to neointimal proliferation, and it can be performed safely and effectively.

REFERENCES

1. Smith WG. Pulmonary hypertension and a continuous murmur due to multiple peripheral stenoses of the pulmonary arteries. *Thorax* 1958;13:194.
2. Franch RH, Gay BB Jr. Congenital stenosis of the pulmonary artery branches: a classification, with postmortem findings in two cases. *Am J Cardiol* 1963;35:512.
3. Rowe RD. Pulmonary arterial stenosis. In: Rowe RD, ed. *Heart disease in infancy and children,* 3rd ed. New York: Macmillan, 1978.
4. Schwalbe E. Morphologie der missbildungen und der tiere. In: Fisher G, ed. Jena, Vol. 1, part 3,1909,426.
5. Fouron JC, Favreau-Ethier M, Marion P, et al. Les sténoses pulmonaires périphériques congénitales: préentation de 16 observations et revue de la littérature. *Can Med Assoc J* 1967;96:1084.
6. Valdes-Cruz LM, Yoganathan AP, Tamura T, et al. Studies *in vitro* of the relationship between ultrasound and laser Doppler velocimetry and applicability of the simplified Bernoulli relationship. *Circulation* 1986;73:300–308.
7. Agustsson MH, Arcilla RA, Giasul BM, et al. The diagnosis of bilateral stenosis of the pulmonary branches based on characteristic pulmonary trunk pressure curves: a hemodynamic and angiocardiographic study. *Circulation* 1962;26:421.
8. Martin EC, Diamond NG, Casarella WJ. Percutaneous transluminal angioplasty in non-atherosclerotic disease. *Radiology* 1980;135:27.

9. Lock JE, Niemi T, Einzig S, et al. Transvenous angioplasty of experimental branch pulmonary artery stenosis in newborn lambs. *Circulation* 1981;64:886.
10. Lock JE, Niemi T, Burke BA, et al. Dilatation angioplasty of congenital cardiac defect: preliminary results. *Circulation* 1982;66:360.
11. Gentles GL, Lock JE, Perry SB. High pressure balloon angioplasty for branch pulmonary artery stenosis: early experience. *J Am Coll Cardiol* 1993;22:867.
12. Lock JE, Castenada-Zuniga WR, Fuhrman BP, et al. Balloon dilatation angioplasty of hypoplastic and stenotic pulmonary arteries. *Circulation* 1983;67:962.
13. Rocchini AP, Keveselis D. The use of balloon angioplasty in the pediatric patient. *Pediatr Clin North Am* 1984;31:1293.
14. Rothman A. Balloon angioplasty of pulmonary artery stenosis. *Prog Pediatr Cardiol* 1992;1:17.
15. Kan JS, Marvin WJ Jr, Bass JL, et al. Balloon angioplasty-branch pulmonary artery stenosis: results from the valvuloplasty and angioplasty of congenital anomalies registry. *Am J Cardiol* 1990; 65:798.
16. Kan JS. Balloon-angioplasty-pulmonic stenosis. In: Doyle EF, et al. *Pediatric cardiology.* New York: Springer-Verlag, 1986.
17. Mitchell SE, Kan JS, White RI Jr. Interventional techniques in congenital heart disease. *Semin Roentgenol* 1985;20:290.
18. Rocchini AP, Kvesekis D, Dick M, et al. Use of balloon angioplasty to treat peripheral pulmonary stenosis. *Am J Cardiol* 1984: 50:1069.
19. Dotter CT, Judkins MP. Transluminal treatment of arteriosclerotic obstruction. *Circulation* 1964;30:654.
20. Dotter CT. Transluminally placed coil spring endarterial tube grafts. *Invest Radiol* 1969;4:329.
21. Palmaz JC, Sibbitt RR, Reuter SR, et al. Expandable intraluminal vascular graft: a feasibility study. *Surgery* 1986;99:199.
22. Palmaz JC, Sibbitt RR, Reuter SR, et al. Expandable intraluminal graft: a preliminary study. *Radiology* 1985;156:73.
23. Sigwart U, Puel J, Mirkovitch V, et al. Intravascular stents to prevent occlusion and restenosis after transluminal angioplasty. *N Engl J Med* 1987;316:701.
24. Mullins CE, O'Laughlin MP, Vick GW 3rd, et al. Implantation of balloon expandable intravascular grafts by catheterization in pulmonary arteries and systemic veins. *Circulation* 1988;77:188.
25. O'Laughlin MP, Perry SB, Lock JE, et al. Use of endovascular stents in congenital heart disease. *Circulation* 1991;83:1923.
26. Shaffer KM, Mullins CE, Grifka RG, et al. Intravascular stents in congenital heart disease: short- and long-term results from a large single-center experience. *J Am Coll Cardiol* 1998;31:661–667.
27. Cheung Y, Sanatari S, Leung MP, et al. Early and intermediate-term complications of self-expanding stents limit its potential application in children with congenital heart disease. *J Am Coll Cardiol* 2000;35:1007–1015.
28. Morrow WR, Palmaz JC, Tio FO, et al. Re-expansion of balloon-expandable stents after growth. *J Am Coll Cardiol* 1993;22:2007.
29. Ing FF, Grifka RG, Nihill MR, et al. Repeat dilation of intravascular stents in congenital heart disease. *Circulation* 1995;92:893–897.
30. Fogelman R, Nykanen D, Smallhorn JF, et al. Endovascular stents in the pulmonary circulation. *Circulation* 1995;92:881.
31. Rothman A, Perry SB, Keane JF, et al. Early results and follow-up of balloon angioplasty for branch pulmonary artery stenosis. *J Am Coll Cardiol* 1990;15:1109–1117.
32. Grifka RG, Vick GW III, O'Laughlin MP, et al. Balloon expandable intravascular stents: aortic implantation and late further dilation in growing minipigs. *Am Heart J* 1993;126:979–984.
33. McMahon CJ, Grifka RG, El Said HG, et al. Intermediate outcome of redilation of endovascular stents in congenital heart defects. *J Am Coll Cardiol* 2000;519a (abst).

Catheter Based Devices: For the Treatment of Non-coronary Cardiovascular Diseases in Adults and Children. Edited by P. Syamasundar Rao and Morton J. Kern, Lippincott Williams & Wilkins, Philadelphia © 2003.

35

ENDOVASCULAR STENTS FOR COARCTATION OF THE AORTA

K. ANITHA JAYAKUMAR
WILLIAM E. HELLENBRAND

Coarctation of the aorta is among the most common congenital heart defects and classically refers to a discrete area of stenosis in the proximal descending thoracic aorta. Over the last several decades it has become increasingly apparent that this seemingly simple anatomic lesion demonstrates remarkable variability in terms of anatomy, physiology, clinical presentation, and outcome.

Surgical repair of coarctation was first described by Crafoord et al. in 1945 (1) and remained standard therapy until 1982, when transcatheter treatment of aortic coarctation was first described by Singer et al. (2) as a less invasive alternative to surgery. Over the years there have been several studies comparing the potential benefits and complications of the various surgical techniques to transcatheter therapy (3). Despite satisfactory immediate results, concerns with angioplasty have persisted regarding long-term outcome, including the risks of recurrent coarctation, aneurysm formation, and aortic dissection (4–6).

Immediate gradient reduction appears similar following either surgery or balloon angioplasty, although the incidence of restenosis with angioplasty is variable, depending on both the anatomy and the age of the patient (7). The role of balloon angioplasty in the management of native coarctation in neonates and infants has remained controversial because of a higher incidence of restenosis, but in children and adults it is more universally accepted, and indeed it is the recommended treatment of choice for recurrent coarctation (8–10). Currently, aneurysm formation with angioplasty is an unusual event (11–13).

Endovascular stent placement has been performed since the mid-1980s and has been used increasingly in adults for coronary artery and peripheral vascular disease. In patients with congenital heart disease, endovascular stents have been used in systemic veins, pulmonary arteries and pulmonary veins, aortopulmonary shunts, stenosed right-ventricle-to-pulmonary artery conduits, and more recently, coarctation of the aorta (14–20). Stents serve as a scaffold and hence provide superior wall support conducive to endothelial cell growth with a reduced incidence of restenosis (21). Stents minimize the extension of wall tears by providing apposition of the torn vessel intima to the media with a possible reduction in aneurysm formation (22–24). Despite concerns regarding acquired stenosis secondary to growth, recent studies have demonstrated the feasibility of further enlargement of the stent years after implantation (10,25,26).

In older children and adults, endovascular stent placement has proven to be an effective and superior alternative to either surgery or balloon angioplasty in the management of simple aortic coarctation either in its native form or after previous surgery or balloon angioplasty (22,27). Although surgery remains the mainstay of therapy in the management of neonatal coarctation, complex aortic coarctation, including long-segment stenosis and transverse arch hypoplasia, can be effectively treated with endovascular stents.

PERCUTANEOUS BALLOON ANGIOPLASTY

Percutaneous balloon angioplasty has become a safe and effective alternative to surgery since the earliest descriptions by Sos, Singer, Lock, and their associates (2,28,29). There have since been numerous reports outlining the techniques and the short-, intermediate-, and long-term results of balloon angioplasty both in native coarctation and in recoarctation. In neonates with complex coarctation and ductal-dependent circulation, surgery is frequently preferred. However, some investigators have demonstrated that in neonates with classical coarctation, the results of balloon angioplasty were comparable to those of surgery with

K. Anitha Jayakumar: Instructor in Pediatrics, Department of Pediatrics, Columbia University College of Physicians and Surgeons; Pediatric Cardiologist, Department of Pediatric Cardiology, Children's Hospital of New York, New York, New York

William E. Hellenbrand: Professor of Clinical Pediatrics, Department of Pediatrics, Columbia University College of Physicians and Surgeons; Director, Pediatric Cardiac Catheterization Laboratory, Children's Hospital of New York, New York, New York, New York

respect to mortality and immediate- and long-term follow-up (7,12,13). Nevertheless, we believe the procedure of choice in neonates should be surgery.

Following balloon angioplasty, the incidence of restenosis has been quoted by varying groups as between 15% and 57%, (13,24,30–35), often attributed to elastic recoil of the vascular wall immediately after balloon deflation. Restenosis has been associated with early infant age and isthmus hypoplasia, the latter frequently accounting for the poor immediate results. Restenosis could also be related to ductal constriction or recoil, intimal hyperplasia due to smooth muscle cell proliferation, and matrix protein production followed by a degree of arterial remodeling (5).

Aneurysm formation follows injury to the vascular intima and media following successful angioplasty and occurs more frequently with native coarctation. The incidence of aneurysms following angioplasty has been reported to be between 4% and 11.5%, and acute aortic disruption has been reported in 1% to 4 % of patients (8,10,31–34). Acute aneurysm formation appears to have little consistent correlation with balloon size or coarctation diameter, suggesting an intrinsic abnormality of the vessel wall (32).

In contrast to its controversial use in neonatal native coarctation, angioplasty has been considered the preferred choice to surgery in older children and adults and in patients with recurrent coarctation (3).

ENDOVASCULAR STENTS

Over the last decade, endovascular stents have been increasingly considered an effective therapeutic modality in the management of native aortic coarctation and recurrent coarctation. The use of endovascular stents in preference to balloon angioplasty has gained acceptance, since these rigid devices provide greater vessel wall support by serving as a framework for endothelial growth that will then maintain the increase in diameter. Stents therefore circumvent some of the problems associated with balloon angioplasty, such as restenosis due to vessel recoil, unfavorable anatomy in the form of long tubular narrowing, hypoplasia of the isthmus or mild discrete obstruction, and acute aortic rupture or aneurysm formation caused by vessel wall disruption. Stent placement has been successful in the management of severe (27) and mild coarctation, including recoarctation (10). The latter group with minimal obstruction at rest often includes patients with increased left ventricular mass, increased obstruction with exercise, and diastolic dysfunction that may be less amenable to conventional balloon dilatation as compared with stent placement (10). Currently, balloon-expandable stent implantation is the only technique available that restores normal anatomy with the least disruption of the vessel histology.

METHOD OF IMPLANTATION

The technique for stent implantation has been well described (17). The procedure was performed under general anesthesia in all but one patient, in whom it was done under conscious sedation. After obtaining access to the femoral artery and vein, intravenous heparin (100 U/kg) was administered to keep the activated clotting time more than 220 seconds, which was maintained throughout the procedure. A complete right and left heart hemodynamic study was performed and the cardiac index was determined using the Fick method and/or thermodilution.

The coarctation site was then crossed in a retrograde fashion and the peak and mean pressure gradients were measured by pullback or by simultaneous ascending and descending aortic pressure recording. Biplane aortography was performed initially in the straight anteroposterior and lateral projections, with a second angiogram in the left anterior oblique projection when the anatomy was not well profiled. Correcting for magnification and using the known diameter of the catheter, measurements were made, including the narrowest diameter and length of the coarctation, the diameter of the isthmus and or transverse arch, and the diameter of the descending aorta at the level of the left atrium. Balloon predilation was not done in most patients before stent implantation.

A long transseptal sheath and dilator were advanced through the femoral artery over a superstiff guide wire across the coarctation site. The tip of the wire was positioned either in the left subclavian artery (LSCA), if the coarctation was in the descending aorta (DAo) distal to the LSCA, or in the right subclavian artery (RSCA), if the coarctation was in the transverse arch (TAR) or just proximal to the LSCA. The wire and therefore the balloon were always kept as straight as possible to prevent balloon rupture during inflation. The dilator was then carefully removed from the sheath, maintaining the sheath and wire in position.

The nature and diameter of the coarctation site, diameter of the isthmus, TAR and DAo with reference to the size of the patient determined the choice of balloon and stent size. The diameter of the first balloon was chosen to be at least twice the diameter of the coarctation in order to stabilize the position of the stent. A second larger balloon was used to inflate the stent to its final diameter. In four patients the stent was crimped onto a balloon-in-balloon (BIB) catheter (NuMED, Inc., Nicholville, NY), which provided extra control to position the stent.

In 33 patients, we used either a Palmaz 308 or a P188 stent (Johnson & Johnson Interventional System, Somerville, NJ). In one patient a 28 Cheatham Platinum (CP) stent (NuMED, Inc., Nicholville, NY) was implanted. The stent was mounted and crimped onto a balloon catheter or a BIB catheter, and the entire system was carefully advanced over the guide wire to be positioned across the coarctation using a digital "roadmap" to identify the anatomic landmarks. Once in position, the sheath was withdrawn to expose the stent and balloon catheter. The balloon was then inflated by hand using dilute contrast up to the recommended inflation pressure. Repeat angiography and pressure measurements were performed.

Before discharge, all patients underwent complete clinical evaluation, echocardiography, and chest films. Patients were asked to follow with their primary cardiologists within 1 to 2 months after discharge from the hospital, then regularly afterward. Initially, the patients were placed on antiplatelet therapy with aspirin for 3 to 6 months after the procedure unless they were on anticoagulation for other reasons. One patient with obstruction in the TAR was maintained on Coumadin for 4 months after the procedure because of proximity of the stent to the left common carotid artery. Currently, no anticoagulation is employed in most patients.

RESULTS

Following encouraging results in animals, Suarez de Lezo et al. reported on the first patient series in 1995 (36), which included ten patients with severe coarctation, ranging in age from 15 days to 43 years. Most of these patients had no associated cardiac anomalies but had an unfavorable anatomy for balloon angioplasty. Following balloon angioplasty alone there was an insignificant change in the gradient and stenosis, whereas following stent placement, the gradient almost disappeared, with a significant decrease in angiographic stenosis. The final stent diameter was chosen to equal the size of the descending aorta at the level of the diaphragm. Aortic wall disruption at the level of the isthmus in an infant was treated with a second stent with satisfactory results. At follow-up 4.4 ± 2.5 months, all patients were asymptomatic with normal blood pressure and no detectable Doppler gradient between the upper and lower extremities. Pulse loss was reported in two patients and reduced in three (36). This was followed by a report on 48 patients who had received stents for aortic coarctation between 1993 and 1998 (27), all of whom were severely hypertensive. Most of these patients had an unfavorable anatomy for balloon angioplasty; this group included 16 patients with recurrent coarctation after surgery and/or balloon angioplasty. Five patients had an associated aneurysm before stent placement, of which one aneurysm was native, two developed after previous balloon angioplasty, and two occurred after surgery. Palmaz stents were deployed, following which the coarctation gradient decreased from 42 ± 12 mm Hg to 3 ± 4 mm Hg and the percent stenosis decreased from 66% ± 15% to 6% ± 15%. Additional short stents were placed in two patients with hypoplastic transverse aor-

tic arches, and the stent acutely migrated in two others. Stent implantation effectively excluded the aneurysm associated with native coarctation in one patient. In four other patients with previous aneurysms, the stent did not obliterate the sac but resulted in a decrease in the size and flow through it. At follow-up 2 to 3 years later, all the patients were normotensive without medication, with no evidence of restenosis in 73%. There was a minor increment in all aortic segments that correlated with the increment in body surface area (BSA) at 2-year follow-up. Two patients (7%) developed new small aneurysms that were coiled. At late follow-up, 30 patients at catheterization had residual gradients secondary to neointimal hyperplasia that was inversely related to age, BSA, and the aortic diameters before and after stent implantation, but was directly related to stented length and the growth of the patient. Stent treatment for coarctation of the aorta provided excellent initial and late results in patients more than 3 years of age but was associated with a greater incidence of endoproliferative restenosis in patients treated as infants (27).

In 1997, Ebeid et al. reported on nine patients with coarctation, all of whom were greater than 10 years of age. Seven had had previous surgical repair, and six had had previous balloon angioplasty. Following stent placement these patients were followed for up to 42 months with no complications. One patient in the group underwent redilation after 3 years for an exercise-induced gradient with no further recurrence. Two patients out of five had residual hypertension.

Marshall et al. recently described the efficacy of stent implantation in 33 patients with mild postoperative coarctation, most of whom also had ventricular diastolic dysfunction that improved following the procedure (10).

Previous studies have demonstrated no mortality following the procedure. Concerns persist about acquired stenosis in growing children because of the fixed diameter of the stent and/or intimal proliferation, despite recent studies that demonstrate the feasibility of stent reexpansion to accommodate for growth without causing significant neointimal injury (10,26,37). Other complications include stent migration, stent fracture, late aneurysm formation, femoral artery damage, and thromboembolic episodes (10,25,27–29,38,39).

Our experience was retrospectively evaluated in an attempt to examine the use of endovascular stents in the management of native and recurrent coarctation as an alternative to surgery or balloon angioplasty. Thirty-four consecutive patients underwent attempted stent implantation for coarctation between May 1993 and July 1999. Twenty-five patients were male and nine were female, between 4 and 36 years of age.

Thirteen patients (38%) had native coarctation (Figure 35.1) and 21 (62%) had recoarctation after surgical repair and/or balloon angioplasty. One patient had a jump graft

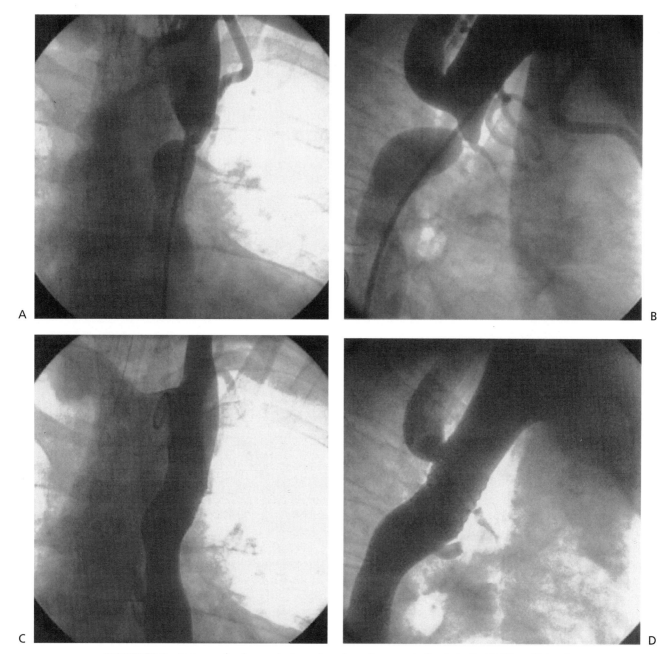

FIGURE 35.1. Aortography demonstrates a discrete native coarctation in both AP (**A**) and lateral views (**B**) in this 20-year-old male with severe upper-extremity hypertension. The gradient across the obstruction was 60 mm Hg and the diameter measured 4 mm. Following stent placement, there was no residual pressure difference and the site was completely opened to 20 mm in diameter (**C, D**).

repair from the transverse arch to the descending aorta to bypass the site of the coarctation as the initial repair and was thus included in the native coarctation group. Eighteen patients (53%) had discrete coarctation versus 16 (47%) who had long-segment coarctation (Figure 35.2). The coarctation was located in the proximal descending aorta in 31 patients (91%) and in the transverse aorta (Figure 35.3) in three patients (9%). Seven patients (21%) had isolated

coarctation and 27 (79%) had associated cardiac defects. Ten patients (26%) were symptomatic, having exercise intolerance with claudication and/or chest pain. Twenty-two patients (65%) were hypertensive and 13 (38%) were on antihypertensive medications.

The stents were successfully implanted in the stenotic area in 37 (97%) of the 38 patients, with a decrease in the peak systolic pressure gradient from 32 ± 12 mm Hg to $4 \pm$

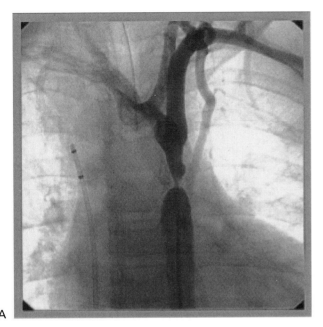

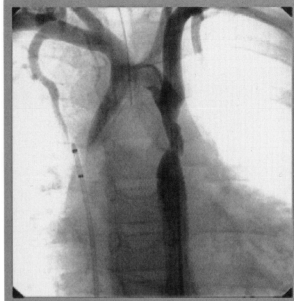

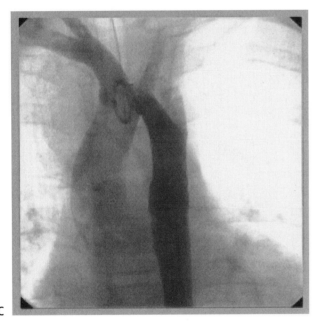

FIGURE 35.2. A: Severe long-segment (native) coarctation in this 8-year-old male in **A**. The pressure difference was 45 mm Hg. **B:** Balloon angioplasty was performed, resulting in a significant intimal tear with residual obstruction. **C:** A stent was then placed over the entire segment with no residual pressure difference and compression of the intimal tear onto the wall of the aorta.

11 mm Hg ($p < .001$) immediately after stent placement. One patient remained with a residual gradient of more than 20 mm Hg. The ratio of final balloon diameter to coarctation diameter before stent placement was 2.7 ± 1.9 (range, 1.4 to 12), whereas the ratio of balloon diameter to DAo diameter was 1.0 ± 0.2 (range, 0.7 to 1.5). The ratio of coarctation diameter to DAo diameter increased by 50% from 0.46 ± 0.16 to 0.92 ± 0.16 ($p < .001$). Final stent diameter at full inflation to balloon diameter ratio was 0.9 ± 0.2 (0.7 to 1.1). Balloons used had a mean diameter of 17 ± 2 mm (range, 12 to 20), while the arterial sheaths used ranged from 8 to 14F. In one adult patient in whom an interposition graft had been placed as a second surgical pro-

cedure, there was significant stenosis at the proximal suture line. A stent was placed across this suture line and fully expanded to the size of the graft with a fall in the gradient from 40 to 0 mm Hg. Another adult had a 4-mm tight coarctation and mild stenosis at the distal end of a jump graft placed between the TAR and the DAo with a 50-mm gradient. Following stent placement across the native coarctation, there was no residual gradient.

Successful outcome was defined as a peak systolic residual gradient after stent implantation of < 20 mm Hg. An unsatisfactory result occurred in one of 33 patients (3%). This patient had a long recoarctation following surgical repair in childhood. Two telescoping stents were placed

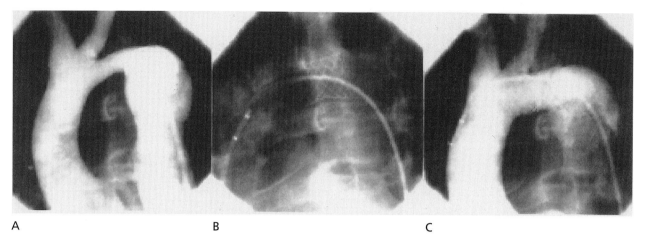

A   B   C

FIGURE 35.3. A: Narrowing of the transverse aortic arch demonstrated by aortography in a 15-year-old patient status post subclavian flap repair for coarctation of the aorta with a peak gradient of 50 mm Hg across the stenosis. **B:** The arch measured 8 mm in diameter. A Palmaz 188 stent was successfully placed across the stenosis and dilated up to 18 mm with complete elimination of pressure difference. **C:** Angiography following stent deployment demonstrates the transverse arch to be widely patent.

but could not be expanded fully despite the use of single- and double-balloon techniques inflated up to 25 atm, with a resultant residual gradient of 60 mm Hg. This patient subsequently had a jump graft placed surgically a month later.

Major complications requiring surgical treatment occurred in two patients (6%), and minor complications developed in four (12%). Major complications included bleeding from the right external iliac artery requiring surgical evacuation of a retroperitoneal hematoma. Another had a fragment of ruptured balloon embolize to the left axillary artery and underwent surgical removal. Minor complications included additional stent placement distal to the coarctation site in three patients after the partially inflated stent migrated and had to be fully expanded in the DAo. One patient developed a small femoral arteriovenous fistula 2 weeks after the procedure that resolved spontaneously. There were no deaths related to the procedure and none of the patients developed acute dissection or aneurysm formation. One 16-year-old patient with Shone's complex with adult respiratory distress syndrome secondary to influenza A sepsis had stent placement for coarctation of the aorta and balloon valvuloplasty of her mitral stenosis to try to improve her low cardiac output state before she was placed on extracorporeal membrane oxygenation (ECMO). She died 2 weeks later from complications related to ECMO. No patient required therapy for paradoxical hypertension.

Four patients underwent repeat cardiac catheterization 16 ± 5 months after their initial stent implantation (range, 10 to 21 months). One of them had a recurrent peak gradient of 24 mm Hg and was successfully dilated from 13 to 17 mm using an 18-mm balloon with a reduction of the peak gradient to 8 mm Hg. This patient was the first to receive a stent for coarctation in this series and large-diameter high pressure balloons were unavailable at the time of the original procedure. Another patient who had stent implantation for both coarctation and branch pulmonary artery stenosis (SVAS syndrome) had a mild gradient of 10 mm Hg and was successfully redilated from 11 to 14 mm. The other two patients had no gradients across the stent. There was no aneurysm formation, stent displacement or fracture, or intimal hyperplasia.

Patients were followed for 29 ± 17 months (median, 28; range, 5 to 81). Follow-up blood pressure and Doppler echocardiographic data are available for 28 of 31 patients. Sphygmomanometric systolic pressure gradients decreased from 39 ± 18 mm Hg to 4 ± 6 mm Hg at follow-up ($p < .001$), and systolic blood pressure decreased from 136 ± 21 to 122 ± 19 mm Hg ($p \leq .002$). Peak Doppler pressure gradients decreased from 51 ± 26 mm Hg to 13 ± 11 mm Hg at follow-up ($p < .001$). Twenty-two of 31 patients (71%) were hypertensive and 13 (42%) were on antihypertensive medications prior to stent implantation. At their last follow-up visit, only eight of 31 (26%) remain hypertensive and on antihypertensive medications ($p < .05$), and all the patients were asymptomatic. For the entire group there was no evidence of recurrent coarctation, aneurysm formation, stent displacement, or fracture identified on follow-up echocardiography, chest x-ray, or MRI. In seven of 31 (23%) patients, a mild gradient in the TAR of 5 to 20 mm Hg became unmasked after the stent was successfully placed in the original coarctation site. They had no pressure differences in the TAR prior to stent implantation. Follow-up of these seven patients has demonstrated persistent mild arch obstruction (≤20 mm Hg) in three patients who also have isthmus and/or arch hypoplasia ($p < .05$). Isthmus and arch hypoplasia are risk factors for early and late failure following balloon angioplasty in coarctation (40).

In our study, early results of stent implantation were comparable to those reported by Suarez de Lezo et al. (27) and Ebeid et al. (25). Although patients with native coarctation had tighter discrete coarctation sites than the recoarctation group, which had longer segments of coarctation (*p* < .05), the early outcomes following stent placement were similar. The results after stent implantation appear satisfactory even in tight coarctation sites compared with the described suboptimal results of balloon angioplasty.

Stent migration is a recognized complication (27) of stent implantation that could be decreased by the use of BIB catheters (NuMED, Inc., Nicholville, NY), which provide more control of the inflation by using the anchoring mechanism of the smaller inner balloon that is inflated first. Stent migration can usually be managed by manipulation of the stent to an area distal to the site of coarctation in the thoracic or abdominal aorta, where it can be expanded to the desired diameter.

In older patients with the coarctation diameter ≤ 4 mm, the stent is opened to 12 to 14 mm at the initial procedure and then fully expanded 6 months later to reduce the risk of rupture and/or aneurysm formation. Residual hypertension occurred in ten of 37 (28%) of our patients, compared with 22% described by Ebeid et al. (25). This was mostly in older children and adults who presented with hypertension and remain on antihypertensive medications at follow-up.

Complications related to arterial access affected 6% (two of 34) in our study, compared with 10% to 19% in those previously reported (27,31,33,34). The vascular complications in our study were not related to the size of the sheaths used but rather to the femoral artery cannulation and could have been prevented. We had no cases of aneurysm formation detected by either echocardiography, repeat catheterization, or MRI, compared with 6% reported by Suarez de Lezo et al. (27).

CONCLUSION

Coarctation of the aorta can be effectively managed with endovascular stents, although some issues regarding its clinical use remain unresolved, such as its role in arch hypoplasia. Its applicability in neonates with a higher incident risk of restenosis secondary to patient growth, and the safety of redilation remain to be defined further. Stent redilation has been successfully performed in animal models and humans several years after initial implantation to accommodate for somatic growth. Follow-up is, however, necessary to demonstrate safety and long-term efficacy.

Endovascular stents when applied in suitable patients can provide an excellent and alternative form of therapy to conventional surgical management. Based on the short- and intermediate-term results of the use of endovascular stents in both native and recurrent coarctation of the aorta in older children and adults, it should be considered the procedure of choice for this group of patients (10,29).

REFERENCES

1. Crafoord C, Nylin G. Congenital coarctation of the aorta and its surgical treatment. *J Thorac Surg* 1945;14:347–361.
2. Singer MI, Rowen M, Dorsey TJ. Transluminal aortic balloon angioplasty for coarctation of the aorta in the newborn. *Am Heart J* 1982;103:131–132.
3. Shaddy RE, Boucek MM, Sturtevant JE, et al. Comparison of angioplasty and surgery for unoperated coarctation of the aorta. *Circulation* 1993;87:793–799.
4. Fletcher SE, Nihill MR, Grifka RG, et al. Balloon angioplasty of native coarctation of the aorta: midterm follow-up and prognostic factors. *J Am Coll Cardiol* 1995;25:730–734.
5. Ino T, Ohkubo M. Dilation mechanism, causes of restenosis and stenting in balloon coarctation angioplasty. *Acta Pediatr* 1997;86:367–371.
6. Rao PS, Thaper MK, Kutayli F, et al. Causes of recoarctation after balloon angioplasty of unoperated aortic coarctation. *J Am Coll Cardiol* 1989;13:109–115.
7. Johnson MC, Canter CE, Strauss AW, et al. Repair of coarctation of the aorta in infancy: comparison of surgical and balloon angioplasty. *Am Heart J* 1993;125:464.
8. Hijazi ZM, Fahey JT, Kleinman CS, et al. Balloon angioplasty for recurrent coarctation of the aorta: immediate and long term results. *Circulation* 1991;84:1150–1156.
9. Maheshwari S, Bruckheimer E, Fahey JT, et al. Balloon angioplasty of postsurgical recoarctation in infants: the risk of restenosis and long term follow-up. *J Am Coll Cardiol* 2000;35:209–213.
10. Marshall AC, Perry SB, Keane JF, et al. Early results and medium-term follow-up of stent implantation for mild residual or recurrent aortic coarctation. *Am Heart J* 2000;139:1054–1060.
11. Yetman AT, Nykanen D, McCrindle BW, et al. Balloon angioplasty of recurrent coarctation: a 12-year review. *J Am Coll Cardiol* 1997;30:811–816.
12. Weber HS, Cyran SE. Initial results and clinical follow-up after balloon angioplasty or native coarctation. *Am J Cardiol* 84:113–116.
13. Mendelsohn AM, Lloyd TR, Crowley DC, et al. Late follow-up of balloon angioplasty in children with a native coarctation of the aorta. *Am J Cardiol* 1994;74:696–700.
14. O'Laughlin MP, Slack MC, Grifka RG, et al. Implantation and intermediate-term follow-up of stents in congenital heart disease. *Circulation* 1993;88:605–614.
15. Pedulla DM, Grifka RG, Mullins CE, et al. Endovascular stent implantation for severe coarctation of the aorta: case report with angiographic and 18-month clinical follow-up. *Catheter Cardiovasc Diagn* 1997;40:311–314.
16. Thanopoulos B, Triposkiadis F, Margetakis A, et al. Long segment coarctation of the thoracic aorta: treatment with multiple balloon-expandable stent implantation. *Am Heart J* 1997;133:470–473.
17. Alcibar J, Cabrera A, Martinez P, et al. Stent implantation in a central aorto-pulmonary shunt. *J Invas Cardiol* 1999;11:506–509.
18. D'Souza SJ, Tsai WS, Silver MM, et al. Diagnosis and management of stenotic aorto-arteriopathy in childhood. *J Pediatr* 1998;132:1016–1022.
19. Sos T, Sniderman KW, Rettek-Sos B, et al. Percutaneous translu-

minal dilation of coarctation of thoracic aorta post mortem. *Lancet* 1979;2:970–971.

20. Brzezinska-Rajszys G, Qureshi SA, Ksiazyk J, et al. Middle aortic syndrome treated by stent implantation. *Heart* 1999;81: 166–170.

21. Slack MC, O'Laughlin MP, Grifka RG, et al. Intravascular stenting versus balloon angioplasty treatment of experimental coarctation of the aorta. *Circulation* 1992;(Suppl)86:I-42.

22. Bulbul ZR, Bruckheimer E, Love JC, et al. Implantation of balloon expandable stents for coarctation of the aorta: implantation data and short term results. *Catheter Cardiovasc Diagn* 1996;39: 36–42.

23. Fletcher SE, Cheatham JP, Froeming S. Aortic aneurysm following primary balloon angioplasty and secondary endovascular stent placement in the treatment of native coarctation of the aorta. *Catheter Cardiovasc Diagn* 1998;44:40–44.

24. O'Laughlin MP, Perry SB, et al. Use of endovascular stents in congenital heart disease. *Circulation* 83:1923–1939.

25. Ebeid MR, Prieto LR, Latson SA, et al. Use of balloon expandable stents for coarctation of the aorta: initial results and intermediate-term follow-up. *J Am Coll Cardiol* 1997;30:1847–1852.

26. Mendelsohn AM, Dorostkar PC, Moorehead CP, et al. Stent redilation in canine models of congenital heart disease: pulmonary artery stenosis and coarctation of the aorta. *Catheter Cardiovasc Diagn* 1996;38:430–444.

27. De Lezo JS, Pan M, Romero M, et al. Immediate and follow-up findings after stent treatment for severe coarctation of the aorta. *Am J Cardiol* 1999;83:400–406.

28. Lock JE, Castaneda-Zuniga WR, Bass J, et al. Balloon dilation of excised aortic coarctations. *Radiology* 1982;143:689–691.

29. Thanopoulos BD, Hadjinikolaou L, Konstadopoulou GN, et al. Stent treatment for coarctation of the aorta: intermediate term follow-up and technical considerations. *Heart* 2000;84:65–70.

30. Grifka RG, Vick GW III, O'Laughlin MP, et al. Balloon expandable intravascular stents: aortic implantation and late further dilation in growing minipigs. *Am Heart J* 1993;126:979–984.

31. Mendelsohn AM. Balloon angioplasty for native coarctation of the aorta. *J Interv Cardiol* 1995;8:487–508.

32. Ovaert C, Benson LN, Nykanen D, et al. Transcatheter treatment of coarctation of the aorta: a review. *Pediatr Cardiol* 1998; 19:27–44.

33. McCrindle BW, Jones TK, Morrow WR, et al. Acute results of balloon angioplasty of native coarctation versus recurrent aortic obstruction are equivalent. *J Am Coll Cardiol* 1996;28: 1810–1817.

34. Rao PS, Galal O, Smith PA, et al. Five- to nine-year follow-up results of balloon angioplasty of native aortic coarctation in infants and children. *J Am Coll Cardiol* 1996;27:462–470.

35. Ray DG, Subramanyam R, Titus T, et al. Balloon angioplasty for native coarctation of the aorta in children and adults: factors determining the outcome. *Int J Cardiol* 1992;36:273–81.

36. De Lezo JS, Pan M, Romero M, et al. Balloon-expandable stent repair of severe coarctation of the aorta. *Am Heart J* 1995;129: 1002–1008.

37. Morrow WR, Smith VC, Ehler WJ, et al. Balloon angioplasty with stent implantation in experimental coarctation of the aorta. *Circulation* 1994;89:2677–2683.

38. Rosenthal E, Qureshi SA, Tynan M. Stent implantation for aortic recoarctation. *Am Heart J* 1995;129:1220–1221.

39. Magee AG, Brzezinska-Rajszys G, Qureshi SA, et al. Stent implantation for aortic coarctation and recoarctation. *Heart* 1999;82:600–606.

40. Kaine SF, Smith EO, Mott AR, et al. Heart disease in the young: quantitative echocardiographic analysis of the aortic arch predicts outcome of balloon angioplasty of native coarctation of the aorta. *Circulation* 1996;94:1056–1062.

Catheter Based Devices: For the Treatment of Non-coronary Cardiovascular Diseases in Adults and Children. Edited by P. Syamasundar Rao and Morton J. Kern, Lippincott Williams & Wilkins, Philadelphia © 2003.

36

DUCTAL STENTS IN THE MANAGEMENT OF CONGENITAL HEART DEFECTS

CARLOS E. RUIZ

One of the most important developments of the last century in the management of ductal-dependent cyanotic heart disease has been the use of prostaglandins (1) to provide ductal patency, allowing stabilization of the critically ill neonate until corrective surgery can be undertaken. In obstructive right heart lesions such as complex pulmonary atresia, tricuspid atresia, and so on, palliation by systemic-to-pulmonary artery shunts has been the standard of care for more than 50 years (2-4). More recently, there have been numerous non-pharmacologic attempts to preserve arterial duct patency. One such technique was the use of formalin infiltration of the arterial duct wall at thoracostomy (5). However, the long-term patency rates were disappointing (6,7), as it did not ensure long-term ductal patency. With the advent of new interventional techniques, balloon angioplasty and thermal balloon dilatation have also been investigated without much improvement on the long-term patency (8–12).

As early as the late 1960s, Dotter (13) introduced the concept of stenting by placing coil grafts in femoral arteries of dogs. Dotter's efforts lay dormant until Maas et al. (14) reintroduced in 1982 the concept with a "double-helix" spiral prosthesis to treat dissecting aortic aneurysms. In the mid-1980s, Julio Palmaz (15) developed the first balloon-expandable stent, and Mullins et al. (16) introduced these stents to pediatric cardiology. In 1991, two groups of investigators (17,18) first reported the experimental use of intravascular stents to maintain ductal patency in an animal model. Indications, techniques, and types of stents used for maintaining ductal patency as an alternative to medical/surgical therapy are reviewed in this chapter.

TYPES OF STENTS

At the present time, more than 80 different stent designs are either approved for clinical use or under investigation in different parts of the world. None of the stents manufactured today are purposely designed for use in the pediatric population with congenital cardiovascular stenotic malformations. Stents that have been used to maintain ductal patency in neonates have been adapted from adult cardiovascular interventional techniques.

There are two major types of stent-expansion mechanisms, self-expandable stents and stents that require a device expansion such as a balloon. The limited experience with ductal stenting has been obtained using balloon-expandable stents designed for coronary artery disease or in some instances mid-range peripheral artery stents used for dilatation of renal arteries. Most of stents used initially were of the slotted-tube design. These were either premounted on a balloon catheter (coronary stents) with an expansion range of 3 to 5 mm or bare stents (biliary stents) that could be mounted on any desired balloon dilatation catheter, with an expansion range of 4 to 7 mm. Foreshortening of this type of stent is quite considerable (>20% at its largest diameter). Therefore precise location of delivery and area of stent coverage are impossible to predict before final delivery. Furthermore, the delivery profile of those early devices was too large to place them safely via an arterial access. This was even more true with the protective sheath, which is used to prevent dislodgment. Another problem with the early stents was their rigidity. This made them very difficult to advance through tortuous vessels.

Currently, there is an extensive selection of balloon-expandable stents (19) with very low delivery profile, excellent flexibility (both before and after deployment), minimal foreshortening (3%), and a variety of lengths that can be more successful and safer than the initial models.

PATIENT SELECTION

The patency of the ductus arteriosus in cyanotic congenital heart disease may serve two purposes: (a) To provide systemic blood flow, as in the case of hypoplastic left heart syndrome (HLHS), and (b) to provide pulmonary blood flow,

Carlos E. Ruiz: Professor of Pediatrics and Medicine, Departments of Pediatrics and Medicine, University of Illinois at Chicago; Chief, Division of Pediatric Cardiology, University of Illinois at Chicago Medical Center, Chicago, Illinois

as in the cases of obstructive right-sided lesions such as critical pulmonary stenosis (with or without hypoplastic right ventricle), pulmonary atresia with intact ventricular septum, tricuspid atresia, and so on. In this section we will explore the different indications and patient selection based on these two types of ducti.

Patients with Ductal-Dependent Systemic Circulation (HLHS)

There is limited experience with the use of stents to maintain ductal flow patency in newborns with HLHS (20–23). Stenting the ductus arteriosus in these patients will maintain ductal patency while awaiting cardiac transplantation, thus shortening hospital stay and expenses. Initial experience has been limited to patients who are awaiting cardiac transplantation and become unresponsive to prostaglandin E_1 (PGE_1). Resistance to PGE_1 occurred mostly due to accidental discontinuation of PGE_1 infusion, such as during transport, resulting in rapid closure of the arterial duct. Until larger studies are conducted confirming the benefits of elective stenting, pharmacologic management of the ductal patency is safe and effective, and should remain the standard of care. Thus elective stenting of the ductus arteriosus in patients with HLHS for the time being cannot be advocated.

Patients with Ductal-Dependent Pulmonary Circulation

Stent implantation into the ductus arteriosus has been proposed as a nonsurgical alternative to aortopulmonary shunt surgery (21–24). It offers the advantages of eliminating initial palliative surgery prior to definitive surgical repair. This approach would also avoid causing distortion of the pulmonary arteries and perhaps maintaining a more physiologic distribution of the pulmonary blood flow.

The morphology of the ductus arteriosus plays a very important role in this type of lesion, since it is much different from the ductus seen in patients with HLHS. It usually is much longer, is more tortuous, and has a tendency to spasm, especially when any type of mechanical stimulus is inflicted.

Based on the anatomy of the congenital heart disease two subgroups could be identified: (a) patients with forward blood flow from the right ventricle into the pulmonary arteries (RV-PA) and (b) patients with the potential to establish RV-PA forward blood flow through interventional procedures, such as perforation of an atretic pulmonary valve. PDA stenting in the first group is usually easy to accomplish, and the success of the patency by and large is a short-term need. This is the case of neonates with critical pulmonary stenosis and dysfunctional right ventricle, or a membranous pulmonary atresia, with a tripartite right ventricle, suitable for a biventricular physiology, that still need aortopulmonary blood flow.

On the other hand, the second subgroup of patients is more controversial. The surgical placement of an aortopulmonary shunt has a good track record of success, despite the complications of thrombosis with the shunt, stenosis at the anastomotic sites, distortion of the pulmonary arteries, and differential pulmonary artery growth (25,26). Stenting the ductus arteriosus in the second group of patients should produce results equal to the surgical shunting procedures, if it is to be advocated as an alternative procedure.

STENT IMPLANTATION TECHNIQUES
Patients with HLHS
Access Site

Although the use of the umbilical vein would theoretically allow preservation of femoral vessels for future needs, this access is not recommended because of the tortuosity of the path toward the ductus. In our experience, the cardiologist needs to have excellent control of the delivery sheath, avoiding any kink that may make advancement of the delivery system difficult. Thus we recommend the femoral vein as the first access of choice. Placement of an arterial line for blood pressure monitoring is also recommended.

Equipment

Of fundamental importance is the availability of a well-equipped cardiac catheterization laboratory with bi-plane fluoroscopy suitable to perform procedures in neonates. The equipment recommended for the deployment of stents is based on difficulties encountered in the early experience. This has transformed the procedure to an easier, safer and less traumatic process at the present time.

1. *Venous delivery sheath.* The most desirable characteristic of the delivery sheath is to facilitate the advancement of the mounted stent into the ductus arteriosus. Thus the sheath must not be likely to cause trauma, be easy to track over the wire with optimal flexibility and maximal resistance to kinking or compression, and offer the minimum friction resistance to the advancement of the device. We found that although there may be others in the market with similar characteristics, the Cook Flexor Check-Flow Introducers (Cook Cardiology, Bloomington, IN) provides many of the desirable features.

The size of the sheath will depend on the stent type and delivery balloon catheter that is to be used. Most of the recommended stents can be delivered through a 5- or 6F sheath.

2. *Support wire.* Given today's stent technology, an extra-support 0.035-inch wire for stent placement in the ductus arteriosus of a patient with HLHS is no longer necessary, since the available stents are very flexible. We recommend

the use of an extra-stiff 0.018-inch wire (such as the Road-Runner, Cook Cardiology, Bloomington, IN). We found that this type of wire causes less strain to the guiding sheath and allows for a nice curve within the right ventricular cavity, causing less tricuspid insufficiency, which is very critical for the hemodynamic stability of the patient during the delivery of the stent.

3. *Stent.* For this type of use, the stent will need to be deployed to diameters varying between 6 and 10 mm., depending on the size of the main pulmonary artery, descending aorta, and ductus arteriosus. Many choices of peripheral (biliary) stents are available today, but we found that balloon-deployed stents are suitable for this application. We have no experience with the self-expandable stents for this application, and therefore we cannot offer a recommendation. The desired features of the stent for this application are low profile, high longitudinal flexibility, high conformability, minimal percent foreshortening, minimal recoil, and good radial force. Given the preceding requirements, there are two types of stents, the premounted ones, such as the Hercu-LINK (Guidant Co., Temecula, CA), with expansion range from 4.5 to 7 mm in diameter and 13 to 23 mm in length; this requires a sheath with an I.D of 2.4 mm. However, this type of premounted stent only accepts a 0.014-inch wire. The second type is bare stents that allow mounting on any desired balloon. One is the NIR (Medinol/SciMed Life, Maple Grove, MN) or NIROYAL (Medinol/SciMed Life, Maple Grove, MN), which are available in diameters from 5 to 12 mm and lengths of 14, 19, and 39 mm, and the Mega-LINK Biliary stent (Guidant Co., Temecula, CA), with diameter capabilities of from 6 to 10 mm and lengths of 18 and 38 mm.

4. *Balloon delivery catheter.* Certainly there is no lack of balloon dilatation catheters; however, for deploying stents the balloon catheters must fulfill certain requirements. They must be low in profile, preferably to accept a 0.021-inch or at least a 0.018-inch wire, with excellent trackability. We prefer the over-the-wire system to the monorail, for better control (especially at the level of the RVOT-PA). The balloon material must have the appropriate surface characteristics to ensure excellent stent retention upon crimping the stent on the balloon, and must be resistant enough to avoid stent puncture, while providing uniform expansion of the stent during deployment. Of critical importance is choosing the appropriate-length balloon for the desired stent, to ensure that the minimal amount of balloon material extends beyond the ends of the crimped stent. This will minimize the chances of the stent perforating the balloon during the crucial deployment time.

In our laboratory, for this type of procedure, we usually use the Thyshak-II balloon catheter (B/Braun Co. Bethlehem, PA), which can be introduced easily through a 5F sheath and will take a 0.021-inch wire, or the Power-Flex Plus (Cordis Co., Miami, FL), which will take up to a 0.035-inch wire. However, it requires at least a 6F sheath.

Procedure

It is best to perform this procedure under general anesthesia. This will enable good control of the ventilation/oxygenation of the neonate during the procedure. The patient is brought to the catheterization laboratory on a prostaglandin (PGE₁) infusion, and this is not discontinued until after the procedure has been successfully completed, with echocardiographic confirmation of correct placement of the stent across the ductus arteriosus. We prefer to have an umbilical or radial arterial line for blood pressure monitoring, as well as blood gas analysis.

The femoral vein is carefully accessed percutaneously and a short (7-cm) sheath is placed. A Berman angiographic catheter is advanced across the ductus arteriosus and a balloon occlusive descending aortogram is performed to best profile the thoracic descending aorta, ductus arteriosus, and transverse aortic arch with all its head vessels. Digital measurements are taken of the diameter of the descending aorta, ductus, and pulmonary artery, as well as the length from the bifurcation of the pulmonary artery to the entry into the descending aorta (Figure 36.1). The Berman catheter is exchanged for a multipurpose catheter that is also brought through the ductus into the mid-abdominal aorta, below the renal arteries, and the 0.018-inch extra-support wire is advanced, leaving the tip above the iliac bifurcation. The delivery sheath is then advanced and the tip is placed in the mid-thoracic aorta. Care must be taken, when placing the sheath, to allow a gentle curve within the right ventricular cavity, to minimize the amount of tricuspid regurgitation (Figure 36.2). Also, gentle manipulation of the sheath will minimize the incidence of arrhythmias and heart block, which could be fatal.

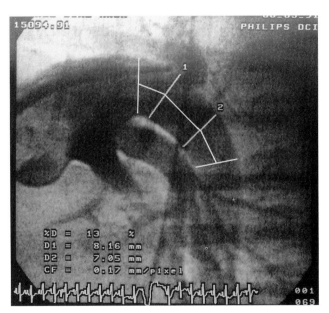

FIGURE 36.1. Digital frame of an aortogram revealing the diameter of the ductus.

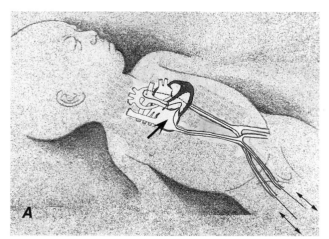
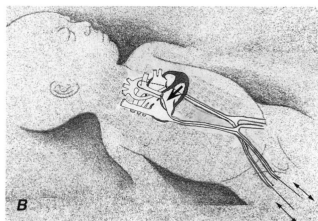

FIGURE 36.2. This diagram shows the exteriorization of the wire introduced through the femoral vein and out of the femoral artery. Maintaining a loose loop of the wire across the tricuspid valve (**A**) toward the cavity of the right ventricle *(black arrows)* minimizes the distortion of the left ventricle. The loop can be tensed (**B**) for short periods of time to facilitate (support) the advancement of the sheath into the descending aorta.

The mounted stent/delivery device is advanced over the wire, while the sheath distal tip remains in the thoracic aorta, and under fluoroscopy, the stent, which usually is highly visible, is positioned across the ductus, still inside the sheath. Then the sheath is carefully pulled back, exposing the stent. Small amounts of diluted contrast material administered through the side arm of the sheath will help position the stent within the desired location (Figure 36.3). One must exercise great deployment control to pre-

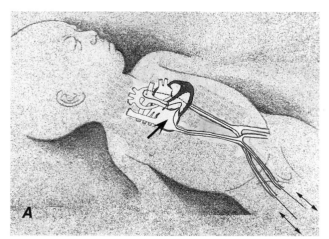

FIGURE 36.3. Final angiogram after stenting of the ductus arteriosus in a patient with hypoplastic left heart syndrome.

vent migration of the stent, which could result in compromised blood flow to the cranial circulation. One-stage deployment may be best and would avoid recrossing the newly deployed stent. The front-loading technique, which consists of passing a balloon catheter through the delivery sheath and then mounting the stent on the balloon, is exteriorized at the distal tip of the sheath. The sheath is advanced over the mounted stent, to protect it. The entire delivery system is then advanced to the desired place over a guide wire. The sheath is pulled back, exposing the stent and allowing the balloon and the stent to expand freely. This technique allowed a smaller sheath but required a tremendous support from the wire, such as extra-stiff 0.035-inch wire that would keep the tricuspid valve more in an opened position, causing severe tricuspid regurgitation and more quickly causing ventricular arrhythmias. This was a very useful technique when the early generation of stents was used; however, with the newer stents it may no longer be needed.

Patients with Ductal-Dependent Pulmonary Circulation

Access Site

The basic technique on how to access vessels is similar to that previously described; however, the access site will depend on the type of congenital anomaly and the location of the ductus. In patients who have forward flow through the pulmonary valve, whether it existed or has been newly created by another interventional procedure, and still need ductal flow, the access for stent placement from the femoral vein, as described for the patients with HLHS, will be the same.

For patients whose anatomy is such that the only pulmonary blood supply is from the ductus, the only possible access to the ductus would be from the aortic side. In some patients, depending on the anomaly, it may be possible to access the aorta from the femoral vein. However, in most instances, this route will make it difficult to ensure good catheter control. Therefore, even if the access to the aorta from the femoral vein is possible, our experience has determined that the arterial, femoral, or axillary access is preferred to obtain maximal catheter control during the procedure.

Equipment

1. *Arterial delivery sheath.* We recommend accessing the desired artery (femoral or axillary) percutaneously and to place a short (7-cm) 4F sheath to first obtain the necessary diagnostic information. After the diameter, length, and configuration of the ductus have been obtained, we exchange the 7-cm, 4F sheath for a 75-cm, 4F sheath (Check-Flow Performer, Cook Cardiology, Bloomington, IN). This sheath will allow safe passage of most of the recommended coronary stents used for this application.

2. *Support wire.* The ductus arteriosus in these types of anomalies tends to be long and tortuous, and tends to spasm upon its manipulation. Therefore crossing the ductus with a wire must be done very delicately and in the most atraumatic manner. We had good success using 0.014-inch high-torque coronary wires. However, there are many new and equally acceptable, if not better, wires on the market. Recommending one over another is a matter of operator experience and preference.

We strongly recommend avoiding wires larger than 0.018 inch to minimize the risk of spasm of the ductus, which may prove fatal.

3. *Stents.* Given that the expansion diameters needed for these applications are much smaller than those for patients with HLHS, existing coronary stents will suffice. We have no experience with self-expandable stents for this application. All coronary stents nowadays come premounted and without a protective sleeve. The desired features of the balloon-expandable stent for these applications are somewhat more demanding than before. Certainly low profile, high longitudinal flexibility, high conformability, minimal percent foreshortening, minimal recoil, and good radial force are still critical. However, a good variety of lengths is of equal importance.

There is a large selection of coronary stents with most of the preceding desired features, and many of them may prove useful, more so in countries outside the United States, where the selection is even larger, but of which we have no experience and cannot comment. From the stents available to us, we had experience mostly with the ACS-Multi Link Tetra (Guidant Co., Temecula, CA) coronary stent and with the NIR coronary stent (Medinol/SciMed

Life, Maple Grove, MN), with very good success. Most of these coronary stents allow diameters ranging from 3 to 5 mm and come in different lengths, ranging from 9 to 38 mm.

Procedure

We perform these types of procedures in neonates under general anesthesia to improve safety and allow the operator to concentrate on the procedure. The arterial access is performed at the location that can offer the highest degree of simplicity from the technical standpoint, to accomplish the stenting of the ductus in safely.

A 7-cm, 4F sheath is advanced in the peripheral artery and an aortogram and selective angiograms of the ductus are taken in different views to profile the ductus. Accurate digital measurements and other necessary information about diameter, length, and conformation of the ductus are obtained so that the appropriate stent size can be chosen. The sheath is replaced with a 75-cm, 4F sheath (internal diameter 5 = 0.068 inch) that will accommodate the stent delivery system. A 0.014-inch coronary wire is advanced through the introducer of the sheath and the introducer is exchanged for a 4F coronary catheter, commonly a JR-2.5. However, the choice of the catheter will depend on the location and the takeoff of the ductus, so as to provide the best support when advancing the wire. In a very careful and gentle manner, the ductus is crossed with the floppy tip wire. Depending on the shape of the ductus and its location, a higher support wire may be needed. If this is the case, the coronary catheter is advanced over the wire and placed distally in the pulmonary artery. Then the wire can be exchanged for one that will give better support to the stent delivery system. To assess the anatomic configuration of the stented duct prior to stent deployment, some investigators recommend a balloon dilatation of the ductus (27); however, this is not necessary with the newer stents that will configure well to the shape of the ductus. The long 4F sheath is then advanced over the coronary catheter into the distal pulmonary artery and the catheter is pulled out. The chosen premounted coronary stent is advanced over the wire, utilizing a similar delivery technique to that described for the patients with HLHS. The stent is placed across the ductus within the sheath, and the sheath is withdrawn to expose the stent, leaving the tip of the sheath at the aortic entry of the ductus for better support of the delivery catheter during balloon inflation (Figure 36.4).

Careful attention must be paid to the angiograms of the ductus after delivery, before the wire is removed, to ensure that the entire length of the ductus has been properly covered by the stent. Otherwise, if there is a segment of ductus that it is not covered by the stent, it could constrict upon discontinuation of the prostaglandins and therefore require a second stent to ensure covering of the entire ductal length.

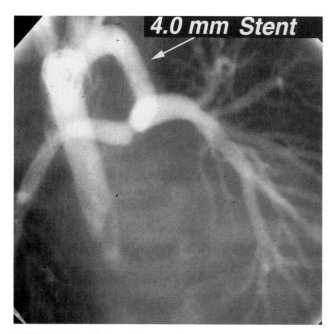

FIGURE 36.4. Final angiogram after stenting of a very elongated and tortuous ductus of a patient with pulmonary atresia intact ventricular septum and right aortic arch.

Patient Management

These patients are given aspirin 1 mg/kg and clopidogrel 1 mg/kg the day before the procedure. They are kept on the same daily dose of aspirin indefinitely and on clopidogrel for at least 8 weeks. All these patients need to be followed for restenosis to anticipate the need for redilatation.

PRESENT AND FUTURE OF DUCTAL STENTING

Currently, there are no pediatric cardiology programs using routine stenting of the ductus for patients with either ductal-dependent systemic circulation or pulmonary circulation.

The need for stenting the ductus in patients with HLHS implies that the patient will undergo cardiac transplantation, since this metal structure will be removed at the time of the transplantation, without much interference with the surgical technique. Therefore programs that contemplate the possibility of ductal stenting in patients with HLHS must have an active cardiac transplantation program. Whether those neonates with HLHS that have been enlisted for cardiac transplantation should undergo ductal stenting routinely has not yet been proven to be of value. It seems prudent at this time to contemplate a prospective randomized study comparing stenting with long-term PGE₁ infusion, to be able to answer this question. If stenting the ductus is as safe and effective as pharmacologic management, we might be able to have those patients await cardiac transplantation as outpatients who could decrease the risk of nosocomial infections and lower the overall cost. However, since there are relatively few centers that have a well-established transplantation program capable of performing such study, this may not be possible.

In the United Kingdom there have been some attempts to stent the ductus arteriosus with simultaneous surgical bilateral pulmonary artery banding and atrial septectomy to control pulmonary blood flow in patients with HLHS undergoing the Norwood procedure (27). Unfortunately, however, even though the stenting procedures were all successful, all patients died. Furthermore, stenting the ductus in patients who will undergo the Norwood operation not only defeats the purpose, but makes the critical balancing of both circulations much more difficult to achieve and could ruin the reconstruction of the neoaorta at a later time.

In patients with ductal-dependent pulmonary circulation, the technique of stent implantation is most challenging. The success varies among different investigators (23,27). However, with the advent of newer stents, this procedure should become more successful. The question is whether this technique will be superior to the standard aortopulmonary shunts. There is no question that from the physiologic standpoint, maintaining ductal patency can provide better distribution of the pulmonary blood flow than a surgical shunt, without the possibility of distorting the integrity of the pulmonary arteries in those patients who will require corrective surgery later. When ductal stenting is performed to provide temporary additional pulmonary blood flow while the right ventricle develops, partial stenting has been proposed (27) of the ductus, with the expectation that intimal proliferation of the nonstented segment will progress to closure after the right ventricle is self-sufficient.

The main problem of a successful ductal stent placement in patients with ductal-dependent pulmonary circulation is the longevity of this patency. Intimal proliferation is almost universal between the first 3 to 6 months, requiring reintervention in most patients (23,27). This does not appear to be a problem in patients with HLHS, because the stented ductus is of a much larger diameter and a matching donor for cardiac transplantation is usually available within a 3-month period.

At the present time, stenting of the ductus arteriosus in patients with ductal-dependent pulmonary circulation remains highly experimental. Perhaps the time has come to consider a prospective multicenter randomized study comparing elective ductal stenting with the traditional aortopulmonary shunt operation.

The future will depend also on the advancements in technology. There has been tremendous improvement in the availability of new stents that are of a much lower profile and are more flexible. Furthermore, new covered coronary stents are being tested. Perhaps the cover will prevent the obstructive effect of the intimal proliferation. Ideally, we should be developing a stent purposely designed for this application that would provide all the necessary requirements to achieve the goal of maintaining ductal patency for the necessary period of time before a corrective surgical procedure. This is unlikely to happen, since the number of stents placed in children per year, even around the world, is infinitesimal, compared with the number of stents currently being placed for coronary or peripheral atherosclerotic application. Thus it would be very difficult to find any company to invest in such a small venture.

REFERENCES

1. Elliott RB, Starling MB, Neutze JM. Medical manipulation of the ductus arteriosus. *Lancet* 1975;1:140.
2. Blalock A, Taussig HB. The surgical treatment of malformations of the heart in which there is pulmonary stenosis or pulmonary atresia. *JAMA* 1945;128:189–202.
3. White BD, McNamara DG, Bauersfeld SR, et al. Five year postoperative results of first 500 patients with Blalock-Taussig anastomosis for pulmonary stenosis or atresia. *Circulation* 1956;14:512–520.
4. Arciniegas E, Blackstone EH, Pacifico AD, et al. Classic shunting operation as part of two-stage repair of tetralogy of Fallot. *Ann Thorac Surg* 1979;27:514–518.
5. Rudolph AM, Heymann MA, Fishman N, et al. Formalin infiltration of the ductus arteriosus: a method for palliation of infants with selected congenital cardiac lesions. *N Engl J Med* 1975;292:1263–1268.
6. Hatem J, Sade RM, Upshur JK, et al. Maintaining patency of the ductus-arteriosus for palliation of cyanotic congenital cardiac malformations: the use of prostaglandin E₁ and formaldehyde infiltration of the ductal wall. *Ann Surg* 1980;192:124–128.
7. Deanfield JE, Rees PG, Bull CM, et al. Formalin infiltration of ductus arteriosus in cyanotic congenital heart disease. *Br Heart J* 1981;45:573–576.
8. Lund G, Cragg A, Rysavy R, et al. Patency of the ductus arteriosus after balloon dilatation: an experimental study. *Circulation* 1983;68:621–627.
9. Walsh KP, Abrams SE, Arnold R. Arterial duct angioplasty as an adjunct to dilatation of the valve for critical pulmonary stenosis. *Br Heart J* 1993;69:260–262.
10. Lund G, Rysavy J, Cragg A, et al. Long-term patency of the ductus arteriosus after balloon dilatation: an experimental study. *Circulation* 1984;69:772–774.
11. Radtke W, Anderson RR, Guerrero L, et al. Creation of a palliative shunt by thermal balloon angioplasty of the ductus arterio-

sus [abstract]. *Proceedings of XXVI Annual General Meeting of the Association of European Pediatric Cardiologists,* Oslo, Norway, June 1990.
12. Abrams SE, Walsh KP, Diamond MJ, et al. Radiofrequency thermal angioplasty maintains arterial duct patency: an experimental study. *Circulation* 1994;90:442–448.
13. Dotter CT. Transluminally placed coilspring endarterial tube grafts. *Invest Radiol* 1969;4:329–332.
14. Maass D, Kropf L, Egloff L, et al. Transluminal implantation of intravascular "double helix" spiral prosthesis: technical and biological considerations. *ESAO Proc* 1982;9:252–256.
15. Palmaz JC, Windeler SA, Garcia F, et al. Atherosclerotic rabbit aortas: expandable intraluminal grafting. *Radiology* 1986;160:723–726.
16. Mullins CE, O'Laughlin MP, Vick GW III, et al. Implantation of balloon-expandable intravascular grafts by catheterization in pulmonary arteries and systemic veins. *Circulation* 1988;77:188–199.
17. Moore JW, Kirby WC, Lovett EJ, et al. Use of an intravascular prosthesis (stent) to establish and maintain short-term patency of the ductus arteriosus in newborn lambs. *Cardiovasc Intervent Radiol* 1991;14:299–301.
18. Coe JY, Olley PM. A novel method to maintain ductus arteriosus patency. *J Am Coll Cardiol* 1991;18:837–841.
19. Serruys PW, Kutryk MJB, eds. *Handbook of coronary stents,* 3rd ed. Martin Dumitz Ltd., 2000.
20. Ruiz CE, Gamra H, Zhang HP, et al. Stenting of the ductus arteriosus as a bridge to cardiac transplantation in infants with the hypoplastic left-heart syndrome. *N Engl J Med* 1993;328:1605–1608.
21. Gibbs JL, Rothman MT, Rees MR, et al. Stenting of the arterial duct: a new approach to palliation for pulmonary atresia. *Br Heart J* 1992;67:240–245.
22. Rosenthal E, Qureshi S, Tynan M. Percutaneous pulmonary valvotomy and arterial duct stenting in neonates with right ventricular hypoplasia. *Am J Cardiol* 1994;74:304–306.
23. Schneider M, Zartner P, Sidiropoulos A, et al. Stent implantation of the arterial duct in newborns with duct-dependent circulation. *Eur Heart J* 1998;19:1401–1409.
24. Siblini G, Rao PS, Singh GK, et al. Transcatheter management of neonates with pulmonary atresia and intact ventricular septum. *Cathet Cardiovasc Diagn* 1997;42:395–402.
25. Tamisier D, Voühe PR, Vermant F, et al. Modified Blalock-Taussig shunt: results in infants less than 3 months of age. *Ann Thorac Surg* 1990;49:797–801.
26. Fermanis G, Ekangaki A, Salmon A, et al. Twelve-year experience with the modified Blalock-Taussig shunt in neonates. *Eur J Cardiothorac Surg* 1992;6:586–589.
27. Gibbs JL, Orhan U, Blackburn MEC, et al. Fate of the stented arterial duct. *Circulation* 1999;99:2621–2625.

Catheter Based Devices: For the Treatment of Non-coronary Cardiovascular Diseases in Adults and Children. Edited by P. Syamasundar Rao and Morton J. Kern, Lippincott Williams & Wilkins, Philadelphia © 2003.

37

STENTS FOR TREATMENT OF SYSTEMIC AND PULMONARY VENOUS OBSTRUCTION

FRANK F. ING

Transcatheter implantation of stents in systemic veins for congenital heart disease was first reported by Mullins in 1988 (1). Since then the use of stents to treat various systemic and pulmonary venous stenoses in children with congenital heart disease has been widely reported, mostly in small series. Although stent treatment for venous stenoses in adults is also well reported, it is important to recognize that the etiology of systemic venous obstructions in the adult (without congenital heart disease) is very different from that in children with congenital heart disease and that, therefore, patient selection, choice of stents, and management strategies may differ. In the adult, systemic veins and vena caval obstructions are usually due to malignancies, hypercoagulable state, thromboembolic events, or thrombosis/fibrosis from radiation therapy or following surgery such as cardiac transplantation and surgically created shunts for hemodialysis. In contrast, mechanisms for systemic venous obstruction in children are almost always associated with congenital heart disease and surgery. Fortunately, obstructions of the venous system in children are relatively uncommon. They include three major central venous systems and their tributaries: the superior vena cava (SVC) and its branches, the inferior vena cava (IVC), and the iliofemoral venous system and the pulmonary veins. In addition, obstructions of surgically created systemic venous baffles following a Mustard or Senning operation or cavopulmonary connections such as the Glenn or Fontan operation are also encountered.

Overall, early results of stent treatment for venous obstructions have been excellent. Furthermore, intermediate-term follow-up for systemic vein stents in several studies have detected no significant in-stent thrombosis (2–6). The intermediate-term results for pulmonary vein stents

have been uniformly poor. The most complete and longest follow-up study of stents implantation in congenital heart disease from Texas Children's Hospital suggested only a few complications, a low rate of restenosis, and excellent intermediate- and long-term results for both systemic venous and venous baffle stenoses (5). In that study 200 patients received stents at various vascular sites with a mean follow-up of 19 ±15 months, the longest being 62 months. Of the 49 patients who received 80 stents in various venous structures, 13 (22 stents) have undergone repeat cardiac catheterization with no significant restenosis, although five stents were further dilated. Several studies showed significant restenosis to range from 1.5% to 9% (3,5,6). Successful further dilation of stents to accommodate growth in children has been reported in both animal and clinical series (3,6–9).

In this chapter we will review current published data on stent treatment of these venous obstructions and focus on specific interventional techniques associated with stent dilation of these vessels.

TYPES OF STENTS

It is important to keep in mind that in a growing child, the stent of choice is one that can be implanted and dilated to an appropriate diameter for that particular-size child and then further dilated over a long period of time to accommodate growth to adult size. Therefore self-expanding stents are seldom used unless the child has no further growth potential. For central large system veins such as the SVC, IVC, proximal pulmonary veins, and even proximal iliac veins, the stents of choice are few and include the Palmaz 308 and 188 stents (Johnson & Johnson Interventional Systems, Warren, NJ) or the new DoubleStrut stents (IntraTherapeutics, Inc., St. Paul, MN), each of which can be progressively dilated to about 18 mm in diameter. For venous tributaries such as the femoral veins and the innom-

Frank F. Ing: Clinical Associate Professor, Department of Pediatrics, University of California; Director, Cardiac Catheterization Laboratory, Department of Pediatric Cardiology, Children's Hospital of San Diego, San Diego, California

inate vein, one of several smaller stents such as the Corinthian series or the Palmaz 154, 204 by J & J, the Bridgestent by Medtronic-AVE, or the NIR stent by Boston Scientific will suffice. In adults with venous obstruction, in addition to the stents described earlier, self-expanding stents such as the Wallstent (Schneider Inc., Minneapolis, MN), Smartstent (Johnson & Johnson Interventional Systems, Warren, NJ), or the Gianturco Z-stents (Cook, Inc., Bloomington, IN) have been used successfully.

SYSTEMIC VEINS

SVC and Branches

The most common causes for SVC obstructions in the pediatric population are due to prolonged indwelling lines, especially in the very sick, small infant, and due to the presence of transvenous pacing wires (10–17). Rarely, SVC obstruction is seen following cannulation for cardiac surgery or extracorporeal membrane oxygenator (ECMO). Obstructions following atrial switch operations for D-transposition of the great arteries or cavopulmonary connections for single-ventricle variants will be discussed at a later section in the chapter. Treatment modalities reported include the use of anticoagulation (18), thrombolytics (19,20), balloon angioplasty (21–25), and surgery (12,26,27), and results have been variable. The largest experience has been in adults with SVC syndrome due to malignancy and postradiation fibrosis (28,29). Rarely, SVC obstruction is a complication following heart transplant (30). While thrombolytics may be useful in thrombotic occlusions, surgical scars, kinks, and fibrotic occlusions associated with surgery for congenital heart disease are not amenable to this mode of therapy (19,20). Although angioplasty of the SVC is well documented, its medium- and long-term effectiveness is suboptimal due to elastic recoil of the vessel or external compression (1,25). Moreover, angioplasty requires using significantly larger balloons or double-balloon techniques—about six to ten times larger than the native obstruction (25). In adults with malignancies and a shortened life expectancy, serial dilations may be acceptable. However, in children, a more aggressive approach with stents should be taken. The use of stents to treat SVC obstruction is well reported but only in small series (2,4,17, 29,31,32). Although studies in adults demonstrate similar results comparing surgery to stent dilation in central venous stenoses (33), there are no known comparison studies for children.

Prolonged indwelling lines from the neck perioperatively can lead to venous obstruction at various levels from the jugular and the subclavian veins to the SVC, especially in the small, sick infant. An obstructed SVC can present with SVC syndrome, which includes head, neck, and upper-body venous congestion. The skin in these regions may have a multitude of superficial engorged veins. Infants with open cranial sutures may present with increasing head circumference or hydrocephalus (4,16). In older patients, headaches may occur. In the case of obstruction of the jugular or subclavian veins alone without involvement of the SVC, patients are usually asymptomatic because there is adequate venous collateralization. The diagnosis of subclavian, jugular, or innominate vein obstruction is often discovered when attempts to cannulate these vessels fail and an angiogram demonstrates the obstruction. While no intervention is necessary to treat obstructions of the branches of the SVC, there is occasionally a need to stent an innominate vein in order to maintain vascular access for implantation of a transvenous pacing wire, or for hemodialysis. Certainly SVC syndrome is an indication for an intervention.

Although most experience with stents in pediatrics involves the J & J Palmaz stent, other stents have been used such as the Wallstent, a flexible, self-expanding stent (34). Vesely reported successful use of Wallstents to treat subclavian and brachiocephalic vein obstructions in adult hemodialysis patients but did require additional angioplasties for in-stent restenosis (35). These self-expanding stents have limited use in the pediatric age group because of the growth potential of the patients and the need for further expansion as the child grows.

One particular group of patients who are at risk for obstruction of the SVC and its tributaries is the group that had transvenous pacing wires implanted for congenital or surgically acquired complete heart block. Over a long period of time, these indwelling wires may lead to obstruction along its vascular course to the heart and may involve the subclavian vein, innominate vein, as well as the SVC. Successful stenting of innominate veins followed by implantation of a transvenous pacing wire in children has been reported (17).

The Palmaz 308 and 188 stents have become the stent of choice for SVC obstruction in children because it can be serially dilated to 18 mm, which approximates the adult size of the SVC. More recently, a new balloon-expandable stent, the DoubleStrut, has been approved for biliary and peripheral stenoses. This stent also can be expanded to 18-mm diameter and is under investigation for use in growing children (36,37).

Standard stent implantation techniques are used for stent implantation. A short-tip superstiff exchange guide wire (Meditech, Inc., Watertown, MA) is passed from the femoral vein into the SVC. A large stent mounted on an appropriately sized balloon is delivered to the site of obstruction for implantation. The size of the balloon is based on the size of the normal caliber of the SVC in the patient. Care is taken to avoid jailing the innominate vein.

Occasionally, in patients with a transvenous pacing system that may need lead revision, vascular obstruction along the course of the pacing lead is encountered. The most common sites are the innominate vein and/or the SVC. Although patients are usually asymptomatic, vascular patency is required for replacement of the pacing lead. If the innominate vein is obstructed but not totally occluded, an 0.035-inch "superstiff" exchange wire can be advanced through the subclavian vein sheath (inserted for the transvenous pacing lead revision) and across the stenotic site and snared in the right atrium with a snare catheter (Microvena Corp., White Bear Lake, MN) inserted through a femoral venous sheath. The exchange wire is withdrawn down the IVC and out of the femoral sheath so that both ends of the wire are exposed for control outside of the body. Alternatively, the exchange wire can be advanced from the femoral vein, snared, and pulled out of the left subclavian vein for the stent procedure. Over the exchange wire, the femoral sheath is exchanged for an 11F long sheath (Cook, Inc., Bloomington, IN)) to traverse the stenotic venous segment. A balloon dilation catheter with a diameter that approximates that of the normal adjacent segment of the affected vessel (usually 12 or 15 mm in diameter) is selected. A Palmaz P308 stent is mounted on the balloon catheter and is advanced through the long sheath to the stenotic site. Angiograms are performed in both the innominate vein and the SVC to optimally position the stent so that it is centered across the stenotic site but not obstruct the right and left jugular venous flow. The balloon is inflated to expand the stent, and then deflated and withdrawn. Additional overlapping stents are often required for relief of long segment stenosis. Poststent pressure measurements and angiograms are performed. If the stent has a residual "waist," a larger balloon or higher-pressure balloon catheter is used to further expand the stent. Figures 37.1A through 37.1K illustrate an example of complete SVC obstruction and the techniques of recannulation and stent implantation to relieve the obstruction.

If complete innominate vein occlusion was found following lead extraction, a 0.035-inch Teflon straight wire, advanced from the femoral vein sheath, can be used to push through the soft thrombus or fibrous material that had filled in the tract of the extracted pacing lead. The Teflon wire is advanced into an introducer sheath placed proximal to the obstruction in the left subclavian vein and then snared and pulled out of the subclavian vein. This wire is exchanged for a 0.035-inch "superstiff" wire for the stent procedure. Intravenous antibiotics (cefazolin 25 mg/kg) are given following stent implantation and continued for 24 hours. Figures 37.2A through 37.2E show a patient with complete innominate vein obstruction following removal of a transvenous pacing lead and subsequent recannulation and stent implantation permitting replacement of the pacing system.

Mullins first reported the use of Palmaz stents in systemic veins in animal experiments in 1988 (1). The same group reported the first pediatric implant in an obstructed SVC after repair of a sinus venosus ASD in 1991 (32). Ing et al. reported a series of eight patients in whom stents were implanted for SVC and/or innominate vein obstructions in order to permit transvenous pacing lead implantation (17). Not only did this technique successfully relieve SVC syndrome in three patients, it also avoided a surgical epicardial approach. Follow-up at mean 1.1 years indicated all stented vessels remained patent. However, subsequent follow-up showed restenosis in two innominate vein stents without clinical symptoms. This technique is particularly useful in patients who are at high risk for systemic venous obstructions and require a pacing system such as those with congenital complete heart block and d-TGA, following a Mustard or Senning operation.

Complications for SVC stents are uncommon. Restenosis is rare because the stents are usually dilated to its maximum size of 18 mm in diameter in the adolescent and adults. Even in the smaller child, the SVC stent can be dilated to 10 mm. The smallest patient reported to receive a SVC stent was 3 months old and weighed 5.5 kg (4). In that case, the patient received a P188 stent and was dilated to a diameter of 10 mm.

To date, there have been no reports of in-stent thrombosis in the SVC of children. However, stented innominate veins with an indwelling endocardial pacing lead have been found to be completely occluded without symptoms (17). Figure 37.3 is a 1-year follow-up angiogram in the innominate vein stent previously shown that demonstrates complete in-stent restenosis. This patient was completely asymptomatic. It is speculated that the combination of a smaller stent lumen, low flow state, and presence of a foreign body (pacing wire) places high risk for restenosis in the innominate vein. Certainly longer-term follow-up and larger series are warranted.

IVC and Iliofemoral Veins

Obstructions of the IVC and its branches are uncommon in children with congenital heart disease. Prolonged indwelling lines and large sheaths or repeated use for cardiac catheterizations are the most common cause of iliofemoral vein obstruction in children with congenital heart disease. When the IVC is involved, the obstruction is usually limited to the infrarenal segment. Rarely, IVC obstruction is seen following surgical repair of congenital heart defects involving the IVC or following heart transplantation. Other rare causes include external compression, malignancy, and obstructed lower-extremity hemodialysis grafts, but these are found more frequently in the adult population (38–42).

In children, iliofemoral vein obstruction is almost always asymptomatic because of adequate paravertebral venous collateral flow. Rarely, acute complete iliac vein obstruction following cardiac catheterization in a very small infant may result in significant venous congestion of the affected leg and in compartment syndrome. In these cases, a surgical approach is indicated. But for the most part, the paravertebral venous collaterals are adequate to drain the venous return from the legs. These collaterals often reenter the IVC

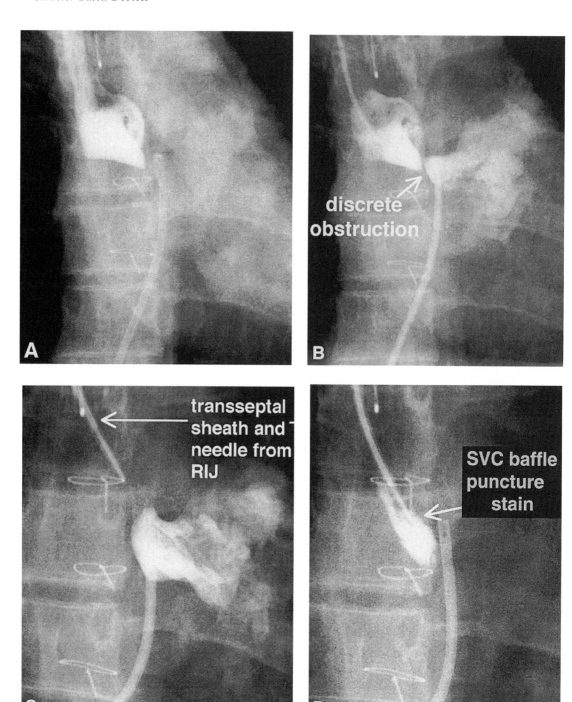

FIGURE 37.1. A: Complete occlusion of the superior vena cava (SVC) baffle is demonstrated in the anterio-posterior (AP) and lateral projection in this 22-year-old patient with d-TGA following a Mustard repair. **B:** Simultaneous injections of contrast from a catheter in the neo-right atrium and in the SVC demonstrated a discrete occlusion *(white arrow)* at the entrance of the SVC. **C:** AP projection of a transseptal sheath, dilator, and needle *(white arrow)* perforating the occluded SVC segment. The needle was directed toward the catheter placed into the neo-right atrium from a femoral vein. It was important to use biplane fluoroscopy during this procedure to ensure proper direction of the transseptal needle. **D:** Hand injection of contrast through the needle during the puncture was used to stain the occluded segment for a roadmap *(white arrow)*. RIJ, right internal jugular vein; SVC, superior vena cava; TG, transposition of the great arteries.

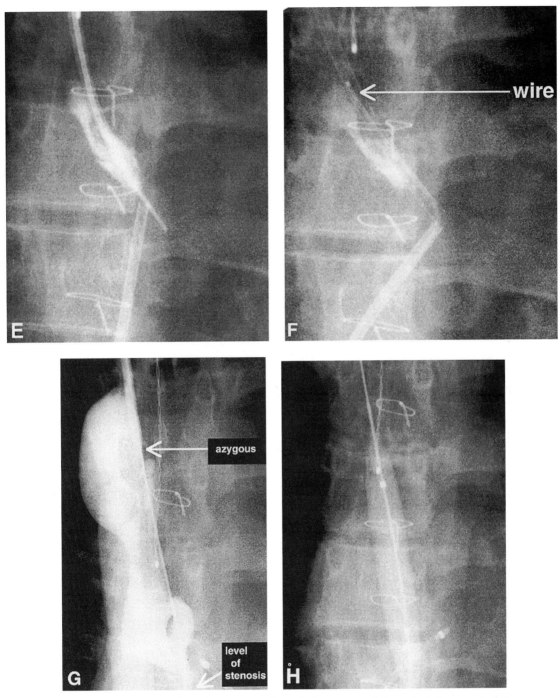

FIGURE 37.1. *(continued)* **E:** The transseptal needle has traversed the occluded segment of the SVC baffle. **F:** An exchange wire *(white arrow)* was passed from an end-hole catheter from the right atrium up into the transseptal sheath. **G:** The wire was pulled out of the transseptal sheath for through-and-through control. Note the dilated azygous *(white arrow)* vein decompressing flow from the obstructed SVC. **H:** A 15-mm-diameter balloon was used to dilate the area of obstruction.
(continues on next page)

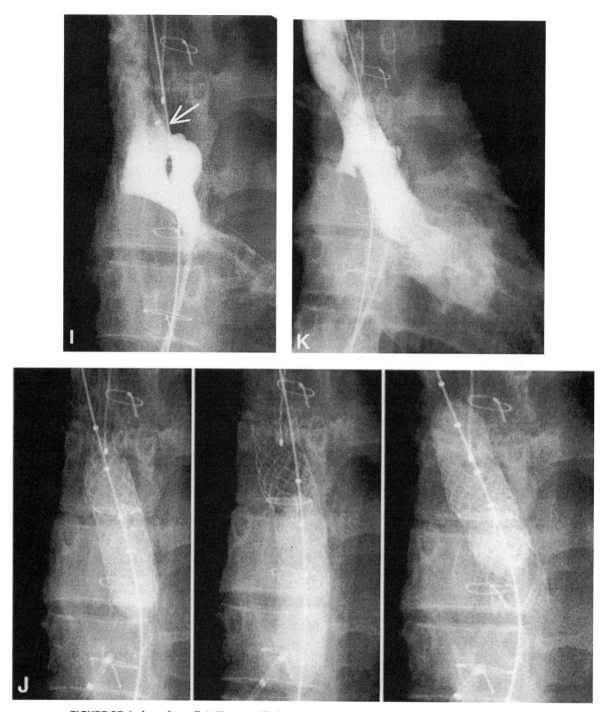

FIGURE 37.1. *(continued)* **I:** The postdilation angiogram showed patency but persistent severe stenosis of the SVC baffle. However, a Cardiomarker catheter easily passed into the SVC from the femoral vein. **J:** Fluoroscopy showed implantation of three overlapping P308 stents along the SVC baffle and dilated to 15-mm diameter. **K:** SVC angiogram following stent implantation demonstrated wide patency. (Sternal wires can also be used as reference points for location of previous stenosis when compared with Figure 37.1A.)

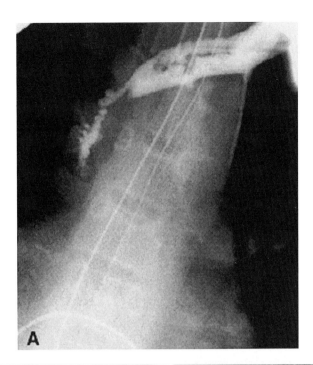

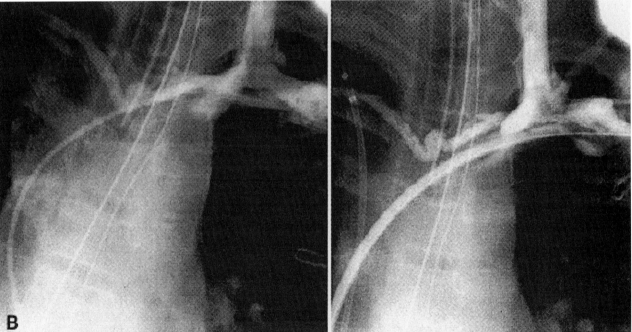

FIGURE 37. 2. A: Left subclavian vein angiogram following transvenous lead extraction demonstrated complete occlusion of the proximal innominate vein in this 15-year-old boy with congenital complete heart block. Thrombus or fibrous material can be seen within the lumen of the innominate vein. **B:** *(Left panel)* A catheter was passed from the femoral vein and through the soft thrombus into the left subclavian vein. *(Right panel)* An exchange guide wire and transseptal sheath traversed the innominate vein obstruction.

(continues on next page)

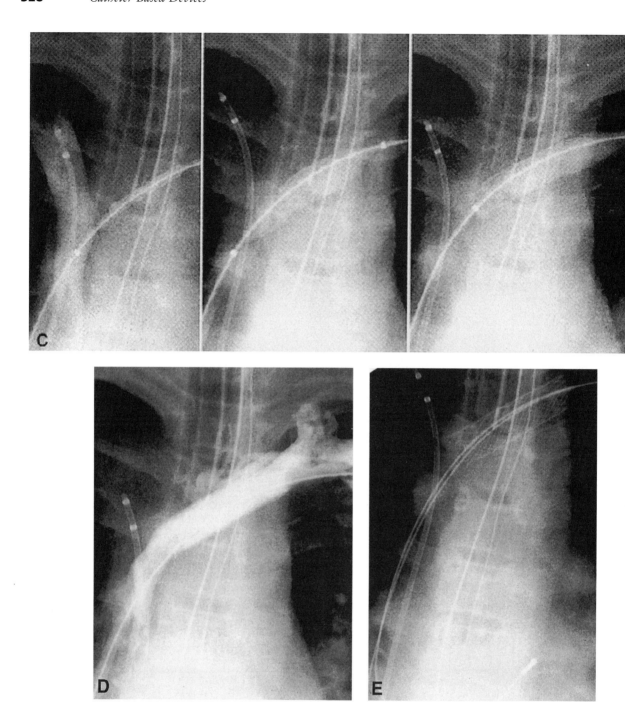

FIGURE 37.2. (continued) C: *(Left panel)* A Palmaz P308 stent mounted on a 12-mm balloon was positioned within the innominate vein obstruction. A second catheter was placed within the right jugular vein for an angiogram to determine the site of its entrance into the SVC for proper stent positioning *(white arrow)*. *(Middle panel)* The stent was implanted just proximal to the right jugular vein/SVC junction. *(Right panel)* A second overlapping stent was implanted. **D:** Following two overlapping stents in the occluded segment of the innominate vein, a repeat angiogram demonstrated wide patency. The catheter in the right jugular vein confirmed that the stents did not cross its orifice in the SVC. **E:** A transvenous pacing lead was implanted through the two overlapping stents.

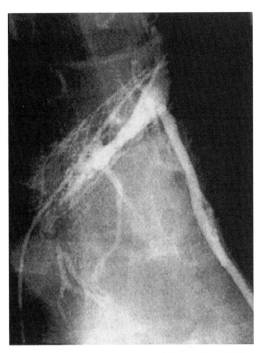

FIGURE 37.3. Follow-up angiogram of the patient in Figure 37.2 1 year later demonstrated complete reocclusion of the innominate vein stents. However, the patient was asymptomatic and no further interventions were performed. With the development of newer methods of lead extraction, including the application of laser energy, it is anticipated that the stent can be recannulated in the future when necessary.

at the level of the renal veins. Diagnosis of iliofemoral vein obstruction is usually made at the time of cardiac catheterization, when the wire cannot be passed into the vein even though there is good venous return from the needle. A hand injection of contrast usually demonstrates significant obstruction with paravertebral venous collateral flow. The indications for stent implantation are not for symptoms, but rather to maintain access for future cardiac catheterization, especially those who need repeated interventions, or for future cardiac surgery (43). Figures 37.4A through 37.4F show a case of a 9-month-old infant after orthotopic heart transplant as a neonate due to dilated cardiomyopathy. This patient was found to have an occluded left femoral vein and severe right femoral vein stenosis. Stent implantation in the right femoral vein permitted a femoral vein approach to her catheterizations. Figures 37.5A through 37.5E demonstrated in-stent reocclusion at her next cardiac catheterization, but the stent provided an excellent target under fluoroscopy for the needle to reenter and recannulate the femoral vein. Using both the AP and lateral projection, one can advance a needle into the occluded vessel lumen as defined by the stent. Access can be achieved without risk of extravasation. This particular patient has undergone multiple catheterizations and biopsies through the stented right femoral vein using this approach.

For stenotic but patent vessels, standard stenting techniques can be used. For complete obstruction of the femoral

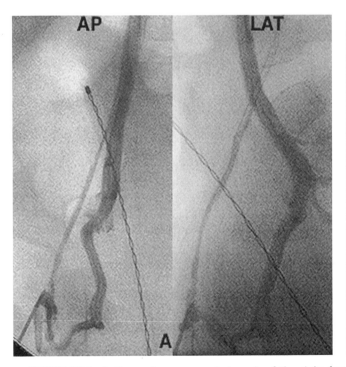
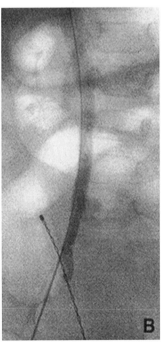

FIGURE 37.4. A: Severe long-segment stenosis of the right femoral vein was found in this 9-month-old infant s/p orthotopic heart transplant for dilated cardiomyopathy. (The left femoral vein was occluded.) The most likely cause of the venous obstruction was due to an indwelling femoral venous line prior to transplant. Because of the need for repetitive cardiac catheterizations and endomyocardial biopsies over a lifetime, it was important to reestablish venous access in at least one femoral vein. **B:** An exchange guide wire traversed the long-segment stenosis and a small injection of contrast demonstrated patency of the iliac vein and inferior vena cava (IVC).

(continues on next page)

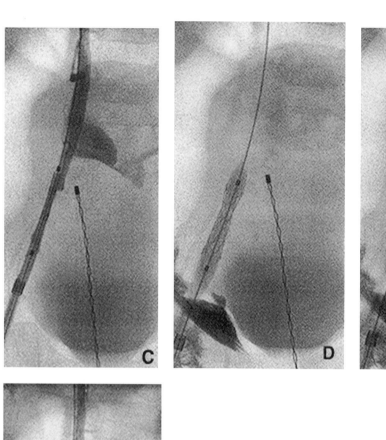

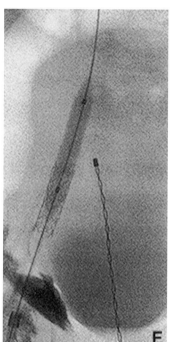

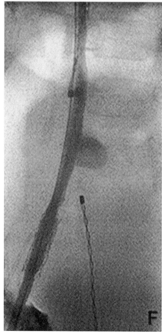

FIGURE 37.4. *(continued)* C: A P294 stent was positioned in the distal femoral vein. **D:** The stent was implanted with a 5-mm-diameter balloon that is slightly larger than the proximal iliac vein. **E:** The balloon was advanced further into the proximal femoral vein/iliac vein in an additional angioplasty. **F:** Poststent angiogram demonstrated wide patency of the right iliofemoral venous system.

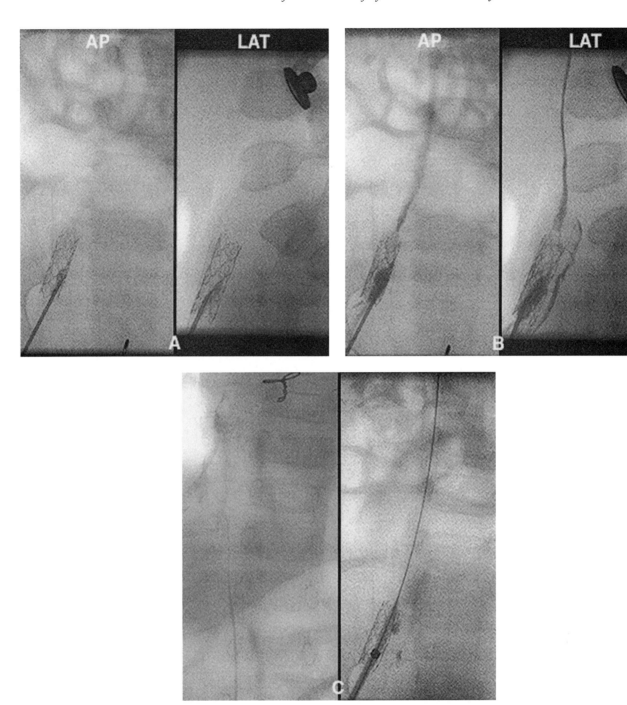

FIGURE 37.5. A: At follow-up catheterization of the patient in Figure 37.4, 3 months later for routine endomyocardial biopsy, as part of the transplant protocol, complete occlusion of the stent was found, most likely due to residual obstruction of the distal femoral vein resulting in inadequate flow and thrombus formation within the stent. Using the stent as a "target" under fluoroscopic guidance in both the anteroposterior and lateral projections, the percutaneous needle was inserted into the stented vessel. **B:** A small hand injection into the needle demonstrated the thrombosed/fibrosed stent with some contrast exiting into the patent proximal femoral vein and iliac vein. **C:** *(Left panel)* Using the stiff end of a guide wire and a 4F stiff dilator, the occluded stent was traversed and a small injection of contrast confirmed that the dilator was within the IVC. *(Right panel)* A Platinum Plus wire was advanced distally into the right atrium and the dilator was exchanged for a 6F sheath for the rest of the catheterization.

(continues on next page)

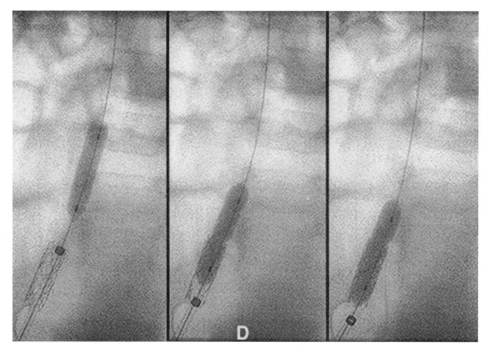

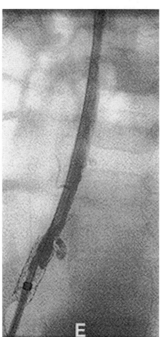

FIGURE 37.5. *(continued)* D: Following the biopsy, a 5-mm-diameter balloon was advanced into the stent and redilated. **E:** Postdilation angiogram demonstrated patency of the proximal stent. At subsequent catheterization, the stent was found again to be occluded, but was recannulated in the same manner without difficulty. At present, we no longer redilate these stents, since success at recannulation is not dependent on stent patency.

veins, these techniques need modification. The first indication of complete obstruction is the inability to pass a wire into the IVC even though there is good blood return out of the needle. A suspected obstruction is first confirmed with a hand-injected angiogram through the femoral vein needle. Careful review of the angiogram in both AP and lateral projections will often reveal a small, tapered remnant of the superficial femoral vein. It is crucial to view the early phase of the injection before superimposition of this remnant by the venous collateral flow. In the lateral projection, the superficial femoral vein can be easily distinguished from the paravertebral venous collaterals by its more anterior position. Once this remnant is identified, a stiff 0.018- or 0.024-inch guide wire such as a straight-tip Glidewire or the stiff back end of a Teflon wire is advanced as far as possible into the remnant vessel. The needle is exchanged for a 4- or 5F tapered dilator. Using a still frame image of the angiogram as a roadmap, the wire can be advanced in small increments followed by the dilator. The stiff dilator prevents proximal buckling of the wire during its advancement. With each advancement, the wire can be removed and a small hand injection of contrast can be given to evaluate extravasation. The injected contrast usually highlights the thrombosed internal lumen of the vessel. These steps are repeated until contrast flows freely into the patent segment of the vessel. Once the dilator is advanced into the patent vessel, an exchange guide wire such as the Platinum Plus (Boston Scientific, Watertown, MA) is advanced through

the dilator into the IVC and the occluded vessel can be serially dilated until the lumen is large enough to accommodate a sheath for stent implantation. Depending on the length of occlusion, single or multiple overlapping stents can be used. Figures 37.6A through 37.6G show angiograms of a 5.3-kg infant with hypoplastic left heart syndrome s/p Norwood I operation who was found to have bilateral femoral vein occlusion extending up to the postrenal vein IVC during his pre-Glenn catheterization. Following recannulation and implantation of seven overlapping stents, the flow was

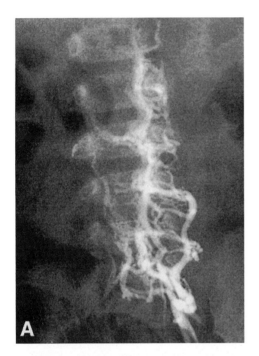

FIGURE 37.6. A: Hand injection of contrast demonstrated complete occlusion of the left iliofemoral venous system in this 5.3-kg infant with hypoplastic left heart syndrome s/p Norwood I operation during a pre-Glenn catheterization. Note contrast entering the paravertebral venous collateral circulation. **B:** *(Left panel)* Careful evaluation of the early phase of the same injection demonstrated a tiny superficial femoral vein remnant *(white arrow)* before filling by the superimposed paravertebral venous collaterals. *(Right panel)* The lateral projection showed the anterior position of the femoral vein remnant *(white arrow)* compared with the posterior paravertebral collateral veins.

(continues on next page)

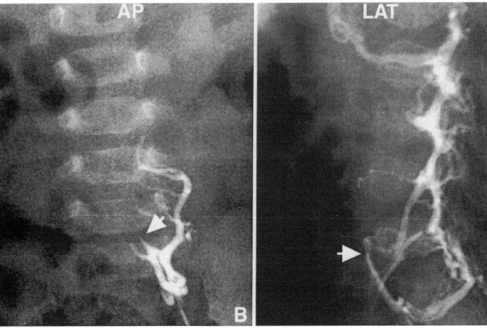

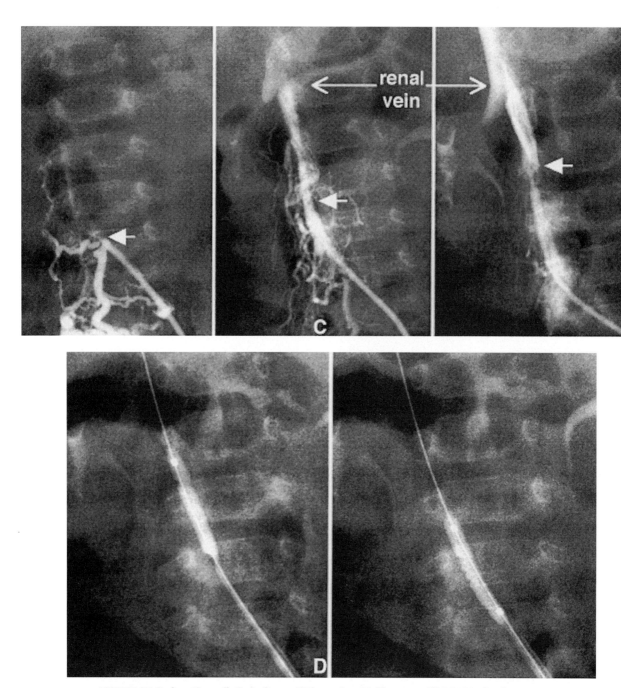

FIGURE 37.6. *(continued)* **C:** *(Left panel)* Through a 4F dilator, a stiff 0.018-inch wire was carefully pushed into the occluded vessel in millimeter increments followed by advancement of the dilator *(white arrow)*. The wire and dilator should follow the expected course of the iliofemoral veins in both AP and lateral projections. *(Middle panel)* Contrast was hand-injected into the dilator after the wire was removed, demonstrating no extravasation. Note the length of the occluded segment that extended from the left superficial femoral vein to the midportion of the IVC just below the renal veins. *(Right panel)* The wire and dilator were advanced beyond the occluded segment. Contrast flowed freely into the patent IVC and the renal veins. **D:** An exchange guide wire was passed across the recannulated vessel and balloon dilation of the entire occluded segment was carried out initially.

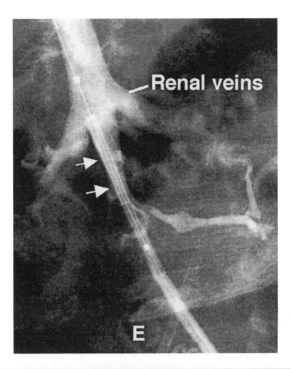

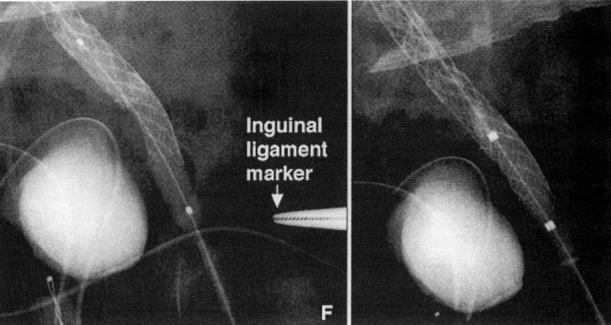

FIGURE 37.6. *(continued)* E: The first stent was positioned just distal to the renal veins. Attention was given to avoid "jailing" the renal veins. **F:** Seven overlapping stents were implanted. A clamp was placed on the surface of the groin corresponding to the level of the inguinal ligament that defined the caudal limit for stent implant. (The three most inferior overlapping stents are shown here.)

(continues on next page)

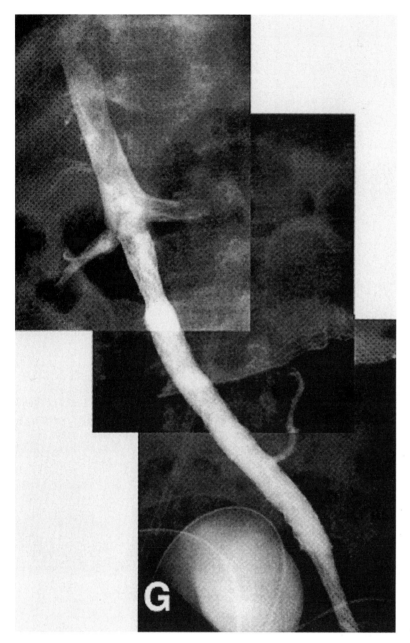

FIGURE 37.6. *(continued)* **G:** Composite of the panned poststent angiogram demonstrating wide patency from the iliofemoral venous system to the proximal IVC. Note the previously seen paravertebral collateral flow was no longer present.

reestablished from the right iliofemoral venous system to the right atrium. This was important since it was anticipated that the patient would require future cardiac catheterizations as well as venous access for future cardiac surgeries.

Special attention should be given to two landmarks: the inguinal ligament and the renal veins. A clamp is placed over the inguinal ligament to help define the most caudal limit for stent position (Figure 37.6F). A percutaneous needle is positioned on the surface of the groin to determine the most caudal level of the vessel that requires stenting in order to permit future access with a percutaneous needle (Figure 37.7). This stent location will allow easy recannula-

tion with a needle should the stent and vessel reocclude in the future as demonstrated in Figures 37.5B through 37.5F. From the lateral projection, the most caudal stent position should not be anterior to the bladder. Hip flexion at the end of the case can be performed under lateral fluoroscopy to evaluate stent position to ensure the absence of movement (Figure 37.8).

In contrast, IVC syndrome can develop following IVC obstructions manifesting with leg pain, edema, ascites, or venous ulcerations (38,40). Renal and hepatic dysfunction as well as Budd-Chiari syndrome have been reported and certainly will require an intervention (44–48). However, if

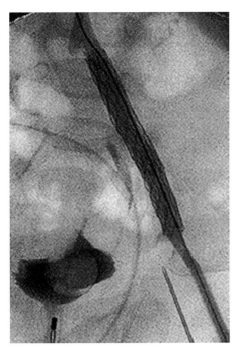

FIGURE 37.7. A percutaneous needle was placed on the skin surface parallel to the femoral vein in order to determine the level at which the most caudal stent must be implanted and still permit access into the stent by the needle. This strategy will permit recanalization of the stent by a needle in the event that it is completely occluded in the future.

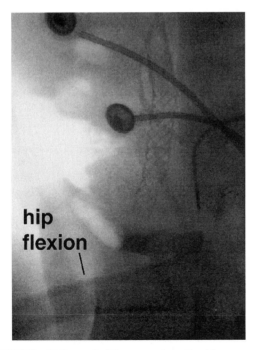

hip
flexion

FIGURE 37.8. At the end of the procedure, the hips were flexed under lateral fluoroscopy to evaluate for potential stent movement. In this patient, five overlapping stents were implanted from the right iliofemoral vein to the IVC. Hip flexion did not change the position of the most caudal stent.

IVC obstruction occurs over a period of time such that adequate venous collateral drainage develops, the patient may be completely asymptomatic. Figures 37.9A through 37.9F are angiograms showing an asymptomatic two-and-one-half-year-old boy following repair for pulmonary atresia and ventricular septal defect (VSD). His VSD was left open due to bilateral hypoplastic branch pulmonary arteries. A stent had been implanted in the left pulmonary artery (LPA) previously at another institution and the plan was to rehabilitate the pulmonary arterial tree before VSD closure. Multiple future catheterizations and interventions were anticipated. However, during follow-up catheterization for additional interventional procedures in the branch pulmonary arteries, his IVC was found to be completely occluded with adequate venous collateralization. Using a stiff end of a wire and a transseptal dilator, the IVC was carefully recannulated and flow was reestablished with implantation of a stent. While this technique did not change the patient's hemodynamics or improve clinical status, it will permit venous access for future interventions in the pulmonary arteries.

In adults with IVC obstruction due to malignancies, various stents, including self-expanding stents, have been used with success to palliate until death. Symptoms of IVC syndrome such as ascites and anasarca can be relieved (40,49–53). In children with growth potential and a longer expected lifespan, the most commonly used stent for the IVC and iliac vein is the Palmaz P308 and P188. For the femoral venous system, the smaller Palmaz stents (P154, 204) can be used. More recently, some have used the more flexible Corinthian stent, and the DoubleStrut stent. Alternatively, the Bridgestent and the NIR stent can also be used in these vessels. For long-segment stenoses, either the longer (4- and 5-cm) stents or overlapping stents can be used.

In stenting infrarenal IVC obstructions, the renal vein orifice must be well defined in order to avoid "jailing" this vessel (Figure 37.6E). Fortunately, most obstructed IVCs in children do not occur at the level of the renal veins due to its high flow. If the IVC obstruction is more proximal, then the hepatic vein drainage needs to be clearly defined before stenting. In completely occluded IVCs, the previously described technique using a dilator and a stiff wire can be used, but occasionally a stiffer transseptal needle may be necessary, and this technique is similar to the one described previously for the occluded SVC.

Early animal experiments with stent implants in the IVC demonstrated success with excellent incorporation of the stent into the caval wall (39). There is extensive experience in stenting of IVC obstructions secondary to malignancies or salvaging lower-extremity hemodialysis access in adults (28,31,39–42,47,50,51,53–62). In the adult literature, the self-expanding Wallstent or the Gianturco Z-stent has been used most frequently. Although stents offer excellent palliation in this group of patients, the reported restenosis rates

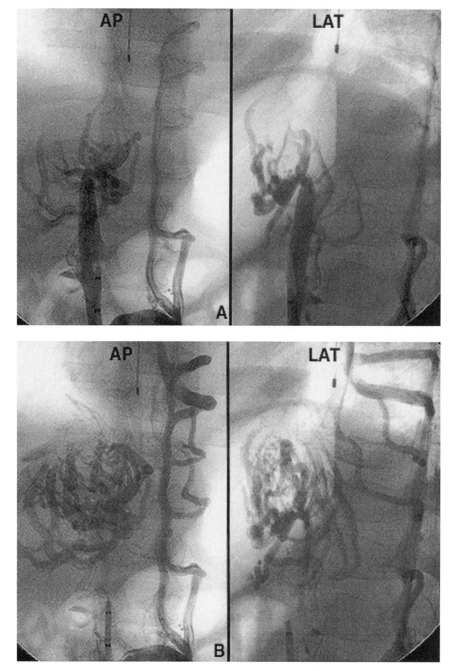

FIGURE 37.9. A: Inferior vena caval (IVC) angiogram of 2-year-old boy with pulmonary atresia, ventricular septal defect (VSD), and discontinuous pulmonary arteries who is s/p unifocalization of the branch pulmonary arteries and a RV to PA homograft. The VSD was left open because of his hypoplastic branch pulmonary arteries. A left pulmonary artery (LPA) stent had been implanted previously at another institution. At follow-up catheterization with the intent to further dilate the LPA stent and possibly place additional stents in the RPA, complete occlusion of the intrahepatic segment of the IVC was found. **B:** Note the development of significant intrahepatic and paravertebral venous collaterals. This patient was asymptomatic and his liver function tests were normal.

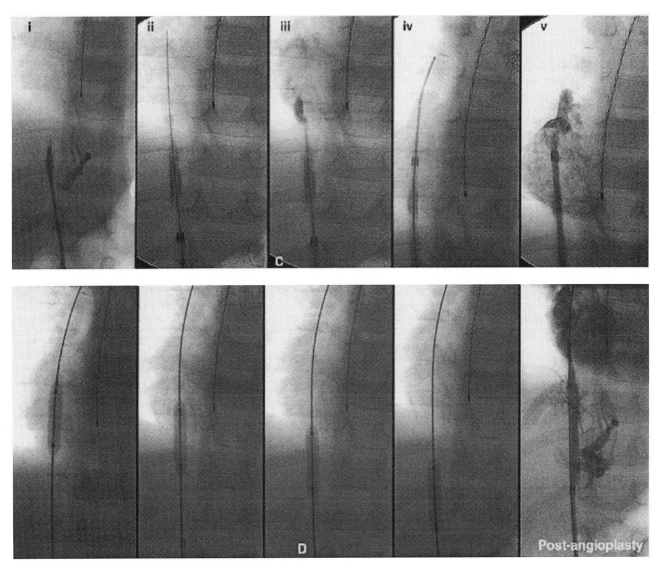

FIGURE 37.9. *(continued)* C: (i) A 5F transseptal dilator was advanced into the IVC as far as possible. A hand injection demonstrated a short distance of complete occlusion. A small amount of contrast entered into the right atrium via intrahepatic venous collaterals. (ii) A stiff end of a guide wire was carefully advanced through the dilator and into the right atrium, and the dilator was exchanged for a 7F transseptal sheath. (iii) The wire was removed and a hand injection of contrast confirmed the position of the sheath and dilator tip in the IVC. Contrast entered into the right atrium with no extravasation. (iv) A new exchange guide wire was advanced into the right atrium followed by advancement of the sheath and dilator into the right atrium. (v) The wire and dilator were removed and a final hand injection through the sheath confirmed successful recannulation of the IVC into the right atrium. **D:** This series of fluoroscopic images demonstrated balloon angioplasty of the recanalized IVC. *(Far right panel)* Postangioplasty angiogram of the IVC demonstrated persistent stenosis. Note the decrease in collateral flow.

(continues on next page)

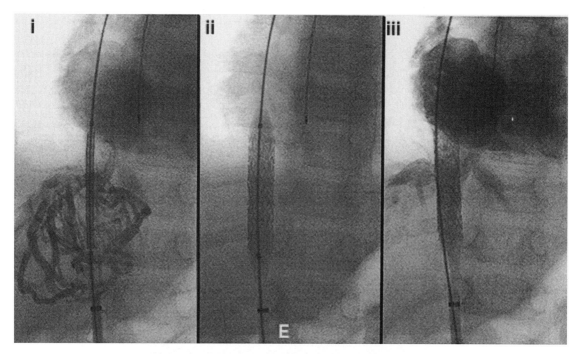

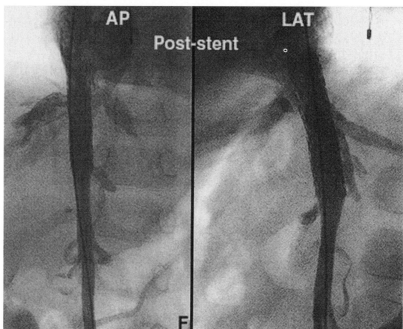

FIGURE 37.9. *(continued)* E: (i) A 36-mm DoubleStrut stent was positioned in the site of obstruction. (ii) The stent is implanted with an 8-mm-diameter balloon. (iii) Follow-up angiogram demonstrated wide patency of the stent. **F:** A final angiogram in the distal IVC demonstrated excellent flow into the right atrium. Note the absence of collateral flow. Contrast also highlighted the unimpeded hepatic venous flow. The hepatic veins appeared to be positioned medial and slightly anterior to the stent.

range from 0 to 50% at intermediate-term follow-up. Long-term outcome has not been well studied.

In a large series by Nazarian there was a 92% success rate using self-expanding stents (Wallstent and Gianturco stents) to treat 59 adults with IVC and/or iliofemoral stenoses (38). Primary patency rate at 1 year was 50%, although sustained symptomatic relief was observed 1 year later in all surviving patients. Overall iliac vein stents have a significantly higher patency rate than femoral stents that is thought to be related to the more extensive disease in the latter group. Also, those with benign disease had a significantly higher patency rate than those with malignancies. Unfortunately, it is difficult to compare adult data to those of children, since the disease processes are different.

Two follow-up studies in children with stented veins are found in the literature: Ing reported the successful use of 85 stents to reconstruct severely obstructed iliofemoral veins ($N = 22$) and IVC ($N = 6$) in 24 patients (43). Most long-segment stenoses required multiple overlapping stents. At mean of 1.7-year follow-up, there was wide patency in seven of nine stented vessels. Interestingly, the two occluded stents were located in the femoral vein and were easily recannulated because the stent offered a visible landmark to aim the percutaneous needle. Ward reported the use of 21 stents in 13 central systemic veins and systemic venous baffles (4). Six of 13 vessels restudied in the catheterization laboratory (mean, 8.8 ± 4.3 months) showed all stents to be patent without evidence of stent fracture or compression and none required redilation. There was only minimal reduction in lumen size from mean 13 ± 4.7 mm to 11 ± 4.7 mm diameter. No gradients were found.

In general, stenting of the IVC and the iliofemoral venous system in children is highly efficacious with low restenosis rate. When femoral vein stents occlude, recannulation can be achieved easily at subsequent cardiac catheterization. However, larger series and longer follow-up studies are warranted.

Postsurgical Systemic Venous Baffles

Postsurgical systemic venous baffle stenosis is seen in two major categories: following a Mustard or Senning repair for d-transposition of the great arteries and cavopulmonary anastomosis (Glenn or Fontan operation) for single-ventricle repairs. Both can result in significant morbidity and mortality if not treated.

Ten percent to 30% of patients with an atrial switch develop baffle obstruction (63–68). In Mustard or Senning baffle obstructions, either or both of the superior and inferior limbs can be involved, resulting in SVC and/or IVC syndrome. Cavopulmonary obstructions can be particularly devastating. In addition to SVC or IVC syndrome, these patients can develop persistent/prolonged pleural or pericardial effusions, protein-losing enteropathy, severe cyanosis due to the development of venous collaterals to the left

heart, or increasing right-to-left shunt through a Fontan fenestration. Increased left-to-right shunting can also occur due to the formation of aortopulmonary collaterals. In the catheterization laboratory, it is important to recognize that even mild gradients in these surgically created venous baffles can result in significant hemodynamic derangements and should be treated aggressively. The results of angioplasty alone are mixed and may depend on the cause of the stenosis (kink, intimal hyperplasia, fibrosis, infiltration, or external compression). In addition, angioplasty often requires very large balloons or double-balloon techniques to adequately dilate the stenosis (69–71). Restenosis can occur due to recoil or external compression (70,72). O'Laughlin first reported the use of stents to treat obstructions in Fontan and Mustard baffles (32). There are several case reports and small series demonstrating the efficacy of implanting Palmaz stents into Mustard and Senning baffles (4,32,66,72–76) as well as cavopulmonary anastomoses (5,32,77). Occasionally, stenting is the only option, as described by Chatelain in a case of successful relief of IVC and SVC Mustard baffle obstruction following unsuccessful surgery and angioplasty (66).

Stent implantation in the obstructed Mustard and Senning baffles or the Glenn and Fontan baffles is quite simple. Unlike stenting a branch pulmonary artery, the vascular course to the baffle obstruction is less tortuous and does not traverse a ventricle. Several key points should be emphasized. For stenting superior-limb baffle obstruction in the Mustard and Senning, it is important to evaluate pulmonary venous flow with a test balloon dilation of the SVC baffle to ensure no pulmonary vein obstruction after a stent has been implanted. This can be performed in two ways. With a balloon inflated along the SVC stenosis, a second catheter is advanced into the ipsilateral pulmonary artery for an angiogram to evaluate the pulmonary venous flow. Alternatively, a transseptal procedure is performed and a second catheter is placed directly into the ipsilateral pulmonary vein for pressure measurements and an angiogram. This maneuver will ensure wide patency of the pulmonary veins after stent implantation into the SVC baffle obstruction. The transseptal technique for Mustard/Senning and Fontan baffles has been well described in the literature by El-Said et al. (78). Figures 37.10A through 37.10E show a patient with obstruction of the SVC or superior limb of a Mustard baffle. Simultaneous injections into the baffle and the right upper pulmonary vein indicate pulmonary venous return is not located near the site of baffle obstruction and stent implantation would not impede pulmonary venous flow.

If there is total occlusion of the SVC, simultaneous injections of contrast from above and below the occluded site are performed to evaluate the length of the occluded segment. This is performed by simultaneously placing catheters from the femoral vein and from the SVC to the site of obstruction. Both AP and lateral projections are used

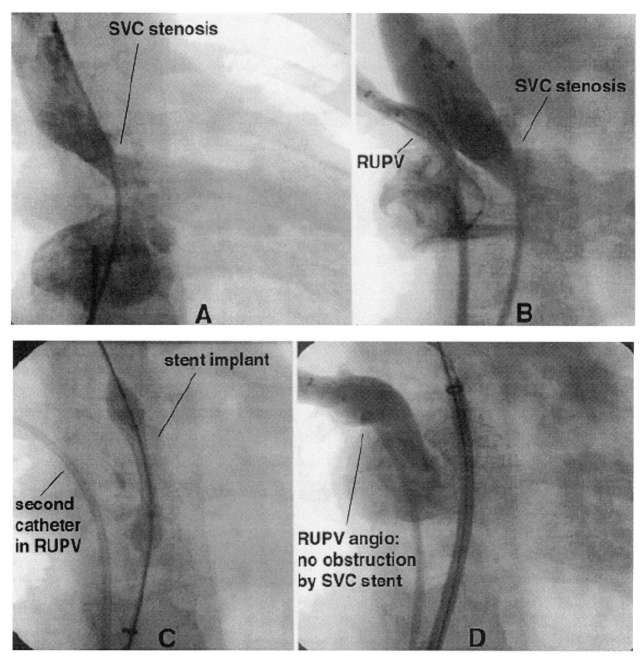

FIGURE 37.10. A: Significant stenosis was noted at the SVC baffle in this post-Mustard patient. **B:** A transseptal across the Mustard baffle was carried out and a second catheter was positioned in the right upper pulmonary vein (RUPV). Simultaneous injection of contrast demonstrated the position of the RUPV relative to the SVC stenosis, confirming that stent dilation of the SVC would not obstruct right upper pulmonary venous flow. **C:** Implantation of a P308 stent was carried out at the SVC obstruction. The second catheter was left in the RUPV to ensure proper position of the stent. **D:** Follow-up angiogram in the RUPV confirmed no flow obstruction by the SVC stent.

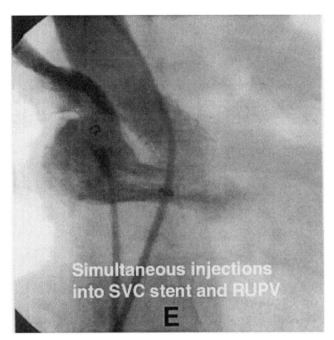

FIGURE 37.10. *(continued)* **E:** Poststent angiograms taken in the RUPV and the SVC confirmed wide patency of the stent and good flow from both vessels into their respective atria.

to precisely evaluate the spatial relationship of the obstruction and the systemic venous atrium. Leaving the femoral venous catheter in the systemic venous atrium as a reference, the catheter and sheath from the SVC are exchanged for a transseptal sheath, dilator, and needle, which are advanced to the occluded site. The needle is carefully advanced across the occluded segment, always directed toward the target reference catheter in the systemic venous right atrium until it traverses the obstruction and enters the atrial cavity. Both AP and lateral views are used to ensure proper alignment of the transseptal needle to the systemic venous atrium. A very small hand injection of contrast (0.1 to 0.2 mL) through the needle is used to stain the occluded segment for a "roadmap." Additional hand injections help to navigate the puncture by demonstrating flow of contrast within the vascular space and not extravasation into the surrounding fibrous tissue or the pericardial space. Once the occluded segment is traversed with the transseptal needle, the transseptal sheath and dilator are advanced over the needle into the systemic venous atrium. The needle and dilator are withdrawn, and a superstiff exchange wire is advanced through the transseptal sheath. The femoral venous catheter is exchanged for a snare, which is used to pull the superstiff wire through and through between the right internal jugular and a femoral vein. A balloon dilatation catheter is used to expand the occluded site to allow placement of the 11- to 12F long sheath, as well as to determine whether that stenotic segment is amenable to further stent dilatation. Usually, severe stenosis persists despite apparently adequate balloon dilatation, and a stent is neces-

sary to maintain vascular patency in the long run. Figures 37.1A to 37.1K illustrate the technique of recannulation through an occluded SVC/Mustard baffle.

Stent implantations for Glenn and Fontan baffle obstructions are quite straightforward since there is no right ventricle to traverse before reaching the branch pulmonary arteries. For Glenn obstructions, the right internal jugular vein is the vessel of choice for access, although the subclavian route has also been reported (77). Patients who develop pulmonary artery distortion following the Glenn operation also can be successfully treated with stents (77). Care should be taken to avoid jailing the branch pulmonary arteries. Figures 37.11A and 37.11B illustrate a 10-year-old boy with tricuspid and pulmonary atresia and discontinuous pulmonary arteries after a classic right-sided Glenn shunt with significant stenosis before and after stent implantation. Figures 37.12A through 37.12C demonstrate an 11-year-old boy with dextrocardia, mitral and pulmonary valve atresia status post (following) lateral tunnel Fontan with significant Fontan obstruction despite only a 3 mm Hg gradient across the stenosis. The patient had protein-losing enteropathy that completely resolved after stent implantation and relief of the obstruction. Figure 37.13 shows a 4-year-old patient double-outlet right ventricle and mitral atresia following an extracardiac conduit Fontan developed significant conduit obstruction also with a small gradient (3 mm Hg). She presented with bilateral pleural effusions and ascites. Her symptoms were also relieved with stent dilation of the Fontan conduit.

O'Laughlin et al. first reported the use of stents to dilate obstructed Fontan and Glenn anastomoses in 1991 (32). Others have also reported excellent results. The primary stents used in these surgical baffles in children have been the J & J 188 and 308 series. However, in older children and adults, self-expanding Wallstents have also been used successfully. Brown reported a series of 11 adult-sized patients with obstructed Mustard baffles who failed balloon angioplasty alone and were successfully treated with Wallstents (79). In his series, ten stents were implanted in the IVC baffles and eight stents were implanted in the SVC baffles. There was a 68% to 71% increase in diameter with significant relief of gradient. Intermediate follow-up (mean, 1.7 years) showed no restenosis.

In a 6-year experience from a single institution, corresponding to the FDA Phase I and II clinical trial of the Palmaz stent in congenital heart disease, Shaffer reported successful stent implants in twenty-two Fontan, nine Glenn, and seven Mustard/Senning baffles (5). In his series of venous stents (which included ten additional patients with SVC and other systemic vein obstructions), a total of 80 stents were implanted in 48 patients. The mean gradient decreased from 7 ± 6.4 mm Hg to 1 ± 1.9 mm Hg. The diameters increased from 2.8 ± 3.6 mm to 12.5 ± 3.9 mm. Among these venous obstructions, there were 12 (18%) with complete occlusion before recannulation and stent

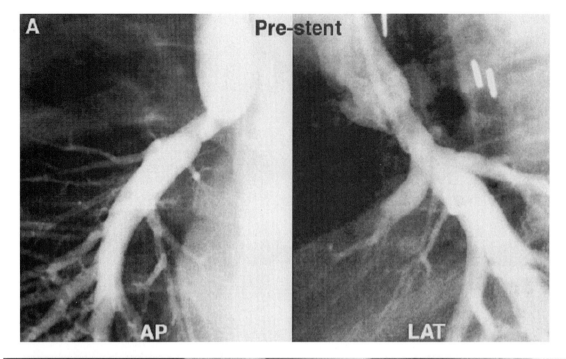

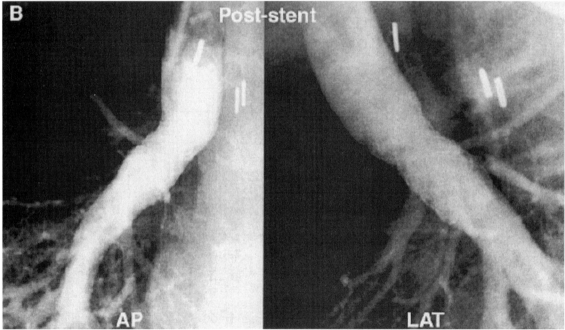

FIGURE 37.11. **A:** Significant stenosis was noted in the classic right Glenn shunt of this 10-year-old boy with tricuspid and pulmonary atresia and discontinuous pulmonary arteries. **B:** Following implantation of a P308 stent, the gradient decreased from 4 to 0 mm Hg.

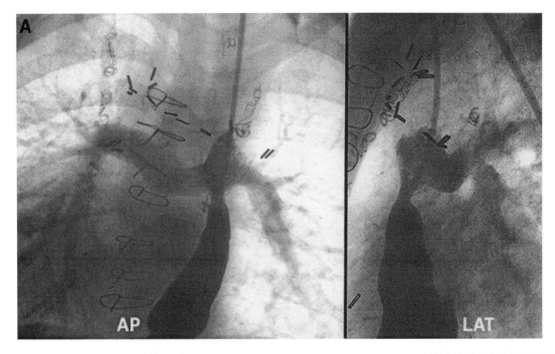

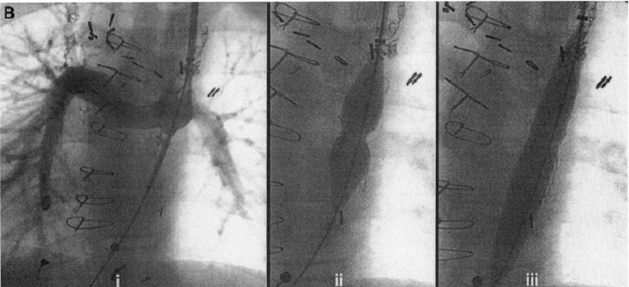

FIGURE 37.12. A: Angiograms of this 11-year-old girl with dextrocardia, mitral and pulmonary atresia s/p a lateral tunnel Fontan operation demonstrated severe battle obstruction just below the pulmonary arteries. Despite only a gradient of only 3 mm Hg, she presented with protein-losing enteropathy. **B:** (i) A pulmonary angiogram was performed to confirm proper position of a P308 stent at the site of obstruction. (ii) The stent was implanted with a 14-mm-diameter balloon. A residual waist was noted. (iii) The waist was further dilated with a 10-mm high-pressure balloon.

(continued on next page)

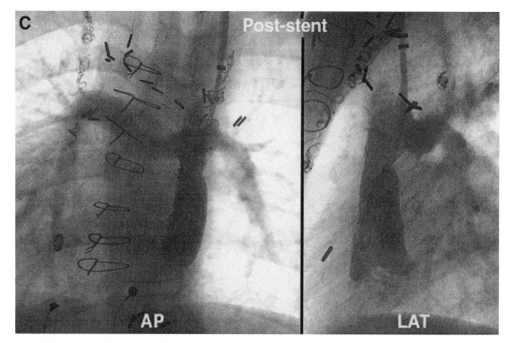

FIGURE 37.12. *(continued)* C: Poststent angiograms demonstrated marked improvement of the Fontan baffle. The minimum diameter increased from 4.5 to 9.7 mm and the gradient was abolished.

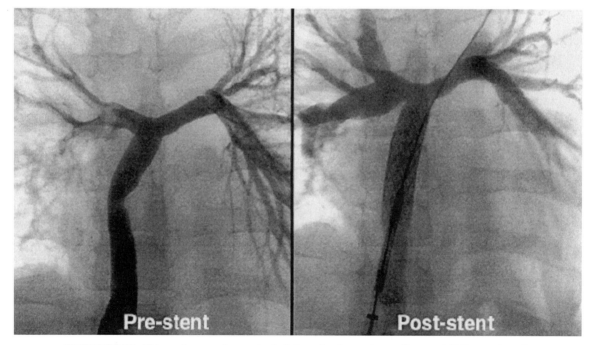

FIGURE 37.13. This angiogram demonstrated stenosis of an extracardiac conduit Fontan in a 4-year-old girl with double-outlet right ventricle and mitral atresia. Despite the appearance of mild stenosis and a gradient of only 3 mm Hg, she presented with persistent bilateral pleural effusions and ascites. Following implantation of a P308 stent, the gradient was eliminated and her symptoms rapidly resolved.

implantation. At follow-up catheterization of 13 patients (22 stents), there was no significant change in the gradient or the lumen diameter. Early in their experience, there were three patients with a stent implanted into their cavopulmonary anastomosis who developed a thrombus in the stent. Interestingly, two of the three revealed significant pulmonary vein stenosis noted only after stent implantation. The third patient has a previously diagnosed right atrial thrombus that extended into the stent after implantation despite anticoagulation.

Stent dilation for surgically created systemic venous baffles has proven to be safe and effective, and probably superior to surgery or angioplasty alone. At the present time, there is no consensus regarding antiplatelet therapy or anticoagulation following the Glenn or Fontan operation, but in the context of an implanted stent in a low-flow situation, lifetime therapy with either aspirin or Coumadin should be considered.

PULMONARY VEINS

Although animal experiments indicate no intrinsic difference in response of pulmonary veins to the presence of a stent when compared with pulmonary arteries (80), clinical experience of restenosis of pulmonary veins is more the rule

than the exception. Pulmonary vein stenosis may either be congenital or be associated with surgical repair of anomalous pulmonary veins. Congenital pulmonary vein stenosis presents a particularly difficult management problem and represents 0.4% to 0.6% of cardiac anomalies in autopsy series (81–83). Progressive pulmonary vein stenosis presents with increasing pulmonary venous congestion, resulting in pulmonary hypertension, right ventricular failure, and ultimately death. There are no good management options because of the high incidence of restenosis. Long-term results from surgical repair (81,84,85,87–91); intraoperative stenting (92–94); and transcatheter approaches, including balloon dilation alone (88) or stenting (94–97), remain uniformly poor. In the context of a univentricular heart or other associated cardiac lesions, the prognosis is particularly dismal (86), and bilateral disease is often lethal (84,90). Figure 37.14 illustrates progressive pulmonary vein stenosis despite adequate stenting. This 3-year-old patient with double-inlet left ventricle s/p Fontan operation was found to have mild left upper pulmonary vein stenosis and no interventions were performed. Two years later, he developed significant stenosis of the left lower pulmonary vein (LLPV). Following implantation of a P188 stent into the LLPV orifice, the gradient decreased from 9 mm Hg to 0 mm Hg and the diameter increased from 5.3 to 10 mm. However, despite adequate relief, at follow-up catheriza-

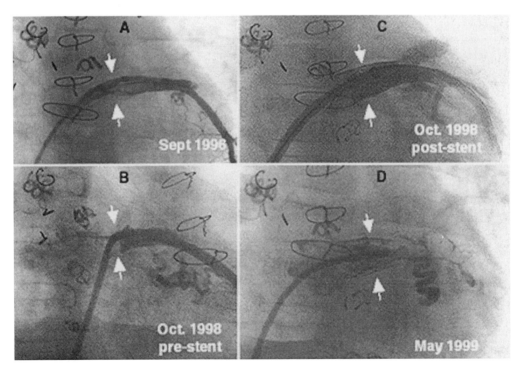

FIGURE 37.14. A: This angiogram demonstrated mild left lower pulmonary vein (LLPV) stenosis in a 3-year-old boy with double-inlet left ventricle s/p Fontan operation. **B:** Two years later, there was progressive stenosis of this pulmonary vein. **C:** Implantation of a P188 stent (dilated with a 10-mm-diameter balloon) resulted in wide patency of this vein. **D:** Seven months later, progressive intimal proliferation of the intraparenchymal pulmonary veins resulted in severe restenosis.

tion only 7 months later, there was significant progressive stenosis of the intraparenchymal segments of the pulmonary vein with intimal proliferation encroaching into the distal aspect of the implanted stent.

Several proposed mechanisms of restenosis include medial fibrosis and intimal proliferation that may occur within the stent and into the distal smaller branches of the pulmonary veins, resulting in diffuse intraparenchymal pulmonary venous obstruction. Pathologic studies suggest some forms of pulmonary vein stenosis also involve diffuse pulmonary venous hypoplasia (98). Studies have shown the intima to be composed of collagen and disorganized elastic fibers with loss of intima and media definition (69). Sadr reported a recent histopathologic study of surgical specimens of ten infants with isolated pulmonary vein stenosis indicating restenosis resulting from myofibroblastic proliferation (99). Postsurgical restenosis of pulmonary veins may be due to low-grade residual venous obstruction following surgery, resulting in reactive fibrosis and self-perpetuating stenosis (100). Smallhorn noted that the presence of echocardiographic findings of turbulence within the pulmonary veins after repair was associated with restenosis (101). Several operations have been designed to eliminate any local turbulence with a sutureless technique and to remove virtually all foreign material and that might be the substrate for restenosis (84,89,90). Although this radical surgical approach shows good short-term results, long-term results remain to be seen. Caldarone reported their surgical experience with pulmonary vein stenosis following total anomalous pulmonary venous return and repair in 170 patients. Thirteen (7.6%) patients developed pulmonary vein stenosis; in this group 17 reoperations were performed (84). Six of nine patients with bilateral involvement died. Two of three survivors were repaired with a novel technique creating a sutureless neoatrium without restenosis at 1.8 years follow-up. They concluded that bilateral disease was lethal whereas unilateral disease was survivable. A new approach using immunosuppressive chemotherapy following radical resection or stent is currently under investigation. The theory of using chemotherapy to reduce hyperplasia of the pulmonary venous vasculature is attractive, but actual data are still lacking. Angioplasty alone is uniformly not effective (69). Mendeloff et al. have recommended lung transplantation for congenital pulmonary vein stenosis (102). They reported a small series of three patients with good short- and intermediate-term follow-up in a disease that is otherwise fatal. Presently, most view stent implantation of pulmonary vein stenosis as a palliation and a bridge to lung transplant.

Stent implantation for pulmonary vein stenosis is relatively more difficult than for other vascular lesions. A transseptal approach is necessary if the atrial septum is intact. This technique is well described in the literature (78) and will not be discussed here. In pulmonary vein stenosis following the Mustard or Senning repair or intracaval baf-

fling of an anomalous pulmonary vein to the left atrium, it is important to assess SVC flow with a test dilation of the pulmonary vein obstruction prior to stent implantation. This will help to ensure no compromise in SVC flow when the pulmonary vein is stented. During test dilation, the balloon should be kept inflated in the pulmonary vein while a SVC angiogram is performed. Pressure gradients across the SVC should also be assessed with the balloon still inflated in the pulmonary vein. The technique of implanting stents in the pulmonary veins under direct vision in the operating room has also been documented (92–94,103).

O'Laughlin reported the first use of stents to dilate pulmonary vein stenosis in one patient in 1991 (32). Since then, several series have been reported, all with poor long-term results. The largest series of pulmonary vein stents in the literature comes from Boston Children's Hospital, which reported 24 stents implanted in 17 patients (95). The mean diameter increased from 4.9 to 10.4 mm with a respective gradient drop from 15.4 to 1.4 mm Hg. Although early results were excellent, restenosis was seen subsequently in 22 out of 24 stents, resulting in nine deaths. Others have reported similar results in smaller series (92–94,96). Driscoll reported eight patients with congenital pulmonary vein stenosis, of which three underwent balloon dilation and one underwent pulmonary venoplasty (88). Although angioplasty provided excellent immediate relief, restenosis occurred later. The surgical patient died. His review of 28 previously reported cases indicated 22 died. Of six patients who underwent surgical repair, four survived. The average age of those who underwent surgery was 8.8 years, compared with 10 months in those who died at operation. The average age of death in those who did not have surgery was 4.1 years. He concluded that the older survivors most likely had less severe disease than those who died early in life.

Coles reported intraoperative stenting of pulmonary veins in a series of five patients in which four developed restenosis, which resulted in death in 3 patients with bilateral pulmonary vein stents (92). Similarly, Ungerleider reported intraoperative stenting of stenotic pulmonary veins in five patients (93). Only one of five had a successful outcome. Four had progressive pulmonary vein restenosis despite stents and two died.

While pulmonary vein stenting can be performed safely with excellent early results, this procedure should be viewed as a palliation and a bridge to lung transplant. Nevertheless review of the literature indicates a minority of cases where stent implantation has resulted in long-term relief of pulmonary vein stenosis. Van de Wal, in his series, observed that obstruction strictly localized to the site of the surgical anastomosis carries a better prognosis than the obstruction located at the individual pulmonary veins (103). At present, the predictive factors of good long-term outcome remain elusive.

REFERENCES

1. Mullins CE, O'Laughlin MP, Vick GW, et al. Implantation of balloon expandable intravascular grafts by catheterization in pulmonary arteries and systemic veins. *Circulation* 1988;77: 188–199.
2. O'Laughlin MP, Slack MC, Grifka RG, et al. Implantation and intermediate-term follow-up of stents in congenital heart disease. *Circulation* 1993;88:605–614.
3. Ing FF, Grifka RG, Nihill MR, et al. Repeat dilation of intravascular stents in congenital heart disease. *Circulation* 1995;92:893–897.
4. Ward CJB, Mullins CE, Nihill MR, et al. Use of intravascular stents in systemic venous and systemic venous baffle obstructions: short-term follow-up results. *Circulation* 1995;91: 2948–2954.
5. Shaffer KM, Mullins CE, Grifka RG, et al. Intravascular stents in congenital heart disease: short- and long-term results from a large single-center experience. *J Am Coll Cardiol* 1998;31: 661–667.
6. McMahon CJ, El Said H, Grifka RG, et al. Intermediate term outcome of redilation of endovascular stents. *J Am Coll Cardiol* 2000;35(Suppl A):519A(abst).
7. Morrow WR, Palmaz JC, Tio FO, et al. Re-expansion of balloon-expandable stents after growth. *J Am Coll Cardiol* 1993; 22:2007–2013.
8. Grifka RG, Vick W, O'Laughlin MP, et al. Balloon expandable intravascular stents: aortic implantation and later further dilation in growing minipigs. *Am Heart J* 1993;126:979–984.
9. Trerotola SO, Lund GB, Samphilipo MA, et al. Palmaz stent in the treatment of central venous stenosis: safety and efficacy of redilation. *Radiology* 1994;190:379–385.
10. Ali MK, Ewer MS, Balakrishman PV, et al. Balloon angioplasty for superior vena cava obstruction. *Ann Intern Med* 1987;1076: 856–857.
11. Brady HR, Fitzcharles B, Goldberg H, et al. Diagnosis and management of subclavian vein thrombosis occurring in association with subclavian cannulation for hemodialysis. *Blood Purif* 1989;74:210–217.
12. Goudevenos JA, Reid PG, Adams PC, et al. Pacemaker-induced superior vena cava syndrome; report of four cases and review of the literature. *Pacing Clin Electrophysiol* 1989;12:1890–1895.
13. Grace AA, Sutters M, Schofield PM. Balloon dilatation of pacemaker induced stenosis of the superior vena cava. *Br Heart J* 1991;654:225–226.
14. Mazzetti H, Dussaut A, Tentori C, et al. Superior vena cava occlusion and/or syndrome related to pacemaker leads. *Am Heart J* 1993;125:831–837.
15. Sherry CS, Diamond NG, Meyers TP, et al. Successful treatment of superior vena cava syndrome by venous angioplasty. *Am J Roentgenol* 1986;147:834–835.
16. Walpole HT Jr., Lovett KE, Chuang VP, et al. Superior vena cava syndrome treated by percutaneous transluminal balloon angioplasty. *Am Heart J* 1988;1156:1303–1304.
17. Ing FF, Mullins CE, Grifka RG, et al. Stent dilation of superior vena cava/innominate vein obstructions permits transvenous pacing lead implantation. *Pacing Clin Electrophysiol* 1998;21: 1517–1530.
18. Gundersen T, Abrahamsen AM, Jorgensen I. Thrombosis of superior vena cava as a complication of transvenous pacemaker treatment. *Acta Med Scand* 1982;212:85–88.
19. Blackburn T, Dunn M. Pacemaker-induced superior vena cava syndrome: consideration of management. *Am Heart J* 1988; 116:893–896.
20. Katz PO, Hackshaw BT, Barish CF, et al. Venous thrombosis as a cause of superior vena cava syndrome: rapid response to streptokinase. *Arch Intern Med* 1983;143:1050–1052.
21. Benson LN, Yeatman L, Laks H. Balloon dilatation for superior vena cava obstruction after the Senning procedure. *Cardiovasc Diagn* 1985;11:63–68.
22. Spittell PC, Vlietstra RE, Hayes DL, et al. Venous obstruction due to permanent transvenous pacemaker electrodes: Treatment with percutaneous transluminal balloon venoplasty. *Pacing Clin Electrophysiol* 1990;13:271–274.
23. Sunder SK, Ekong EA, Sivalingam K, et al. Superior vena cava thrombosis due to pacing electrodes: successful treatment with combined thrombolysis and angioplasty. *Am Heart J* 1992;123: 790–792.
24. Cooper SG, Sullivan ID, Bull C, et al. Balloon dilatation of pulmonary venous pathway obstruction after Mustard repair for transposition of the great arteries. *J Am Coll Cardiol* 1989;14: 94–98.
25. Lock JE, Bass JL, Castenada-Zuniga W, et al. Dilation angioplasty of congenital or operative narrowing of venous channel. *Circulation* 1984;70:457–464.
26. Yoon J, Koh KK, Cho SK, et al. Superior vena cava syndrome after repeated insertion of transvenous pacemaker. *Am Heart J* 1993;126:1014–1015.
27. Alimi YS, Gloviczki P, Vrtiska TJ, et al. Reconstruction of the superior vena cava: benefits of postoperative surveillance and secondary endovascular intervention. *J Vasc Surg* 1998;27: 287–301.
28. Rosch J, Uchida BT, Hall LD, et al. Gianturco-Rosch expandable Z-stents in the treatment of superior vena cava syndrome. *Cardiovasc Interv Radiol* 1992;15:319–327.
29. Solomon NS, Wholey MH, Jarmolowski CR. Intravascular stents in the management of superior vena cava syndrome. *Catheter Cardiovasc Diagn* 1991;23:245–252.
30. Sze DY, Robbins RC, Semba CP, et al. Superior vena cava syndrome after heart transplantation: percutaneous treatment of a complication of bicaval anastomoses. *J Thorac Cardiovasc Surg* 1998;116:253–261.
31. Elson JD, Becker GJ, Wholey MH, et al. Vena caval and central venous stenoses: management with Palmaz balloon-expandable intraluminal stents. *J Vasc Interv Radiol* 1991;22:215–223.
32. O'Laughlin MP, Perry SB, Lock JE, et al. Use of endovascular stents in congenital heart disease. *Circulation* 1991;83: 1923–1939.
33. Wisselink W, Money SR, Becker MO, et al. Comparison of operative reconstruction and percutaneous balloon dilation for central venous stenosis. *Am J Surg* 1993;166:200–205.
34. Redington AN, Hayes AM, Ho SY. Transcatheter stent implantation to treat aortic coarctation in infancy. *Br Heart J* 1993;69: 80–82.
35. Vesely TM, Hovsepian DM, Pilgram TK, et al. Upper extremity central venous obstruction in hemodialysis patients: treatment with Wallstents. *Radiology* 1997;204:343–348.
36. Ing FF, Mathewson JW, Cocalis M, et al. The new DoubleStrut stent: *in vitro* evaluation of stent geometry following over dilation and initial clinical experience in congenital heart disease. *J Am Coll Cardiol* 2001;37(Suppl A):467A.
37. Rutledge JM, Grifka RG, Nihill MR, et al. Initial experience with IntraTherapeutics DoubleStrut LD stents in patients with congenital heart disease. *J Am Coll Cardiol* 2001;37(Suppl A): 461A.
38. Nazarian GK, Bjarnason H, Dietz CA, et al. Iliofemoral venous stenosis: effectiveness of treatment with metallic endovascular stents. *Radiology* 1996;200:193–199.
39. Charnsangavej C, Carrasco CH, Wallace S, et al. Stenosis of the

vena cava: preliminary assessment of treatment with expandable metallic stents. *Radiology* 1986;161:295–298.

40. Fletcher WS, Lakin PC, Pommier RF, et al. Results of treatment of inferior vena cava syndrome with expandable metallic stents. *Arch Surg* 1998;133:935–938.

41. Razavi MK, Hansch EC, Kee ST, et al. Chronically occluded inferior venae cavae: endovascular treatment. *Radiology* 2000; 214:133–138.

42. Funaki B, Szymski GX, Leef JA, et al. Treatment of venous outflow stenoses in thigh grafts with Wallstents. *Am J Roentgenol* 1999;172:1591–1596.

43. Ing F, Fagan TE, Grifka RG, et al. Reconstruction of stenotic or occluded iliofemoral veins and inferior vena cava using intravascular stents: Re-establishing access for future cardiac catheterization and cardiac surgery. *J Am Coll Cardiol* 2001;37:251–257.

44. Rector WG, Xu YH, Goldstein L, et al. Membranous obstruction of the inferior vena cava in the United States. *Medicine* 1985;64:134–143.

45. Mitchell MC, Boitnott JK, Kaufman S, et al. Budd-Chiari syndrome: etiology, diagnosis and management. *Medicine* 1982;61: 199–218.

46. Okuda H, Yamagata H, Obata H, et al. Epidemiological and clinical features of Budd-Chiari syndrome in Japan. *J Hepatol* 1995;22:1–9.

47. Helmy T, Ware DL, Patterson C, et al. Focal elastic obstruction on the inferior vena cava. *Catheter Cardiovasc Diagn* 2000;51: 494–499.

48. Yang XL, Cheng TO, Chen CR. Successful treatment by percutaneous balloon angioplasty of Budd-Chiari syndrome caused by membranous obstruction of inferior vena cava: 8-year follow-up study. *J Am Coll Cardiol* 1996;28:1720–1724.

49. Hartley JW, Awrich AE, Wong J, et al. Diagnosis and treatment of the inferior vena cava syndrome in advanced malignant disease. *Am J Surg* 1986;152:70–74.

50. Furui S, Sawada S, Irie T, et al. Hepatic inferior vena cava obstruction: treatment of two types with Gianturco expandable metallic stents. *Radiology* 1990;176:665–670.

51. Furui S, Sawada S, Kuramoto K, et al. Gianturco stent placement in malignant caval obstruction: analysis of factors for predicting the outcome. *Radiology* 1995;195:147–152.

52. Oudkerk M, Heystraten FMJ, Stoter G. Stenting in malignant vena caval obstruction. *Cancer* 1993;71:142–146.

53. Irving JD, Dondelinger RF, Reidy JF, et al. Gianturco self-expanding stents: clinical experience in the vena cava and large veins. *Cardiovasc Interv Radiol* 1992;15:328–333.

54. Kaul U, Agarwal R, Jain P, et al. Management of idiopathic obstruction of the hepatic and suprahepatic inferior vena cava with a self-expanding metallic stent. *Catheter Cardiovasc Diagn* 1996;39:252–257.

55. Chang TC, Zaleski GX, Lin BH, et al. Treatment of inferior vena cava obstruction in hemodialysis patients using Wallstents: early and intermediate results. *Am J Roentgenol* 1998;171: 125–128.

56. Putnam JS, Uchida BT, Antonovic R, et al. Superior vena cava syndrome associated with massive thrombosis: treatment with expandable wire stents. *Radiology* 1988;167:727–728.

57. Carrasco CH, Charnsangavej C, Wright KC, et al. Use of the Gianturco self-expandable stent in stenoses of the superior and inferior venae cavae. *J Vasc Interv Radiol* 1992;3:409–419.

58. Quinn SF, Schuman ES, Hall L, et al. Venous stenoses in patients who undergo hemodialysis: treatment with self-expandable endovascular stents. *Radiology* 1992;183:499–504.

59. Antonucci F, Salomonowitz E, Stuckmann G, et al. Placement of venous stents: clinical experience with a self-expanding prosthesis. *Radiology* 1992;183:493–497.

60. Sawada S, Fujiwara Y, Toyama T, et al. Application of expand-

able metallic stents to the venous system. *Acta Radiol* 1992;33: 156–159.

61. Walker HS, Rholl KS, Register TE, et al. Percutaneous placement of a hepatic vein stent in the treatment of Budd-Chiari syndrome. *J Vasc Interv Radiol* 1990;1:23–27.

62. Lopez RR Jr, Benner KG, Hall L, et al. Expandable venous stents for treatment of the Budd-Chiari syndrome. *Gastroenterology* 1991;10051:1435–1441.

63. Godman MJ, Friedli B, Pasternac A, et al. Hemodynamic studies in children four to ten years after Mustard operation for transposition of the great arteries. *Circulation* 1976;53: 532–538.

64. Stark J, Silove ED, Taylor JFN, et al. Obstruction to systemic venous return following the Mustard for transposition of the great arteries. *J Thorac Cardiovasc Surg* 1974;68:742–749.

65. Stark J, Tynan MJ, Ashcroft KW, et al. Obstruction of pulmonary veins and superior vena cava after the Mustard operation for transposition of the great arteries. *Circulation* 1972; 45(Suppl 1):I-116–I-120.

66. Chatelain P, Meier B, Friedle B. Stenting of superior vena cava for symptomatic narrowing after repeated atrial surgery for D-transposition of the great vessels. *Br Heart J* 1991;66:466–468.

67. Egboff LP, Greed MD, Dirk M, et al. Early and late results with the Mustard operation in infancy. *Ann Thorac Surg* 1987;26: 474–488.

68. Trusler GA, Williams WG, Izukawa F, et al. Current results with the Mustard operation in isolated transposition of the great arteries. *J Thorac Cardiovasc Surg* 1990;80:381–389.

69. Lock JE, Bass JL, Castaneda-Zuniga W, et al. Dilatation angioplasty of congenital or operative narrowing of venous channel. *Circulation* 1984;70:457–464.

70. Coulson JD, Jennings RB Jr., Johnson DH, Pulmonary venous atrial obstruction after the Senning procedure: relief by catheter balloon dilatation. *Br Heart J* 1990;64:160–162.

71. Cooper SG, Sullivan ID, Bull C, et al. Balloon dilation of pulmonary venous pathway obstructions after Mustard repair for transposition of the great arteries. *J Am Coll Cardiol* 1989;14: 194–198.

72. Hosking M, Murdison K, Duncan W. Transcatheter stent implantation for recurrent pulmonary venous pathway obstruction following Mustard procedure. *Br Heart J* 1994;72:85–88.

73. Abdulhamed JM, Alyousef SA, Mullins C. Endovascular stent placement for pulmonary venous obstruction after Mustard operation for transposition of the great arteries. *Heart* 1996;75: 210–212.

74. Michel-Behnke I, Hagel KJ, Bauer J, et al. Superior caval venous syndrome after atrial switch procedure: complete venous obstruction by gradual angioplasty and placement of stents. *Cardiol Young* 1998;8:443–448.

75. Santoro G, Ballerini L, Bialkowski J, et al. Stent implantation for post-Mustard systemic venous obstruction. *Eur J Cardiothorac Surg* 1998;14:332–334.

76. Bu'Lock FA, Tometzki AJ, Kitchiner DJ, et al. Balloon expandable stents for systemic venous pathway stenosis after the late Mustard's operation. *Heart* 1998;79:225–229.

77. Moore JW, Spicer RL, Perry JC, et al. Percutaneous use of stents to correct pulmonary artery stenosis in young children after cavopulmonary anastomosis. *Am Heart J* 1995;130: 1245–1249.

78. El-Said HG, Ing FF, Grifka RG, et al. 18-year experience with transseptal procedures through baffles, conduits and other intra-atrial patches. *Catheter Cardiovasc Interv* 2000;50: 434–439.

79. Brown SC, Eyskens B, Mertens L, et al. Self-expandable stents for relief of venous baffle obstruction after the Mustard operation. *Heart* 1998;79:230–233.

80. Hosking M, Redmond M, Allen L, et al. Responses of systemic and pulmonary veins to the presence of an intravascular stent in a swine model. *Catheter Cardiovasc Diagn* 1995;36: 90–96.

81. Park SC, Neches WH, Lenox CC, et al. Diagnosis and surgical treatment of bilateral pulmonary vein stenosis. *J Thorac Cardiovasc Surg* 1974;67:755–761.

82. Bridges ND, Mallory GB Jr. Huddleston CB, et al. Lung transplant in children and young adults with cardiovascular disease. *Ann Thorac Surg* 1995;59:813–821.

83. Edwards JE, Congenital stenosis of the pulmonary veins: pathologic and developmental considerations. *Lab Invest* 1960;9: 46–50.

84. Calderone CA, Hajm HK, Kadletz M, et al. Relentless pulmonary vein stenosis after repair of total anomalous pulmonary venous drainage. *Ann Thorac Surg* 1998;66:1514–1520.

85. Sade RM, Freed MD, Matthews EC, et al. Stenosis of individual pulmonary veins: review of the literature and report of a surgical case. *J Thorac Cardiovasc Surg* 1974;67:953–962.

86. Calderone CA, Hajm HK, Kadletz M, et al. Surgical management of total anomalous pulmonary venous drainage: impact of coexisting cardiac anomalies. *Ann Thorac Surg* 1998;66: 1521–1526.

87. Binet JP, Bouchard F, Langlois J, et al. Unilateral congenital stenosis of the pulmonary veins: a very rare cause of pulmonary hypertension. *J Thorac Cardiovasc Surg* 1972;63:397–402.

88. Driscoll DJ, Hesslein PS, Mullins CE. Congenital stenosis of individual pulmonary veins: clinical spectrum and unsuccessful treatment by transvenous balloon dilation. *Am J Cardiol* 1982; 49:1767–1772.

89. Lacour-Gayet F, Eey C, Planche C. Pulmonary vein stenosis: description of a sutureless surgical technique using the *in situ* pericardium. *Arch Mal Coeur Vaiss* 1996;89:633–636.

90. Lacour-Gayet F, Zoghbi J, Serraf AE, et al. Surgical management of progressive pulmonary venous obstruction after repair of total anomalous pulmonary venous connection. *J Thorac Cardiovasc Surg* 1999;117:679–687.

91. Hyde JA, Stumper O, Barth MJ, et al. Total anomalous pulmonary venous connection: outcome and surgical correction and management of recurrent venous obstruction. *Eur J Cardiothorac Surg* 1999;15:735–740.

92. Coles JG, Yemets I, Najm HK, et al. Experience with repair of congenital heart defects using adjunctive endovascular devices. *J Thorac Cardiovasc Surg* 1995;110:1513–1520.

93. Ungerleider RM, Johnson TA, O'Laughlin MP, et al. Intraoperative stents to rehabilitate severely stenotic pulmonary vessels. *Ann Thorac Surg* 2001;71:476–481.

94. Mendelsohn AM, Bove EL, Lupinetti FM, et al. Intraoperative and percutaneous stenting of congenital pulmonary artery and vein stenosis. *Circulation* 1993;88:210–217.

95. Revekes WJ, Wiedman MU, Lock JE, et al. Implantation and follow-up of endovascular stents in pulmonary vein stenosis. *J Am Coll Cardiol* 1999;33(Suppl A):527A.

96. Zahn EM, Houde C, Smallhorn JS, et al. Use of endovascular stents in the treatment of pulmonary vein stenosis. *Circulation* 1992;86(Suppl I):I-632.

97. Coulson JD, Bullaboy CA. Concentric placement of stents to relieve an obstructed anomalous pulmonary venous connection. *Catheter Cardiovasc Diagn* 1997;42:201–204.

98. Nakib A, Moller J, Kanjuh V, et al. Anomalies of the pulmonary veins. *Am J Cardiol* 1967;20:77–90.

99. Sadr IM, Tan Puay, Kieran MW, et al. Mechanism of pulmonary vein stenosis in infants with normally connected veins. *Am J Cardiol* 2000;86:577–579.

100. Wilson WR, Ilbawi MN, DeLeon SY, et al. Technical modifications for improved results in total anomalous pulmonary venous drainage. *J Thorac Cardiovasc Surg* 1992;103:861–871.

101. Smallhorn JF, Burrows P, Wilson G, et al. Two-dimensional and pulsed Doppler echocardiography in the postoperative evaluation of total anomalous pulmonary venous connection. *Circulation* 1987;76:298–305.

102. Meddeloff EN, Spray TL, Huddleston CB, et al. Lung transplantation for congenital pulmonary vein stenosis. *Ann Thorac Surg* 1995;60:903–907.

103. Van de Wal HJCM, Hamilton DI, Godman MJ, et al. Pulmonary venous obstructions following correction for total anomalous pulmonary venous drainage: a challenge. *Eur J Cardiothorac Surg* 1992;6:545–549.

Catheter Based Devices: For the Treatment of Non-coronary Cardiovascular Diseases in Adults and Children. Edited by P. Syamasundar Rao and Morton J. Kern, Lippincott Williams & Wilkins, Philadelphia © 2003.

38

NuMED CHEATHAM PLATINUM STENTS: ROLE IN THE MANAGEMENT OF CONGENITAL HEART DEFECTS

JOHN P. CHEATHAM

Successful balloon angioplasty of pulmonary artery stenosis associated with congenital heart disease was initially described by Lock and colleagues in 1981 (1,2). During the next decade there were many reports of similar successes for other vascular obstructions (3–7). However, failure of balloon angioplasty may occur for several reasons. Early failures are seen with lesions that are too rigid to be dilated, from elastic recoil or external compression of the vessel wall, from aortic thrombosis, or from intimal tears or flaps. Later failures typically occur from restenosis of successfully dilated lesions.

Balloon-expandable intravascular stents designed to support the vessel wall can improve early and late angioplasty results, except in lesions too rigid for balloon dilation. The concept of intravascular stent implantation was first introduced by Dotter in 1969 (8). However, extensive clinical trials were not carried out until the late 1980s after improvements in stent design and technology were made. By and large, these trials involved stent implantation in adults with peripheral vascular or coronary artery obstructions. The balloon-expandable Palmaz stent (Johnson & Johnson, Cordis Division, Warren, NJ), designed by Palmaz, was used for iliac, biliary, and renal artery stenoses, as well as for an intrahepatic portacaval shunt (9–11). Later, Schatz modified the stent (Palmaz-Schatz) for use in coronary artery stenosis (12). In 1988, Mullins reported the experimental results of implanting the Palmaz stent into pulmonary arteries and systemic veins in the canine animal model (13). After this initial successful report, the Palmaz stent was used to treat virtually all vascular obstructions associated with congenital heart disease over the next decade (14–104). Unfortunately, in the United States, after nearly 10 years of clinical trials under an FDA-sponsored Investigational Device Exemption (IDE) with Mullins as the principal investigator, no premar-

ket approval application was filed. Therefore no FDA-approved balloon-expandable intravascular stent is currently available to treat vascular obstructions associated with congenital heart disease.

However, "off-label" implantation of the slot-designed, stainless steel Palmaz stent at sites other than their original FDA approved sites (i.e., peripheral vessels and coronary arteries) was commonly performed by the pediatric interventionalist and uncovered certain limitations and disadvantages in stent design. The "medium-sized" Palmaz stent (P-104, 154, 204, and 394) has a "manufacturer's recommended expanded diameter" range of from only 4 to 9 mm, whereas the "large stents" (P-128, 188, and 308) have expanded diameters that range from 8 to 12 mm. Unfortunately, most of the target lesions associated with congenital heart disease will have an eventual adult diameter that ranges from 15 to 24 mm (i.e., pulmonary arteries, systemic veins, aorta, extracardiac conduits, etc.), which places the Palmaz stent as a less than ideal endoprosthesis. Pediatric interventionalists routinely "overexpanded" the Palmaz stent up to 18 mm to treat large-vessel stenosis but found the stent to shorten up to 50% of its original length. Not only will the stent be too short for many of the long-segment stenotic lesions, but the inability to expand to diameters greater than 18 mm may lead to vessel stenosis in later adulthood. Outside of the United States, an "extra-large" Palmaz stent (P-4015, 5015) has been available for several years that expands to 24 mm but is manufactured only in 40- or 50-mm lengths. This eliminates its use in shorter stenotic lesions or tortuous vessels. Within the past year the "extra-large" Palmaz stents have been made available in the United States (P-4010 and P-5010). So, although routinely used by pediatric interventionalists, some of the limitations and disadvantages of the Palmaz stent are as follows:

1. Designed for adult peripheral vascular obstructions, not congenital heart disease (CHD).
2. Rigid, sharp-edged, stainless steel endoprosthesis that is difficult to deliver in tortuous vessels and has a tendency

John P. Cheatham: Professor, Department of Pediatrics, Ohio State University Medical Center; Director, Cardiac Catheterization and Interventions, The Heart Center at Columbus Children's Hospital, Columbus, Ohio

to rupture the delivery balloon catheter and traumatize the vessel.

3. A slot design that causes significant stent shortening during "overdilation" that may lead to unnecessary and costly multiple stents with suboptimal results.

4. Limited range of expanded stent diameters and lengths.

BACKGROUND

Development of the NuMED Cheatham Platinum Stent

Rather than continue to use a stent that was not designed, or FDA approved, for the treatment of obstructive vascular lesions associated with CHD, we designed the NuMED Cheatham Platinum (CP) stent (NuMED, Inc., Nicholville, NY). Early in the stent design and developmental phase, we established several goals:

1. The stent should be expandable from 8 to 24 mm to allow for adult somatic growth.
2. A wide selection of stent lengths should be available to meet the demands of variable target lesions.
3. The stent should shorten ≤20% at full expansion.
4. The stent must have atraumatic, round leading and trailing edges to minimize delivery balloon and vessel trauma.
5. The stent should be more "flexible" yet stronger than the Palmaz stent.
6. The stent should maintain the current, or no more than 1F larger, introducer sheath for delivery.

In November of 1996, we embarked upon a collaborative effort and designed a handmade stent composed of heat-tempered 90% platinum and 10% iridium 0.013-inch

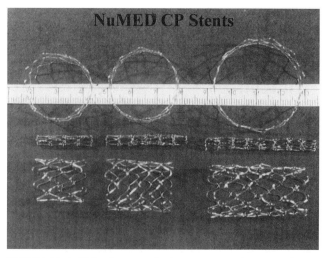

FIGURE 38.1. This photograph demonstrates the "zig" design of the NuMED Cheatham Platinum stent. The rows of zigs are laser-welded together, allowing a variety of stent lengths. Note that at maximum expanded diameters, the shortening of the stent is 20%.

wire arranged in a "zig" pattern (Figure 38.1). The number of zigs in a row can be varied and will impact on the strength, eventual expanded diameter, and percent shortening of the stent, whereas the row of zigs are laser-welded together and will determine the length of the stent. We have chosen to vary the number of zigs per row from six to eight zigs to allow the lowest stent profile with maximum expanded diameters from 15 to 24 mm. We have set a goal of ≤20% stent shortening at maximum expansion. Therefore if the patient is small and the target lesion is a vessel with an adult diameter of ≤15 mm, then a six-zig pattern is chosen to give the lowest profile. If the eventual adult target vessel diameter is between 16 and 24 mm, then an

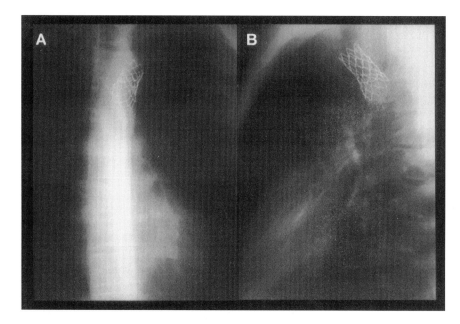

FIGURE 38.2. A PA and lateral chest x-ray demonstrating the superior radiopacity of platinum in the Cheatham Platinum stent compared with the stainless steel Palmaz stent is shown here.

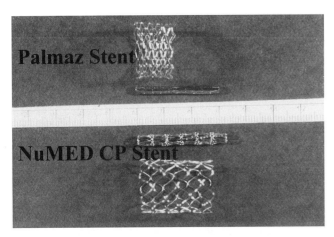

FIGURE 38.3. This photograph demonstrates ≈ 50% shortening of the Palmaz-308 stent when "overdilated" to 18 mm, compared with an eight-zig, 34-mm Cheatham Platinum stent expanded to the same diameter.

eight-zig CP stent is preferable to minimize stent shortening. A custom-made ten-zig stent will allow expansion to 30 mm with ≤20% stent shortening. However, the profile and necessary introducer sheath will be larger. The length of the stent can be manufactured by varying the number of rows and is a multiple of the height of the zigs (≈ 5.6 mm) (i.e., two rows = 11 mm length, three rows = 16 mm, four rows = 22 mm, five rows = 28 mm, six rows = 34 mm, seven rows = 39 mm, eight rows = 45 mm, nine rows = 50 mm, etc.).

The advantages of the NuMED CP stent compared to the Palmaz stent are as follows:

1. Superior radiopacity secondary to the platinum composition (Figure 38.2).
2. Superior "compression" or radial hoop strength secondary to the tempered wire and zig design.
3. Less rigidity because of the malleability of the tempered platinum-iridium wire.
4. Less potential trauma to the delivery balloon and target vessel secondary to the rounded edges of the zig pattern.
5. Wider range of expanded diameters from 8 to 24 mm (ten-zig can be expanded to 30 mm) while maintaining ≤20% stent shortening.
6. Superior selection of stent lengths to meet the demands of a wide range of target lesions. and
7. Maximal stent shortening of ≤20% will minimize chances of missing the target site or need of multiple serial stents (Figure 38.3).

Development of the NuMED BIB Catheter

It became obvious during the development of the CP stent that the conventional single-balloon delivery catheter used for Palmaz stent delivery was less than ideal. A noncompliant, thick-walled balloon is required to expand the stent to avoid balloon rupture during partial expansion of the sharp-edged stent. Entrapment of the punctured balloon catheter is a significant complication that may lead to urgent surgical removal of the stent and catheter. The delivery balloon is typically chosen to be longer than the stent length to avoid stent migration during delivery. Unfortunately, this choice results in the balloon initially expanding proximally and distally to the unexpanded stent. This leads to a series of undesirable events that may lead to procedural complications:

1. Excessive flaring of the ends of the stent, which, in the case of the Palmaz stent, allows the sharp edges of the stainless steel to traumatize the delivery balloon and/or the target vessel wall (Figure 38.4). This leads to a ruptured balloon during partial stent expansion and may aggravate the intimal or medial tear occurring during angioplasty.
2. The ends of the balloon expanded first allows the entire delivery system to act as a "flotation" catheter during the critical time of stent expansion, which causes unwanted catheter–stent movement.
3. The uneven action of balloon expansion at one end of the catheter predisposes to "milk" the stent off the balloon catheter, leading to stent embolization before full expansion.
4. A single balloon delivery catheter does not allow repositioning of the stent during deployment.

In an effort to minimize these problems, some pediatric interventionalists have recommended using very short balloons while delivering the Palmaz stent [i.e., the delivery balloon would actually be shorter than the stent length (personal communication, Dr. Charles Mullins)]. However, this technique has an inherent risk of stent migration and embolization during deployment if the stent moves during delivery. With the Palmaz stent design possessing some of the disadvantages already mentioned, a less-than-ideal balloon delivery catheter potentially exaggerates these problems. Therefore, we not only sought to develop an improved balloon-expandable stent in the NuMED CP stent, but also modified an existing angioplasty catheter to improve the efficacy and safety of stent deployment.

In November 1997, the NuMED balloon-in-balloon (BIB) catheter was designed (NuMED, Inc., Nicholville, NY) with an inner Tyshak II balloon and an outer Z-Med balloon. The inner balloon is very low-profiled and expands to one-half the outer balloon diameter, while the length is 1 cm shorter than the outer balloon (Figure 38.5). The BIB outer balloon diameters range from 8 to 24 mm with variable balloon lengths, while the shaft of the catheter is either 8F or 9F to ensure acceptable inflation and deflation times of the inner and outer balloons. The desired diameter to expand the target lesion is measured and matched to the outer Z-Med balloon diameter, whereas the length of the CP stent to treat the target stenotic site is matched to the inner balloon length, which is chosen to be *shorter* than the

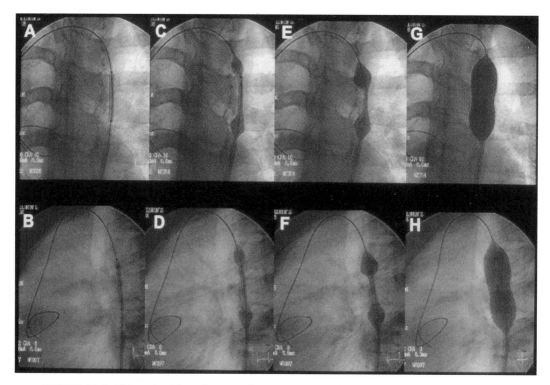

FIGURE 38.4. This series of angiograms demonstrates the flaring action of the Palmaz stent when delivered on a conventional single long balloon catheter. One can readily see how this delivery system could act as a "flotation" catheter, causing unwanted movement during stent deployment.

stent length. For example, if a stenotic pulmonary artery requires an expanded stent diameter of 18 mm and length of 35 mm, an eight-zig, 39-mm CP stent is chosen and placed on a BIB catheter with an inner balloon diameter of 9 mm that is 3.5 cm long, with the outer balloon diameter being 18 mm and the length being 4.5 cm. Therefore the inner balloon is shorter than the stent and the outer balloon is longer than the stent. The inner balloon is *always* inflated

first using a twisting action of the locked endoflator that expands the stent to one-half of the target vessel diameter without flaring of ends of the stent, since the balloon is shorter than the stent. Because the stent is still in contact with the unexpanded outer balloon material, the entire stent–balloon delivery catheter system can be repositioned before final deployment by expanding the outer balloon.

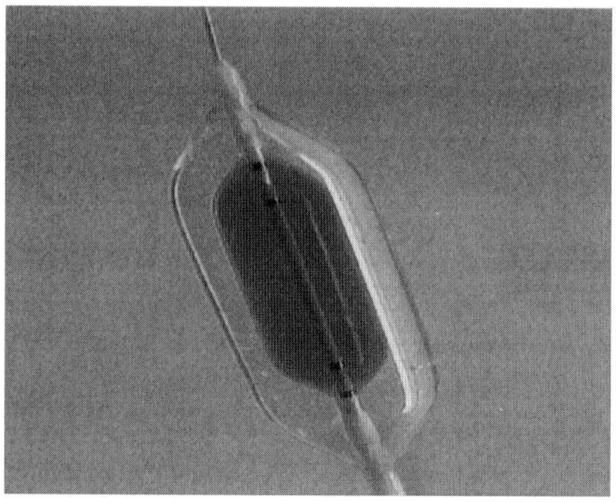

Bench and Animal Testing

Previous biocompatibility, corrosion, and fatigue testing on the 90% platinum, 10% iridium wire was performed on 0.007-inch wire used for a coronary stent. In addition, bench testing of compression strength (radial hoop strength), percent stent shortening at specific expanded diameters using a six-zig and eight-zig pattern (custom ten-zig), and determination of necessary introducer sheath sizes were performed. Initially, the CP stent and BIB delivery catheter were tested *in vitro* in isolated canine and porcine hearts, great arteries, and systemic veins. Then acute and 6-month chronic studies were performed in the canine animal model under an approved Institutional Animal Care and Use Committee (IACUC) protocol (Figure 38.6). We initially implanted four CP stents mounted on BIB catheters acutely to assess the feasibility of stent design and delivery methods with target sites in the main pulmonary artery, left pulmonary artery, superior

FIGURE 38.5. This is a picture of the NuMED balloon-in-balloon, or BIB, catheter demonstrating the inner balloon inflated while the outer balloon is also expanded. Note the inner balloon is one-half the diameter of the outer balloon and 1 cm shorter.

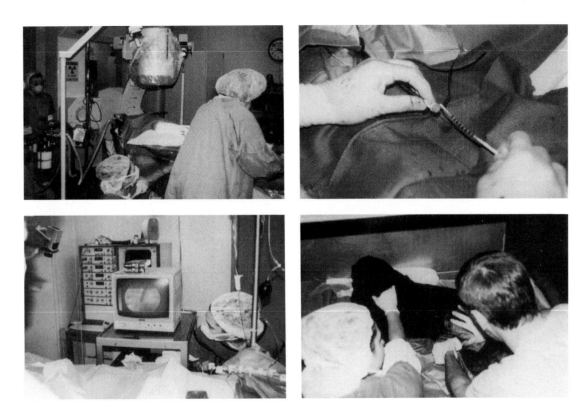

FIGURE 38.6. The four panels in this photograph demonstrate the cardiovascular research laboratory at the University of Nebraska Medical Center. The canine animal model was used for the acute and chronic studies involving the development of the NuMED Cheatham Platinum stent and balloon-in-balloon catheter.

vena cava, and left subclavian artery. Next, we implanted a total of 27 CP stents, including seven ePTFE and polyurethane-covered stents, in four dogs over a 6-month study period. Implanted stents ranged from six-zig 22-mm to eight-zig 45-mm, and BIB catheters ranged from 8 to 24 mm. Some of the CP stents were reexpanded using larger-diameter balloon catheters during the study. Sites of implantation included right pulmonary artery, left pulmonary artery, main pulmonary artery, superior vena cava, inferior vena cava, aortic arch and isthmus, descending aorta, and left subclavian artery. All animals were euthanized as per protocol and gross and microscopic pathology studies were performed by the University of Nebraska Medical Center cardiovascular pathology staff, using hematoxylin and eosin and elastin staining along with electron microscopy (Figure 38.7).

Clinical Trials

The initial results and success of bench testing and animal studies justified initiating clinical trials. From August 1998 through August 1999, 45 patients (25 males and 20 females) underwent CP stent implantation. Their age ranged from 1.8 to 60 years, with an average of 19, whereas weight varied from 10 to 93.2 kg, with an average of 54.1. Twenty-five patients with coarctation of the aorta (CoA)

underwent stent placement, 17 with native and eight with recurrent obstruction. As expected, those patients with pulmonary artery branch stenosis after surgical repair of CHD, especially tetralogy of Fallot, comprised the next largest subgroup of patients. There were five with isolated right pulmonary artery (RPA) stenosis, two with isolated left pulmonary artery (LPA) stenosis, and six with bilateral branch stenosis requiring simultaneous delivery of "kissing stents." Four patients had recurrent right-ventricle-to-pulmonary-artery (RV-PA) homograft stenosis, and one each had right Blalock-Taussig shunt stenosis, multiple sites of left-to-right shunt inside a lateral tunnel Fontan repair, and an obstructed superior vena cava (SVC) baffle limb after Mustard repair for transposition of the great arteries (TGA).

A total of 57 NuMED CP stents was implanted in the 45 patients. Forty-eight of the stents deployed were composed of eight zigs per row, with lengths varying between 22 and 50 mm. Seven stents with six zigs per row and lengths of 22 or 28 mm were used, and one seven-zig, 45-mm CP stent was implanted. We covered four stents by sewing pre-stretched ePTFE material to the outside of the partially expanded stent and then recrimped it on the BIB catheter. In three cases the covered stent was used to prevent significant aortic injury in treating CoA. One patient had post-operative CoA with complete aortic obstruction after

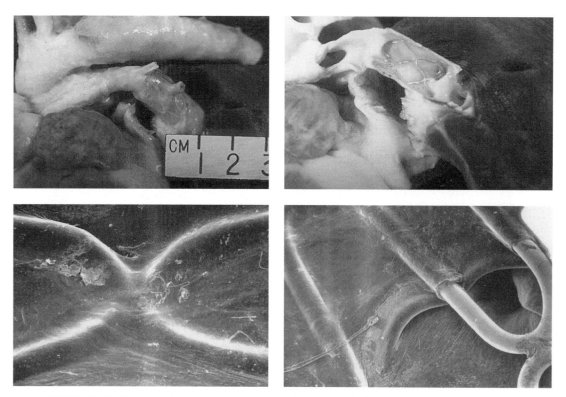

FIGURE 38.7. The upper two panels demonstrate the gross pathology of the Cheatham Platinum stent implanted into the aorta and pulmonary artery. The electron-microscopic appearance of an "endothelialization" process covering the zig design of the Cheatham Platinum stent is shown in the lower two panels. Note there is no endothelial covering of the stent at branching vessels or venous valves.

"jump" tube graft insertion, another had severe native CoA (<2 mm), and the third patient was postoperative CoA repair with a tube graft flap causing obstruction. In the fourth child receiving a covered stent, a ten-zig, 117-mm-long CP stent was implanted inside a "dehisced" lateral tunnel causing hypoxemia after Fontan repair. In the study, BIB catheter outer balloon diameters ranged from 10 to 24 mm during initial implant, with reexpansion of the stent to 30 mm in one patient. The long, Mullins-type introducer sheaths ranged from 9 to 14F. The large covered CP stent mounted on a 22-mm BIB catheter required an 18- and 22F sheath.

Method of Implantation

After informed consent and IRB or Ethical Committee approval, standard hemodynamic and angiographic studies were performed. The target lesion and surrounding vessels were measured and the ultimate diameter and length of the CP stent were determined. The appropriate BIB catheter was chosen and prepared, being careful to "dry-prep" the inner balloon first, followed by the outer balloon. It is very important that the operator remember to center the stent over the inner and outer balloon radiopaque markers and confirm the stent's position under fluoroscopy *before* crimping. We recommend

crimping using gentle finger pressure (avoiding bending or twisting the stent) with a "rolling action" applied along the entire length of the stent. With the heat-tempered platinum-iridium wire and BIB catheter design, it is unnecessary to press hard during the crimping process, as was commonly necessary to ensure that the stainless steel Palmaz stent adhered to the balloon. We then apply undiluted contrast media, affectionately known as "Mullins glue," to coat and to promote adhesiveness of the stent to the balloon prior to delivery. The inner balloon is *always* inflated first using a twisting action of the locked endoflator to maintain positive pressure and avoid loss of balloon–stent contact. The stent is still repositionable at this stage and small hand injections of contrast through the delivery sheath or second catheter may be performed for precise stent placement. The outer balloon is then inflated to expand the stent to the desired diameter, with minimal stent flaring or catheter movement. After deflating both balloons, we found that reinflating the outer balloon alone was helpful in fully expanding the stent. Using the preceding technique of BIB catheter delivery, we believe it unnecessary to use pharmaceutical agents, such as Adenosine, to temporarily stop the heart while the stent is expanded. We think electively stopping the heart in the catheterization laboratory is a bad thing. (It sometimes happens without trying!)

RESULTS

Immediate Results

The results of CP stent implantation are as follows. The peak systolic gradient was reduced in 17 patients with native CoA from 56.2 to 4.6 mm Hg, whereas in the eight patients with recurrent aortic obstruction, the gradient was reduced from 41.8 to 0.9 mm Hg, both of which are statistically significant at $p < .001$ using paired t tests (Figures 38.8 to 38.10). Isolated RPA and LPA stenoses were also effectively treated with peak systolic gradient reductions from 54.6 to 5 mm Hg and 52.5 to 6.5 mm Hg, respectively, ($p < .001$) (Figure 38.11). In the six children with combined RPA and LPA stenoses, "kissing stents" reduced the peak systolic gradients from 43.5 and 45 mm Hg to 6.8 and 6.0 mm Hg, respectively

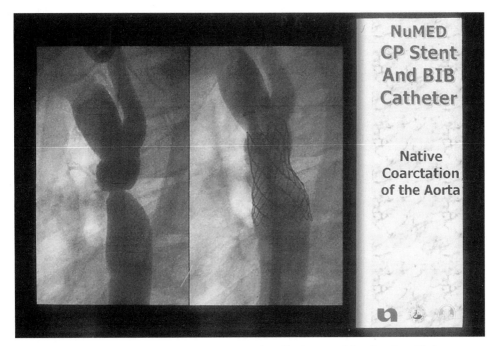

FIGURE 38.8. These two angiograms demonstrate the effective use of the Cheatham Platinum stent in the treatment of native aortic coarctation. There was no residual peak systolic gradient after stent deployment.

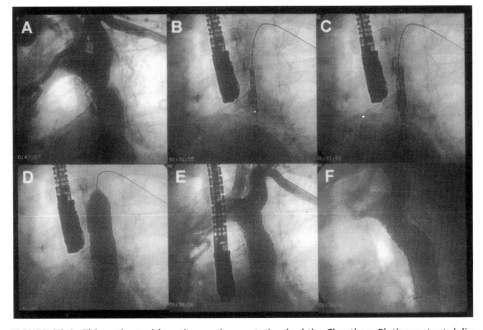

FIGURE 38.9. This patient with native aortic coarctation had the Cheatham Platinum stent delivered on a BIB catheter with the use of transesophageal echocardiography (TEE).

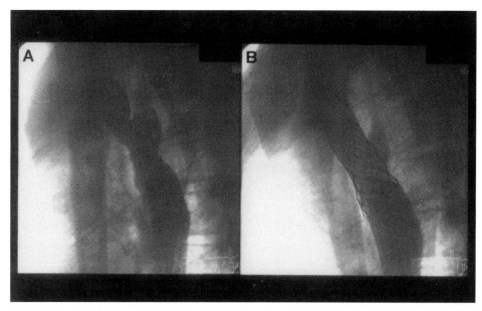

FIGURE 38.10. This teenage boy had recurrent CoA after the Teles surgical procedure where the left subclavian artery (LSCA) is relocated. Note the two areas of residual obstruction proximal and distal to the origin of the LSCA and how effectively the lesions are treated with an eight-zig, 50-mm-long Cheatham Platinum stent. The LSCA remains patent despite the stent crossing the origin of the vessel.

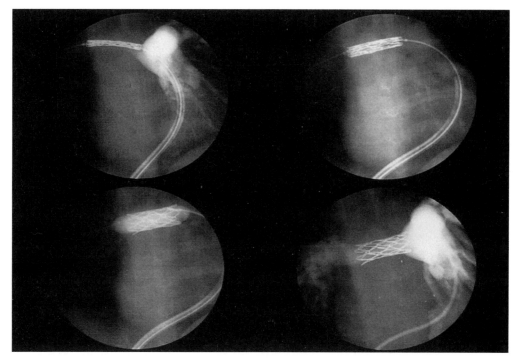

FIGURE 38.11. The four panels in this photograph nicely demonstrate a six-zig, 22-mm-long Cheatham Platinum stent effectively treating severe right pulmonary artery stenosis after a Blalock-Taussig shunt for complex cyanotic congenital heart disease in a 2-year-old. Note the inner and outer balloon deployment of the highly radiopaque Cheatham Platinum stent using the balloon-in-balloon delivery catheter.

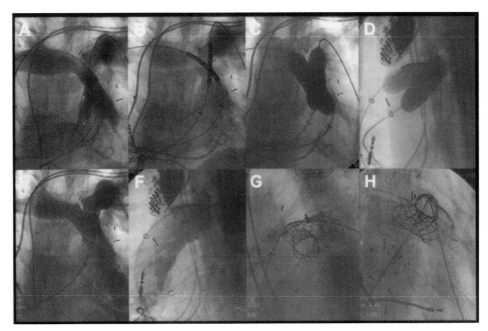

FIGURE 38.12. **A** through **H** demonstrate the technique of simultaneous delivery of Cheatham Platinum stents for bilateral proximal pulmonary branch stenoses involving the main pulmonary artery in a patient after tetralogy of Fallot repair, so-called kissing stents. Note how the stents overlie each other to provide continued access into both pulmonary branches **(G, H)**.

($p < .01$) (Figure 38.12). The four patients with recurrent RV-PA homograft obstruction also had effective relief of their gradients from 55 to 14.3 mm Hg ($p < .01$) (Figure 38.13). After stenting the stenotic right Blalock-Taussig shunt in the young man with complex cyanotic CHD, O2 saturations increased from 78% to 88%. The implantation of the long, covered CP stent was also clinically effective in treating the young man with multiple leaks in the lateral tunnel by improving resting O2 saturations from 80% to 96% (Figures 38.14 and 38.15). Finally, the

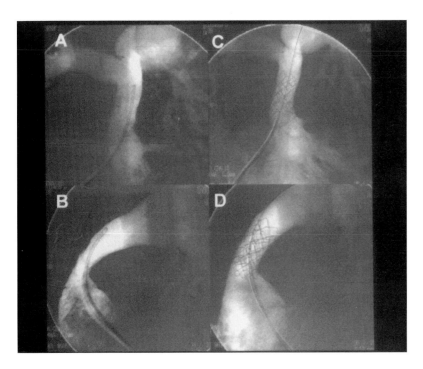

FIGURE 38.13. In this series of angiograms, recurrent RV-to-PA homograft obstruction is nicely demonstrated in **A** and **B,** whereas effective relief of obstruction is shown after two eight-zig, 39-mm CP stents were placed coaxially RV, right ventricle; PA, pulmonary artery.**(C,D)**.

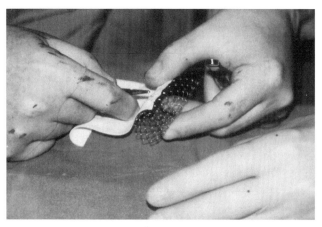

FIGURE 38.14. This photograph demonstrates sewing the pre-stretched ePTFE material to the ten-zig 117-mm-long CP stent to be implanted inside a dehisced lateral tunnel after Fontan repair.

9 mm Hg mean gradient across the obstructed SVC baffle after Mustard's repair was completely eliminated (Figure 38.16).

Complications

During the initial clinical trials, two procedural complications were reported. In one man with severe native CoA requiring a covered stent, there was transient left hemotho-

rax. There was also traumatic stent fracture during attempted entry of the long, covered CP stent in the Fontan patient using a modified "front-load" technique. The stent was inadvertently pushed out of the delivery sheath in the groin with the first row of ten zigs being traumatized and fractured. Both procedural complications were considered avoidable, and there were no further sequelae.

Follow-up

There has been limited follow-up thus far because of the relative short study period and large number of institutions involved. Stent fatigue fracture and fragment embolization have occurred in two patients with recurrent RV-PA homograft obstruction and previously failed Palmaz stents. This is a recognizable problem with balloon-expandable metal stents being compressed externally. More recently, there was a report of possible fatigue fracture in a stent placed in the SVC–right atrial junction that may have been related to improper crimping technique. Two patients with severe native CoA and stenoses of less than 2 mm had immediate residual gradients of 20 and 25 mm Hg secondary to limited stent expansion to avoid excessive vessel trauma and possible aneurysm formation with planned stent redilation later. One patient had a 30-mm Hg residual aortic gradient 10 months after implant secondary to an intimal flap that was successfully treated with a second CP stent. All patients are currently taking antiplatelet medication and are reportedly doing well.

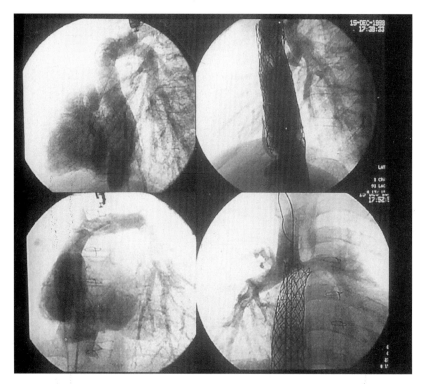

FIGURE 38.15. The top left (lateral) and bottom left (AP) panels demonstrate significant right-to-left shunting through the dehisced lateral tunnel in a 10-year-old boy after Fontan repair for complex single ventricle. Note there is virtually no residual right-to-left shunt after implantation of the ePTFE-covered Cheatham Platinum stent with excellent flow into both the right and left pulmonary arteries as demonstrated in the two panels on the right.

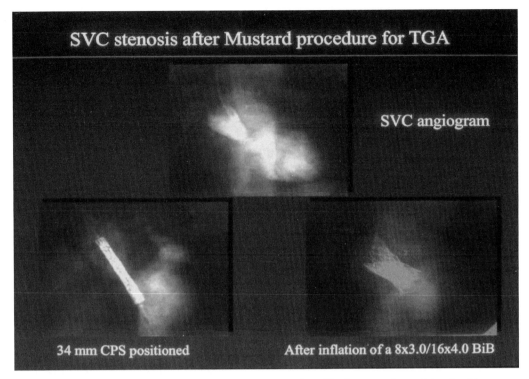

FIGURE 38.16. The three angiograms demonstrate the effective use of an eight-zig, 34-mm Cheatham Platinum stent in treatment of severe baffle obstruction of the SVC limb after Mustard repair for TGA.

CONCLUSION

In conclusion, the NuMED CP stent offers an effective, nonsurgical treatment for a wide variety of vascular obstructions associated with congenital heart disease. The heat-tempered, platinum-iridium wire and zig design improves stent strength, radiopacity, and "flexibility" compared with the Palmaz stent. The CP stent design also minimizes stent shortening and vessel/balloon trauma while offering a wide range of expanded diameters (8 to 30 mm) and variable lengths (11 to 117 mm) in this study—both clearly superior to the Palmaz stent.

The NuMED BIB catheter is an innovative concept that has significantly improved operator control during intravascular stent delivery. It minimizes stent flaring, migration, and shortening while effectively eliminating catheter movement during deployment. It also allows the partially expanded stent to be repositioned before final expansion, which is a significant benefit to the interventionalist to maintain control and precisely position the stent. We currently use the BIB catheter for all stents, including the Palmaz and the new IntraStent DoubleStrut stents (IntraTherapeutics, Inc., St. Paul, MN), if the target vessel diameter is ≥8 mm. Although more data and longer follow-up are required, the NuMED CP stent and BIB delivery catheter offer great promise in the future treatment of children and adults with congenital heart disease. FDA submission for approval under the Humanitarian Device Exemption (HDE) and application for CE Mark are currently under way.

THE FUTURE

Although covering the CP stent with stretched ePTFE is possible, more investigation and refinement in design are needed. We are currently testing an ultrathin ePTFE material that can be applied to the CP stent using biodegradable adhesives, eliminating the tedious task of sewing the material to the stent at the time of delivery (Figure 38.17). In addition, biocompatible polyurethane and silicone coatings are being tested (Figure 38.18). After the recent reports of stent fracture and embolization, further metallurgy and fatigue testing were performed at NuMED facilities and abroad. An experimental design change to eliminate the laser welds (i.e., laser cutting the stent from a solid heat-tempered, platinum-iridium tube instead of being hand-made from round, 013-inch wire) was tested but reintroduced "sharp edges" that could traumatize the delivery balloon and target vessels, which we believe are undesirable characteristics. Instead, the laser welds of the stent were

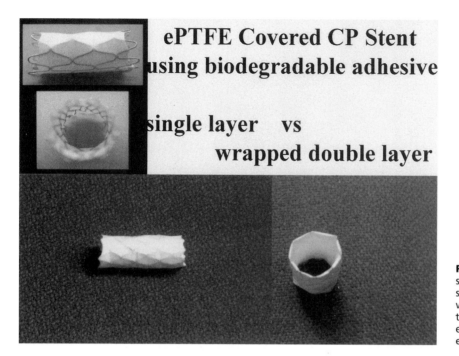

FIGURE 38.17. This photograph demonstrates two covered Cheatham Platinum stents using ultrathin ePTFE material applied with a biodegradable adhesive, avoiding the tedious task of sewing the prestretched ePTFE material to the stent. ePTFE, superelastic polytetra fluroethylene.

altered in order to resist stent fragmentation and embolization while maintaining stent integrity and strength during external compression testing. The CP stent remained "stronger" than the Palmaz stent after these modifications.

The XL Palmaz stent (P-4010, 5010, and soon 3110) has recently been introduced in the United States, but the slot design, sharp edges, and stent shortening are still present. In addition, the long, rigid lengths of only 40 and 50 mm (soon 31 mm) limits its usefulness in many vascular obstructions associated with CHD. Cordis, Johnson & Johnson Interventions, has recently introduced the Genesis peripheral vascular stent to replace the Palmaz stent. The

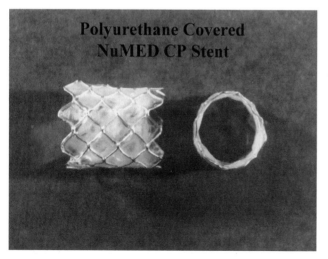

FIGURE 38.18. The low profile of a polyurethane-coated NuMED Cheatham Platinum stent is demonstrated in this photograph.

Genesis stent has flexible joints to allow for better tracking and placement in tortuous vessels. The stents are manufactured in lengths of 19, 25, 29, 39, and 59 mm, but can only be "overexpanded" to 18 mm, similar to the Palmaz stent. This remains a limitation when treating coarctation of the aorta, or in other large diameter vessels. The recently FDA-approved biliary IntraStent DoubleStrut and LD stents offer some promise with their "open-cell" design to improve flexibility to treat tortuous obstructive lesions and to minimize stent shortening (Figure 38.19). There is a greater choice in stent lengths (i.e., 16, 26, 36, 56, and 76 mm) than with the Palmaz stent, although not as many as with the NuMED CP stent. However, the FDA-approved manufacturer's recommended maximum expanded diameter of 12 mm remains problematic and requires the interventionalist to "overdilate" to 18 mm with no hope of dilating to 24 mm to accommodate adult growth. We currently use the IntraStent to treat small infants with tortuous vascular obstructions (i.e., pulmonary artery stenosis), using a new, custom-made front-load delivery system (105).

The development of the NuMED CP stent has led to other projects and ideas that will continue to push pediatric transcatheter therapy to new heights. In addition to the development of the NuMED BIB delivery catheter, the NuMED Pulmonary Valved Stent designed by Dr. Philipp Bonhoeffer (Necker Children's Hospital, Paris, France) was possible because of the CP stent design (Figure 38.20). The covered CP stent has been redesigned using e-PTFE applied by a biodegradable adhesive to allow transcatheter options in the treatment of complex congenital heart disease, including a combined transcatheter and surgical version of the "Norwood Procedure." We have initial results using custom made

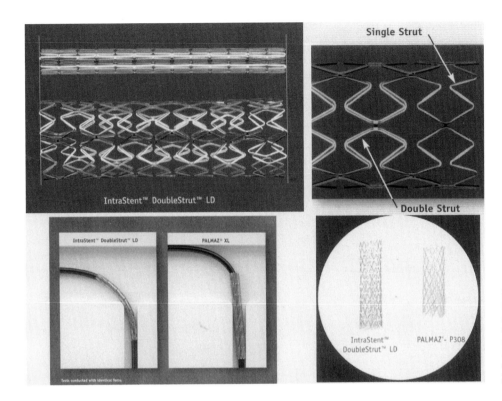

FIGURE 38.19. The new IntraStent DoubleStrut LD design is shown here and demonstrates the open-cell design that allows greater flexibility of the stent to treat tortuous vascular obstruction. Note the significant difference between the rigid Palmaz XL design and the flexible IntraStent.

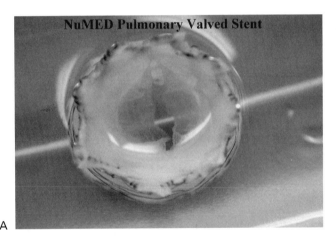

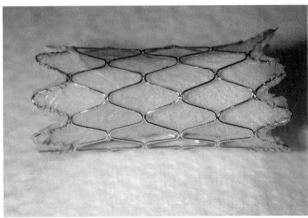

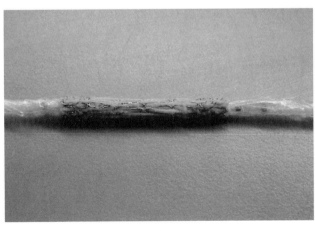

FIGURE 38.20. A: The NuMED Pulmonary Valved Stent is shown viewed with the valve partially opened. **B:** Philipp Bonhoeffer's design uses the bovine jugular vein and accompanying valve that is hand-sewn to the partially expanded Cheatham Platinum stent. **C:** The entire stent is then hand-crimped onto a BIB delivery catheter for percutaneous implantation.

Amplatzer pulmonary artery flow restrictors and PDA stents as initial palliation for newborns with hypoplastic left heart syndrome. This has been modified to a combined surgical RPA and LPA bands followed by PDA stenting and balloon atrial septostomy. Stage II is a "comprehensive" surgical palliation, while Stage III is a transcatheter approach using a covered CP stent to complete the Fontan circuit by connecting the IVC to the pulmonary artery. Indeed, the future of stent therapy for CHD remains bright, but we must continue to improve stent design and technology.

ACKNOWLEDGMENTS

Mr. Allen Tower, President, NuMED, Inc., and Doug J. Villnave and Richard Normile (NuMED), for their technical support and creativity; Ms. Mary Mercer, for her clerical assistance; and the following investigators: Asad Arain, Kaleem Aziz, Luigi Ballerini, Jack Bandel, Ramon Bermudez-Canete, Antonio Carvalho, Francisco Chamie, Luiz Christiani, Cesar Esteves, Roberto Formigari, Yousef Goussous, Fakhri Hakim, Leopoldo Hernandez, Akham Hiari, Ziyad Hijazi, Larry Latson, Chuck Mullins, Helder Pauperio, Jose Pulido, Shakeel Qureshi, Carlos Ruiz, Steven Shapiro, MD; Leo Solarewicz, William Torres, and Neil Wilson.

REFERENCES

1. Lock JE, Niemi T, Enzig S, et al. Transvenous angioplasty of experimental branch pulmonary artery stenosis in newborn lambs. *Circulation* 1981;64:886.
2. Lock JE, Castaneda-Zuniga WR, Fuhrman BP, et al. Balloon dilation angioplasty of hypoplastic and stenotic pulmonary arteries. *Circulation* 1983;67:962.
3. Rocchini AP, Kveselis D, Dick M, et al. Use of balloon angioplasty to treat peripheral pulmonary stenosis. *Am J Cardiol* 1984;54:1069.
4. Lababidi Z, Wu J, Walls JT. Percutaneous balloon aortic valvuloplasty: results in 23 patients. *Am J Cardiol* 1984;53:194.
5. Lock JE, Bass JL, Amplatz K, et al. Balloon dilation angioplasty of aortic coarctations in infants and children. *Circulation* 1983;68:109.
6. Driscoll DJ, Hesslein PS, Mullins CE. Congenital stenosis of individual pulmonary veins: clinical spectrum and unsuccessful treatment by transvenous balloon dilation. *Am J Cardiol* 1982;49:1767.
7. Coulson JD, Pitlick PT, Miller DC, et al. Severe superior vena cava syndrome and hydrocephalus after the Mustard procedure: findings and a new surgical approach. *Circulation* 1984;70:I-47.
8. Dotter CT. Transluminally placed coil spring endarterial tube grafts: long-term patency in canine popliteal artery. *Invest Radiol* 1969;4:329.
9. Palmaz JC, Richter GM, Noeldge G, et al. Intraluminal stents in atherosclerotic iliac artery stenosis: preliminary report of a multicenter study. *Radiology* 1988;168:727.
10. Palmaz JC, Windeler SA, Garcia F, et al. Atherosclerotic rabbit aortas: expandable intraluminal grafting. *Radiology* 1986;160: 723.
11. Palmaz JC, Sibbit RR, Reuter SR, et al. Expandable intrahepatic portacaval shunt stents: early experience in the dog. *Am J Radiol* 1985;145:821.
12. Schatz RA, Palmaz JC, Tio FO, et al. Balloon-expandable intracoronary stents in the adult dog. *Circulation* 1987;76:450.
13. Mullins CE, O'Laughlin MP, Vick GW III, et al. Implantation of balloon-expandable intravascular grafts by catheterization in pulmonary arteries and systemic veins. *Circulation* 1988;77:188.
14. O'Laughlin MP, Perry SB, Lock JE, et al. Use of endovascular stents in congenital heart disease. *Circulation* 1991;83:1923.
15. O'Laughlin MP, Slack MC, Grifka RG, et al. Implantation and intermediate-term follow-up of stents in congenital heart disease. *Circulation* 1993;88:605.
16. Perry SB, O'Laughlin MP, Mullins CE, et al. Endovascular stents in congenital heart disease. *Prog Pediatr Cardiol* 1992;1: 35.
17. Ing FF, Grifka RG, Nihill MR, et al. Repeat dilation of intravascular stents in congenital heart defects. *Circulation* 1995;92: 893.
18. Cheatham JP. Pulmonary stenosis. In: Garson A Jr, Bricker JT, Fisher DJ, et al., eds. *The science and practice of pediatric cardiology.* Baltimore: Williams & Wilkins, 1998:1207.
19. McCrindle BW, Jones TK, Grifka RG, et al. Factors associated with immediate results after balloon dilation of pulmonary artery stenoses. *Circulation* 1997;96:374.
20. Saidi AS, Lovalchin JP, Fisher DJ, et al. Balloon pulmonary valvuloplasty and stent implantation. For peripheral pulmonary artery stenosis in Alagille syndrome. *Tex Heart Inst J* 1998;25:79.
21. O'Laughlin MP. Catheterization treatment of stenosis and hypoplasia of pulmonary arteries. *Pediatr Cardiol* 1998;19:48.
22. Chau AK, Leung MP. Management of branch pulmonary artery stenosis: balloon angioplasty or endovascular stenting. *Clin Exp Pharmacol Physiol* 1997;24:960.
23. Trant CA Jr, O'Laughlin MP, Ungerleider RM, et al. Cost-effectiveness analysis of stents, balloon angioplasty, and surgery for the treatment of branch pulmonary artery stenosis. *Pediatr Cardiol* 1997;18:339.
24. Zeevi S, Berant M, Blieden LC. Midterm clinical impact versus procedural success of balloon angioplasty for pulmonary artery stenosis. *Pediatr Cardiol* 1997;18:101.
25. Hijazi ZM, al-Fadley F, Geggel RL, et al. Stent implantation for relief of pulmonary artery stenosis: immediate and short-term results. *Catheter Cardiovasc Diagn* 1996;38:16.
26. Hatai Y, Nykanen DG, Williams WG, et al. Endovascular stents in children under I year of age: acute impact and late results. *Br Heart J* 1995;74:689.
27. Moore JW, Spicer RL, Perry JC, et al. Percutaneous use of stents to correct pulmonary artery stenosis in young children after cavopulmonary anastomosis. *Am Heart J* 1995;130:1245.
28. Oyen WJ, van Oort AM, Tanke RB, et al. Pulmonary perfusion after endovascular stenting of pulmonary artery stenosis. *J Nucl Med* 1995;36:2006.
29. Fogelman R, Nykanen D, Smailhorn JF, et al. Endovascular stents in the pulmonary circulation: clinical impact on management and medium-term follow-up. *Circulation* 1995;92:881.
30. Morrow WR, Palmaz JC, Tio FO, et al. Re-expansion of balloon-expandable stents after growth. *J Am Coll Cardiol* 1993; 22:2007.
31. Morriss MJH, McNamara DG. Coarctation of aorta and interrupted aortic arch. In: Garson A Jr, Bricker JT, Fisher DJ, et al., eds. *The science and practice of pediatric cardiology.* Baltimore: Williams & Wilkins, 1998:1317.
32. Suarez de Lezo J, Pan M, Romero M, et al. Immediate and follow-up findings after stent treatment for severe coarctation of aorta. *Am J Cardiol* 1999;83:400.
33. Ledesma M, David F, Jimenez S, et al. Stents in aortic coarcta-

tion: immediate results and short follow-up. *J Am Coll Cardiol* 1999;33:519A.

34. Morrow WR, Srnith VC, Ehier WJ, et al. Balloon angioplasty with stent implantation in experimental coarctation of the aorta. *Circulation* 1994;89:2677.

35. Suarez de Lezo J, Pan M, Rornero M, et al. Balloon-expandable stent repair of severe coarctation of the aorta. *Am Heart J* 1995; 129:1002.

36. Ing FF, Goldberg B, Siegel DH, et al. Arterial stents in the management of neurofibromatosis and renovascular hypertension in a pediatric patients: case report of a new treatment modality. *Cardiovasc Intervent Radiol* 1995;18:414.

37. Diethrich EB, Heuser RR, Cardenas JR, et al. Endovascular techniques in adult aortic coarctation: the use of stents for native and recurrent coarctation repair. *J Endovasc Surg* 1995;2:183.

38. Rosenthal E, Oureshi SA, Tynan M. Stent implantation for aortic recoarctation. *Am Heart J* 1995;129:1220.

39. Mendelsohn AM, Dorostkar PC, Moorehead CP, et al. Stent redilation in canine models of congenital heart disease: pulmonary artery stenosis and coarctation of the aorta. *Catheter Cardiovasc Diagn* 1996;38:430.

40. Buibul ZR, Bruckheimer E, Love JC, et al. Implantation of balloon-expandable stents for coarctation of the aorta: implantation data and short-term results. *Catheter Cardiovasc Diagn* 1996;39:36.

41. Ruiz CE, Zhang HP. Stenting coarctation of the aorta: promising concept but primitive technology. *Catheter Cardiovasc Diagn* 1996;39:43.

42. Harrison DA, McLaughlin PR. Interventional cardiology for the adult patient with congenital heart disease: the Toronto Hospital experience. *Can J Cardiol* 1996;12:965.

43. Thanopoulos BV, Triposkiadis F, Margetakis A, et al. Long segment coarctation of the thoracic aorta: treatment with multiple balloon-expandable stent implantation. *Am Heart J* 1997;133: 470.

44. Pedulla DM, Grifka RG, Mullins CE, et al. Endovascular stent implantation for severe recoarctation of the aorta: case report with angiographic and 18-month clinical follow-up. *Catheter Cardiovasc Diagn* 1997;40:311.

45. lno T, Ohkubo M. Dilation mechanism, causes of restenosis and stenting in balloon coarctation angioplasty. *Acta Paediatr* 1997;86:367.

46. Ebeid MR, Prieto LR, Latson LA. Use of balloon-expandable stents for coarctation of the aorta: initial results and intermediate-term follow-up. *J Am Coll Cardiol* 1997;30:1847.

47. Ovaert C, Benson LN, Nykanen D, et al. Transcatheter treatment of coarctation of the aorta: a review. *Pediatr Cardiol* 1998; 19:27.

48. D'Souza SJ, Tsai WAS, Silver MM, et al. Diagnosis and management of stenotic aorto-arteriopathy in childhood. *J Pediatr* 1998;132:1016.

49. Fletcher SE, Cheatham JP, Froemming S. Aortic aneurysm following primary balloon angioplasty and secondary endovascular stent placement in the treatment of native coarctation of the aorta. *Catheter Cardiovasc Diagn* 1998;44:40.

50. Ruiz CE. Stenting coarctation of the aorta: forget ye not-better is the evil of good. *Catheter Cardiovasc Diagn* 1998;44:45.

51. Redington AN, Hayes AM, Ho SY. Transcatheter stent implantation to treat aortic coarctation in infancy. *Br Heart J* 1993;69:80.

52. Cheatham J, Tower A, Ruiz C, et al. The transcatheter treatment of coarctation of the aorta using balloon expandable intravascular stents: development of the NuMED Cheatham Platinum (CP) stent and Balloon-in-Balloon (BIB) catheter. Abstract presentation at the 11 International Symposium on Diseases of the Aorta, Sao Paulo, Brazil, 1999.

53. Sawada S, Fujiwara Y, Koyama T, et al. Self-expandable metal-lic stent for use in venous occlusions. *Nippon lgaku Hoshasen Gakkai Zasshi* 1990;50:599.

54. Lindstrom F, Lunderquist A, Jakobsson P. Endoprosthetic dilatation of the vena cava eliminates obstruction in superior vena cava syndrome. *Lakartidningen* 1991;88:52.

55. Sawada S, Fujiwara Y, Koyama T, et al. Application of expandable metallic stents to the venous system. *Acta Radiol* 1992;33:156.

56. Edwards RD, Cassidy J, Taylor A. Case report: superior vena cava obstruction complicated by central venous thrombosis-treatment with thrombolysis and Gianturco-Z stents. *Clin Radiol* 1992;45:278.

57. Eng J, Sabanathan S. Management of superior vena cava obstruction with self-expanding intraluminal stents. Two case reports. *Scand J Thorac Cardiovasc Surg* 1993;27:53.

58. Watkinson AF, Hansell DM. Expandable Wallstent for the treatment of obstruction of the superior vena cava. *Thorax* 1993;48: 915.

59. Rosenblum J, Leef J, Messersmith R, et al. Intravascular stents in the management of acute superior vena cava obstruction of benign etiology. *J Parent Enteral Nutr* 1994;18:362.

60. Nicholason AA, Ettles DF, Arnold A, et al. Treatment of malignant superior vena cava obstruction: metal stents or radiation therapy. *J Vasc lnterv Radiol* 1997;8:781.

61. Benito F, Sanchez C, Oliver J. Stent implantation in systemic venous baffle obstruction after Mustard-type operation repair in an adult. *Rev Esp Cardiol* 1997;50:904.

62. Ing FF, Mullins GE, Grifka RG, et al. Stent dilation of superior vena cava and innominate vein obstructions permits transvenous pacing lead implantation. *Pacing Clin Electrophysiol* 1998; 21:1517.

63. Ward CJB, Mullins CE, Nihill MR, et al. Use of intravascular stents in systemic venous and systemic venous baffle obstructions. *Circulation* 1995;91:2948.

64. Rosenthal E, Qureshi SA, Tynan M, et al. Percutaneous pacemaker lead extraction and stent implantation for superior vena cava occlusion due to pacemaker leads. *Am J Cardiol* 1996;77: 670.

65. Abdulhamed JM, Yousef SA, Khan MAA, et al. Placement of endovascular stents for systemic venous obstruction after the Mustard operation. *Cardiol Young* 1994;4:390.

66. Schranz E, Michel-Behnke I, Schmid FX, et al. Gradual angioplasty and stent implantation to treat complete superior vena cava occlusion after Mustard procedure. *Catheter Cardiovasc Diagn* 1996;38:87.

67. O'Laughlin MP. Gradual angioplasty and stent implantation to treat complete superior vena cava occlusion after Mustard procedure. *Catheter Cardiovasc Diagn* 1996;38:91.

68. Powell AJ, Lock JE, Keane JF, et al. Prolongation of RV-PA conduit life span by percutaneous stent implantation. *Circulation* 1995;92:3282.

69. Hosking MCK, Benson LN, Nakanishi T, et al. Intravascular stent prosthesis for right ventricular outflow obstruction. *J Am Coll Cardiol* 1992;20:373.

70. Hayes AM, Nykanen DG, McCrindle SW, et al. Use of balloon expandable stents in the palliative relief of obstructed right ventricular conduits. *Cardiol Young* 1997;7:423.

71. Gibbs JL, Uzun O, Blackburn ME, et al. Right ventricular outflow stent implantation: an alternative to palliative surgical relief of infundibular pulmonary stenosis. *Heart* 1997;77:176.

72. Hijazi ZM. lnterventionalists: watch out for coronary arterial anomalies in tetralogy of Fallot (Editorial). *Catheter Cardiovasc Diagn* 1997;42:408.

73. Moore JW, Kirby WC, Lovett EJ, et al. Use of an intravascular endoprothesis (stent) to establish and maintain short-term patency of the ductus arteriosus in newborn lambs. *Cardiovasc lntervent Radiol* 1991;14:299.

74. Ruiz GE, Gamra H, Zhang HP, et al. Brief report: stenting of the ductus arteriosus as a bridge to cardiac transplantation in infants with the hypoplastic left heart syndrome. *N Engl J Med* 1993;328:1605.

75. Abrams SE, Walsh KP. Arterial duct morphology with reference to angioplasty and stenting. *Int J Cardiol* 1993;40:27.

76. Ruiz CE, Zhang HP, Larsen RL. The role of interventional cardiology in pediatric heart transplantation. *J Heart Lung Transplant* 1993;12:S164.

77. Gibbs JL, Wren C, Watterson KG, et al. Stenting of the arterial duct combined with banding of the pulmonary arteries and atrial septectomy or septostomy: a new approach to palliation for the hypoplastic left heart syndrome. *Br Heart J* 1993;69:551.

78. Slack MC, Kirby WC, Towbin JA, et al. Stenting of the ductus arteriosus in hypoplastic left heart syndrome as an ambulatory bridge to cardiac transplantation. *Am J Cardiol* 1994;74:636.

79. Zahn EM, Chang AC, Aldousany A, et al. Emergent stent placement for acute Blalock-Taussig shunt obstruction after Stage I Norwood surgery. *Catheter Cardiovasc Diagn* 1997;42:191.

80. Coles JG, Yemets I, Najm HK, et al. Experience with repair of congenital heart defects using adjunctive endovascular devices. *J Thorac Cardiovasc Surg* 1995;110:1513.

81. Gibbs JL, Rothman MT, Rees MR, et al. Stenting of the arterial duct: a new approach to palliation for pulmonary atresia. *Br Heart J* 1992;67:240.

82. Zahn EM, Lima VC, Benson LN, et al. Use of endovascular stents to increase pulmonary blood flow in pulmonary atresia with ventricular septal defect. *Am J Cardiol* 1992;70:411.

83. McLeod KA, Blackburn ME, Gibbs JL. Stenting of stenosed aortopulmonary collaterals: a new approach to palliation in pulmonary atresia with multifocal aortopulmonary blood supply. *Br Heart J* 1994;71:487.

84. Redington AN, Somerville J. Stenting of aortopulmonary collaterals in complex pulmonary atresia. *Circulation* 1996;94:2479.

85. Vance MS. Use of Palmaz stents to palliate pulmonary atresia with ventricular septal defect and stenotic aortopulmonary collaterals. *Catheter Cardiovasc Diagn* 1997;40:387.

86. Brown SC, Eyskens B, Mertens L, et al. Percutaneous treatment of stenosed major aortopulmonary collaterals with balloon dilatation and stenting: what can be achieved? *Heart* 1998;79:24.

87. Driscoll DJ, Hesslein PS, Mullins CE. Congenital stenosis of individual pulmonary veins: clinical spectrum and unsuccessful treatment by transvenous balloon dilation. *Am J Cardiol* 1982;49:1767.

88. Hosking M, Redmond M, Allen L, et al. Responses of systemic and pulmonary veins to the presence of an intravascular stent in a swine model. *Catheter Cardiovasc Diagn* 1995;36:90.

89. Santoro G, Formigari R, Mazzera E, et al. Intraoperative stent implantation in congenital stenosis of pulmonary veins. *G Ital Cardiol* 1996;26:201.

90. Mendelsohn AM, Bove EL, Lupinetti FM, et al. Intraoperative and percutaneous stenting of congenital pulmonary artery and vein stenosis. *Circulation* 1993;88:210.

91. Hosking MC, Murdison KA, Duncan WJ. Transcatheter stent implantation for recurrent pulmonary venous pathway obstruction after the Mustard procedure. *Br Heart J* 1994;72:85.

92. Coulson JD, Bullaboy CA. Concentric placement of stents to relieve an obstructed anomalous pulmonary venous connection. *Catheter Cardiovasc Diagn* 1997;42:201.

93. Cheatham J, Tower A, Ruiz C, et al. Initial experience using the NuMED Cheatham Platinum (CP) stent and a new balloon delivery catheter in children and adults with congenital heart disease. *Catheter Cardiovasc Interv* 1999;47:122.

94. Bandel JW, Tortoledo F, Izabuirre L, et al. Primera experiencia en el pais con un Cheatham platinum NuMED stent (CP stent) para el tratamiento de la coartacion de aorta. *Gac Med Caracas* 2000;108:35.

95. Jain A, Ramee SR, Culpepper WR, et al. Intravascular ultrasound-assisted percutaneous angioplasty of aortic coarctation. *Am Heart J* 1992;123:514.

96. Benson LN, Ovaert C, Nykanen D, et al. Nonsurgical management of coarctation of the aorta. *J Interv Cardiol* 1998;11:345.

97. Suarez de Lezo J, Pan M, Romero M, et al. Immediate and follow-up findings after stent treatment for severe coarctation of the aorta. *Am J Cardiol* 1999;83:400.

98. Gunn J, Cleveland R, Gaines P. Covered stent to treat co-existent coarctation and aneurysm of the aorta in a young man. *Heart* 1999;82:351.

99. Magee AG, Brzezinska-Rajszys G, Qureshi SA, et al. Stent implantation of aortic coarctation and recoarctation. *Heart* 1999;82:600.

100. Brzezinska-Rajszys G, Qureshi SA, Ksiazyk J, et al. Middle aortic syndrome treated by stent implantation. *Heart* 1999;81:166.

101. Marshall AC, Perry SB, Keane JF, et al. Early results and medium-term follow-up of stent implantation for mild residual or recurrent aortic coarctation. *Am Heart J* 2000;139:1054.

102. Thanopoulos BD, Hadjinikolaou L, Konstadopoulou GN, et al. Stent treatment for coarctation of the aorta: intermediate term follow-up and technical considerations. *Heart* 2000;84:65.

103. Ruiz CE, Zhang HP, Butt AI, et al. Percutaneous treatment of abdominal aortic aneurysm in a swine model. *Circulation* 1997;96:2438.

104. Gibbs JL. Treatment options for coarctation of the aorta. *Heart* 2000;84:11.

105. Cheatham JP. Initial use of the IntraTherapeutics, Inc. IntraStent DoubleStrut biliary endoprosthesis in the treatment of congenital heart disease. The 3rd World Congress of Pediatric Cardiology and Cardiac Surgery, Poster Presentation, May 2001.

39

NEWER STENTS IN THE MANAGEMENT OF VASCULAR STENOSES IN CHILDREN

P. SYAMASUNDAR RAO

The concept of stenting a vascular wall to treat stenotic lesions was developed in the 1960s. Experimental work in the 1980s established the feasibility and potential for clinical benefit of such prosthesis. Clinical studies in the late 1980s and early 1990s suggested that stents are useful in the treatment of stenotic lesions of coronary arteries, iliac arteries, and renal arteries in adults (1–4). Pediatric applications followed (5). The utility of stents in treating obstructive lesions of the branch pulmonary arteries (5–7), systemic (8,9) and pulmonary (10) veins, and aorta (11) is well established. Stents have also been employed in the treatment of right ventricular outflow tract obstruction (12). The use of stents to keep the ductus open in order to provide systemic blood flow in hypoplastic left heart syndrome patients has been described (13). Stents have also been used to provide/augment pulmonary blood flow in pulmonary atresia patients either by stenting the ductus arteriosus (14,15) or stenotic aortopulmonary collateral vessels (16). Two types of stents (i.e., balloon-expandable and self-expandable) have been used. Of these, balloon-expandable Palmaz stents are most commonly used (5–18). The utility of Palmaz stents has been discussed in detail in the preceding chapters. Despite good results in relieving the obstruction, the Palmaz stents have a number of disadvantages, including the need for a large delivery sheath, balloon rupture, stent displacement, and difficulty in traversing a tortuous course. For these reasons we (19) and others (20,21) have tried other types of stents, which are more flexible and are likely to circumvent some or most of the problems observed with Palmaz stents. These are Bridge (Medtronic AVE, Santa Rosa, CA), NuMED CP (NuMED, Hopkinton, NY), IntraStent (IntraTherapeutics, St. Paul, MN), and Corinthian (Cordis Endovascular, Warren, NJ) stents. The NuMED CP stent was dis-

cussed in a preceding chapter. The remaining stents will be reviewed in this chapter.

BRIDGE STENTS

The Stent

The stent is composed of 2-mm-long stainless steel sinusoidal elements connected to each other by laser fusion. The elliptorectangular strut design of the sinusoidal elements imparts strength to the stent. The dual-helical fusion of the sinusoidal elements increases longitudinal flexibility. The edges of the stent are smooth, so that injury to the balloon is minimized. The stents are mounted on the delivery balloon by a combination of heat and pressure by creating "pillows" of the balloon material to fill spaces between the struts of the stent along its entire length (Figures 39.1 and 39.2). This stent retention mech-

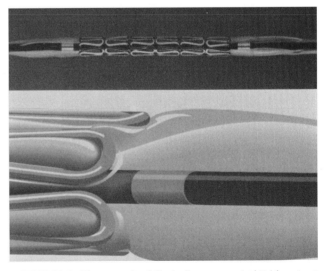

FIGURE 39.1. Photograph of the balloon-mounted Bridge stent (top) and of the stent-retaining system showing "pillows" in between the stent struts (bottom). (Courtesy of Medtronic Arterial Vascular Engineering, Santa Rosa, CA.)

P. Syamasundar Rao: Professor of Pediatrics, Medicine, and Cardiology, Department of Pediatrics, University of Texas-Houston Medical School; Director, Division of Pediatric Cardiology, Memorial Hermann Children's Hospital, Houston, Texas

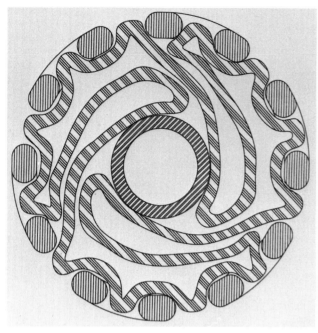

FIGURE 39.2. Cross-sectional view of the balloon-mounted stent demonstrating the method of folding the balloon and how "pillows" of the balloon between struts of the stent are secured. (Courtesy of Medtronic Arterial Vascular Engineering, Santa Rosa, CA.)

anism prevents displacement/dislodgment of the stent from the balloon while traversing a tortuous course. Photographs of the stent are shown in Figures 39.1 and 39.3. The balloon-mounted stents are manufactured in different diameters (6 to 10 mm in 1-mm increments) and lengths (28, 40, and 60 mm) as shown in Table 39.1. At the time of stent expansion, there is minimal foreshortening of the stent (Table 39.1).

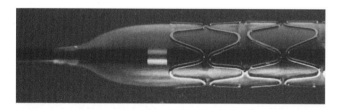

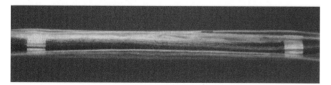

FIGURE 39.3. Photograph of an inflated balloon with stent expanded (top) and the balloon catheter after the stent has been deployed (bottom). (Courtesy of Medtronic Arterial Vascular Engineering, Santa Rosa, CA.)

TABLE 39.1. DIAMETERS AND LENGTHS OF BRIDGE STENTS

S No.	Diameter (mm)	Length (mm)	Length after Implantation (mm)
1	6	28*	27
2	7	28*	27
3	8	28*	26
4	9	28†	25
5	10	28†	24
6	6	40*	40
7	7	40*	40
8	8	40*	39
9	9	40†	38
10	10	40†	37

*60-mm-long stents are also available. They will shorten to 59 mm on deployment.
†60-, 80-, and 100-mm-long stents are also available. The deployed length is 1 to 3 mm shorter than the original length.

Implantation Procedure

Informed consent from the patient/parents, as appropriate, is obtained for off-label use of bridge stents. The procedure is performed under conscious sedation. Cardiac catheterization is performed to confirm the clinical and echocardiographic diagnosis and to exclude other associated lesions. Pressure gradients across the stenotic lesion and selective cineangiography to demonstrate the stenotic lesion are initially obtained. Measurements are made of (a) diameters of the stenotic site and of the vessel proximal and distal to the obstructive lesion, (b) the diameter of the contralateral pulmonary artery in branch pulmonary artery (BPA) stenoses, and (c) "stentable" length of the vessel in two orthogonal views and averaged. These data are used in the selection of expanded diameter and length of the stent. An arterial line, to monitor the blood pressure and blood gas values, is inserted before stenting. Heparin 100 U/kg is administered, and activated clotting times are monitored and maintained between 200 and 250 seconds by administering additional doses as necessary.

A 5F multi-A2 (Cordis, Miami, FL) or 7F balloon wedge (Arrows International, Reading, PA) is positioned across the stenotic lesion, usually with the aid of a straight 0.035-inch Benston guide wire (Cook, Bloomington, IN). The guide wire is then replaced with either an extra-stiff exchange length 0.035-inch Amplatz (Cook) or a super-stiff, short-tipped Amplatz (Meditech, Natick, MA) guide wire and the catheter is removed. An appropriate-sized long blue Cook sheath (Cook) with a multipurpose curve and a radiopaque marker at the tip is introduced over the stiff guide wire. Once the tip of sheath is past the region intended to be stented, the dilator is removed and the sheath is flushed appropriately to prevent inadvertent air entry. In some cases a short sheath (see results section) is introduced. The stent-mounted catheter is advanced over stiff guide wire, but within the sheath and is positioned across the site of obstruction, and the tip of the sheath is withdrawn proximal to the site of obstruction, based on bony landmarks. In cases where a long blue Cook sheath is inserted, contrast is injected via the side arm of the sheath. The position of the stent is adjusted as needed. The balloon is inflated at the manufacturer-recommended pressure. Additional balloon inflations, either with the same or with a larger balloon catheter, are performed as necessary. Following deployment of the stent, the balloon is removed and a multitrack catheter (Braun, Bethlehem, PA) is positioned over the wire and pressure pullback recordings and cineangiogram are performed to assess the result of stent placement. The effect of heparin is not reversed, nor is additional heparin administered. Three doses of cefazolin 25 mg/kg/dose are administered at 6- to 8-hour intervals. The first dose is given in the catheterization laboratory. Platelet-inhibiting doses of aspirin (5 to 10 mg/kg) are administered daily for a total of 6 weeks. Chest roentgenograms, two-dimensional and Doppler echocardiographic studies, and quantitative pulmonary perfusion scan (in BPA stenosis cases) are obtained on the morning following the procedure. Follow-up clinical, chest x-ray, and echocardiographic studies are performed 1, 6, and 12 months after the procedure and yearly thereafter.

Case Material

The patients presented in this section include the cases reported previously by us (19). The patient characteristics and results will be described separately for each lesion.

Branch Pulmonary Artery Stenosis

Patient and Lesion Characteristics

There were eight patients in this group. Their ages were 0.4 to 13 years, with a median of 10 years. They weighed 6.1 to 48.2 kg, with a median of 25 kg. Complex congenital heart disease with pulmonary atresia or severe stenosis was present in seven patients. Six had total surgical correction, but significant branch pulmonary artery stenosis persisted. The seventh patient had a bidirectional Glenn procedure but had severe long-segment left pulmonary artery stenosis. The eighth patient had a diaphragmatic hernia repaired in infancy and had severe narrowing of the left pulmonary artery.

Decreased perfusion in the ipsilateral lung was observed by quantitative pulmonary perfusion scans: 22.8% ± 9.4% (range, 12% to 34%; median, 19%). The stenotic segments measured 1 to 4.8 mm in diameter, with a median of 3.9 mm. The peak-to-peak systolic pressure gradient across the stenosed pulmonary artery varied between 20 and 41 mm Hg, with a median of 23 mm Hg.

Procedural and Stent Data

An 8F long blue Cook sheath was used for stent deployment in five patients. In the remaining three children, 8- or 7F short sheaths were used. Six- to 10-mm-diameter stents were used. Six stents were 40 mm long and two were 28 mm long.

Immediate Results

The peak-to-peak systolic pressure gradient across the stenotic lesion decreased ($p < .01$) from 29 ± 11 to 10 ± 10 mm Hg following stent deployment. Similarly, stenotic diameter of the vessel increased ($p < .01$) from 3.7 ± 1.4 to 9 ± 2 mm. Angiographic examples are shown in Figures 39.4 to 39.7. Ipsilateral pulmonary flow, determined by quantitative pulmonary perfusion scans improved ($p < .05$) from 23% ± 9% to 41% ± 15%.

Complications

Dislodgment of a left pulmonary artery stent toward the main pulmonary artery was observed immediately following the removal of the deflated balloon was seen in one patient. It could not be repositioned into the left pulmonary artery, but it could be repositioned into the normal right pulmonary artery, where it was expanded and implanted. Immediately thereafter, a Palmaz stent (Cordis Endovascular, Warren, NJ) mounted on a BIB (NuMED, Hopkinson, NY) catheter was successfully implanted at the intended site. No other complications were encountered.

Follow-up Results

Follow-up data, 6 to 12 months following the procedure were available in all eight patients. Peak instantaneous Doppler gradient, which decreased ($p < .01$) from 59 ± 16 mm Hg to 16 ± 7 mm Hg immediately after stent placement, remained unchanged (19 ± 10 mm Hg; $p > .1$) at follow-up. Follow-up catheterization and angiography was undertaken in three children. No change in angiographic or hemodynamic data was observed. Redilatation of one stent was successfully performed in one child; there was constriction of the stent at the time of implantation. One infant with complex cardiac disease with single-ventricle physiology (Figure 39.7) underwent uneventful bidirectional Glenn procedure 4 months after stent deployment. No complications related to the stent were observed during follow-up.

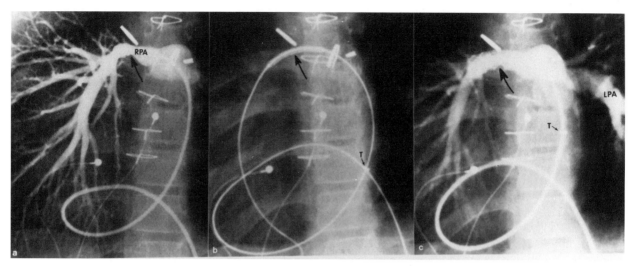

FIGURE 39.4. Selected cine frames from 30-degree right anterior oblique view demonstrating **(a)** narrowed right pulmonary artery (RPA) *(arrow)*, **(b)** position of the stent before implantation *(large arrow)* and **(c)** improved size of the pulmonary artery following stent deployment. Note the tortuous course of the catheter in a patient with dextrocardia and morphologic left ventricle to pulmonary artery conduit (not shown). The position of the tip of the long blue Cook sheath (T) is shown. Because of its length (65 cm), it could not be advanced any further, but the stent catheter could easily be maneuvered across the stenotic RPA. LPA, left pulmonary artery; RPA, right pulmonary artery. (From Rao PS, Balfour IC, Singh GK, et al. Bridge stents in the management of obstructive vascular lesions in children. *Am J Cardiol* 2001;88:699–702, with permission.)

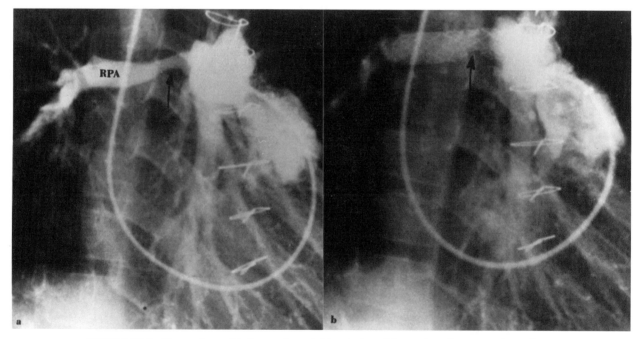

FIGURE 39.5. Cineangiographic frames in a right anterior oblique view demonstrating a long segment *(arrow)* narrowing of the right pulmonary artery (RPA) **(a)** which is expanded following stent placement **(b)**. There is mild residual constriction *(arrow* in **b**). This child has infrahepatic interruption of the inferior vena cava with azygous continuation and therefore the stent was implanted via transjugular approach. In this patient, the procedure was performed without the use of a long sheath.

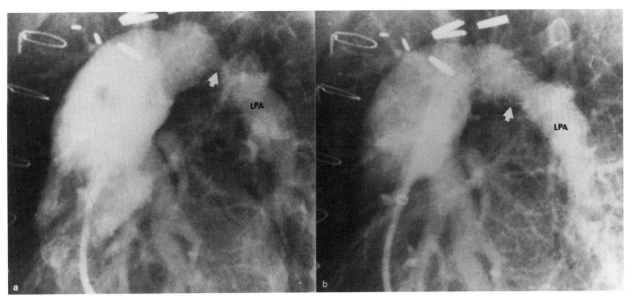

FIGURE 39.6. Left pulmonary artery (LPA) stenosis prior to (**a**) and following (**b**) stent implantation demonstrating wide-open LPA. Both cine frames are obtained in a left anterior oblique view. (From Rao PS, Balfour IC, Singh GK, et al. Bridge stents in the management of obstructive vascular lesions in children. *Am J Cardiol* 2001;88:699–702, with permission.)

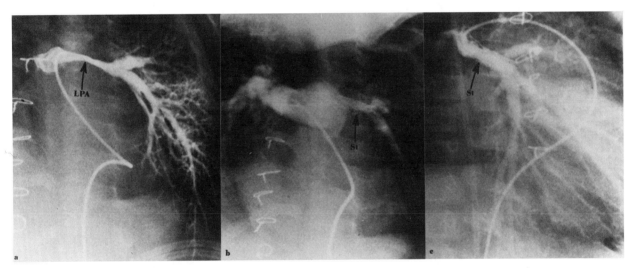

FIGURE 39.7. Selected cineangiographic frames in a "sitting-up" view demonstrating a long-segment, hypoplastic left pulmonary artery (LPA) in **a** that was enlarged by a stent (St) shown in **b.** Restudy 4 months later (**c**) continues to show patency of the stent. Mild neointimal proliferation is seen at the proximal end of the St. Successful bidirectional Glenn was performed following the last study.

Right Ventricular Outflow Obstruction

Two children, ages 5.5 and 6.0 years, who had truncus arteriosus repaired in infancy with a right-ventricular-to-pulmonary-artery aortic homograft, developed obstruction of the conduit. Peak systolic pressure gradients across the calcified homograft during cardiac catheterization were 64 and 60 mm Hg, respectively. A 10-mm-diameter, 40-mm-long

Bridge (Medtronic AVE, Santa Rosa, CA) stent was implanted across the stenosed conduit (Figure 39.8). The conduit was then expanded with a 12-mm-diameter XXL balloon (Meditech, Boston, MA). The lower end of the stent was expanded to a 16-mm (Figure 39.9) balloon. The peak gradients, immediately after implantation of the stent, were reduced to 25 and 20 mm Hg, respectively. Follow-up for 6 months in one child revealed peak instantaneous

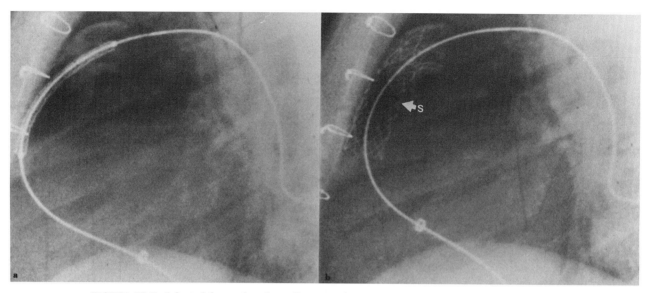

FIGURE 39.8. Selected frame for cineradiograms demonstrating position of the unexpanded stent across the stenotic conduit (**a**) and of the expanded stent (S) following its implantation (**b**).

Doppler gradient of 36 mm Hg. The other child has so far been followed for 18 months with a Doppler peak instantaneous gradient of 50 mm Hg. None of the patients has so far required replacement of the conduit.

Coarctation of the Aorta

Two patients, both 15 years old, developed aortic recoarctation after surgical repair of their coarctations in infancy. Systemic hypertension was present. Stent was implanted in one patient via an 8F long blue Cook sheath introduced through the right femoral artery percutaneously. The second patient had bilateral femoral artery blockage by previous procedures. Iliac artery cut-down was performed by the general surgery group and an 8F short sheath was placed into it, and the hub of the sheath was exteriorized. A 10-mm-diameter, 40-mm-long Bridge stent was implanted via the 8F short sheath initially. The stent was then dilated with a 14-mm diameter XXL balloon catheter (Meditech). The peak-to-peak systolic pressure gradients were 25 and 30 mm Hg, respectively, and the

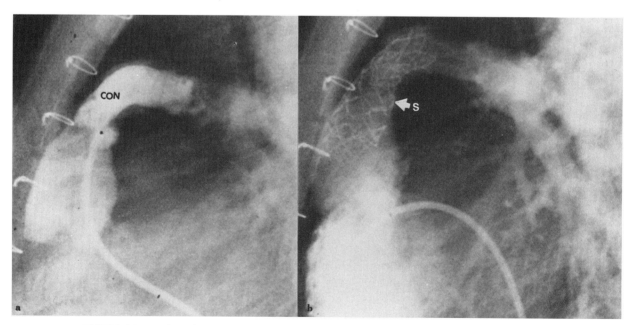

FIGURE 39.9. Selected cineangiograms showing stenotic conduit (CON) prior to (**a**) and following (**b**) stent (S) placement and enlargement. Note the lower end is wider because it was dilated with a larger balloon.

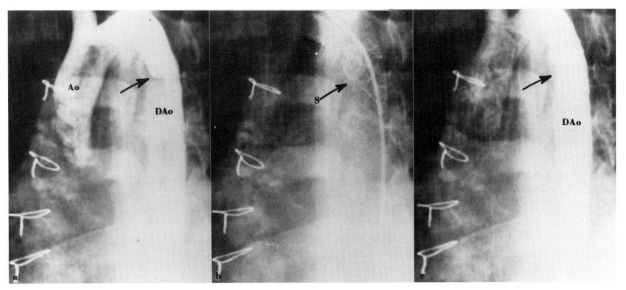

FIGURE 39.10. Aortic arch cineangiographic frames in a left anterior oblique view demonstrating aortic coarctation *(arrow)* (**a**) that is completely abolished following stent placement (**c**). Cineradiographic frame (**b**) showing the stent (S) shown in the middle. Ao, aorta; DAo descending aorta. (From Rao PS, Balfour IC, Singh GK, et al. Bridge stents in the management of obstructive vascular lesions in children. *Am J Cardiol* 2001;88:699–702, with permission.)

gradients were abolished following stent deployment. Angiographically (Figure 39.10), there was improvement. Follow-up clinical and echocardiographic studies performed 6 months after the procedure suggested no residual obstruction.

Superior Vena Caval Stenosis

Surgical repair of sinus venous atrial septal defect with partial anomalous pulmonary venous return was performed at age 16 months. At age 2 years, this child developed signs of

superior vena caval obstruction. Two-dimensional and Doppler echocardiographic studies revealed obstructed superior vena cava. Cardiac catheterization and angiography (Figure 39.11A) confirmed severe superior vena caval stenosis. The mean gradient across the obstruction was 19 mm Hg. A 10-mm-diameter, 28-mm-long Bridge stent was implanted (Figure 39.11B) via a long 8F blue Cook sheath introduced via the right femoral vein. The pressure gradient was completely abolished, and there was remarkable angiographic improvement (Figure 39.11C). At the latest follow-

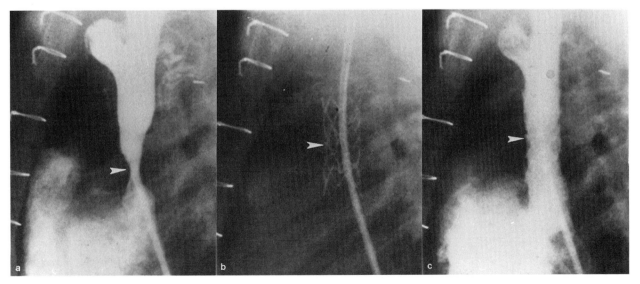

FIGURE 39.11. Superior vena caval (SVC) cineangiographic frame (**a**) in lateral view demonstrating narrowed *(arrow)* SVC. The stent is shown in the middle panel (**b**). Following stent deployment (**c**), the SVC constriction is completely relieved. RA, right atrium.

up 6 months after stent placement, there was no clinical or Doppler evidence for superior vena caval obstruction.

Comments

The data presented in this group of patients, though small, demonstrate feasibility, safety, and efficacy of Bridge stents in the management of stenotic vascular lesions in the pediatric population.

Implantation of the stents via small-caliber sheaths is feasible. Also, it was feasible to implant the stents without a long sheath. This is particularly useful in situations where a long sheath could not be introduced. The stents could be passed through tortuous courses (e.g., Figure 39.4). Indeed, in this particular patient (Figure 39.4), prior attempts to place a Palmaz stent resulted in balloon rupture. We were able to maneuver this stent into the iliac vein, where it was implanted. The ability to pass through tortuous courses may be related to the flexibility of the stent. Displacement of the stent from the balloon did not occur in any case. This may be related to creation of "pillows" of the balloon material in between the struts of the stent (Figures 39.1 and 39.2). No balloon ruptures occurred; this may be related to smooth edges of the stent. Perforation and vessel wall injury, such as seen with Palmaz stent (22,23), is unlikely to be seen with this stent because of rounded edges of the stent and uniform expansion without flaring edges (23).

The effectiveness of the stent in relieving the pulmonary arterial obstruction appears to be similar to that observed with the Palmaz stent (5–7). Despite calcification of the conduit, no balloon rupture was observed during stent deployment in the conduit stenosis patients. So far, prolongation of conduit life has been achieved, as has been demonstrated with Palmaz stents (24). Relief of systemic venous obstruction is also similar to that seen after implantation of Palmaz stents (8,9). Relief of coarctation of the aorta is also similar to that reported with Palmaz stents (11,25–27).

Only one complication occurred; there was displacement of the stent after implantation. This may have been related to entrapment of balloon material onto the stent, which might have pulled the stent while withdrawing the balloon. In this patient, only a short sheath was used. If a long sheath had been used, the tip of the sheath could have been advanced into the stent over the deflated balloon (28) to prevent inadvertent displacement of the stent. We therefore advocate using a long delivery sheath routinely, unless it is not feasible to do so, such as in the aortic coarctation case cited earlier.

The major disadvantage of the Bridge stent is lack of availability of larger-diameter stents (e.g., 12-, 14-, 16-, 18-, and 20-mm diameters).

In conclusion, the data, though limited, suggested feasibility, safety, and effectiveness of Bridge stents in relieving vascular obstructive lesions in children. These stents may serve as an excellent alternative to Palmaz stents (19). Availability of larger-diameter stents will make this stent more useful than it is now.

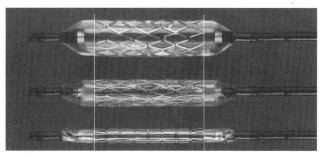

FIGURE 39.12. Photograph of an IntraStent DoubleStrut Para-Mount stent mounted on a balloon unexpanded *(bottom)* and expanded to varying diameters *(middle and top)* demonstrating no shortening. (Courtesy of IntraTherapeutics, St. Paul, MN.)

INTRASTENT STENTS

The Stent

This is a DoubleStrut (Intra Therapeutics, St. Paul, MN) stent cut from 316L stainless steel tube by laser. It has a good radial strength and is flexible, allowing it to traverse tortuous courses. The unique cell design and parallel struts allow distribution of stress over a wider area and thus uniformly support the vessel lumen. When expanded, there is no shortening of the stent (Figures 39.12 and 39.13). The manufacturer uses a "Micro-Grip" internal finish of the stent by creating better surface tension. This is presumed to minimize stent slippage from the balloon. The stents are available in both balloon-mounted [IntraStent DoubleStrut ParaMount (Figure 39.12)] and unmounted [IntraStent DoubleStrut LD (Figure 39.13)]. Balloon-mounted stents are available in 5- to 8-mm-diameter sizes, in 1-mm increments. Several lengths and sizes are available, 16 and 36 mm (Table 39.2). Unmounted stents are also available in various lengths (Table 39.2). The most useful sizes for pediatric use are 16, 26, and 36 mm long. The manufacturer

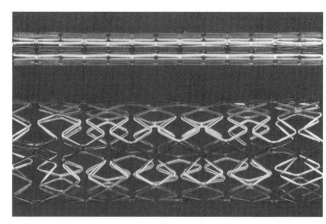

FIGURE 39.13. Photographs of a preexpanded IntraStent DoubleStrut LD stent *(top)* and following expansion *(bottom)* demonstrating no shortening. (Courtesy of IntraTherapeutics, St. Paul, MN.)

TABLE 39.2. DIAMETERS AND LENGTHS OF INTRASTENTS

S No.	Diameter (mm)	Length (mm)*
	IntraStent DoubleStrut ParaMount (Balloon-Mounted)	
1	5	16
2	6	16
3	7	16
4	8	16
5	5	36
6	6	36
7	7	36
8	8	36
	IntraStent DoubleStrut LD (Not Balloon-Mounted)	
9	9, 10, 11, and 12	16
10	9, 10, 11, and 12	26
11	9, 10, 11, and 12†	36
12	9, 10, 11, and 12	56
13	9, 10, 11, and 12	76

*There is no discernible shortening of the stents on expansion.
†We were able to expand these stents up to 18 and 20 mm without evidence of loss of vessel wall support.

does not recommend expansion above 12 mm, although we have expanded it up to 20 mm without any problem.

Implantation Procedure

The procedure of stent implantation is similar to that described for the Bridge stents. The unmounted stents, however, need to be mounted on delivery balloon of appropriate size. We have used BIB balloons (NuMED, Hopkinton, NY) for this purpose. The size of the sheath for stent delivery should be one French size larger than that required for BIB catheter.

Results

There is only limited experience with this stent. Data reported in an abstract form by Rutledge (20), Ing (21), and their associates and our personal experience will be reviewed.

Rutledge and her associates (20) reported IntraStent implantation in 13 patients with branch pulmonary artery stenosis, aortic coarctation and vena caval stenoses. The patients were 1.4 to 32 (median 10) years of age and weighed 11 to 88 (median 22) kg. Stented vessel diameter increased from 5.7 ± 3.7 to 11.6 ± 3.3 mm ($p < .001$). Data on gradient reduction were not given. They did not observe any complications. They concluded that these stents are safe and effective in treatment of vascular stenoses associated with congenital heart defects.

Ing and his associates (21) also report their experience with these stents in 13 patients, ages 0.4 to 21.3 (median, 3) years. They weighed 5.4 to 68.2 (median, 24.9) kg. Fol-

lowing stent implantation, the peak-to-peak systolic pressure gradient decreased from 28.8 ± 14.8 to 4.8 ± 4.9 mm Hg ($p < .05$) and stented vessel diameter increased ($p < .05$) from 5.1 ± 2.6 to 8.9 ± 3.2 mm. They reported two complications, one circumferential balloon rupture before full expansion of the stent, requiring surgical removal, and another, a pinpoint balloon rupture after full expansion, not requiring additional interventions. The authors attribute the circumferential balloon rupture to heavily calcified homograft rather than to the stent. Neither of the preceding groups reported follow-up data.

Our personal experience at Cardinal Glennon Children's Hospital is limited to nine patients and includes branch pulmonary artery stenosis ($N = 5$), aortic coarctation ($N = 3$), and right ventricular outflow conduit stenosis ($N = 1$). Reduction of pressure gradients and increase in stenotic vessel diameter occurred in each case. The most important finding in our series is that we were able to expand the stent up to 18 and 20 mm without any problem.

Comments

Based on these limited data, the IntraStent appears to be useful in relieving obstructive vascular lesions associated with congenital heart disease and may serve as an effective alternative to Palmaz stents. These stents may have an advantage over Bridge stents, mainly because of the availability of larger-diameter stents.

OTHER STENTS

Corinthian IQ stents (Cordis Endovascular) have been used in a limited number of patients and to date there are no publications on its use. Palmaz Genesis stents (Cordis Endovascular) are another group of flexible stents under development. These stents have been approved since initial drafting of this chapter. Our personal experience in six patients is excellent and comparable to that described in the preceding sections.

CURRENT STATUS

Bridge, IntraStent, and Corinthian stents are available for off-label use. These stents are approved by the FDA for biliary and/or peripheral arterial use. The NuMED CP stent is available only at institutions participating in clinical trials.

SUMMARY AND CONCLUSION

Palmaz stents have been used in the past for treatment of vascular obstructive lesions in children. Because of some problems with the stent, mainly balloon ruptures and longitudinal rigidity, a number of investigators studied the utility of more flexible stents. Available data on Bridge, IntraStent, Palmaz Genesis, and NuMED$_{cp}$ stents suggest their feasibility, safety, and effectiveness in relief of obstructive vascular lesions, and these stents may serve as alternatives to Palmaz stents. Other stents are in development. A larger experience with follow-up data, preferably comparative studies, is necessary to identify the best stent for pediatric or congenital heart disease use.

REFERENCES

1. Sigwart W, Puel J, Mirkowich V, et al. Intravascular stents to prevent occlusion and restenosis after transluminal angioplasty. *N Engl J Med* 1987;316:701–706.
2. Palmaz JC, Richter GM, Noeldge G, et al. Intraluminal stents in atherosclerotic iliac artery stenosis: preliminary report of a multicenter study. *Radiology* 1988;168:727–731.
3. Levine MJ, Leonard BM, Burke IA, et al. Clinical and angiographic results of balloon-expandable intracoronary stents in right coronary artery stenosis. *J Am Coll Cardiol* 1990;16:332–339.
4. Rees CR, Palmaz JC, Becker CJ, et al. Palmaz stents in atherosclerotic stenosis involving the ostia of the renal arteries: preliminary report of a multicenter study. *Radiology* 1991;181:507–514.
5. O'Laughlin MP, Perry SB, Lock JE, et al. Use of endovascular stents in congenital heart disease. *Circulation* 1991;83:1923–1939.
6. Hijazi ZM, Al-Fadley F, Geggel RL, et al. Stent implantation for relief of pulmonary artery stenosis: immediate and short-term results. *Catheter Cardiovasc Diagn* 1996;38:16–23.
7. Shaffer KM, Mullins CE, Grifka RG, et al. Intravascular stents in congenital heart disease: short- and long-term results from a large single-center experience. *J Am Coll Cardiol* 1998;31:661–667.
8. Chatelain P, Meier B, Friedle B. Stenting of superior vena cava and inferior vena cava for symptomatic narrowing after repeated atrial surgery for D-transposition of the great arteries. *Br Heart J* 1991;66:466–468.
9. Brown SC, Eyskens B, Mertens L, et al. Self-expandable stents for relief of venous baffle obstruction after the Mustard procedure. *Heart* 1998;79:230–233.
10. Hosking MCK, Murdison KA, Duncan WJ. Transcatheter stent implantation for recurrent pulmonary venous pathway obstruction after Mustard procedure. *Br Heart J* 1994;72:85–88.
11. Suarez de Lezo J, Pan M, Romero M, et al. Balloon expandable stent repair of severe coarctation of the aorta. *Am Heart J* 1995;129:1002–1008.
12. Hosking MCK, Benson LN, Nakanishi T, et al. Intravascular stent prosthesis for right ventricular outflow obstruction. *J Am Coll Cardiol* 1992;20:373–380.
13. Ruiz CE, Gamra H, Zhang HP, et al. Stenting of ductus arteriosus as a bridge to cardiac transplantation in infants with the hypoplastic left heart syndrome. *N Engl J Med* 1993;328:1605–1608.
14. Gibbs JL, Rothman MT, Rees MR, et al. Stenting of the arterial duct: a new approach to palliation for pulmonary atresia. *Br Heart J* 1992;67:240–245.
15. Siblini G, Rao PS, Singh GK, et al. Transcatheter management of neonates with pulmonary atresia and intact ventricular septum. *Catheter Cardiovasc Diagn* 1997;42:395–402.
16. Brown SC, Eyskens B, Mertens L, et al. Percutaneous treatment of stenosed major aortopulmonary collaterals with balloon dilatation and stenting: what can be achieved? *Heart* 1998;79:24–28.
17. Redington AN, Weil J, Somerville J. Self-expanding stents in congenital heart disease. *Br Heart J* 1994;72:378–383.
18. Chandar JS, Wolfe SB, Rao PS. Role of stents in the management of congenital heart defects. *J Invasive Cardiol* 1996;8:314–325.
19. Rao PS, Balfour IC, Singh GK, et al. Bridge stents in the management of obstructive vascular lesions in children. *Am J Cardiol* 2001;88:699–702.
20. Rutledge JM, Grifka RG, Nihill MR, et al. Initial experience with Intra-Therapeutics DoubleStrut LD stents in patients with congenital heart disease. *J Am Coll Cardiol* 2001;37:461A(abst).
21. Ing FF, Mathewson JW, Cocalis M, et al. New double strut stent: *in vitro* evaluation of stent geometry following overdilatation and initial clinical experience in congenital heart disease. *J Am Coll Cardiol* 2001;37:467A(abst).
22. Evans J, Saba Z, Rosenfeld H, et al. Aortic laceration secondary to Palmaz stent placement for treatment of superior vena caval syndrome. *Catheter Cardiovasc Interv* 2000;49:160–162.
23. Cheatham JP. A tragedy during Palmaz stent implant for SVC syndrome: was it the stent or was it the balloon delivery system? (Editorial). *Catheter Cardiovasc Interv* 2000;49:163–166.
24. Powell AJ, Lock JE, Keane JF, et al. Prolongation of RV-PA conduit life span by percutaneous stent implantation: intermediate-term results. *Circulation* 1995;92:3282–3288.
25. Bulbul ZR, Bruckheimer E, Love JC, et al. Implantation of balloon expandable stents for coarctation of the aorta: implantation data and short-term results. *Catheter Cardiovasc Diagn* 1996;39:36–42.
26. Ebeid MR, Preito LR, Latson LA. The use of balloon expandable stents for coarctation of the aorta: initial results and intermediate-term follow-up. *J Am Coll Cardiol* 1997;30:1847–1852.
27. Rao PS. Stents in the treatment of aortic coarctation (Editorial). *J Am Coll Cardiol* 1997;30:1853–1855.
28. Recto MR, Ing FF, Grifka RG, et al. A technique to prevent newly implanted stent displacement during subsequent catheter and sheath manipulation. *Catheter Cardiovasc Interv* 2000;49:297–300.

40

PERCUTANEOUS REVASCULARIZATION IN PERIPHERAL VASCULAR DISEASE

PETER R. VALE
RIYAZ BASHIR
KENNETH ROSENFIELD

The peripheral vasculature is complex and fascinating in its biology and dynamic in its function, associated with many unique disease states. Although their primary focus remains in the diagnosis and treatment of cardiac disorders, many cardiovascular specialists are no longer limiting themselves to treatment of coronary artery disease (CAD). Instead, they are adopting a "global vascular management" strategy for their patients that also involves attention to noncoronary manifestations of atherosclerosis, based on the fact that the coronary and noncoronary circulations are inseparable and interdependent. They may each cause disabling or life-threatening symptoms, are affected by the same disease processes, commonly coexist, frequently influence the treatment of either condition, and often require the same treatment modalities.

The increasing popularity of percutaneous therapy for peripheral arterial disease (PAD) underscores the importance for vascular specialists and interventionalists to have a comprehensive understanding of the mechanisms of angioplasty, the indications for intervention, the expected short- and long-term outcome for a given revascularization procedure, and the potential complications. To provide some of the necessary resources, this chapter focuses on catheter-based interventional techniques. Following a basic discussion of general principles pertaining, in particular, to lower-extremity arterial disease, regional areas of interest will be discussed in detail, specifically aortoiliac, femoropopliteal, mesenteric, and thoracic great vessels. Specific chapters will focus on percutaneous revascularization of the carotid and renal arteries and abdominal aortic aneurysms.

Peter R. Vale: Departments of Vascular Medicine and Cardiology, St. Elizabeth's Medical Center, Tufts University School of Medicine, Boston, Massachusetts

Riyaz Bashir: Assistant Professor of Medicine, Department of Internal Medicine, Director of Cardiovascular Diseases, Medical College of Ohio, Toledo, Ohio

Kenneth Rosenfield: Director, Cardiac and Vascular Invasive Services, Cardiology Division, Massachusetts General Hospital, Boston, Massachusetts

GENERAL CONSIDERATIONS

Disease of the peripheral arteries remains a leading cause of morbidity and mortality in the world. Atherosclerosis of the peripheral arteries is the most common cause of symptomatic obstruction in the peripheral arterial tree. It is present in more than 5.5% of women more than 65 years of age and in more than 20% of men and women combined more than 75 years of age (1). An aging population, however, guarantees that the prevalence will continue to increase. The pathophysiologic basis of atherosclerotic PAD is identical to that which occurs in coronary artery atherosclerosis. Likewise, the same risk factors are associated, including tobacco smoking, diabetes mellitus, hypertension, hyperlipidemia, a positive family history, and advanced age. Other disease states that affect the noncoronary circulation include thromboangiitis obliterans (Buerger's disease), the vasculitides, vasospastic disorders, atheroembolic syndromes, and the hypercoagulable states, but these are beyond the scope of this chapter.

The clinical presentation of patients with PAD is highly variable and depends on the involved vascular territory. Symptoms range from mild lower-extremity discomfort during intense exercise, to the presence of constant rest discomfort, painful ulceration, or frank gangrene. Claudication is described variably as pain, tightness, aching, soreness, hardness, or heaviness that occurs in the calf, buttocks, or arch of the foot during ambulation and resolves with rest, similar to the pattern of exertional angina in CAD. Although intermittent claudication can be mild and nondisabling, it can become severely disabling. Pain at rest occurs if the impairment of blood flow is severe enough that oxygen and nutrient supply falls below the resting requirements of the distal tissue. Where the level of tissue ischemia is severe, cell injury and death will occur, leading to tissue breakdown, clinically manifested as ulceration and/or gangrene. Neither of these is likely to resolve without restoration of nutrient (usually pulsatile) flow to the affected extremity. Similar symptoms occur in the hand and/or forearm of patients with severe atherosclerosis of vessels supplying the upper extremities. In mesenteric vessels, however, the extensive collateral circulation generally does not cause symptoms until several major vessels are occluded, at which point abdominal angina or bowel infarction may ensue.

As is the case in CAD, symptoms related to PAD rarely occur until the atherosclerotic process has narrowed the vessel diameter by at least 50%. However, the presence of one or more lesions ≥50% does not imply that the patient will be symptomatic. Indeed, a large number of patients with PAD remain asymptomatic, even in the presence of severe and extensive disease. Patients with complete occlusion of the major blood supply to a limb or organ may have few symptoms if an ample collateral supply is present. Rutherford and colleagues (2), by defining the signs and symptoms according to their intensity, and combining these with non-invasive data, have developed a series of categories to describe the severity of chronic limb ischemia (Table 40.1). Such standardization has greatly enhanced the ability of investigators to perform meaningful comparative analyses of treatment strategies. Furthermore, it has facilitated decision-making for clinicians regarding optimal therapy for a given level of limb ischemia.

In patients with PAD an important consideration in any treatment strategy is the natural history and the uninterrupted clinical course of patients with both symptomatic and asymptomatic disease. The course of lower-extremity arterial disease is usually one of slow progression of symptoms over time (3). Approximately 70% of patients will remain unchanged or less symptomatic after 5 to 10 years. Fewer than 30% will progress to require intervention, and fewer than 10% will need amputation. In addition, patients with diabetes mellitus, who comprise a large percentage of patients with PAD, are a unique subgroup in terms of prognosis and natural history of the disease. Diabetics have a high likelihood of developing critical limb ischemia; indeed, their amputation rate is seven times greater than that in nondiabetic patients with PAD.

Insofar as PAD is a marker for systemic atherosclerosis, a secondary goal is to reduce the incidence of coronary and cerebrovascular events. Therapeutic options include conservative measures, percutaneous intervention, and surgery. With respect to noninvasive measures, risk factor modification (cessation of smoking is paramount) should thus be an important part of any treatment plan and may reduce progression of disease. Because limb ischemia may stimulate collateral growth, formal exercise training in a supervised setting may increase claudication-free walking distance by approximately twofold in patients with mild or moderate symptoms. Those with severe claudication, rest pain, or tissue loss (e.g., Rutherford category ≥3) are less likely to benefit from exercise.

Patients with PAD mostly receive drug treatment for coexisting disease (e.g., hypertension), for risk factor modification (e.g., hyperlipidemia), and as prophylaxis against thrombotic events associated with atherosclerosis (e.g., antiplatelet drugs), predominantly to reduce associated cardiac and cerebrovascular morbidity and mortality. No pharmacologic agent has proved efficacious enough to produce significant improvement in symptoms of PAD to gain widespread acceptance or use. Two established drugs, however, have gained FDA approval despite the fact that controlled trials evaluating efficacy compared with placebo have produced variable results. Pentoxyphylline (Trental), a rheolytic agent, has shown up to a 21% increase over

TABLE 40.1. CLINICAL CATEGORIES OF CHRONIC LIMB ISCHEMIA

Grade	Category	Clinical Description	Objective Criteria
0	0	Asymptomatic	Normal treadmill/stress test
	1	Mild claudication	Completes treadmill exercise,* ankle pressure after exercise <50 mm Hg but >25 mm Hg less than brachial
I	2	Moderate claudication	Between categories 1 and 3
	3	Severe claudication	Cannot complete treadmill exercise and ankle pressure after exercise <50 mm Hg
II	4	Ischemic rest pain	Resting ankle pressure <60 mm Hg, ankle or metatarsal pulse volume recording flat or barely pulsatile; toe pressure <40 mm Hg
	5	Minor tissue loss—nonhealing ulcer, focal gangrene with diffuse pedal ischemia	Resting ankle pressure <40 mm Hg, flat or barely pulsatile ankle or metatarsal pulse volume recording; toe pressure <30 mm Hg
III	6	Major tissue loss—extending above transmetatarsal level, functional foot no longer salvageable	Same as category 5

*Five minutes at 2 mph on a 12% incline.
From Rutherford RB, Flanigan DP, Guptka SK. Suggested standards for reports dealing with lower extremity ischemia. *J Vasc Surg* 1986;4:80, with permission.

placebo in walking distance in recent trials, and patients most likely to benefit were those with symptoms for longer than 1 year and an ankle/brachial index (ABI) < 0.80. However, most investigators agree that Trental is of little overall value in the treatment of symptomatic PAD (4,5). On the other hand, in a recent clinical trial, cilastazol (Pletal), a phosphodiesterase III inhibitor with vasodilator and antiplatelet activity, demonstrated a 47% increase in walking distance compared to placebo (13%) and improved quality of life (6). Prostaglandins have been used in several studies of patients with critical limb ischemia with some success (7). A number of vasodilator (e.g., Ca²⁺ channel blockers, alphaadrenergic antagonists, and others), antiplatelet (e.g., aspirin, ticlopidine, clopidogrel) and metabolic agents (L-carnitine, L-arginine) have been studied, but none has been conclusively demonstrated to improve symptoms related to PAD.

Another novel form of "medical" or "noninvasive" therapy currently under investigation in early Phase I and II clinical trials is the use of growth factors to treat critical limb ischemia (8,9). The premise behind this treatment is that the obstructed main vessel may not require recanalization if flow can be augmented by the development of more collateral vessels, a process termed *therapeutic angiogenesis.* Angiogenic cytokines [e.g., basic fibroblast growth factor (bFGF) and vascular endothelial growth factor (VEGF)] can be administered as recombinant protein or as gene encoding for that protein, either by direct intravascular infusion or by site-specific intramuscular injection.

INTERVENTIONAL STRATEGIES

General Concepts

Significant technological advances over the past 10 years now enable more safe and efficacious invasive treatment of atherosclerotic PAD. However, the slow progression of symptoms should generally temper aggressive recommendations for invasive therapy in PAD. Intervention is therefore only indicated in selected patients with intermittent claudication in whom exercise treatment has failed; except in two unique subgroups:

1. *Patients with diabetes mellitus,* who have a higher likelihood of developing critical limb ischemia, and progress to amputation at seven times the rate of nondiabetic patients with PAD. Accordingly, a more aggressive approach is taken when a diabetic shows initial signs of deterioration.
2. *Patients with acute limb ischemia* (ALI), which occurs most commonly as a result of embolic arterial occlusion in which the source is cardiac in more than 75% of cases, with atrial fibrillation the primary cause.

ALI may also be caused by *in situ* thrombosis of diseased native-extremity vessels or bypass grafts. When it occurs spontaneously, especially in the absence of an underlying high-grade stenosis, the possibility of a previously unrecognized hypercoagulable state must be entertained. The clinical presentation of acute limb ischemia is typically a dramatic one. There is the sudden onset of severe pain, followed shortly by paresthesia and, ultimately, motor dysfunction (e.g., paralysis). On examination the extremity is cool, pale, and pulseless. Rutherford and colleagues (10) described a series of clinical categories of limb ischemia, with well-defined diagnostic criteria that help determine whether the affected limb is viable, in imminent jeopardy (e.g., "threatened"), or already irreversibly damaged (Table 40.2). As is the case for the standardized Rutherford criteria for chronic limb ischemia, evaluation based on these criteria forms the basis for therapeutic decisions in the setting of ALI. Whether a given patient will present with one category or another depends upon many factors, including the duration, level, and etiology of the occlusion; the status of the underlying vessels; and general factors (blood pressure, cardiac output, diabetes, 02 saturation). Paradoxically, it is the patient with less underlying atherosclerotic PVD and poorly developed collateral circulation (e.g., the patient

TABLE 40.2. CLINICAL CATEGORIES OF ACUTE LIMB ISCHEMIA

Category	Description	Capillary Return	Muscle Weakness	Sensory Loss	Doppler Signals	
					Arterial	Venous
Viable	Not immediately threatened	Intact	None	None	Audible (ankle pressure >30 mm Hg)	Audible
Threatened	Salvageable if promptly treated	Intact, slow	Mild, partial	Mild, incomplete	Inaudible	Audible
Irreversible	Major tissue loss, amputation regardless of treatment	Absent (marbling)	Profound, paralysis	Profound, anesthetic	Inaudible	Inaudible

From Rutherford RB, Flanigan DP, Guptka, SK. Suggested standards for reports with lower extremity ischemia. *J Vasc Surg* 1986;4:80–94, with permission.

with atrial fibrillation who embolically occludes a normal common femoral or popliteal artery) that develops the most acute ischemia.

Once the indications for invasive therapy are clear and the anatomic substrate has been defined, the choice will be between conventional surgery and catheter-based techniques. Surgical strategies typically involve placement of natural (saphenous vein) or prosthetic (Dacron or PTFE) materials to bypass or substitute for the diseased native artery. In some situations, such as the common femoral artery, the native vessel is treated by surgical removal of the obstructing atheroma (i.e., endarterectomy). In general, these operations are undertaken using general anesthesia, with significant blood loss and fluid shifts, in patients who may have profound involvement of other critical organ supply (e.g., extensive CAD). When it is possible to provide a similar level of correction and durability of benefit with catheter-based (endovascular) treatments, risk and disability may be minimized.

Major innovative advances have facilitated safer and more effective angioplasty since the pioneering work of Dotter, Judkins, Gruentzig, and others (11,12) more than 35 years ago. These include lower-profile catheters (limiting complications related to vascular access), novel materials for balloon and guide wire construction facilitating passage through occluded vessels, debulking techniques such as directional and rotational atherectomy for atheroma that are eccentric or heavily calcified, and endovascular stents that have dramatically improved both short-term and long-term outcomes (13,14) (Figure 40.1). Subsequently, results have been overwhelmingly positive, and consequently per-cutaneous revascularization has become increasingly popular as the first line of therapy for PAD.

Innovations and improvements in imaging techniques have also resulted in better appreciation of the acute results of percutaneous interventions. Paramount among these has been digital enhancement of conventional contrast images and on-line intraprocedural imaging using intravascular ultrasound (IVUS) (15–17), providing better comprehension of the mechanisms responsible for successful angioplasty. Concomitantly, the volume of contrast required during a given intervention has been reduced.

ANATOMIC REGIONS OF INTEREST

Technical features, likelihood of success, and chances for clinical improvement, however, vary in degree according to the region of interest within the peripheral circulation. Weighted consideration of these individual issues is required to determine the appropriateness of nonsurgical revascularization. Vascular specialists must therefore have a comprehensive understanding of all aspects of a given revascularization procedure: (a) the indications for intervention, (b) the therapeutic alternatives available and their expected outcomes, (c) the techniques employed during an intervention, and (d) the potential complications. Table 40.3 summarizes the current recommendations for revascularization at various peripheral sites.

Nonetheless, it is important to realize that, although the degree of disability is obviously a prime consideration, anticipated short- and long-term clinical benefit is the

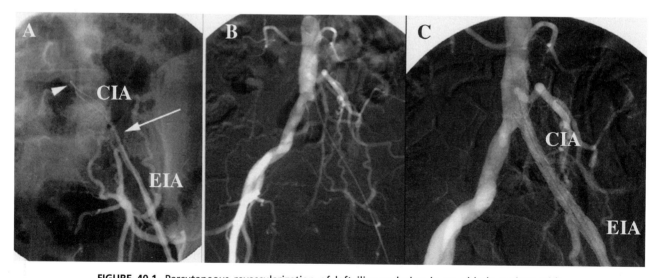

FIGURE 40.1. Percutaneous revascularization of left iliac occlusion in an elderly patient with limb ischemia. **A:** Access was obtained via the left common femoral artery and initial angiography demonstrated total occlusion of the left iliac artery *(arrow)*. The occlusion was traversed with a glide wire *(arrowhead)*. **B:** Aortoiliac angiography demonstrated occlusion at the ostium of the left common iliac artery. The right iliac artery and aorta were normal. **C:** Following angioplasty and stent deployment in the common iliac (CIA) and proximal external iliac arteries (EIA), flow was reestablished to the left lower extremity.

TABLE 40.3. REVASCULARIZATION STRATEGY BASED ON ANATOMIC REGIONS OF INTEREST

Arterial Site and Lesion Type	Revascularization Strategy					Clinical Indication (e.g., Rutherford Category/Other)*	
	Percutaneous						
	Balloon Angioplasty (PTA)	Adjunctive Therapy			Surgery	Percutaneous	Surgery
		Stent	Thrombolysis	Other			
Infrarenal Aorta and Iliac							
A. Stenosis	Treatment of choice.	Approved for suboptimal PTA result. Useful for unfavorable lesions. Role of primary stenting controversial but likely improves results and reduces restenosis.		Preliminary experience with early endografts not better than bare stent.	Reserved for cases of severe diffuse disease deemed inappropriate for PTA/stent.	≥2/3	≥3
B. Occlusion	Appropriate for short occlusion. Lengthy occlusions also may respond, especially with adjunctive thrombolysis or primary stenting.	Primary stenting indicated.	Essential for Rx of recent occlusion (<1 month). Also may be used for chronic occlusions.	Preliminary experience with early endografts not better than bare stent.	Useful for lengthy occlusion, especially if distal aorta is stenosed or occluded.	≥2/3	≥2/3
Common Femoral	Reserved for patients with severe fibrosis due to previous surgery. Some reports of PTA as first line of therapy in selected patients.	Not approved. Flexible stents may be employed under certain "salvage" situations.			Preferred treatment, especially if in association with proximal/distal bypass.	≥2/3	≥2/3
Profunda Femoris	Reserved for cases of severe or limb-threatening ischemia with no good surgical options. Stakes high if SFA occluded already.	Not approved. Little experience reported thus far, but anecdotal acute success.			Preferred treatment for proximal disease (endarterectomy + patch). Mid/distal vessel not easily accessed.	≥4	≥3

(continued)

TABLE 40.3. *(continued)*

Arterial Site and Lesion Type	Balloon Angioplasty (PTA)	Stent	Thrombolysis	Other	Surgery	Percutaneous	Surgery
			Revascularization Strategy			**Clinical Indication (e.g., Rutherford Category/Other)***	
			Percutaneous				
			Adjunctive Therapy				
SFA/ Popliteal							
A. Stenosis	Treatment of choice for short lesions. Can be utilized in lengthy lesions as initial treatment. Long-term results less favorable, but risk < surgery.	Not approved. Useful for "bail-out" indication.	Useful only if nonocclusive thrombus present, or recent occlusion < 6 weeks old.	a. Directional atherectomy may be useful to debulk focal/ eccentric stenoses, but no clear-cut long-term improvement over PTA alone. b. Rotational atherectomy occasionally useful for calcified plaque. c. Trials under way using covered stents.	Reserved for cases of diffuse disease deemed inappropriate for percutaneous therapy.	≥2/3	≥3
B. Occlusion	Treatment of choice for short (<7 cm) occlusion.	Approved for bail-out indication.	Use highly recommended for recent (<1 month) thrombosis/ occlusion. Some operators also prefer for chronic occlusion. May convert short or long occlusion into focal or segmental stenosis, facilitating treatment.		Treatment of choice for lengthy (e.g., >10 cm) occlusion.		
Infrapopliteal	Appropriate choice for treatment of discrete stenosis or focal occlusion.	Not approved. Useful to salvage failed PTA.	Useful for recent thrombosis or thrombo-embolism.	a. Rotational atherectomy may be useful to debulk calcified lesions. b. Excimer laser may be used as adjunctive Rx.	Treatment of choice for lengthy diffuse disease/ long occlusion(s), and not suitable or high-risk for percutaneous Rx.	≥3/4 (?2)	≥4

(continued)

TABLE 40.3. *(continued)*

Arterial Site and Lesion Type	Revascularization Strategy					Clinical Indication (e.g., Rutherford Category/Other)*	
	Percutaneous						
		Adjunctive Therapy					
	Balloon Angioplasty (PTA)	Stent	Thrombolysis	Other	Surgery	Percutaneous	Surgery
Subclavian/ Inominate Stenosis/ Occlusion	Preferred treatment for stenosis. Successful in most occlusions.	Stents useful to optimize PTA results.	Indicated for recent occlusion (<1 month). May facilitate PTA in chronic occlusion, but little published experience.		Reserved for PTA non-candidates or failures who have severe symptoms.	Moderate to severe arm claudication, subclavian steal syndrome, or coronary steal syndrome, or coronary steal via internal mammary artery.	Severe arm claudication, and/or subclavian steal syndrome.
Mesenteric	Reasonable first line of therapy, but untested compared with surgery.	Probable treatment of choice for ostial lesions.			Previously accepted standard but PTA + stent may be equal with less risk.	Significant clinical evidence of mesenteric ischemia.	Clear-cut evidence of mesenteric ischemia and PTA/ stent not feasible.

*Indications vary widely, depending on risk–benefit ratio of a given procedure in a given patient. These are intended to be general guidelines only.

CHF, congestive heart failure; DA, directional atherectomy; Med Rx, medical therapy; NA, not applicable; POBA, plain old balloon angioplasty; PTA, percutaneous transluminal angioplasty; Rx, treatment; SFA, superficial femoral artery.

major determinant of the role of catheter techniques in the management of PAD. Stents are the latest major advance to impact endovascular treatment of PAD, and stented endografts are evolving rapidly. However, to appreciate the role of endovascular stents fully, it is important to know the indications and results of percutaneous transluminal angioplasty (PTA) of the targeted vascular bed.

Furthermore, the preferred interventional technique for particular types of lesions also needs to be addressed. However, because the management of an individual lesion in a particular patient depends on a number of factors, any classification or categorizing of recommendations is difficult (18). The remainder of this chapter reviews percutaneous revascularization applied to specific regions of interest in the peripheral vasculature.

AORTOILIAC OBSTRUCTIVE DISEASE

Most disease in the infrarenal abdominal aorta and iliac arteries is atherosclerotic in origin. Since Gruentzig's origi-

nal report (19) describing an 87% 2-year patency rate with PTA for iliac stenoses, several series have demonstrated that the outcomes of aortoiliac PTA have been consistently among the most favorable (20–23). In fact, these excellent procedural and long-term results, enhanced recently by the addition of endovascular stenting, are so predictable that the physical finding of a diminished femoral pulse is a useful sign for identifying patients who are likely to benefit from a percutaneous approach.

Surgical revascularization for aortoiliac disease commenced with endarterectomy in the 1940s and bypass surgery in the 1950s. Long-term patency in the range of 90% at 1 year, 75% to 80% at 5 years, and 60% to 70% at 10 years can be expected. However, in the best of hands, the mortality rate for these patients with high likelihood of coexisting coronary artery disease is 2% and 3%, associated significant morbidity notwithstanding. Accordingly, the threshold for surgical intervention has remained high, reserved for patients with critical limb ischemia or advanced degrees of disability (Rutherford category 3 or above).

Indications for Revascularization

Aortoiliac revascularization is recommended for

1. Relief of symptomatic lower-extremity ischemia, including claudication, rest pain, ulceration or gangrene, or embolization causing blue-toe syndrome (24) (Figure 40.2).
2. Restoration and/or preservation of inflow to the lower extremity in the setting of preexisting or anticipated distal bypass (25,26) (Figure 40.3).
3. Procurement of access to more proximal vascular beds for anticipated invasive procedures (e.g., cardiac catheterization/PTCA, intraaortic balloon insertion) (27).
4. Rescue flow-limiting dissection complicating access for other invasive procedures (Figure 40.4).

Balloon Angioplasty

Isolated Aortic Lesions

Relatively few studies exist that examine the outcome of PTA in isolated aortic segments, due to the relatively uncommon occurrence of this entity. Early reports of PTA for atherosclerotic aortic disease had been mostly limited to discrete, focal lesions less than 2 cm long (28). Successful dilation of these lesions has been accomplished using either side-by-side simultaneously inflated balloons or a single large balloon, with favorable results in greater than 90% (Figure 40.5). More recently, Audet and colleagues (29) reported technical success and clinical improvement in 85% of patients, and primary and secondary clinical

patency rates of 76% and 88% at 5 years and 72% and 76% at 10 years, respectively.

Aortic Bifurcation and Iliac Lesions

Most atherosclerotic aortic disease includes plaque that extends into the iliac arteries. The need for revascularization at the aortic bifurcation itself using either "kissing balloons" or "kissing stents" (30) is much more frequent than with balloon dilation of isolated aortic lesions (Figure 40.6). In addition, patients with aortic stenoses usually have disease below the aorta that is considered to limit flow more, and therefore to be more responsible for the ischemic syndrome (Figure 40.5). Over the past 15 years, the revascularization strategy for this disease has changed significantly. A threefold increase in aortoiliac PTA and a concurrent decrease in aortobifemoral bypass grafting have been noted (31). However, in spite of the changing patterns and overwhelming evidence supporting a less invasive strategy of balloon angioplasty (with or without stenting), considerable controversy remains in some circles concerning the "optimal" treatment (32) with interventionalists generally supporting a primary strategy of angioplasty and stenting and vascular surgeons generally supporting a more traditional approach of "definitive" revascularization with aortobifemoral bypass, especially in young patients or those with advanced or diffuse disease (33).

The results of balloon angioplasty for iliac stenoses, particularly focal lesions, are excellent, with acute technical and clinical success in excess of 90% (21,34). One-, 3-, and 5-year patency rates range from approximately 75% to 95%,

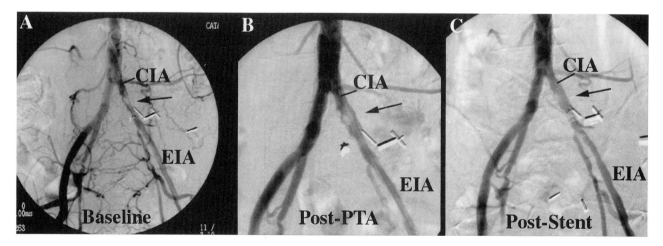

FIGURE 40.2. PTA/Stent for iliac stenosis in a 54-year-old patient with Rutherford Category II claudication and "blue-toe syndrome." **A:** Baseline angiogram demonstrates a focal stenosis in the left common iliac artery (CIA) resulting from a large, calcified, and ulcerated plaque that was the likely source of the distal embolization. **B:** Persistence of the plaque following balloon angioplasty; a suboptimal result despite some increase in luminal diameter. Rocklike calcium plaque remains a source of emboli. **C:** Exclusion of calcified plaque burden and restoration of full luminal patency following deployment of endovascular stent.

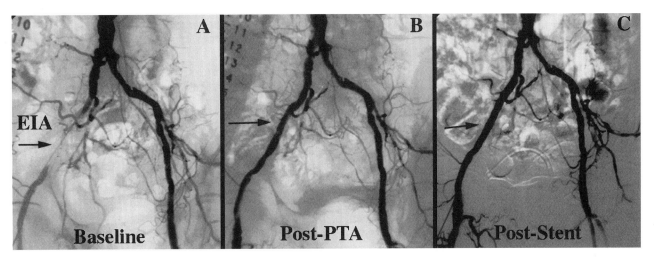

FIGURE 40.3. Percutaneous revascularization of external iliac artery (EIA) occlusion in a 75-year-old patient with distal disease and a nonhealing ulcer. Patient had significant coronary artery disease and previous abdominal surgery. Surgical risk of abdominal vascular reconstruction was therefore reduced by sequential PTA/stent and surgical distal bypass. **A:** Access obtained in the ipsilateral common femoral artery and the occlusion traversed with a glide wire. Angiography, in the left anterior oblique projection, demonstrates a lengthy (5-cm) occlusion of the right EIA, moderate disease of the contralateral common iliac artery, and right superficial femoral artery occlusion. **B:** Luminal patency was restored with balloon angioplasty. **C:** Final angiography following stent deployment demonstrates excellent result. Femoropopliteal bypass facilitated healing of the ulcer and resolution of symptoms.

60% to 90%, and 55% to 85%, respectively. Factors associated with good results include short, focal lesions; large vessel size; common iliac (as opposed to external iliac); single lesion (as opposed to multiple serial lesions); male gender; lesser Rutherford category (claudication as opposed to critical limb ischemia); and the presence of good runoff. The results in patients with diffuse disease, smaller vessels, diabetes mellitus, female gender, critical limb ischemia, and poor runoff are less favorable. Nonetheless, patients in these categories may still benefit from PTA.

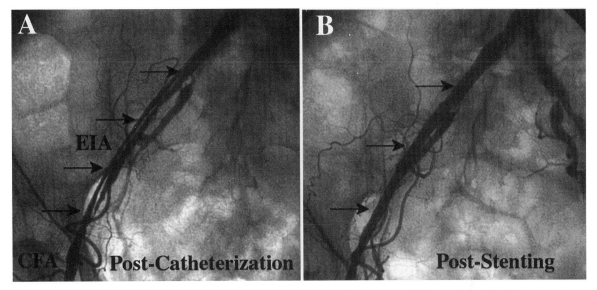

FIGURE 40.4. Eighty-four-year-old female complaining of increasing right leg pain and coolness during cardiac catheterization. **A:** Following cardiac catheterization, iliac angiogram demonstrates flow-limiting, lengthy spiral dissection *(arrows).* **B:** Flow was restored after treatment with PTA and Wallstent. When encountering new symptoms of lower-extremity ischemia during catheterization, angiographic delineation of the cause is preferable to removing the sheath and hoping for restoration of flow. CFA, common femoral artery; EIA, external iliac artery.

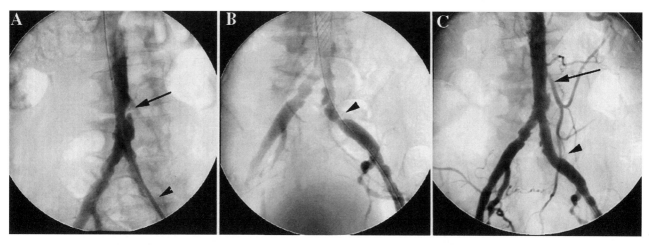

FIGURE 40.5. Balloon angioplasty (PTA) and stent deployment of aortoiliac lesions for Rutherford Category III claudication in a 74-year-old male. Access was obtained in the left common femoral artery with an 8F sheath. **A:** Baseline aortoiliac angiography demonstrated a large ulcerated plaque in the distal aorta *(arrow)* with more than 70% narrowing of the lumen by intravascular ultrasound. A critical stenosis was demonstrated in the left common iliac *(arrowhead)* with partial occlusion by a (long 35-cm) sheath employed to facilitate delivery of the stent. **B:** Initial PTA with a 9-mm balloon followed by successful deployment of a Palmaz P-308 endovascular stent that was postdilated to 12 mm. The sheath was withdrawn into the left external iliac artery and PTA was performed on the common iliac artery with a residual stenosis *(arrowhead)*. **C:** Final angiographic image following deployment of a balloon-expandable (Palmaz) stent in the common iliac artery *(arrowhead)* demonstrating excellent flow and luminal patency of the aorta and iliac system.

PTA can also be performed for aortoiliac *occlusions,* though the results are less favorable. Initial technical success rates between 70% and 98% have been reported (21,22,35,36). Long-term outcome is also less favorable, with patency rates at 1 and 3 years of approximately 55% to 95% and 50% to 85%. Thrombolytic therapy (37–40), recent advances in guide wire (e.g., hydrophilic) and catheter technologies, and the availability of stents (and potentially stent-grafts) have led to an increased ability to primarily traverse even lengthy, chronic occlusions (Figure 40.1). Furthermore, the ability of stents to scaffold the plaque, affix the thrombus to the vessel wall, and thus reduce the likelihood of distal embolization, provides the opportunity to recanalize these occlusions with more primary efficacy and improved results.

Endovascular Stents

Since the approval (for use in iliac arteries) of the Palmaz balloon-expandable stent (P-308 series) in 1993 and the self-expanding Wallstent prosthesis in 1996 for failed PTA (residual mean gradient of greater than or equal to 5 mm Hg), residual stenosis of more than 30%, or presence of a flow-limiting dissection (41,42), many investigators (43–47) have documented the extent to which stents have dramatically changed both short-term (by improving the immediate hemodynamic results of PTA) and long-term (by effectively managing recoil and PTA related flow-limiting dissections) results. This is particularly true in chronic

iliac artery occlusions, in which PTA alone often fails because of dissection and marked elastic recoil with reobstruction of the lumen and a residual pressure gradient. These studies have demonstrated acute technical success rates in the range of 90% to 100%. Average 1- and 3-year patency rates have also improved over PTA alone for both stenoses and occlusions, to 90% versus 72% and 75% versus 64%, respectively (18). This compares favorably with results of surgical recanalization of aortoiliac disease in which primary patency at 1, 5, and 10 years is 85% to 90%, 75% to 80%, and 60% to 70%, respectively. Richter and colleagues (48) suggested that significant improvements in long-term patency may be achieved in patients randomized to PTA-and-stent versus PTA alone (clinical success rate of 96% versus 68% and 2-year patency of 96% versus 79%), respectively. Furthermore, the angiographic patency (93%) in these patients studied at 5-year follow-up rivals the best clinical patency reported at a similar time interval in patients undergoing operative revascularization.

As a result of these superior cosmetic and hemodynamic outcomes, a strategy of primary stent deployment for aortoiliac disease has been advocated recently (36,49,50). However, to date, there have been no prospective, randomized, controlled trials that support a primary stenting strategy. The Dutch Iliac Stent Trial (51) reported clinical success, hemodynamic success (based on ABI), and patency (based on color Duplex) rates for primary stenting versus PTA plus selective stenting of 78% versus 76%, 85% versus 85%, and 71% versus 70%, respectively. These rates are

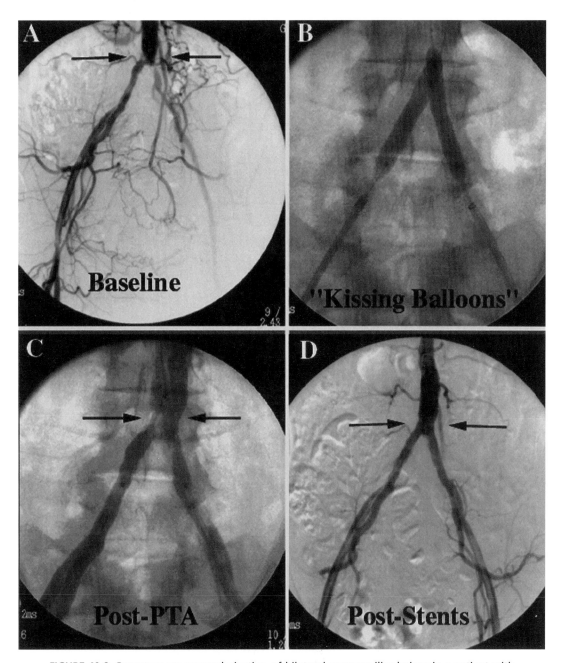

FIGURE 40.6. Percutaneous revascularization of bilateral common iliac lesions in a patient with disabling buttock and thigh claudication, and chronic myocardial ischemia. **A:** Baseline angiography demonstrates bilateral common iliac ostial stenoses *(arrows)*. **B:** Balloon angioplasty using "kissing balloons." **C:** Residual lesions *(arrows)* with dissection following PTA. **D:** Deployment of "kissing stents" resulted in normal patency of iliac vessels *(arrows)* and excellent distal flow with abolishment of pressure gradients. Percutaneous revascularization avoided potential high morbidity/mortality associated with surgical reconstruction.

comparable to those of many surgical series of aortobifemoral bypass. A metaanalysis (34) on 14 studies involving more than 2,100 patients undergoing aortoiliac PTA versus aortoiliac stenting showed greater immediate success rate for stents than for PTA alone (96% versus 91%). For patients with claudication, 4-year primary patency rates for occlusions were 61% for stents versus 54% for PTA (compared with rates for stenotic lesions of 77% for stenting versus 65% for PTA alone). Thus stenting yielded better acute results and reduced the relative risk of 4-year failure by nearly 40% over PTA alone.

For complex aortoiliac stenoses and for occlusions, stenting is the preferred primary therapy of most interventionalists (42,44,52) (Figures 40.1, 40.2, and 40.6). In a reanalysis of the Palmaz multicenter iliac data, Laborde and colleagues (53) assessed the influence of disease severity on the outcome of revascularization by stenting in 455 patients. In patients with only focal aortoiliac or common iliac lesions (40% patients), the rates for complete relief of symptoms and 3-year persistent clinical benefit were 88% and 92%, respectively. In patients with external iliac disease, the rates were 85% and 98%, respectively. For patients with multilevel disease involving the infrainguinal vessels, the rates were 60% and 61%, respectively, and this extent of disease was the most powerful predictor of unsatisfactory early outcome in iliac stenting. In addition, they demonstrated that female gender predicted unsatisfactory clinical outcome and higher periprocedural complications.

Treatment Strategies and Technical Aspects

Before undertaking aortoiliac PTA, careful consideration should be given to the issue of arterial access. Baseline angiograms and/or noninvasive studies form the basis of decisions regarding access. With unilateral disease that ends above the common femoral artery, ipsilateral retrograde access provides the most direct approach to the stenotic (or occlusive) lesion, and facilitates stent deployment (Figure 40.2). The contralateral approach has become more popular with the advent of "cross-over" sheaths and guiding catheters (54), and is selected when the lesion is located near the common femoral artery or the femoral head, when the ipsilateral groin is scarred or the common femoral artery is heavily calcified, or if more distal revascularization is to be pursued in the same sitting. For iliac occlusions, either retrograde or contralateral access is appropriate, and frequently both are required. For lesions involving the aortic bifurcation, a bilateral retrograde femoral approach is recommended in order to enable placement of "kissing stents."

Role of Pressure Gradients and Intravascular Ultrasound

Pressure gradients are routinely measured across iliac and aortic lesions, but there are few objective data regarding what constitutes a significant hemodynamic stenosis. By convention, a 5-mm Hg mean resting pressure gradient is indicative of a significant residual stenosis. If the resting gradient is borderline, a persistent (e.g., more than 60 seconds) mean pressure gradient of more than 15 mm Hg after administration of vasodilator (200 to 300 µg of nitroglycerin) is considered significant.

Clinical experience has demonstrated that intravascular ultrasound (IVUS) is unequivocally superior to contrast angiography in its ability to demonstrate detailed vessel anatomy (16,55–58) (by direct planimetry of luminal cross sections) and other details that are angiographically "silent," the dimensions of the reference site, the degree of narrow-

ing, and the characteristics of the vessel wall (e.g., calcium). IVUS can be of great utility during aortoiliac angioplasty by identifying plaque at sites of hemodynamically significant stenoses that are typically underestimated by conventional diagnostic angiography, including tortuous common and external iliac arteries (15,55,57,58), at the ostium of the common iliac artery, the common iliac bifurcation, or eccentric lesions in the distal aorta. Furthermore, when used in conjunction with physiologic indices including intraarterial measurement of translesion pressure gradient and/or intraarterial Doppler measurement flow velocity (59), IVUS can identify those lesions that are appropriate for revascularization, thereby obviating the often required multiple, angulated angiographic views.

Thrombolytic Therapy

For occlusions in peripheral vessels, catheter-directed thrombolysis is much more effective than systemic fibrinolysis. The technical aspects of use vary among investigators. There is agreement that the catheter must penetrate into the occlusion in order for the thrombolytic agent to have any effect. Some prefer going one step further and crossing the occlusion primarily, in order to "lace" the thrombolytic agent throughout the occlusion and enhance the efficiency of thrombolysis. Others prefer crossing the occlusion and administering the thrombolytic in "pulsed spray" fashion, a technique that may accelerate clot dissolution, but is associated with a slightly higher incidence of distal embolization. Urokinase has been the agent of choice with alternatives being tPA (40) and Retavase (Figure 40.7).

Use of Aortoiliac PTA/Stenting in Conjunction with Surgery

In some patients with claudication and in rare patients with limb ischemia, the iliac lesion coexists with more distal disease (SFA and/or infrapopliteal vessels) (60). Improved inflow by iliac revascularization secondarily improves outflow, either via the profunda in the case of an occluded SFA or by increasing perfusion pressure to that segment of the infrainguinal circulation that remains patent. Implicit in this strategy is the lesser degree of technical difficulty, high incidence of procedural success, and low rate of restenosis associated with iliac PTA. Moreover, PTA avoids the complication of iatrogenic postoperative impotence, reported to complicate 10% to 25% of aortoiliac operations (61).

Similarly, in patients undergoing surgical treatment of distal disease (60), percutaneous revascularization of an iliac lesion may facilitate patency of a downstream femoral-popliteal conduit designed to bypass an occluded SFA (Figure 40.3). Alternatively, nonsurgical revascularization of an aortoiliac or isolated iliac lesion in patients with coronary heart disease and aortoiliac occlusive disease may permit surgical revascularization to be adjusted one level caudal, thereby

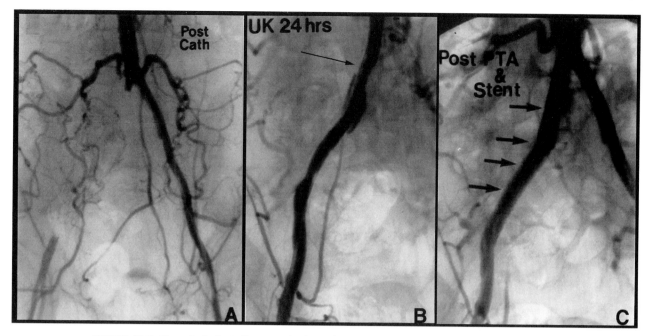

FIGURE 40.7. Thrombolysis, balloon angioplasty (PTA), and stent deployment to the right iliac artery in a patient with acute limb ischemia. **A:** Initial access was achieved via the left common femoral artery, and baseline angiography demonstrated long occlusion of the right common iliac and external iliac arteries with reconstitution at the level of the right femoral artery. The occlusion was traversed with a glide wire from the right femoral artery, followed by initiation of a urokinase infusion via a Fountain catheter. **B:** Following 24 hours of lytic therapy, the iliac artery was patent with no residual thrombus. A stenosis *(arrow)* was noted in the common iliac artery. **C:** Final angiography following PTA and stent deployment demonstrated excellent luminal patency and normal flow.

reducing the risk of a marked increase in cardiac morbidity and mortality (62,63). Similarly, in the patient, for example, with a lengthy unilateral occlusion of one iliac artery and less extensive obstruction of the contralateral side, higher-risk aortofemoral bypass surgery may be obviated by percutaneous treatment of the less diseased iliac artery, followed by a cross-femoral graft to the contralateral femoral artery.

Occasionally, even when anticipating the need for cross-femoral grafting, treatment of the contralateral artery may enable better collateralization and unexpectedly remove the need for surgery altogether. As surgeons become more proficient in endovascular techniques, they are bringing these techniques into the operating room and employing them in conjunction with more conventional bypass procedures. Several reports describe the technique of common femoral artery cutdown, intraoperative balloon angioplasty, and stent deployment of iliac arteries, followed by fem-pop or fem-fem bypass in the same sitting. This approach is a natural extension of the use of endovascular techniques to minimize morbidity and mortality, and to maximize the benefit for the patient. Likewise, revascularization may be staged with proximal PTA first, followed by surgery some 3 to 4 weeks later. Each of these strategies carries merit. Approaches will vary from institution to institution, depending upon available resources and expertise.

Current Recommendations

PTA is generally applied to more focal disease of the distal aorta, common iliac arteries, and external iliac arteries. The technical and initial clinical success of PTA of iliac stenosis in all series ranges from 90% to 100%. The technical success rate of recanalization of segmental (external or common) iliac occlusions is 80% to 85%. Long-term patency rates in patients with intermittent claudication are close to 80% at 1 year and 60% at 5 years. Once an iliac artery occlusion has been recanalized successfully, the patency rate does not differ from that for patencies after PTA for stenosis. However, complications are higher after recanalization of occlusions (6%) than after standard PTA of stenosis (3.6%).

The current consensus is that stents are appropriate for use in aortoiliac disease in the following instances:

- Significant elastic recoil following PTA based on residual pressure gradient causing insufficient hemodynamic result.
- Flow-limiting dissection.
- Lengthy or complex lesions where balloon angioplasty has been shown to yield suboptimal results and where primary stenting may give more satisfactory results.
- Restenotic aortoiliac lesion after previously performed PTA.

- Reconstruction of the aortoiliac bifurcation.
- Iliac artery ulceration associated with symptoms.
- Revascularization of "donor artery," in preparation for more distal fem-fem or fem-distal bypass.
- Primary therapy for aortoiliac chronic occlusion.

Several issues, however, remain outstanding. First, the role of primary stent deployment for *uncomplicated* iliac lesions is yet to be defined. Many interventionalists believe this strategy is warranted, given the positive aspects and the absence of significant complications associated with stenting at this level. Second, the usefulness and cost-effectiveness of multiple stents also remains to be established.

COMMON FEMORAL ARTERY

Indications for Intervention and Results

Revascularization of the common femoral artery (CFA) has long been considered to be exclusively within the purview of the vascular surgeon for several reasons:

- Access is easily achieved through a local incision and often under local anesthesia.
- The results of endarterectomy and/or patch angioplasty are outstanding.
- Access via the percutaneous approach can be problematic if the contralateral and/or brachial sites are unavailable.

In addition, the propensity for this vessel to demonstrate elastic recoil and the concern about dissecting or thrombosing the only site of inflow to the entire leg raise the level of concern about dilating this vessel. Although there is good evidence now that balloon angioplasty can be judiciously employed, with excellent results and minimum complications, large series of common femoral angioplasty are not available.

Lesion characteristics play a significant role in determining the success of PTA. Lesions that tend to respond better are focal, concentric, or bandlike, with less extensive plaque burden. This might include iatrogenic lesions resulting from either single or repeated arterial puncture. On the other hand, more complex lesions, including those with "cauliflower," calcified plaque, or a large plaque burden extending into the origins of the superficial femoral and profunda femoris arteries tend not to respond as well. In general, the more calcification that is present, the less responsive the common femoral lesion is to balloon angioplasty.

The use of stents in the common femoral artery is ill advised, as their placement may preclude future surgical procedures or compromise future attempts at percutaneous access. However, concern that PTA-induced plaque fractures could propagate into the common femoral bifurcation, leading to potential compromise of both SFA and profunda, implicitly suggests that PTA of the common femoral artery must be undertaken with considerable caution, especially given the ease of surgical access in this location.

Treatment Strategies and Technical Aspects

PTA is typically done via the contralateral approach, using a crossover-guiding catheter or sheath or from the

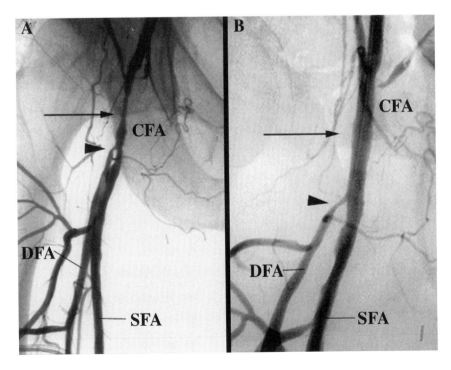

FIGURE 40.8. Balloon angioplasty (PTA) of common femoral artery in a patient with multiple previous right leg surgical interventions, resulting in severe scarring of right groin. **A:** High-grade, diffuse stenosis *(arrow)* in right common femoral artery (CFA) extending to the origins *(arrowhead)* of the profunda femoris (DFA) and superficial femoral artery (SFA). Revascularization with PTA was performed via the contralateral approach. **B:** Final angiogram demonstrates excellent patency of the CFA and proximal SFA, with mild recoil at the origin of the DFA. Patient's claudication symptoms resolved, and he continues to be minimally symptomatic 4 years later.

brachial approach. In occasional instances, the lesion will be far enough from the sheath insertion site that ipsilateral access is possible, though technically more challenging. Complex angioplasty is often required when the lesion involves the bifurcation of the CFA into profunda femoris and SFA branches, which is frequently the case (Figure 40.8). In this situation, accommodation must be made to enable the passage of two balloons simultaneously (large enough contralateral sheath to accommodate two balloons), as "kissing" balloons must occasionally be used. We encourage active discussion with surgical colleagues before undertaking a complex angioplasty involving the common femoral and its bifurcation. Rarely, these cases may need surgical "rescue." However, in a moderately large series at our institution, we have not yet encountered a situation where urgent surgery was required. Occasionally, directional atherectomy, via an ipsilateral approach, is utilized to reduce the chance of recoil and provide a better cosmetic result than PTA alone. Furthermore, there is also theoretical benefit to using a debulking strategy with rotational atherectomy.

The biggest impediment to successful long-term outcome following CFA revascularization is that of restenosis. There are no long-term studies, but the restenosis rate is widely accepted to be greater than 50%. Patients often may experience persistent relief of critical symptoms, even in the face of moderate or moderately severe restenosis. It is important to realize that, in this site, one does not need to achieve perfection to have a beneficial clinical outcome.

Profunda Femoris Artery

Indications for Intervention and Results

The profunda femoris or deep femoral artery (DFA) is the main source of collaterals to the lower extremity. In occlusion of the SFA or of a femoropopliteal bypass graft, the DFA alone becomes responsible for maintaining viability of the lower extremity (Figure 40.9). Traditionally, bypass surgery is performed for occlusive disease in the DFA, which almost always occurs in conjunction with SFA disease. For disease involving the ostia of the SFA and profunda, endarterectomy and patch angioplasty can be performed.

Technically satisfactory results of profunda PTA have been described previously (64). A more recent series by Silva and colleagues (65) suggests that this is a relatively safe procedure. However, because of the potential for producing limb-threatening ischemia or limb loss, in the event that the vessel thromboses or occludes, caution should be exercised when considering PTA for these lesions. For the present, PTA is reserved for situations of severe ischemia (Rutherford category 4, 5, or 6) and in which surgery is absolutely contraindicated. In addition, critical lesions involving the middle or distal portions of the descending branch of the profunda may occasionally warrant treatment with PTA, since they are less accessible to the surgeon.

Treatment Strategies and Technical Aspects

Angioplasty of the profunda, similar to that for the CFA, is best performed from the contralateral side. Antegrade

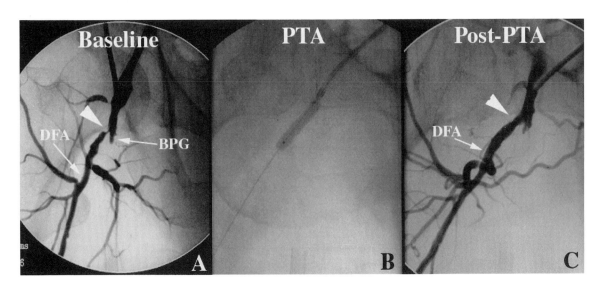

FIGURE 40.9. Balloon angioplasty (PTA) for profunda femoris disease in a 50-year-old patient with multiple previous percutaneous interventions, including endovascular stenting, for recurrent femoropopliteal bypass graft occlusion (chronic SFA occlusion). A below-knee amputation was required for critical limb ischemia. **A:** Critical stenosis *(arrow)* of the profunda femoris artery (DFA) causing stump ischemia, and chronic occlusion of a femoropopliteal graft (BPG). A stent is present in the middle portion of the graft. **B:** Balloon angioplasty performed at low inflation pressure using the antegrade approach. **C:** Final angiographic image demonstrating restoration of luminal patency.

access is sometimes appropriate, depending upon the location of the stenosis and the condition of the CFA. If the lesion is immediately adjacent to the common femoral, then it may be problematic to treat, although directional atherectomy of this site must be performed in an antegrade fashion. Since the profunda is the "vessel of last resort" for maintaining blood flow to the lower extremity, we advocate a conservative posture with respect to balloon size and inflation pressure. The outcome of stenting in the profunda is unknown, much like the long-term outcome of balloon angioplasty alone. Accordingly, stenting is reserved for cases of true flow-limiting dissection after balloon angioplasty, wherein patency of the vessel and viability of the limb might be threatened without maintaining an open vessel.

SUPERFICIAL FEMORAL AND POPLITEAL ARTERIES

Previous experience has failed to document any significant difference in either acute or long-term results for revascularization of the SFA versus the popliteal artery. Accordingly, as has traditionally been the case, these vessels will be considered together.

In contrast to iliofemoral disease, disease in the SFA/popliteal arteries typically occurs in older patients, is associated more closely with the presence of CAD (66,67), and involves symptoms twice as often or more. Patients with SFA/popliteal disease usually present with claudication. Less frequently, the presentation is critical limb ischemia. However, even in cases of SFA occlusion, symptoms may be minimal in the presence of a patent DFA with well-developed collaterals.

An important caveat in the management of patients with symptomatic SFA/popliteal disease is the issue of restenosis. While acute procedural success for percutaneous revascularization of lesions in the SFA using conventional guide wires and standard PTA is well in excess of 90% (see later), published reports have established that restenosis may complicate the clinical course of as many as 60% of patients undergoing PTA for SFA/popliteal disease. The cause of the high restenosis rate, which plagues intervention in this vascular segment, is an enigma. Its occurrence raises fundamental questions as to whether the biology and pathophysiology of plaque formation in the SFA/popliteal is in some way different from that in other vessels. The disappointing durability of PTA for SFA lesions has serious implications. Although bypass surgery often may be used to treat successfully these patients, such surgery is not risk-free, particularly in a population of patients with a high frequency of comorbid diseases, including coronary and carotid disease. Consequently, any enthusiasm for reducing symptoms in these patients must be tempered by the reduced likelihood of long-term success, with both percutaneous and surgical approaches, and weighted consideration must be given to the potential for risks and benefits of interventions in this high-risk population.

Indications for Revascularization

Decisions regarding intervention for infrainguinal disease must take into account several factors: the degree to which the patient is disabled, the presence of comorbid factors, and the anticipated outcome and benefit (both acute and long term) from intervention, whether surgical bypass or PTA. In general, patients with mild, nondisabling claudication should not undergo interventional therapy for SFA/popliteal disease. Conservative treatment with an exercise program may be expected to augment collateral flow and increase walking distance in most of these patients. Less than a quarter of these patients will progress to the point of developing more disabling symptoms or a threatened limb. Once a threatened limb or severely disabling claudication is present, therapy is indicated. There remains considerable controversy, as in the case of more advanced aortoiliac disease, as to the relative role of percutaneous therapy versus surgery (68,69). Analysis of the results of each of these strategies sheds some light on this issue.

Balloon Angioplasty

The results of balloon angioplasty, which has been performed in the SFA for nearly 20 years, have improved over time with respect to the acute results. Early results from patients undergoing PTA of femoral-popliteal stenoses and occlusions, most of whom were patients with intermittent claudication, disclosed acute technical success rates between 82% and 96% (70–77). Primary patency rates at 1, 3, and 5 years were, on average, approximately 60%, 50%, and 45%.

In a recent comprehensive report utilizing a prospective analysis of PTA of 208 lesions in 140 limbs, Matsi and colleagues reported an overall acute angiographic success rate of 88% and a successful immediate clinical outcome in 91% of SFA lesions (77). Systematic, prospective long-term follow-up of all study patients using ankle-brachial indices and clinical symptoms revealed primary patency rates of 47%, 44%, and 43% in patients evaluated at the 1-, 2-, and 3-year marks, respectively. Secondary patency was 63% at 1 year and 59% at 2 and 3 years. Predictors of long-term patency included fewer stenoses, shorter lesion length, better runoff, and concentric morphology. In another recent review, Murray and colleagues (73) noted that the technical success improved from 70% to 91%. Among their own patients, they demonstrated excellent acute and long-term efficacy in dilating lesions greater than 10 cm in length.

Factors that influence long-term outcome following SFA/popliteal PTA include claudication as the presenting symptom, presence of a more severe lesion at baseline, presence of stenosis versus occlusion (78), presence of two- or three-vessel runoff (70–73,77–79), absence of residual stenosis following angioplasty, and restoration of an ABI to greater than 0.9 at 24 hours *post procedure* (80). Factors that negatively influence long-term patency include the presence of diabetes, threatened limb loss, or diffuse atherosclerotic vascular disease (72).

In making decisions about therapy for revascularization in SFA/popliteal disease, the recent analysis of Hunink and colleagues (81) is perhaps the most comprehensive and useful. These investigators analyzed the relative benefit and cost-effectiveness of PTA versus bypass surgery by evaluating 5-year outcomes in approximately 4,800 PTA and 4,500 bypass procedures performed since 1995. Their conclusion was that, for patients with *disabling claudication* due to femoral-popliteal stenosis *or* occlusion, PTA is the preferred initial treatment. For patients in whom *chronic critical ischemia* was present secondary to femoral-popliteal *occlusion,* bypass surgery, if feasible, is the preferred treatment.

Stenoses of the SFA and/or Popliteal Artery

The acute procedural success that may be currently achieved using conventional guide wires and standard PTA in *nonocclusive* (i.e., stenotic) lesions in the SFA is similar to that reported for iliac stenoses, and approaches 100% (Figure 40.10). This contrasts with results of earlier reports (70,78,82,83) describing acute success rates as low as 72%. Long-term patency in the SFA, however, is clearly inferior to that which may be expected in iliac stenoses. Five-year primary patency rates varying from 43% to 70% have been reported for revascularization of SFA stenoses (70,75, 76,83).

Occlusions of the SFA and/or Popliteal Artery

Among patients studied angiographically for consideration of revascularization, *occlusions* are more prevalent than stenoses. The success rate in crossing occluded segments of the SFA/popliteal has improved dramatically in recent years, implying that, although the long-term implications for revascularization of SFA are associated with a high likelihood of recurrence (1,2,3,4,7), the chances of achieving short-term patency (i.e., acute procedural success) are higher for SFA occlusions. This is the case even for long (>10 cm) SFA occlusions and is due largely to two technical modifications. The first is the use of thrombolytic therapy (see later) (Figure 40.11). The second advance, which has contributed to improved procedural success in recanalizing SFA occlusions, is the use of hydrophilic (so-called glide) guide wires. Among 190 consecutive patients at our institution in whom the glide wire was used to attempt percutaneous revascularization of SFA total occlusions, the glide wire successfully traversed the segment in 180 (95%). PTA alone or in combination with directional atherectomy and/or laser angioplasty was then used to complete the percutaneous revascularization in all 107 patients (84) (Figure 40.12). The ankle brachial index improved from 0.48 before to 0.82 after revascularization. Improvement in Rutherford class by one or more grades was observed in 94% patients seen at 1-month follow-up. This experience was noteworthy for two reasons in particular. First, 21 of these occlusions were more than 20 cm long, and mean occlusion length was 9.8 cm. Second, IVUS examination during these procedures demonstrated, in approximately one-third of patients, a subintimal route of recanalization (85), which had no obvious effect on acute success or long-term patency.

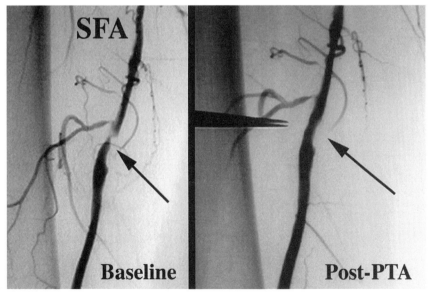

FIGURE 40.10. Balloon angioplasty (PTA) of the superficial femoral artery in a patient with disabling claudication. **A:** Baseline angiography demonstrated a focal lesion in the superficial femoral artery (SFA). PTA was performed with a short, low-profile balloon. **B:** Final angiography disclosed patency and normal flow, with complete resolution of symptoms.

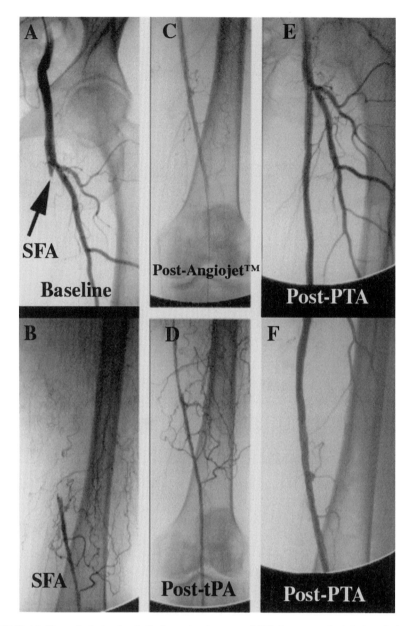

FIGURE 40.11. Thrombolysis, rheolytic thrombectomy, and PTA for acute limb ischemia in an 87-year-old female with polycythemia. Baseline angiogram demonstrates **(A)** occlusion of the proximal superficial femoral artery (SFA), with reconstitution via collaterals from the profunda **(B)** at the adductor canal. The occlusion was traversed with a glide wire and partially recanalized **(C)** with rheolytic thrombectomy (Angiojet). Luminal patency was reestablished with thrombolytic therapy (tPA), revealing moderate disease in the mid-SFA **(D)**. Following balloon angioplasty, final angiographic images **(E)** and **(F)** demonstrated widely patent SFA with normal flow/caliber.

However, despite these favorable acute, procedural results in patients with chronic total occlusion, the role of percutaneous revascularization is still evolving. Certainly for patients with nonhealing lesions and/or threatened limb loss in whom the risks of surgery are considered prohibitive, or in whom veins are unavailable for distal bypass, percutaneous revascularization of even lengthy, occluded segments may facilitate healing. In patients with rest pain or severe claudication, PTA may be employed at a lower risk than conventional surgical reconstruction. All attempts to optimize acute procedural results in patients with lengthy total occlusions of the SFA, however, must be tempered by the high frequency of restenosis following percutaneous revascularization of such lesions (70,78,82,83,86). Therefore in patients with less severe symptoms, improved ability to revascularize does not itself constitute a sufficient basis for routine invasive therapy.

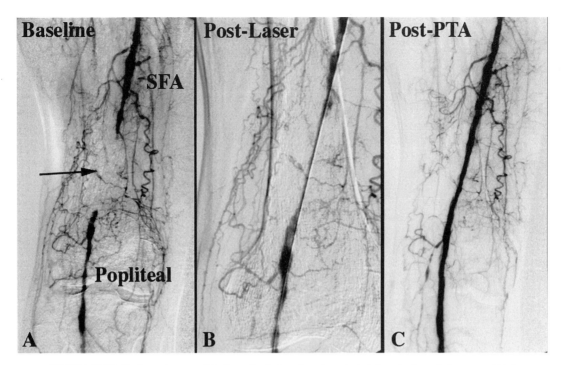

FIGURE 40.12. Excimer laser-assisted angioplasty of a chronic total occlusion of the superficial femoral artery in an elderly diabetic patient with necrotic foot ulceration and threatened limb. **A:** Baseline angiogram demonstrates a total occlusion *(arrow)* in the superficial femoral artery (SFA) and diffuse disease of the popliteal artery. **B:** The occlusion was traversed with glide wire, followed by excimer laser angioplasty. **C:** Balloon angioplasty resulted in complete patency of the SFA and popliteal artery, with complete healing of the ulcer over 6 months.

Endovascular Stents

In contrast to the documented benefits achieved by endovascular stents for iliac PTA, experience thus far in the SFA has been less favorable. The most troublesome lesions for SFA/popliteal PTA include eccentric stenoses, long-segment stenoses (and occlusion), and stenoses due to intimal hyperplasia at graft anastomosis. PTA can fail because of elastic recoil or obstructing intimal flaps caused by extensive dissection. Stents can dramatically enhance acute outcome, especially when they are needed to rescue a flow-limiting dissection resulting from PTA. However, while the immediate and early results have been excellent, restenosis caused by intimal hyperplasia in the stented segment is quite common in the first 3 to 6 months. Consequently, studies from a variety of stent designs in the SFA (43,87–91) have all failed to show a significant reduction in restenosis. Primary 1- and 3-year patency rates were in the range of 22% to 81% and 18% to 72%, respectively. In further contrast to results reported for iliac applications, the use of stents in the SFA has been complicated by an unpredictable incidence of subacute thrombosis, and thus uncertainty regarding the need for short-term, and even possibly long-term, anticoagulation (87).

Uncontrolled studies employing the Palmaz stent (92) and the Wallstent (93) demonstrated modest improvement in intermediate-term patency when compared with historical controls using PTA alone. Not surprisingly, these preliminary, nonrandomized studies indicate that, much like PTA alone, the most favorable long-term results are seen with stents in the proximal SFA. Not unexpectedly, the fate of stents placed at the adductor canal or below is more sobering. The descriptions of deformation or compression of stents placed within the adductor canal (94), a finding that led to the premature termination of a randomized trial between SFA stent implementation and PTA alone, suggest that balloon-expandable stents may be suboptimal for use in this vessel and that self-expandable stents are advisable.

Three trials highlight the current perspective on the correct role of stents in the SFA/popliteal artery. In the study by Gray and colleagues (88), stenting was used only as a fallback procedure, to salvage the results of a suboptimal PTA (defined as the presence of a flow-limiting dissection, residual pressure gradient of greater than 15 mm Hg, or stenosis greater than 30%). Lesions were lengthy (mean, 16.5 cm), and endpoints for primary patency were strict (restenosis greater than 50%, reocclusion, or decrease in postprocedure ABI by more than 0.15). When taking into account the poor substrate of patients who received stents, the 46% 1-year patency rate is an acceptable outcome for procedures that were, before stenting, doomed to failure. In a recent trial by Cejna (95), patients

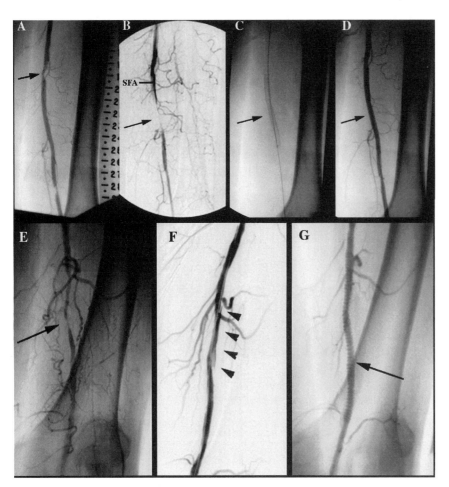

FIGURE 40.13. Stents deployed for complication of balloon angioplasty to the superficial femoral artery following in patients with claudication. **A:** Baseline angiography disclosed a focal lesion *(arrow)* in the middle superficial femoral artery (SFA). **B:** Balloon angioplasty resulted in flow-limiting dissection and occlusion. **C:** Deployment of self-expanding endovascular stent was required. **D:** Final angiography demonstrated complete patency and normal flow. **E:** Baseline angiography in a second patient disclosed focal critical stenosis *(arrow)* in the SFA at the adductor canal with patent popliteal artery. **F:** Balloon angioplasty resulted in a lengthy flow-limiting dissection *(arrowhead)*. **G:** A Vascucoil endovascular prosthesis *(arrow)* was deployed repairing the dissection and preserving luminal patency. Patient has remained asymptomatic at 2-year follow-up.

were randomized between PTA and primary (Palmaz) stent deployment. Results showed that, although the 6-month primary patency rate for stents was superior (86% versus 79%), the 2-year follow-up results were equivalent. Damaraju and colleagues (96) deployed Wallstents in iliac and femoral locations. By both univariate and multivariate analysis, the location of stents in the femoral artery was a harbinger of poor long-term patency. In fact, despite 100% initial success, the primary patency for femoral stents was only 49% at 1 year and 41% at 2 years. This stands in contrast to the 86% and 82% 1- and 2-year patency rates, respectively, of iliac Wallstents. Recent pooled data from 11 studies (585 patients) of stents in both femoropopliteal stenoses and occlusions revealed weighted average technical success, 1- and 3-year-patency rates of 98%, 67%, and 58%, respectively (18).

These data underscore the difficulty of obtaining good results for stenting in the femoral artery. Consequently, there seems to be no long-term benefit to femoral-popliteal stenting at the present time. However, there appears at least to be an acute hemodynamic benefit for treatment of a flow-limiting dissection and for failed balloon angioplasty (18) (Figure 40.13). If stents are to be placed for this indication, they should be of the self-

expanding variety. Balloon-expandable stents should particularly be avoided within the adductor canal. The only current formal FDA-approved stent for the SFA/popliteal is that employing the Intrastent VascuCoil (Figure 40.13). This is a spring-shaped, self-expanding Nitinol stent that has the capability of flexing in excess of 90 degrees without compromising its integrity. Future studies will determine whether this or the other Nitinol stents [Smart stent (Figure 40.13), Symphony stent, and Memotherm stent] offer any advantage over the previous stainless steel designs in the SFA/popliteal arteries.

Adjunctive Therapies

A variety of other technologies, including directional atherectomy, rotational atherectomy, laser angioplasty, and other novel therapies, have been investigated as means of improving long-term patency and reducing restenosis in the SFA.

Directional atherectomy (DA) has the unique capability of resecting intact atherosclerotic plaque, which can be used for a variety of laboratory analyses (97). However, the superiority of DA from a therapeutic standpoint remains less clear. In patients with short, eccentric lesions, DA (with or without adjunctive PTA) seems to offer satisfactory acute results, similar to those reported for PTA (79,98,99). The impact of DA on subsequent restenosis, however, remains controversial. For the present, there is no evidence to support the use of DA as a means of preventing restenosis (100). We reserve its use for lesions resistant to balloon dilation and for fibrotic lesions with significant recoil (e.g., graft anastomoses).

Rotational atherectomy (101,102) has not thus far been demonstrated to have an advantage for SFA/popliteal revascularization, save for those rare patients in whom the extent of calcific deposits renders the lesion refractory to alternative techniques. Furthermore, to impact significantly upon a vessel the size of the SFA, the disproportionately large introducer sheath required to accommodate appropriately sized devices represents a distinct disadvantage for SFA rotational atherectomy. In the smaller popliteal artery, the debulking effect of rotational atherectomy may ultimately prove to offer some benefit over balloon angioplasty alone.

The role of *laser angioplasty* in SFA/popliteal revascularization remains controversial and unproven. A variety of laser sources have been investigated for this application, including thermal ("hot-tip") systems (103,104), continuous wave (CW) lasers such as Nd:YAG (105), and pulsed laser systems using either visible (flash-lamp-pumped dye) (106,107), infrared (holmium) (108), or ultraviolet (excimer) (109) wavelengths. No trial has thus far demonstrated any definitive benefit of this device at this level. Our own clinical experience with the excimer has been more favorable than that with the alternative wavelengths, particularly in completion of revascularization that was refractory to conventional techniques (Figure 40.12). Although there is preliminary evidence (110) to suggest that the thrombolytic properties of excimer laser radiation may be exploited to reduce the need for thrombolytic therapy in selected patients, this application requires further confirmation. Evidence that excimer laser angioplasty can reduce restenosis remains the subject of ongoing studies. A trial (PELA) that employs the strategy of debulking using excimer laser, followed by balloon angioplasty for revascularization of lengthy SFA occlusions, has recently begun.

For SFA/popliteal occlusions, the use of *thrombolytic therapy* in advance of PTA is controversial and the exact role remains unknown. Thrombolytic therapy can be successful in some patients even with chronic total occlusion, because the occlusion in lower-extremity arteries is often characterized by a lengthy, gelatin-like thrombus superimposed upon a high-grade atherosclerotic lesion (39,111) (Figure 40.11). Thus thrombolytic therapy can convert a long occlusion to one that is either shorter or not occlusive. Notwithstanding these good results, data from the multicenter STILE trial (Surgery and Thrombolysis for Ischemia of the Lower Extremity) (37) suggest that reestablishing patency by this approach is not as durable as fem-pop bypass. Some also argue that direct recanalization with PTA alone for SFA/pop occlusions may be as effective (technical and cost)

as pretreatment with thrombolytic therapy. Regarding the use of thrombolytic therapy for acute (≤14 days duration) occlusions, both the STILE trial and a similar randomized investigation by Ouriel and associates (112) demonstrated that thrombolysis was equivalent to surgery for restoration of patency and limb salvage but showed reduced in-hospital complications and 12-month mortality compared with the surgical group.

Preliminary use of *rheolytic thrombectomy* devices (113,114) (Possis, Angiojet), either in lieu of or in conjunction with thrombolytic therapy, has demonstrated encouraging results for treatment of acute and chronic thrombus in the SFA/pop (as well as other sites) and highlighted the potential for this device to reduce procedure time, hospital stay, and risks associated with prolonged infusion of thrombolytic therapy (Figure 40.11). A direct comparison between mechanical and pharmacologic thrombolysis seems warranted in light of these promising initial results.

Restenosis

Despite the fact that PTA has been used widely and successfully to treat atherosclerotic obstructions in the peripheral and coronary circulations, restenosis following PTA of the SFA/popliteal artery continues to be a frustrating, and consequently expensive, complication of this otherwise efficacious intervention, more so than for any other vessel in the body. As indicated earlier, stents may ameliorate the flow-limiting complications of PTA acutely, but thus far they have been shown to have no significant impact on long-term patency.

Several promising strategies lie on the horizon for treating this vexing problem. First is the concept of gene transfer of angiogenic cytokines. Isner and colleagues have effectively transferred genetic material in animals to accelerate reendothelialization of the disrupted endovascular surface and inhibit intimal hyperplasia, thereby reducing restenosis (115). An ongoing Phase I trial in humans undergoing SFA/popliteal PTA has thus far demonstrated similar encouraging results, though these findings are preliminary (116).

Second, the concept of endovascular brachytherapy (117,118), which is currently being tested in coronary arteries, is also undergoing studies (PARIS trial) in conjunction with SFA/popliteal PTA. Preliminary results are also encouraging from this trial, but enrollment is ongoing.

Third, the use of covered stents for SFA/popliteal disease has been proposed as a mechanism to prevent intimal proliferation, which is the predominant cause of reocclusion within current SFA stents. Clinical trials of the Gore Hemobahn device and the Cragg Endopro system for this application are currently under way. Finally, other areas of research, including local drug delivery of agents that might reduce restenosis, are being contemplated (119,120).

Treatment Strategies and Technical Aspects

The most common route of access has been the antegrade approach, although the incidence of complications is slightly higher than that with retrograde access. Direct manipulation is facilitated and more steerablilty and support are available for traversing complex lesions or occlusions. Liabilities include the possibility that the lesion may involve the origin of the SFA, which may not be accessible if the antegrade puncture is immediately proximal or superimposed. Contralateral access permits imaging of the CFA bifurcation and allows iliac and infrainguinal disease to be treated in the same sitting, and has become increasingly popular with the development of curved (Cobra, LIMA) or retroflexed (Sos Omni, Simmons) catheters that allow easier access to the contralateral common iliac artery, and kink-resistant sheaths that maintain access around the aortic bifurcation. However, the requirement of lengthy wires and balloons, and the lack of support make traversal of critically narrowed or occluded sites problematic. The retrograde popliteal approach (121) is reserved for rare cases where the conventional approaches fail to enable traversal of a narrowed or occluded segment. The brachial approach, while providing better radiation protection, requires the use of lengthy wires and devices. The choice of access is ultimately based on all the information available, including prior angiographic examination, current duplex study, and physical findings of disease along the planned access route.

Current Recommendations for Superficial Femoral and Popliteal Disease

The acute technical success of balloon angioplasty for SFA/popliteal stenosis or occlusion is currently in the range of 90% to 100%. The principal factors in long-term patency are governed by the status of the runoff vessels and the presence of occlusion. Long-term patency of 50% can be anticipated at 5 years; this is significantly less than that of iliac angioplasty. Thus the threshold for intervention below the inguinal ligament should be higher. However, for patients with claudication severe enough to warrant intervention, PTA is the preferred initial treatment. This applies to both stenoses and occlusions that are amenable to revascularization. Lengthy, flush occlusions of the SFA may not be approachable. Rotational atherectomy can be applied in rare instances where there is extremely heavy calcification and resistance to dilation. Directional atherectomy can be used for very focal lesions or, if necessary, for removal of a flap that is limiting flow (flap atherectomy). Endovascular stents as a primary approach are not indicated. However, at present they have a role in salvage of acute PTA failures or complications. For chronic critical ischemia, or even acute limb-threatening ischemia, surgery is the preferred modality. However, one caveat to that is in the case of patients in

whom the need for coronary bypass grafting is anticipated; in these patients, as long as instrumentation does not preclude future surgical intervention, PTA may be preferred, in order to preserve the leg veins for future coronary bypass surgery.

INFRAPOPLITEAL ARTERIES

Published clinical experience involving percutaneous revascularization of the anterior tibial, tibioperoneal trunk, posterior tibial, and peroneal arteries has been far more limited than that for aortoiliac and SFA sites. This is related to several issues, including the fact that claudication is rarely due to isolated disease of the infrapopliteal arteries; knee-to-foot patency of one of the three major branches is generally regarded as sufficient to prevent critical lower limb ischemia; restenosis rates in these vessels have typically been the highest of any of the lower-extremity sites; and obstructive disease in these arteries is often occlusive or diffuse and complicated by heavy calcific deposits. Furthermore, diabetics have a high incidence of infrapopliteal disease, which is associated with diffusely atretic vessels that respond poorly to balloon dilation.

The ability to treat infrapopliteal disease has improved with technologic advances, including low-profile, high-pressure balloons and atraumatic guide wires, and the application of techniques employed for coronary arterial revascularization has consequently resulted in a more widespread application of percutaneous revascularization for infrapopliteal disease (122) (Figure 40.14). Despite this many of the patients treated with infrapopliteal angioplasty to date have been those who were too high risk or otherwise unqualified for bypass surgery. The latter is still considered the standard of care for patients with critical limb ischemia due to infrapopliteal disease. Regardless of the conduit (reversed vein, *in situ* vein, or prosthetic material) patency rates are inferior to those of more proximal reconstruction. The long-term clinical outcome of percutaneous therapy may ultimately equal that of distal bypass grafting. Over the past decade, reports have documented that stenotic and even short occlusions of one or more infrapopliteal arteries can be revascularized percutaneously with a high degree of efficacy and at extraordinarily low risk (123–126), particularly for critical limb ischemia as opposed to claudication (Figure 40.14). These studies have demonstrated technical and clinical success rates in the range of 80% to 95%. (The success rate in stenoses is superior to that in occlusions.)

It must be emphasized that the goals of infrapopliteal revascularization often differ from those of above-the-knee therapy and vary with clinical presentation. In most patients with claudication, for example, below-knee angioplasty is unnecessary, as treatment of coexisting proximal disease alone is often sufficient for symptomatic relief. There is a subset of patients who claudicate solely because

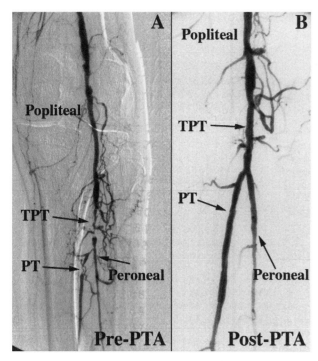

FIGURE 40.14. PTA of occluded tibioperoneal trunk and posterior tibial arteries in a patient with foot ulceration and threatened limb loss. **A:** Baseline angiogram demonstrates 2-cm occlusion of the tibioperoneal trunk (TPT) and focal subtotal occlusion of the proximal posterior tibial artery (PT). The anterior tibial artery was occluded at the origin. Segments were recanalized with glide wire, followed by PTA alone. **B:** Final angiogram post-PTA demonstrates widely patent tibioperoneal trunk, posterior tibial artery, and peroneal artery.

One point concerning percutaneous infrapopliteal revascularization requires special emphasis: the incidence of restenosis, which remains high, should not be a factor in the decision to employ a percutaneous approach for what is, in many of these patients, a short-term problem. If uninterrupted patency of even one vessel can be achieved, the improvement in antegrade nutrient flow is typically adequate to facilitate limb salvage. Once healed, most patients will do satisfactorily, even in the face of documented restenosis, if they can avoid subsequent foot trauma. This strategy is further supported by the fact that both the short-term and long-term outcomes of distal surgical reconstruction for infrapopliteal disease are likewise imperfect. It is also conceivable that both of these revascularization strategies will be supplemented in many instances by the strategy of therapeutic angiogenesis (9,128).

When performing infrapopliteal PTA, care should be taken to ensure that subsequent surgical options are not compromised. For example, overdilation and disruption of a distal, previously uncompromised vessel may prohibit subsequent bypass to that site. Although this rarely occurs, a conservative strategy is encouraged to avoid "burning a bridge" to a subsequent surgical intervention. Rotational atherectomy or excimer laser angioplasty can be useful as adjunctive therapy to angioplasty. Specifically, lesions that have unfavorable morphology, such as total occlusions, heavy calcification, and ostial disease, may benefit from these "niche" devices (129–131). Endovascular stents are not recommended for infrapopliteal vessels.

LOWER-EXTREMITY BYPASS GRAFTS

Stenosis in a lower-extremity bypass graft can threaten the patency of the graft and shorten its life. The etiology of bypass graft stenoses is variable. Stenoses that occur within the first few weeks of graft placement usually indicate a technical problem, which is best treated by repeat surgery and graft revision. Graft failure within a slightly later time frame (months to 1 year) can be due to myointimal hyperplasia, atherosclerosis, or progressive fibrosis of a poor venous conduit. Several other factors may contribute to graft failure, including the presence of poor inflow or poor outflow, low cardiac output, presence of a hypercoagulable state, compression of the graft due to patients crossing their legs or assuming other compromised positions, and external compression of the graft by sclerosis and fibrosis (e.g., from a scarred groin). Prosthetic conduits are more likely to present with abrupt occlusion, whereas native venous conduits tend to present with a progressive downhill course. Of course, even in the case of the latter, abrupt thrombosis and acute limb ischemia can occur.

Graft failure, or impending graft failure, is often not heralded by increasing clinical symptoms. Accordingly, a strategy of regular graft surveillance using duplex ultrasonogra-

of infrapopliteal disease, for whom percutaneous therapy is becoming more popular. Such a strategy should be reserved, at least for the present, for patients who have severe symptoms (Rutherford category 3). Infrapopliteal PTA may also be justified in claudicants who undergo proximal revascularization (with either surgery or PTA), in whom the runoff is severely impaired, as outflow may be the principal determinant of long-term patency for femoropopliteal revascularization.

In patients with rest pain or ischemic ulceration, restoration of uninterrupted patency of at least one of the three major infrapopliteal arteries is generally required to obviate symptoms and/or heal a distal ischemic lesion (Figure 40.14). In this group of patients, aggressive application of percutaneous revascularization may achieve extremely gratifying results, even in patients with calcified and/or lengthy total occlusions. If uninterrupted patency of even the one vessel can be achieved, the improvement in antegrade nutrient flow is typically adequate to facilitate limb salvage. Once healed, most patients will do satisfactorily, even in the face of documented reocclusion or restenosis. This strategy is further supported by the fact that both short- and long-term outcomes of distal surgical reconstruction for infrapopliteal disease are likewise imperfect (127).

phy is recommended to preserve and extend the life of the graft. For impending graft failure, detected by duplex ultrasonography or by increasing symptoms, immediate arteriography is recommended, followed by either surgical or percutaneous revascularization. Some series in the surgical literature suggest that, while PTA can be acutely successful, the long-term patency is inferior to that associated with surgical revision (132). Nonetheless, surgical revision may be complicated by imperfect long-term patency as well. In a recent study by Avino and colleagues (80), duplex scan surveillance was used to detect vein graft stenoses, and was employed to direct the revascularization strategy. In general, PTA was used primarily for cases with myointimal hyperplasia, vein fibrosis, sclerotic valves, and focal lesions less than 4 cm in length. For more extensive lesions, such as lengthy sclerotic vein segments, multiple-graft stenoses, and perianastomotic lesions, surgical interposition or jump graft techniques were employed. Of the 118 primary and 26 recurrent stenotic sites treated, 67 were addressed percutaneously. One-year stenosis-free patency for PTA was 66%, and for surgery was 76%. Notably, the PTA procedures were performed with on-line duplex monitoring, in order to ensure an optimal hemodynamic result. Long-term assisted graft patency was 91% at 1 year, and 80% at 3 years, remarkably high for grafts that have already required a first intervention. In another report from the same group, Gonsalves identified lesion characteristics that correlated with successful PTA outcome, including vein size greater than or equal to 3.5 mm, lesion length less than 2 cm, and occurrence of the lesion more than 3 months from surgery. If lesions fulfilled those criteria, the requirement for reintervention during 21-month follow-up was significantly reduced. The recommendations of the AHA task force in

1993 (133) were that focal lesions of the distal anastomosis of a femoropopliteal or femorotibial graft are amenable to PTA. Other lesions that are likely amenable include focal stenoses of proximal graft anastomoses (Figure 40.15) or short-segment lesions (3 cm or less) occurring within the bypass graft. Lengthy lesions (especially more than 10 cm) and stenoses associated with anastomotic aneurysms are recommended to undergo surgical revision.

For patients presenting with graft occlusion, the choices are more difficult. As indicated earlier, based on results from the Stile trial (37), the Rochester trial (112), and the recently completed TOPAS trial, patients presenting with acute or subacute thromboses (less than 14 days) are best treated with catheter-directed thrombolysis. An alternative is balloon embolectomy, though the latter strategy may be associated with a higher morbidity and mortality over the ensuing year (112). The one exception to this is the recently placed graft that fails almost immediately, which should return immediately to the operating room for surgical thrombectomy and revision. For patients with long-standing grafts that fail, determination of the factors responsible requires reestablishing enough flow to visualize the graft angiographically. Review of previous angiograms, including baseline (pregraft) and completion (postgraft) studies, often provides a clue as to the factors that may have contributed to thrombosis. In cases of early graft failure, reexamination of these angiographic studies may provide clues previously overlooked, such as stenosis of an inflow vessel, poor or inadequate distal runoff, or the presence of a venous side branch that was not sutured.

For patients presenting with impending graft failure based on a duplex study, access should be obtained to optimize the therapeutic alternatives. For example, after angiog-

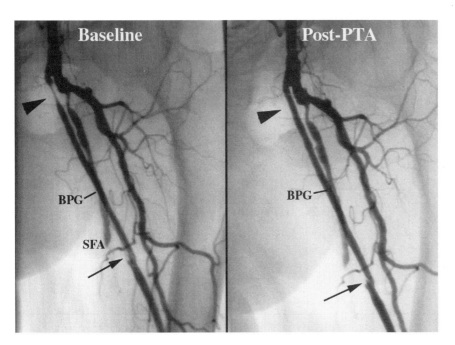

FIGURE 40.15. Right anterior oblique view of critical stenosis *(arrowhead)* at origin of femoropopliteal graft (BPG) and moderate irregular lesion *(arrow)* at distal end of jump-graft placed during previous graft revision. SFA is occluded proximally. Lesions were detected during routine surveillance (patient asymptomatic). Because of the proximity of lesions to the ipsilateral common femoral artery, contralateral access may be preferred. Post PTA, stenoses is eliminated, but regular surveillance will be essential to prevent graft failure.

raphy documents the presence of a proximal or distal anastomotic lesion, it is conceivable that the lesion could be resistant to balloon dilation alone. In these cases directional atherectomy is a useful tool for salvaging the graft and improving the outcome of the percutaneous intervention (134). Reported technical success rates in excess of 90% and 2-year patency rates of 80% are favorable compared with historical results of balloon angioplasty alone, especially for anastomotic lesions, and appear to be comparable to those of surgical revision, although direct comparison has not been performed. Likewise, although stents have been advocated for use in failing vein grafts, their utility has not been studied in any formal trials to date.

SUBCLAVIAN AND INNOMINATE ARTERIES

Indications for Intervention and Results

The vast majority of supraaortic disease in these vessels is due to atherosclerosis. However, giant cell arteritis, Takayasu's arteritis, and fibromuscular disease (FMD) can also cause clinically relevant disease (135–137). These patients may present with vertebrobasilar insufficiency, upper limb claudication (subclavian steal syndrome), or digital embolization. Routine examination (measurement of cuff pressure and palpation of pulses in both upper extremities, plus auscultation over the supra- and subclavicular areas) uncovers patients with asymptomatic subclavian disease. Initially, such patients do not require treatment, but they should be followed closely for progression or development of related symptoms, especially if coronary bypass surgery is anticipated. In such a patient, consideration should be given to empirical treatment of a critical

subclavian stenosis to preserve the option of using the internal mammary conduit.

Current clinical indications for subclavian revascularization are

- Symptomatic ischemia of the posterior fossa (e.g., vertebrobasilar insufficiency) and/or upper extremity, with or without subclavian steal syndrome (Figure 40.16).
- Preservation of flow, where thrombosis or progressive stenosis could have devastating consequences, especially in the case of CABG surgery utilizing the internal mammary arteries (e.g., ischemia in L [left] internal mammary artery [IMA]/right (R) IMA LIMA/RIMA territory with or without coronary-subclavian steal syndrome) (Figure 40.16).
- Preservation of inflow to axillary graft or dialysis conduit.
- "Blue-digit" syndrome (embolization to fingers).

Until recently, surgical treatment (carotid-subclavian or axilloaxillary bypass, endarterectomy, or aortosubclavian bypass) was considered the treatment of choice for subclavian disease. PTA has potential advantages over surgery: it eliminates the need for general anesthesia, shortens hospital stay, is less invasive, and reduces overall morbidity. It also avoids concern about potential stenosis in the carotid artery, which serves as the donor for carotid-subclavian bypass.

Most published series of subclavian PTA report technical success and complication rates of more than 90% and less than 10%, respectively (138–140). Complications are generally minor and infrequent, but include problems related to femoral or brachial access, inadvertent "jailing," dissection, and embolization of the vertebral or LIMA. Direct comparison between surgery and PTA for subclavian disease is ham-

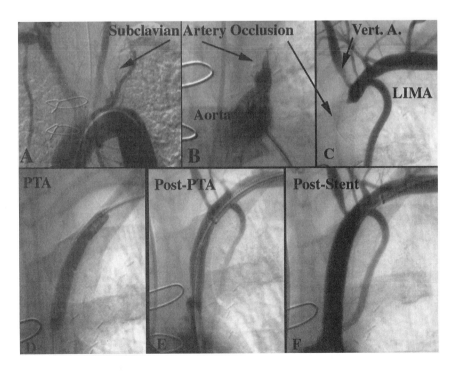

FIGURE 40.16. Subclavian artery revascularization for disabling upper limb claudication and coronary steal syndrome in an elderly patient who developed recurrent angina 10 years following coronary artery bypass surgery with left internal mammary artery (LIMA) graft to the left anterior descending coronary artery. Arch aortogram (**A**) discloses short-segment occlusion of the left subclavian artery (SCA) 1 cm from the origin, with reconstitution distally. SCA filling is predominantly via patent LIMA (coronary steal). Radionuclide imaging disclosed mild stress-induced anterior wall ischemia. **B:** Selective cannulation of SCA demonstrates a "beaklike" obstruction. **C:** Angiography via brachial artery access demonstrates reconstitution proximal to the LIMA and vertebral artery (vert). **D:** PTA performed after lesion traversed with a glide wire from the arm and resulted in restoration of luminal patency with residual stenosis. **E:** Stent deployment was successfully performed proximal to the vertebral artery to include the origin of the SCA with relief of angina and upper limb claudication.

pered by the absence of randomized controlled studies. For *focal subclavian stenoses,* one multicenter analysis compared primary subclavian stenting (in 108 patients) to 2,496 surgical patients (reported in the surgical literature between 1966 and 1998) (141). The surgical series had a stroke rate of 3%, mortality of 2%, and complications in 13%, whereas the stent series reported no strokes, no deaths, and 6% overall complications. Recurrence rates were 12% in surgical patients and 3% in stent patients. In contrast, PTA alone for *occlusive* disease has a lower chance of success (50% to 75%) and increased potential to embolize thrombus or atheroma into the cerebral, upper-extremity, or coronary circulation. Recent series indicate that primary stenting has emerged as an appropriate initial strategy for symptomatic patients and may further improve the results (139,142–145) (Figure 40.16).

Treatment Strategies and Technical Aspects

Noninvasive testing with duplex ultrasound before undertaking subclavian or brachiocephalic angioplasty is essential with determination of the direction of flow in the vertebral arteries (antegrade or retrograde, the latter indicating the presence of a steal syndrome), and documentation as to the presence or absence of carotid disease. If vasculitis is suspected clinically, the erythrocyte sedimentation rate should be measured. Premedication with aspirin is standard, with the optional addition of clopidogrel (Plavix, Bristol-Meyers Squibb, Hillside, NJ) or ticlopidine (Ticlid, Roche Laboratories, Nutley, NJ). In cases of subclavian occlusion, because nascent thrombus may occur in the segment immediately beyond the occlusion, patients may benefit from anticoagulation (in conjunction with antiplatelet therapy) for a period of several weeks before revascularization.

The femoral approach is used most commonly but requires careful catheter manipulation in a diseased aortic arch, to avoid atheroembolic complications. The brachial approach, described by Dorros (139), may be useful for total occlusions, especially for those that are "flush" with the aorta. However, it should be noted that a higher percentage of complications has been reported when using the brachial site, whether cut down or percutaneous. A nonselective aortic arch angiogram, using a multiple side-hole catheter, such as a pigtail, should be obtained before gaining selective access into the subclavian or innominate artery. It may be possible to steer a guide wire directly across a stenosis from the sheath before advancing a selective catheter, thus minimizing contact with the diseased aortic wall. However, selective cannulation of the vessel with a diagnostic catheter (e.g., JR4, cobra, Simmons) is usually required in the case of occlusion.

No stent has yet received specific approval by the FDA for use in the subclavian artery; however, both balloon-expandable and self-expanding steel or Nitinol stents have been used. Predilation is performed with an undersized

(usually 4 to 5 mm in diameter) balloon. Most left subclavian lesions are located proximal to the vertebral artery, where use of either balloon-expandable or self-expanding stents is reasonable. For lesions located beyond the internal mammary artery, self-expanding stents should be used to avoid the potential for late stent compression by extravascular structures at the thoracic outlet. If the lesion is adjacent to or spans across the origins of the vertebral and/or IMA, attempts should be made to avoid placing these vessels into "stent jail." When stenting the innominate artery, care should be taken to avoid encroaching upon the origin of the right common carotid artery. Stents should be post-dilated with care to minimize the risk of dissection that might extend into the vertebral artery or internal mammary artery; such dissections can often be salvaged by stenting the origin of the affected branch vessel.

No data exist regarding the use of Plavix or Ticlid, though many maintain this regimen for 4 weeks after the procedure. During clinical follow-up, the resolution of symptoms should be documented, equalization of blood pressures in both upper extremities should be confirmed, and the duplex study should show triphasic brachial waveforms with restoration of normal antegrade flow in the vertebral arteries. Restenosis within subclavian arteries occurs in 10% to 20% of patients and may be treated by stenting (if not stented initially) or balloon angioplasty (for in-stent restenosis). Stent "compression" should be treated by balloon reexpansion and placement of a self-expanding stent within the old device.

MESENTERIC ARTERIES

Indications for Treatment and Results

Stenosis of mesenteric vessels is a frequent finding during routine angiographic studies of the abdominal aorta, but ischemic consequences of those stenoses occur infrequently. When they do occur, their presentation may be quite subtle and not always easy to ascribe to mesenteric ischemia. The classic syndrome of postprandial abdominal pain, gas, diarrhea, food avoidance, and weight loss is uncommon and is most likely to occur in the setting of severe global compromise of blood supply to the mesentery, such as occlusion of two out of three mesenteric vessels, and a critical stenosis in the third. There are syndromes with lesser degrees of ischemia, wherein patients will present with variable symptoms, including mild postprandial aching or discomfort, diarrhea, nausea, or gaseousness, in which two mesenteric vessels are patent, but both with severe narrowing. Occasionally, even a single critically narrowed vessel can cause these symptoms.

The angiographic diagnosis can be as ambiguous and difficult as the clinical manifestations. Because the mesenteric vessels originate on the anterior wall of the aorta and project anteriorly, the origins of these vessels are rarely seen during a conventional "AP" angiogram. Therefore extremely angulated and/or lateral views are required to define aortoostial lesions in these vessels.

As is the case with many other vascular sites, the standard of therapy for mesenteric disease has been surgical (endarterectomy or bypass), with a mortality rate that approaches 6% (146). In the current era, however, balloon angioplasty can be effective in restoring acute patency, though restenosis rates are 50% or more, due to the ostial location of these lesions. Although prospective studies of long-term outcome following PTA/stenting have yet to be done, early indications suggest that stents reduce acute recoil and may lead to a better long-term patency (147, 148). The biggest dilemma in patients with mesenteric disease is deciding who is likely to benefit. Certainly, the incidental finding of a mesenteric vessel during routine angiography for other reasons does not necessarily indicate the need for treatment. A conservative approach is indicated in situations where symptoms of mesenteric ischemia are absent. At the other extreme, the percutaneous approach is ill advised in patients with acute mesenteric ischemia, and in whom bowel infarction has already taken place. These patients are better served by surgical repair and intestinal resection.

Treatment Strategies and Technical Aspects

Aortoostial mesenteric disease is similar in most respects to aortoostial renal artery disease. Therefore the approach to balloon angioplasty and stenting is identical. Thus far, there are no controlled trials, nor are any large series reported using stents in mesenteric arteries. Anecdotally, the results are similar to those for renal stenting, but three things distinguish mesenteric vessels from the renal arteries: First, the celiac and superior mesenteric arteries both tend to arise off the aorta at more of a downward angle than the renal arteries, making access more difficult from below. Second, visualization of the target vessel and lesion site may be more difficult in these vessels than for the renal arteries and often dictates the need for a lateral projection. Third, the complications related to failure and/or embolization into these arteries can have severe consequences, including bowel infarction, sepsis, and death. Therefore extreme caution must be used.

HEMODIALYSIS CONDUITS

Patients dependent on hemodialysis number in excess of 120,000. Recent evidence shows this number to be increasing at a rate of 10% per year (149). As the population of patients on dialysis expands and life expectancy on dialysis increases, preservation of vascular access sites has become increasingly important. Repeated large-gauge needle punc-

tures three times per week, increased sheer forces and intraluminal pressure during dialysis, and postdialysis compression of puncture sites are all factors that may contribute to the high incidence of stenosis and thrombosis that occur in dialysis conduits, be they arteriovenous (AV) fistulas or Gortex grafts. AV fistulas tend to develop fibrous strictures at, and proximal to, sites of repeated puncture. Gortex grafts develop stenoses principally localized to the venous and arterial anastomoses; accumulation of pseudointima within the body of the graft may also predispose to graft failure. Surgical revision typically involves several days of hospitalization and placement of temporary access. A more important consequence of surgical revision, however, is the use of proximal vein, which may limit options for future surgical management. PTA has played an increasingly important role in maintaining the functional status of hemodialysis access conduits (Figure 40.17). The use of PTA for dialysis conduits requires a different perspective from PTA at other sites. Because the patency of dialysis conduits is problematic, regardless of whether surgery or other approaches are utilized, restenosis is tolerated at a higher frequency than nearly all other circumstances.

Percutaneous treatment of stenotic or occluded grafts or fistulae is usually technically straightforward. Acute success rates of 70% to 95% have been reported (149–151). However, primary restenosis rates are higher than those for PTA in most other vascular beds, up to 60% and 80% at 1 and 2 years, respectively (151,152). *Secondary* patency, however, has been quite acceptable (>70% at 2 years) in series where the investigators closely monitored graft function and performed early angiography and repeat PTA in cases of recurrent stenosis (151). Thus, although the average graft may only remain functional for 4 to 6 months after a single PTA, as opposed to 14 to 18 months after surgical revision (149), close monitoring of graft function and appropriately timed intervention can enhance the results of the percutaneous strategy and delay the need for graft revision.

Angioplasty of offending lesions in dialysis conduits often requires use of high-pressure (up to 20 atm) inflation, because of the fibrotic nature of the strictures within the venous system and at the graft anastomosis. IVUS is particularly useful for determining the reference diameter and quantifying the extent of recoil. Even aggressive angioplasty using oversized balloons, however, is often insufficient, in which case adjunctive treatment with directional atherectomy may be useful to "cut" the fibrous band. Endovascular stents have also been investigated, but their role remains to be determined.

Management of dialysis conduits requires the cooperative efforts of a team, consisting of nephrologists, vascular surgeons, and interventionalists. The nephrologists and dialysis nursing staff must pay close attention to the hemodynamic function of access sites during dialysis. Increase in venous pressure, decrease in arterial flow, increase in recirculation, and poor dialysis efficiency are all factors that

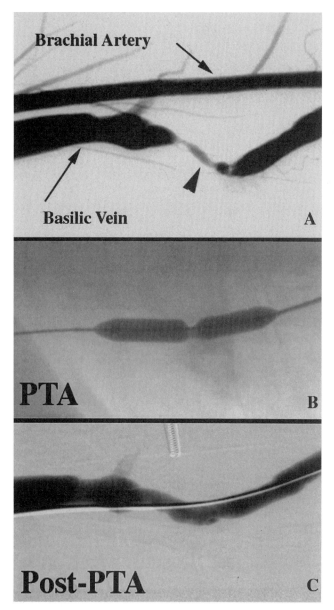

FIGURE 40.17. Percutaneous revascularization (PTA) of a hemodialysis conduit (arteriovenous fistula) in an elderly patient with chronic renal failure. **A:** Diagnostic fistulogram, obtained because of poor dialysis efficiency (high venous pressures) demonstrated a high-grade, focal stenosis *(arrowhead)* in the mid-portion of the basilic vein. **B:** Angioplasty was performed using a noncompliant balloon. **C:** Final angiographic image demonstrated acute technical success with resolution of the stenosis and minimal elastic recoil.

should trigger the request for a diagnostic angiogram. Focal stenoses can be treated initially using PTA and, for resistant lesions, directional atherectomy. Thereafter patients should be monitored particularly closely, as one can expect a high incidence of restenosis. Repeated percutaneous interventions, in the interest of preserving the access site and avoiding the need to sacrifice an additional vein, are appropriate. However, in cases of recurrent early failure and/or extensive graft degeneration, surgical revision becomes necessary.

ACKNOWLEDGMENTS

The authors would like to thank the expert assistance of Mr. Andre Griben for preparation of the figures, Mrs. Judith Soressi for preparation of the manuscript, and the nursing and support staff of the Division of Vascular Medicine at Saint Elizabeth's Medical Center for their dedication in caring for the patients undergoing peripheral vascular interventions.

REFERENCES

1. Creager MA, Halperin JL, Coffman JD. Raynaud's phenomenon and other vascular disorders related to temperature. In: Loscalzo J, Creager MA, Dzau VJ, eds. *Vascular medicine: a textbook of vascular biology and diseases.* Boston: Little, Brown, 1996:965–997.
2. Rutherford RB, Flanigan DP, Guptka SK. Suggested standards for reports dealing with lower extremity ischemia. *J Vasc Surg* 1986;4:80–94.
3. European Working Group on Critical Leg Ischemia. Second European consensus document on chronic critical leg ischemia. *Circulation* 1991;84(Suppl IV):IV-1.
4. Spittell JA. Pentoxifylline and intermittent claudication (Editorial). *Ann Intern Med* 1985;102:126–127.
5. Creager MA. Can claudication be treated medically? *J Vasc Med Biol* 1989;1:269–271.
6. Money SR, Herd JA, Isaacsohn JL, et al. Effect of cilastazol on walking distances in patients with intermittent claudication caused by peripheral vascular disease. *J Vasc Surg* 1998;27:267–275.
7. Hiatt WR. Current and future drug therapies for claudication. *Vasc Med* 1997;2:257–262.
8. Isner JM, Baumgartner I, Rauh G, et al. Treatment of thromboangiitis obliterans (Buerger's disease) by intramuscular gene transfer of vascular endothelial growth factor: preliminary clinical results. *J Vasc Surg* 1998;28:964–975.
9. Baumgartner I, Pieczek A. Manor O. Constitutive expression of phVEGF†165 following intramuscular gene transfer promotes collateral vessel development in patients with critical limb ischemia. *Circulation* 1998;97:1114–1123.
10. Rutherford RB, Becker GJ. Standards for evaluating and reporting the results of surgical and percutaneous therapy for peripheral arterial disease. *Radiology* 1991;181:277–281.
11. Gruentzig AR. Transluminal dilatation of coronary artery stenosis (letter to editor). *Lancet* 1978;1:263.
12. Dotter CT, Judkins MP. Transluminal treatment of arteriosclerotic obstruction: description of a new technique and a preliminary report of its application. *Circulation* 1964;30:654–670.
13. Isner JM, Rosenfield K. Redefining the treatment of peripheral artery disease: role of percutaneous revascularization. *Circulation* 1993;88:1534–1557.
14. Long AL, Page PE, Raynaud AC, et al. Percutaneous iliac artery stent: angiographic long-term follow-up. *Radiology* 1991;180:771–778.
15. Losordo DW, Rosenfield K, Pieczek A, et al. How does angioplasty work? Serial *in vivo* morphometric analysis of mechanisms of angioplasty in humans using intravascular ultrasound. *Circulation* 1992;86:1845–1858.
16. Rosenfield K, Isner JM. Intravascular ultrasound in patients undergoing coronary and peripheral arterial revascularization. In: Topol EJ, ed. *Textbook of interventional cardiology.* Philadelphia: WB Saunders, 1994:1153–1185.

17. Rajachandran M, Rosenfield K, Schainfeld R, et al. Is there a role for intravascular ultrasound in carotid artery stenting? *J Am Coll Cardiol* 1997;29:363A(abst).

18. Dormandy JA, Rutherford RB. Management of peripheral arterial disease. *J Vasc Surg* 2000;31:S1–S296.

19. Gruntzig A., Kumpe D.A. Technique of percutaneous transluminal angioplasty with the Gruntzig balloon catheter. *Am J Roentgenol* 1979;132:547–552.

20. Tegtmeyer CJ, Hartwell GD, Selby JB, et al. Results and complications of angioplasty in aortoiliac disease. *Circulation* 1991; 83(Suppl I):I-53–I-60.

21. Johnston KW. Iliac arteries: reanalysis of results of balloon angioplasty. *Radiology* 1993;186:207–212.

22. Blum U, Gabelmann A, Redecker M, et al. Percutaneous recanalization of iliac artery occlusions: results of a prospective study. *Radiology* 1993;189:536–540.

23. Martin EC. Percutaneous therapy in the management of aortoiliac disease. *Semin Vasc Surg* 1994;7:17–27.

24. O'Keeffe ST, Woods BO, Breslin DJ, et al. Blue toe syndrome: causes and management. *Arch Intern Med* 1992;152: 2197–2202.

25. Lopez-Galarza LA, Ray LI, Rodriguez-Lopez J, et al. Combined percutaneous transluminal angioplasty, iliac stent deployment, and femorofemoral bypass for bilateral aortoiliac occlusive disease. *J Am Coll Surg* 1997;184:249–258.

26. Schroder A, Muckner K, Riepe G, et al. Semiclosed iliac recanalisation by an inguinal approach: modified surgical techniques integrating interventional procedures. *Eur J Vasc Endovasc Surg* 1998;16:501–508.

27. Cooper CJ, Moore JA, Burket MW. Intraaortic balloon pump insertion after percutaneous revascularization in patients with aortoiliac stenosis. *Circulation* 1998;98:I-444.

28. Tadavarthy AK, Sullivan WA Jr, Nicoloff D, et al. Aorta balloon angioplasty: 9-year follow-up. *Radiology* 1989;170:1039–1041.

29. Audet P, Therasse E, Oliva VL, et al. Infrarenal aortic stenosis: long-term clinical and hemodynamic results of percutaneous transluminal angioplasty. *Radiology* 1998;209:357–363.

30. Mendelsohn FO, Santos RM, Crowley JJ, et al. Kissing stents in the aortic bifurcation. *Am Heart J* 1998;136:600–605.

31. Whiteley MS, Ray-Chaudhuri SB, Galland RB. Changing patterns in aortoiliac reconstruction: a 7-year audit. *Br J Surg* 1996; 83:1367–1369.

32. Brewster MD. Current controversies in the management of aortoiliac occlusive disease. *J Vasc Surg* 1997;25:365–379.

33. Pentecost J.J. The use of angioplasty, bypass surgery, and amputation in the management of peripheral vascular disease (letter). *N Engl J Med* 1992;326:413.

34. Bosch JL, Hunink MG. Meta-analysis of the results of percutaneous transluminal angioplasty and stent placement for aortoiliac occlusive disease. *Radiology* 1997;204:87–96.

35. Gupta AK, Ravimandalom K, Rao VRK. Total occlusion of iliac arteries: results of balloon angioplasty. *Cardovasc Intervent Radiol* 1993;16:165–177.

36. Henry M, Amor M, Ethevenot G, et al. Percutaneous endoluminal treatment of iliac occlusions: long-term follow-up in 105 patients. *J Endovasc Surg* 1998;5:228–235.

37. The STILE Investigators. Results of a prospective randomized trial evaluating surgery versus thrombolysis for ischemia of the lower extremity. *Ann Surg* 1994;220:251–268.

38. Ouriel K, Veith FJ, Sasahara, AA. A comparison of recombinant urokinase with vascular surgery as initial treatment for acute arterial occlusion of the legs. *N Engl J Med* 1998;338:1105–1111.

39. Working Party on Thrombolysis in the Management of Limb Ischemia. Thrombolysis in the management of lower limb peripheral arterial occlusion-a consensus document. *Am J Cardiol* 1998;81:207–218.

40. Weaver FA, Comerota AJ, Youngblood M, et al. Surgical revascularization versus thrombolysis for nonembolic lower extremity native artery occlusions: results of a prospective randomized trial. *J Vasc Surg* 1996;24:513–523.

41. Palmaz JC, Richter GM, Noeldge G. Intraluminal stents in atherosclerotic iliac artery stenosis: preliminary report of multicenter study. *Radiology* 1988;168:727–731.

42. Murphy TP, Webb MS, Lambiase RE, et al. Percutaneous revascularization of complex iliac artery stenoses and occlusions with use of Wallstents: three-year experience. *J Vasc Interv Radiol* 1996;7:21–27.

43. Martin EC, Katzen BT, Benenati JF, et al. Multicenter trial of the Wallstent in the iliac and femoral arteries. *J Vasc Interv Radiol* 1995;6:843–849.

44. Treiman GS, Schneider PA, Lawrence PF, et al. Does stent placement improve the results of ineffective or complicated iliac artery angioplasty? *J Vasc Surg* 1998;28:104–112.

45. Murphy KD, Encarnacion CE, Le VA, et al. Iliac artery stent placement with the Palmaz stent: follow-up study. *J Vasc Interv Radiol* 1995;6:321–329.

46. Rees CR, Palmaz JC, Garcia O, et al. Angioplasty and stenting of completely occluded iliac arteries. *Radiology* 1989;172: 953–959.

47. Sapoval MR, Long AL, Pagny JY, et al. Outcome of percutaneous intervention in iliac artery stents. *Radiology* 1996;198: 481–486.

48. Richter GM, Roeren T, Brado M. Further update of the randomized trial: iliac stent placement versus PTA-morphology, clinical success rates, and failure analysis. *J Vasc Interv Radiol* 1993;4:30.

49. Onal B, Ilgit ET, Yucel C, et al. Primary stenting for complex atherosclerotic plaques in aortic and iliac stenoses. *Cardiovasc Intervent Radiol* 1998;21:386–392.

50. Sullivan TM, Childs MB, Bacharach JM, et al. Percutaneous transluminal angioplasty and primary stenting of the iliac arteries in 288 patients. *J Vasc Surg* 1997;25:829–838.

51. Tetteroo E, van Engelen AD, Spithoven JH, et al. Stent placement after iliac angioplasty: comparison of hemodynamic and angiographic criteria. *Radiology* 1996;201:155–159.

52. Vorwerk D, Gunther RW, Schurman, et al. Aortic and iliac stenoses: follow-up results of stent placement after insufficient balloon angioplasty in 118 cases. *Radiology* 1996;198:45–48.

53. Laborde JC, Palmaz JL, Rivera FJ, et al. Influence of anatomic distribution of atherosclerosis on the outcome of revascularization with iliac stent placement. *J Vasc Intervent Radiol* 1995;6: 513-521.

54. White CJ, Nguyen M, Ramee, SR. Use of a guiding catheter for contralateral femoral artery angioplasty. *Catheter Cardiovasc Diagn* 1990;21:15–17.

55. Isner JM, Rosenfield K, Losordo DW, et al. Combination balloon-ultrasound imaging catheter for percutaneous transluminal angioplasty: validation of imaging, analysis of recoil, and identification of plaque fracture. *Circulation* 1991;84:739–754.

56. Rosenfield K, Kaufman J, Pieczek A, et al. Human coronary and peripheral arteries: on-line three-dimensional reconstruction from two-dimensional intravascular US scans. *Radiology* 1992;184:823–832.

57. Rosenfield K, Losordo DW, Ramaswamy K, et al. Three-dimensional reconstruction of human coronary and peripheral arteries from images recorded during two-dimensional intravascular ultrasound examination. *Circulation* 1991;84:1938–1956.

58. Isner JM, Rosenfield K, Kelly S, et al. Percutaneous intravascular ultrasound examination as an adjunct to catheter-based interventions: preliminary experience in patients with peripheral vascular disease. *Radiology* 1990;175:61–70.

59. Isner JM, Kaufman J, Rosenfield K, et al. Combined physio-

logic and anatomic assessment of percutaneous revascularization using a Doppler guidewire and ultrasound catheter. *Am J Cardiol* 1993;71:70D–86D.

60. Veith FJ, Gupta SK, Wengerter KR, et al. Changing arteriosclerotic disease patterns and management strategies in lower-limb-threatening ischemia. *Ann Surg* 1990;212:402–414.

61. Kumpe DA, Rutherford RB. Percutaneous transluminal angioplasty for lower extremity ischemia. In: Rutherford RB, ed. *Vascular surgery*, 3rd ed. Philadelphia: WB Saunders, 1992:759–761.

62. Eagle KA, Coley CM, Newell JB, et al. Combining clinical and thallium data optimizes preoperative assessment of cardiac risk before major vascular surgery. *Ann Int Med* 1989;110:859–866.

63. Lalka SG, Sawada SG, Dalsing MC, et al. Dobutamine stress echocardiography as a predictor of cardiac events associated with aortic surgery. *J Vasc Surg* 1992;15:831–842.

64. Varty K, London NJM, Ratliff DA, et al. Percutaneous angioplasty of the profunda femoris artery: a safe and effective endovascular technique. *Eur J Vasc Surg* 1993;7:483–487.

65. Silva JA, White CJ, Ramee SR. Percutaneous profundoplasty in the treatment of severe lower extremity ischemia: results of long-term surveillance. *Therapy* 2001;8:75–82.

66. Smith GD, Shipley MJ, Rose G. Intermittent claudication, heart disease risk factors, and mortality: the Whitehall Study. *Circulation* 1990;82:1925–1931.

67. Criqui MH, Langer RD, Fronek A, et al. Mortality over a period of 10 years in patients with peripheral arterial disease. *N Engl J Med* 1992;326:381–386.

68. Porter JM. Endovascular arterial intervention: expression of concern. *J Vasc Surg* 1995;21:995–997.

69. Moore WS. Therapeutic options for femoropopliteal disease. *Circulation* 1991;83(Suppl 1):I-91–I-93.

70. Krepel VM, van Andel HJ, van Erp WFM, et al. Percutaneous transluminal angioplasty of the femoropopliteal artery: initial and long-term results. *Radiology* 1985;165:325–328.

71. Gallino A, Mahler F, Probst P, et al. Percutaneous transluminal angioplasty of the arteries of the lower limbs: a 5-year follow-up. *Circulation* 1984;70:619–623.

72. Capek P, McLean GK, Berkowitz HD. Femoropopliteal angioplasty: factors influencing long-term success. *Circulation* 1991; 83:I-70–I-80.

73. Murray JG, Apthorp LA, Wilkins RA. Long-segment (≥10 cm) femoropopliteal angioplasty: improved technical success and long-term patency. *Radiology* 1995;195:158–162.

74. Jeans WD, Armstrong S, Cole SEA. Fate of patients undergoing transluminal angioplasty for lower-limb ischemia. *Radiology* 1990;177:559–564.

75. Johnston KW. Femoral and popliteal arteries: reanalysis of results of balloon angioplasty. *Radiology* 1992;183:767–771.

76. Hunink MG, Donaldson MC, Meyerovitz MF, et al. Risks and benefits of femoropopliteal percutaneous balloon angioplasty. *J Vasc Surgery* 1993;17:183–184.

77. Matsi PJ, Manninen JI, Vanninen RL, et al. Femoropopliteal angioplasty in patients with claudication: primary and secondary patency in 140 limbs with 1–2-year follow-up. *Radiology* 1994;191:727–733.

78. Johnston KW, Rae M, Hogg-Johnston SA. Five year results of a prospective study of percutaneous transluminal angioplasty. *Ann Surg* 1987;206:403–413.

79. Gordon IL, Conroy RM, Tobis JM, et al. Determinants of patency after percutaneous angioplasty and atherectomy of occluded superficial femoral arteries. *Am J Surg* 1994;167: 115–119.

80. Avino AJ, Bandyk DF, Gonsalves AJ, et al. Surgical and endovascular intervention for infrainguinal vein graft stenosis. *J Vasc Surg* 1999;29:60–71.

81. Huink MGM, Wong JB, Donaldson MC, et al. Revascularization for femoropopliteal disease: a decision and cost-effectiveness analysis. *JAMA* 1995;274:165–171.

82. Zeitler E, Richter EI, Roth FJ, et al. Results of percutaneous transluminal angioplasty. *Radiology* 1983;146:57–60.

83. Hewes RC, White RI, Murray RR. Long-term results of superficial femoral artery angioplasty. *Am J Roentgenol* 1986;146: 1025–1029.

84. Pieczek AM, Langevin RE Jr, Razvi S, et al. Successful percutaneous revascularization of 180/190 (95%) consecutive peripheral arterial total occlusions using hydrophilic ("glide") wire. *Circulation* 1992;86:I-704(abst).

85. Rosenfield K, Losordo DW, Ramaswamy K, et al. Three-dimensional reconstruction of intravascular ultrasound images recorded in 68 consecutive patients following percutaneous revascularization of totally occluded arteries: *in vivo* evidence that the neolumen frequently includes subintimal component. *Circulation* 1991;84:II-686(abst).

86. Morgenstern BR, Getrajdman GI, Laffey KJ, et al. Total occlusions of the femoropopliteal artery: high technical success rate of conventional balloon angioplasty. *Radiology* 1989;172: 937–940.

87. Sapoval MC, Long AL, Raynaud AC, et al. Femoropopliteal stent placement: long-term results. *Radiology* 1992;184: 833–839.

88. Gray BH, Sullivan TM, Childs MB, et al. High incidence of restenosis/reocclusion of stents in the percutaneous treatment of long-segment superficial femoral artery disease after suboptimal angioplasty. *J Vasc Surg* 1997;25:74–83.

89. Gray BH, Olin JW. Limitations of percutaneous transluminal angioplasty with stenting for femoropopliteal arterial occlusive disease. *Semin Vasc Surg* 1997;10:8–16.

90. White GH, Liew SC, Waugh RC, et al. Early outcome and intermediate follow-up of vascular stents in the femoral and popliteal arteries without long-term anticoagulation. *J Vasc Surg* 1995;21:270–279.

91. Strecker EP, Boos IB, Gottmann D. Femoropopliteal artery stent placement: evaluation of long-term success. *Radiology* 1997;205:375–383.

92. Henry M, Amor M, Ethevenot G, et al. Palmaz stent placement in iliac and femoropopliteal arteries: primary and secondary patency in 310 patients with 2–4-year follow-up. *Radiology* 1995;197:167–174.

93. Do DD, Triller J, Walpoth BH, et al. A comparison study of self-expandable stents vs balloon angioplasty alone in femoropopliteal artery occlusions. *Cardiovasc Intervent Radiol* 1992; 15:306–312.

94. Rosenfield K, Schainfeld R, Pieczek A, et al. Restenosis of endovascular stents due to stent compression. *J Am Coll Cardiol* 1997;29:328–338.

95. Cejna M, Illiasch H, Waldenberg P, et al. PTA vs Palmaz stent in femoropopliteal obstructions: a prospective randomised trial—long-term results. *Radiology* 1998;209:492.

96. Damaraju S, Cuasay L, Le D, et al. Predictors of primary patency failure in Wallstent self-expanding endovascular prostheses for iliofemoral occlusive disease. *Tex Heart Inst J* 1997;24: 173–178.

97. Pickering JG, Weir L, Jekanowski J, et al. Proliferative activity in peripheral and coronary atherosclerotic plaque among patients undergoing percutaneous revascularization. *J Clin Invest* 1993;91:1469–1480.

98. Dorros G, Lyer S, Lewin R, et al. Angiographic follow-up and clinical outcome of 126 patients after percutaneous directional atherectomy (Simpson AtheroCath) for occlusive peripheral vascular disease. *Catheter Cardiovasc Diagn* 1991;22:79–84.

99. Haji-Aghaii M, Fogarty TJ. Balloon angioplasty, stenting, and role of atherectomy. *Surg Clin North Am* 1998;78:593–616.

100. Vroegindeweij D, Tielbeek AV, Buth J, et al. Directional atherectomy versus balloon angioplasty in segmental femoropopliteal artery disease: two-year follow-up with color-flow duplex scanning *J Vasc Surg* 1995;21:255–269.

101. Dorros G, Lyer S, Zaitoun R, et al. Acute angiographic and clinical outcome of high speed percutaneous rotational atherectomy (Rotablator). *Catheter Cardiovasc Diagn* 1991;22:157–166.

102. White CJ, Ramee SR, Escobar A, et al. High-speed rotational ablation (Rotablator) for unfavorable lesions in peripheral arteries. *Catheter Cardiovasc Diagn* 1993;30:115–119.

103. Seeger JM, Abela GS, Silverman SH, et al. Initial results of laser recanalization in lower extremity arterial reconstruction. *J Vasc Surg* 1989;9:10–17.

104. Sanborn TA, Cumerland DC, Greenfield AJ. Percutaneous laser thermal angioplasty: mitral results and 1-year follow-up in 129 femoropopliteal lesions. *Radiology* 1988;168:121–125.

105. Lammer J, Karnel F. Percutaneous transluminal laser angioplasty with contact probes. *Radiology* 1988;168:733–737.

106. Murray A, Mitchell DC, Grasty M, et al. Peripheral laser angioplasty with pulsed dye laser and ball-tipped optical fibers. *Lancet* 1989;2:1471–1474.

107. Huppert PE, Duda SH, Helber U, et al. Comparison of pulsed laser-assisted angioplasty and balloon angioplasty in femoropopliteal artery occlusions. *Radiology* 1992;184:363–367.

108. White CJ, Ramee SR, Collins TJ, et al. Recanalization of arterial occlusions with a lensed fiber and a holmium:YAG laser. *Lasers Surg Med* 1991;11:250–256.

109. Isner JM, Donaldson RF, Deckelbaum LI, et al. The excimer laser: gross, light microscopic, and ultrastructural analysis of potential advantages for use in laser therapy of cardiovascular disease. *J Am Coll Cardiol* 1985;6:1102–1109.

110. Rosenfield K, Pieczek A, Losordo DW, et al. Excimer laser thrombolysis for rapid clot dissolution in lesions at high risk for embolization: a potentially useful new application for excimer laser. *J Am Coll Cardiol* 1992;19:104A(abst).

111. Earnshaw JJ, Birch P. Peripheral thrombolysis: state of the art. *Cardiovasc Surg* 1995;3:357–367.

112. Ouriel K, Shortell CK, DeWeese JA, et al. A comparison of thrombolytic therapy with operative revascularization in the initial treatment of acute peripheral arterial ischemia. *J Vasc Surg* 1994;19:1021–1030.

113. Silva JA, Ramee SR, Collins TJ, et al. Rheolytic thrombectomy in the treatment of acute limb-threatening ischemia: immediate results and six-month follow-up of the multicenter AngioJet Registry. *Catheter Cardiovasc Diagn* 1998;45:386–393.

114. Mathie AG, Bell SD, Saibil EA. Mechanical thromboembolectomy in acute embolic peripheral arterial occlusions with use of the AngioJet rapid thrombectomy system. *J Vasc Intervent Radiol* 1999;10:583–590.

115. Isner JM, Walsh K, Rosenfield K, et al. Arterial gene therapy for restenosis. *Human Gene Ther* 1996;7:989–1011.

116. Vale PR, Wuensch DI, Rauh GF, et al. Arterial gene therapy for inhibiting restenosis in patients with claudication undergoing superficial femoral artery angioplasty. *Circulation* 1998;17:I-66 (abst).

117. Minar E, Pokrajac B, Ahmadi R, et al. Brachytherapy for prophylaxis of restenosis after long-segment femoropopliteal angioplasty: pilot study. *Radiology* 1998;208:173–179.

118. Waksman R. *Textbook of cardiovascular medicine.* Philadelphia: Lippincott Williams & Wilkins, 1999.

119. Vogelzang RL. Future directions in vascular and interventional radiology research. *Radiology* 1998;209:17–18.

120. Gershlick A. Endovascular manipulation to restrict restenosis. *Vasc Med* 1998;3:177–188.

121. McCullough KM. Retrograde transpopliteal salvage of the failed antegrade transfemoral angioplasty. *Australas Radiol* 1993;37:329–31.

122. Bakal CW, Sprayregen S, Scheinbaum K, et al. Percutaneous transluminal angioplasty of the infrapopliteal arteries: results in 53 patients. *Am J Roentgenol* 1990;154:171–174.

123. Bakal CW, Cynamon J, Sprayregen S. Infrapopliteal percutaneous transluminal angioplasty: what we know. *Radiology* 1996;200:36–43.

124. Dorros G, Jaff MR, Murphy KJ, et al. The acute outcome of tibioperoneal vessel angioplasty in 417 cases with claudication and critical limb ischemia. *Catheter Cardiovasc Diagn* 1998;45:251–256.

125. Fraser SC, al-Kutoube MA, Wolfe JH. Percutaneous transluminal angioplasty of the infrapopliteal vessels: the evidence. *Radiology* 1996;200:33–36.

126. Hanna GP, Fujise K, Kjellgren O, et al. Infrapopliteal transcatheter interventions for limb salvage in diabetic patients: importance of aggressive interventional approach and role of transcutaneous oximetry. *J Am Coll Cardiol* 1997;30:664–669.

127. Parsons RE, Suggs WD, Lee JJ, et al. Percutaneous transluminal angioplasty for the treatment of limb threatening ischemia: do the results justify an attempt before bypass grafting? *J Vasc Surg* 1998;28:1066–1071.

128. Isner JM, Walsh K, Symes J, et al. Arterial gene transfer for therapeutic angiogenesis in patients with peripheral artery disease. *Human Gene Ther* 1996;7:959–988.

129. Isner JM, Pieczek A, Rosenfield K. Untreated gangrene in patients with peripheral artery disease. *Circulation* 1994;89:482–483.

130. Henry M, Amor M, Ethevenot G, et al. Percutaneous peripheral atherectomy using the rotablator: a single-center experience. *J Endovasc Surg* 1995;2:51–66.

131. Isner JM, Rosenfield K. Redefining the treatment of peripheral artery disease. *Circulation* 1993;88:1534–1557.

132. Sievert H, Ensslen R, Fach A, et al. Brachial artery approach for transluminal angioplasty of the internal carotid artery. *Catheter Cardiovasc Diagn* 1996;39:421–423.

133. Pentecost MJ, Criqui MH, Dorros G. Guidelines for peripheral percutaneous transluminal angioplasty of the abdominal aorta and lower extremity vessels. *Circulation* 1994;89:511–531.

134. Porter DH, Rosen MP, Skillman JJ, et al. Mid-term and long-term results with directional atherectomy of vein graft stenosis. *J Vasc Surg* 1996;23:554–567.

135. Ozdil E, Krajcer Z, Angelini P. Percutaneous balloon angioplasty with adjunctive stent placement in the mesenteric vessels in a patient with Takayasu's arteritis. *Circulation* 1996;93:1940–1941.

136. Arend WP, Michel BA, Bloch DA, et al. The American College of Rheumatology 1990 criteria for the classification of Takayasu arteritis. *Arthritis Rheum* 1990;33:1129–1134.

137. Tanimoto A, Hiramatsu K. Percutaneous transluminal angioplasty for Takayasu's arteritis. *Semin Interv Radiol* 1993;10:1–7.

138. Millaire A, Trinca ZM, Marache P, et al. Subclavian angioplasty: immediate and late results in 50 patients. *Catheter Cardiovasc Diagn* 1993;29:8–17.

139. Dorros G, Lewin RF, Jamnadas P, et al. Peripheral transluminal angioplasty of the subclavian and innominate arteries utilizing the brachial approach: acute outcome and follow-up. *Catheter Cardiovasc Diagn* 1990;19:71–76.

140. Henry M, Amor M, Henry I, et al. Percutaneous transluminal angioplasty of the subclavian arteries. *J Endovasc Surg* 1999;6:33–41.

141. Hadjipetrou P, Cox S, Piemonte T, et al. Percutaneous revascularization of atherosclerotic obstruction of aortic arch vessels. *J Am Coll Cardiol* 1999;33:1238–1245.

142. Kumar K, Dorros G, Bates CM, et al. Primary stent deploy-

ment in occlusive subclavian artery disease. *Catheter Cardiovasc Diagn* 1995;34:281–285.

143. Ansel GM, Barry SG, Yakubov JS. Primary stenting of symptomatic subclavian artery stenosis. *Circulation* 1996;94(Suppl I): 58.

144. Al-Mubarak N, Liu MW, Dean LS, et al. Immediate and late outcomes of subclavian artery stenting. *Catheter Cardiovasc Interv* 1999;46:169–172.

145. Hebrang A, Maskovic J, Tomac B. Percutaneous transluminal angioplasty of the subclavian arteries: long-term results in 52 patients. *Am J Roentgenol* 1991;156:1091–1096.

146. Johnson KW, Lindsay TF, Walker PM. Early and late results and suggested surgical approach for chronic and acute mesenteric ischemia. *Surgery* 1995;118:1–7.

147. Matsumoto AH, Angle JF, Tegtmeyer CJ. Mesenteric angioplasty and stenting for chronic mesenteric ischemia. In: Perler BA, Becker GI, eds. *Vascular intervention: a clinical approach.* New York: Thieme, 1998:545–556.

148. Khosla S, Zhang SY, Jenkins JS. Endovascular stent revascularization of mesenteric and celiac arteries for the management of chronic mesenteric ischemia. *Circulation* 1997;96:I-275.

149. Gaylord GM, Taber TE. Long-term hemodialysis access salvage: problems and challenges for nephrologists and interventional radiologists. *J Vasc Interv Radiol* 1993;4:103–107.

150. Kumpe DA, Cohen MA, Durham JD. Treatment of failing and failed hemodialysis access sites: comparison of surgical treatment with thrombolysis/angioplasty. *Semin Vasc Surg* 1992;5: 118–127.

151. Turmel-Rodrigues L, Pengloan J, Blanchier D, et al. Insufficient dialysis shunts: improved long-term patency rates with close hemodynamic monitoring, repeated percutaneous balloon angioplasty, and stent placement. *Radiology* 1993;187: 273–278.

152. Glantz S, Gordon DH, Lipkowitz GS, et al. Axillary and subclavian vein stenosis: percutaneous angioplasty. *Radiology* 1988; 168:371–373.

41

CAROTID ARTERY STENTING

SRIRAM S. IYER
JIRI J. VITEK
GISHEL NEW
NADIM AL-MUBARAK
GARY S. ROUBIN

Carotid artery stenting (CAS) is currently being investigated as an alternative treatment to carotid endarterectomy (CEA) (1–6). The goal of both procedures is identical: prevention of stroke from extracranial carotid disease. Carotid stenting offers patients a less invasive and less traumatic means of achieving this goal. The efficacy of carotid stenting in preventing stroke depends on the ability of the operator to produce a complication-free result. The purpose of this chapter is to describe the technical details and patient selection factors that have allowed us to improve the outcomes from this procedure.

CLINICAL PROTOCOL

Patients are admitted the day of the procedure and consent is obtained for brachiocephalic angiography and possible stent placement should the lesion prove to be of significant severity and anatomically suitable for percutaneous intervention (Figure 41.1). All patients are evaluated by board-certified neurologists (independent of the study) to document the periprocedural clinical status and to compute the baseline National Institutes of Health (NIH) and other functional stroke scales. All patients have a computerized tomographic (CT) or magnetic resonance imaging (MRI) scan to document baseline changes. Before stenting, all patients undergo brachiocephalic angiography (if not

recently done). Patients are informed that carotid stenting is considered investigational, does not have Food and Drug Administration approval, and has a favorable outlook for both the medium (2-year) and long term (7). Patients are started on antiplatelet therapy, aspirin 325 mg daily and clopidogrel (Plavix) 75 mg bid (previously ticlopidine, Ticlid), preferably for 3 days before the procedure. In all cases, patients receive either ticlopidine (total dose 500 mg) or clopidogrel (total dose 450 mg) before the intervention.

■ In the clinical protocol (Table 41.1) we place great emphasis on antiplatelet therapy before and after carotid stenting.

Sriram S. Iyer: Clinical Associate Professor, Department of Medicine, New York School of Medicine; Associate Chief, Endovascular Services, Interventional Cardiology, Lenox Hill Hospital, New York, New York

Jiri J. Vitek: Interventional Neuroradiologist, Interventional Cardiology, Lenox Hill Hospital, New York, New York

Gishel New: Associate Professor, Department of Cardiology, Monash University; Director of Cardiology, Department of Cardiology, Box Hill Hospital, Melbourne, Australia

Nadim Al-Mubarak: Associate Professor, Case-Western Reserve University, Director, Endovascular Therapeutics, University Hospital System of Cleveland, Cleveland, Ohio

Gary S. Roubin: Clinical Professor of Medicine, New York University School of Medicine, New York University; Chief, Endovascular Services, Interventional Cardiology, Lenox Hill Hospital, New York, New York

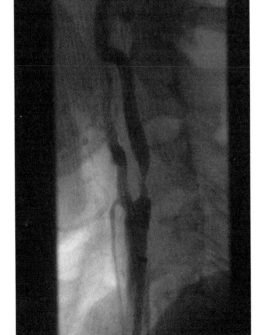

FIGURE 41.1. High-grade asymptomatic left internal carotid artery stenosis.

TABLE 41.1. CLINICAL PROTOCOL

Premeds
ASA 325 mg PO bid × 3 days
Clopidogrel 150 mg PO bid × 3 days
Preprocedure
Carotid duplex ultrasound
CT scan/MRI
Independent neurologic examination
Protocol consent signed
Knowledge of LV Fn
Well hydrated
Procedure
Same-day admit
No sedation
Single procedure
Head restrained by cradle
Four vessel angio
Stent one side if bilateral disease
Squeeze toy in contralateral hand
Neuro evaluation immediately after procedure

LV, left ventricle; PO, per os (by mouth)

The low rates of acute and delayed stent thrombosis and poststenting embolic events are predicated upon correct and compulsive doses of adjunctive antiplatelet therapy.

PROCEDURAL CONSIDERATIONS

Angiography and stenting are performed using local anesthesia at the site of femoral vascular access. Neurologic status (8), electrocardiogram, heart rate, and blood pressure are monitored throughout the procedure. Temporary cardiac pacing is available if required.

TECHNIQUE

The current technique of carotid angioplasty and stenting pioneered and developed by us (SI, GR, JV) while at the University of Alabama at Birmingham and has been adopted (with minor modifications) by most high-volume carotid angioplasty centers around the world. The technical approach can be divided into the following ten steps:

1. Vascular access
2. Angiographic evaluation
3. Carotid sheath placement
4. Crossing the stenosis
   a. Procedure without distal neuroprotection
   b. Procedure with distal neuroprotection
5. Lesion predilatation
6. Stent deployment
7. Postdilatation
8. Removal of neuroprotective device
9. Final angiographic assessment
10. Sheath removal and hemostasis

Vascular Access

Femoral arterial access is the preferred, recommended approach. Direct percutaneous puncture of the carotid artery as a method of vascular access is for the most part contraindicated. The frequent need for general anesthesia, the proximity of the access site to the site of the lesion, problems of local hematoma, and the need for compressing a superficial stented vessel for securing hemostasis are some of the reasons that the direct carotid stick method is no longer used even by physicians who advocated this technique in the past. Femoral venous access is unnecessary, unless it is required for administering fluids and medications (e.g., atropine). We no longer advocate the routine placement of a temporary venous pacemaker.

Diagnostic Angiographic Evaluation

In the vast majority of patients, brachiocephalic angiography is performed using a single, 100-cm 5F Vitek catheter (VTK, Thorocon, NB; Cook Inc., Bloomington, IN). Diagnostic angiography consists of visualization of the origins of the brachiocephalic arteries from the aortic arch (by selective injections) in at least two orthogonal projections of both carotid bifurcations and of both vertebral arteries, and intracranial study of both carotid arteries and the dominant vertebral artery.

The initial complete brachiocephalic angiography has several advantages. It

- Remains the most reliable method for precise assessment of the degree of carotid artery stenosis (9).
- Demonstrates anatomic conditions that are unfavorable for carotid stenting or that increase the difficulty of the procedure (e.g., dilated/extended arch, marked vessel tortuosity, heavily calcified stenosis, lesions with obvious filling defects).
- Provides preprocedural knowledge of contralateral carotid stenosis or occlusion and the status of the intracranial circulation (isolated hemisphere, collateral supply) that could impact the stenting technique (e.g., shorter balloon inflations, choice of neuroprotective device: occlusion versus filter).
- Reliably demonstrates significant flow limiting distal and intracranial internal carotid artery stenosis. Although the bifurcation stenosis may be treatable, the ultimate benefit of stroke reduction may not accrue to the patient because of disease that is more cephalad.
- In case of an intraprocedural neurologic event, the subsequent intracranial angiograms can be compared with the baseline, periprocedural pictures.

The following is a disadvantage of brachiocephalic angiography:

- The main risks relate to the use of iodinated radiographic contrast and the risk of a procedure-related neurologic event. In our group's experience, which includes an experienced neuroradiologist (JV), this risk is very small (0.1% to 0.2%).

Carotid Sheath Placement

Once the diagnostic study is completed and the stenotic internal carotid artery is identified, the 100-cm 5F Vitek diagnostic (VTK) catheter is advanced over a 0.038-inch glide wire into the common carotid artery and positioned just below the carotid bifurcation. The glide wire is removed, the catheter is flushed, and a small quantity of contrast is injected to produce a roadmap of the ipsilateral external carotid artery. Once the origin and the course of the external carotid artery are defined, the 0.038-inch glide wire is placed back into the VTK catheter and used to direct the catheter into the external carotid artery. The glide wire is withdrawn and replaced with a 260-cm extra-stiff Amplatz wire (Cook Inc., Bloomington, IN). The VTK catheter is withdrawn and the 6- or 7F, 90-cm sheath (Shuttle Introducer, Cook, Inc., Bloomington, IN) is advanced into the common carotid artery over the exchange-length Amplatz wire, anchored in the external carotid artery. If the diagnostic angiography has been done previously, the stenting procedure begins by placing the 6- or 7F shuttle sheath, via the femoral approach, into the descending thoracic aorta a short distance below the origin of the left subclavian artery (Figure 41.2). After withdrawing the inner dilator from the Shuttle sheath (Table 41.2), a 125-cm, 5F Vitek diagnostic catheter (VTK Thorocon NB 125 cm, Cook,

TABLE 41.2. STENT DELIVERY "SHUTTLE" SHEATH

Side(ID):	7F (0.100 n.); 6F (0.087 n.)
Length:	90 cm
Delivery tip:	Radioopaque band Easy identification
Inner dilator:	Tapered, flexible Facilitates delivery
Other features:	Large-bore touhy-borst Sheath resists kinking
Delivery:	More than 0.038-in. glide or Extra-stiff Amplatz Up to 10 mm Wallstent
Next generation:	Hydrophyllic coating, soft tip, improved Touhy

Inc., Bloomington, IN) is introduced into the shuttle sheath. Care must be taken not to advance the shuttle sheath too close to the aortic arch because this will compromise the operator's ability to maneuver the VTK catheter. Using a 0.038-inch glide wire, the common carotid artery is accessed with the VTK catheter, and this catheter is advanced into the external carotid artery. (Roadmapping is often helpful at this stage.) Using the appropriate guide wire (0.038-inch glide or extra stiff Amplatz, depending on the degree of unfolding of the aortic arch and the amount of carotid tortuosity), the shuttle sheath is advanced over the VTK catheter into the common carotid artery. If the advancement of the sheath over the VTK catheter is not smooth (i.e., the operator senses that any further push on the Shuttle sheath will be counterproductive and only result in prolapse of the entire system out of the carotid artery), the VTK catheter is exchanged for the inner introducer of the sheath and then advanced into the common carotid artery. As soon as the shuttle sheath is placed into the arterial system, 4,000 to 5,000 U of heparin is administered through the sheath to raise the activated clotting time (ACT) to approximately 225 seconds (Hemotec method). Since the usual procedure time is between 20 and 40 minutes, further heparin administration is rarely required. Larger doses of heparin may increase the risk of catastrophic brain hemorrhage.

The coaxial sheath technique has a number of advantages:

- This technique permits continuous access to the common carotid artery. Once the sheath is in the common carotid below the bifurcation, unfavorable anatomy (elongated arch, tortuosity of the common carotid artery) is no longer an issue influencing technical success.
- When the passage of the guide wire through the stenosis is difficult (eccentric stenosis, ulcerations, internal carotoid artery (ICA) kinks and tortuosities, angulated takeoff of the ICA) or when complications develop (dissection, intracranial embolism), the coaxial configuration has obvious advantages.

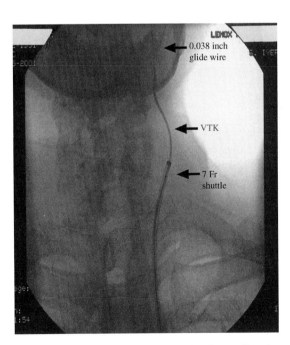

FIGURE 41.2. The 7F Shuttle sheath is in the descending thoracic aorta and contains the 125-cm 5F Vitek catheter.

- The sheath carries a large-bore Tuohy-Bourst valve seal, which permits unimpeded catheter or guide wire introduction. The side arm allows intermittent or continuous flushing and contrast injection and facilitates continuous intraarterial blood pressure monitoring.
- The sheath can also be used as a reference for sizing the internal and common carotid arteries (using online quantitative carotid arteriography [QCA]).

Disadvantages of the coaxial system (sheath or guiding catheter) include the following:

- By placing the 6- or 7F sheath in the common carotid artery (especially if the carotid artery is tortuous), kinks can be created, existing tortuous loops can be exaggerated, and the tortuosity (together with the carotid bifurcation) is displaced cephalad. These disappear once the sheath is withdrawn, but the appearance of "pseudolesions" can complicate the stenting procedure. The exaggeration of existing loops increases the difficulty of negotiating and placement of higher-profile neuroprotective devices.
- On rare occasion, dissection of the innominate or common carotid artery may result following advancement of the sheath over the 5F catheter (see technique—access sheath placement).
- There is always the possibility of embolization during sheath advancement, a part of the procedure that cannot be "neuroprotected." Based on our wide experience, the risk of a clinically obvious embolic event during this phase of the procedure is quite small. The relatively small number of "HITS" (high-intensity transients) on transcranial Doppler sonography (TCD) during sheath placement corroborates this clinical observation. *Placing the stent delivery sheath in the common carotid artery in a safe and expeditious manner is the key to successful carotid angioplasty. Recognizing and appropriately responding to "difficult access situations" constitutes a large and important part of the learning curve!*

Crossing the Stenosis

Using appropriately angled views, baseline angiograms (via the Shuttle sheath) are acquired to show the maximum severity of the stenosis. QCA is performed in this projection to measure the percent diameter of the stenosis and the diameter of the common carotid artery. Note that the optimal angulation for performing the intervention need not be identical to the one displaying the stenosis with maximum severity. Instead, this working projection should maximally separate the internal and external carotid arteries and clearly display bony landmarks. The operator should have a clear idea about the stenosis location in relation to the bony landmarks (Figure 41.1). To continuously monitor neurologic status and particularly strength of the upper extremity, a squeeze toy is placed in the patient's contralateral hand (9).

The next step depends on whether the procedure is being planned without or with a neuroprotective device.

Carotid Stenting Without Neuroprotection

After appropriate shaping of the wire tip, the stenotic lesion is crossed with a steerable 0.014-inch coronary guide wire. Wire selection depends on the severity, location, length, angulation, and eccentricity of the stenosis and the anatomy of the bifurcation (Figure 41.1). A variety of 0.014-inch wires are available. We commonly use an exchange length 0.014-inch Balance Wire (Guidant Inc., Temacula, CA) or 0.014-inch Choice PT Wire (SciMed Inc., Maple Grove, MN). After crossing the stenosis, the tip of the wire is placed close to the skull base. If the internal carotid artery is kinked or has coils or tortuosities, the wire is passed through distally to the level of skull base.

Carotid Stenting Using a Neuroprotective Device

Table 41.3 shows the various neuroprotective devices. Although several of these devices have approval for sale in Europe (CE Mark), at this time none of these devices has been approved for use in the United States. Neuroprotective devices can be classified into two groups: occlusion systems and filters.

Choice of Neuroprotective Device
Distal Occlusion Balloon (Percusurge). Even in the hands of experienced operators, the average time that neuroprotective devices need to be in place is about 10 to 12 minutes. In contrast to the filters, the Percusurge occlusion balloon does not allow flow into the distal bed. Therefore before selecting an occlusion balloon for neuroprotection, it is important to *establish the adequacy of the circle of Willis. Hence the value of an adequately performed and properly interpreted four-vessel angiogram cannot be overstated.*

If the contralateral carotid artery is occluded and flow to that hemisphere is being maintained by crossover collaterals from the index carotid artery or in cases of "isolated hemi-

TABLE 41.3. NEUROPROTECTION DEVICES

GROUP I: Occlusion Systems
  Distal (Guard wire, Percusurge, Sunnyvale, CA)
  Proximal (ArteriA, Tokyo, Japan)
GROUP II: Filters
  Accunet (Guidant, Temacula, CA)
  Angioguard (Cordis, Miami, FL)
  E-Trap (Metamorphics)
  Filter wire (Boston Scientific, Boston, MA)
  Neuroshield (Mednova)
  TRAP (Microvena, White Bear Lake, MN)

sphere" (the hemisphere relies solely on the ipsilateral carotid artery for supply; absent or inadequate collaterals from the vertebrals and contralateral carotid), *neuroprotection using distal occlusion is not an option.*

Filters. Although a device that maintains flow while affording embolic protection is obviously preferable, the crossing profile of all currently available filters is larger than the profile of the "balloon on a wire" distal occlusion Percusurge device. These larger-profile devices are difficult to negotiate through the stenosis and into the distal internal carotid artery in certain anatomic situations (e.g., markedly eccentric and/or severely calcified/fibrotic lesions and marked tortuosity of the distal internal carotid artery).

Proximal Occlusion with Reversal of Flow (Arteria). In proximal occlusion with reversal of flow (Arteria), neuroprotection is conferred by the combination of the inflated common carotid and external carotid balloons. This dual inflation reverses flow in the index carotid artery. Any emboli generated during the procedure will travel in the direction of flow, in this case away from the distal cerebral bed and towards the femoral artery. Two important features differentiate this proximal occlusion system from *all* distal embolic protection systems:

1. The protection feature can be activated before crossing the stenosis in the internal carotid artery. In tortuous anatomies, a fair bit of wire manipulation can be anticipated. The advantage of a system that protects the distal bed from embolization during all stages of internal carotid manipulation is obvious.
2. The carotid angioplasty and stenting procedure can be performed using standard low-profile coronary balloons and wires. Since flow reversal is an integral part of the protection mechanism, anatomies not suitable for the distal occlusion balloon will be unsuitable for proximal occlusion as well.

Placement of Distal Neuroprotective Devices

All currently available distal protection devices are developed on a 0.014-inch wire system. After prepping the protection device, the wire tip is shaped appropriately and the protection device is negotiated through the stenosis (Figure 41.3). The device has to be placed sufficiently cephalad to the stenosis. If the device is placed very close to the stenosis, there will not be adequate room to accommodate the tip of the stent delivery system, and satisfactory coverage of the lesion with the stent will be impossible.

Lesion Predilatation

Cases Without Neuroprotection

For predilatation of the stenosis, we routinely use a Cobra 18, 4 × 40 mm coronary balloon (SciMed Inc., Maple

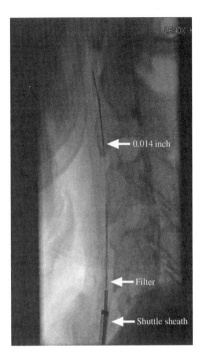

FIGURE 41.3. Carotid stenting with neuroprotection. The lesion is crossed with a filter on a 0.014-inch wire.

Grove, MN), or the Savvy balloon 4 × 40 mm (Cordis Corp., Miami, FL). Both of these over-the-wire balloons accept 0.018-inch wires. If the stenosis is preocclusive, we prefer a gradual step-up during predilatation. The first predilatation is performed with a 2-mm balloon (Ranger 2 × 40 mm, SciMed, Inc., Maple Grove, MN). This is followed by a second predilatation using the 4-mm balloon. Before this dilatation, the balloon catheter is advanced distally into the internal carotid artery and the 0.014-inch wire is changed for 0.018-inch exchange wire (Roadrunner, Cook, Inc., Bloomington, IN). Again, the tip of the 0.018-inch wire should be located close to the skull base and certainly must be passed through all kinks and tortuosities of the internal carotid artery. If the stenosis is smooth and not extremely severe and if the internal carotid artery is not very tortuous, the 0.018-inch roadrunner wire can be used as a primary wire to cross the stenosis. Very rarely and usually in heavily calcified lesions, if the stent does not easily pass through the stenosis after predilatation with the 4-mm balloon, a 5 mm balloon may be needed for additional predilatation. Just before stenting (after predilatation and with the 0.018-inch Nitinol wire in place), a control arteriogram is performed to once again establish the relationship of the stenosis to the bony landmarks.

Cases with Neuroprotection

At the present time, at our center, most carotid stenting procedures are performed using neuroprotection (Figures 41.4 and 41.5). Since all current distal neuroprotective systems

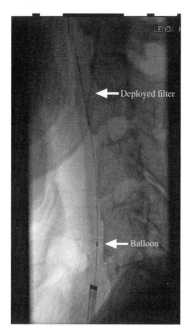

FIGURE 41.4. After deploying the filter, the predilatation balloon is advanced over the 0.014-inch wire that carries the filter in its distal end.

are 0.014-inch wire-based systems, our current practice is to predilate using 0.014-inch compatible balloons (4 × 40 mm Adante Scimed, Inc; Maple Grove, MN). With a neuroprotective device in place it is better to use monorail systems. Not only are exchanges with monorail systems faster than over-the-wire systems, the entire system is much more stable, since the operator has control over both the wire carrying the neuroprotective device and the balloon or stent.

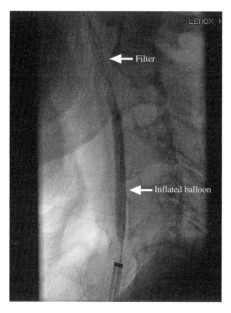

FIGURE 41.5. The lesion is predilated with a 4- × 40-mm monorail, low-profile 0.014-inch compatible coronary balloon.

Such stability is very important since it minimizes the up-and-down movement of the neuroprotective device and reduces the chance of spasm and/or dissection.

Why Predilate?

Experimental work of Ohki et al. (10) demonstrated that embolic debris may be released with "primary stenting" without predilatation and during lesion dilatation with large peripheral (0.035-inch compatible) balloons. We do not practice "primary stenting" without predilatation. We believe that later postdilatation of the constricted stent is associated with more "scissoring" of the stent wires on plaque, with greater risk of embolization. For routine predilatation we use low-profile coronary 4 × 40 mm balloons. These balloons "rewrap well" without residual wings, a desirable feature when the deflated balloon is withdrawn.

Four-millimeter balloon predilatation does not cause major occlusive dissections and is sufficient for passage of the stent (Figure 41.1). The inflation pressure is 8 to 10 atm, and the balloon must be fully deflated before withdrawal. The longer length of the balloon (40 mm) also is advantageous: it prevents the balloon from sliding in and out of the stenosis during inflation ("watermelon seed effect"), and the operator gets a good idea of where the stent will be when deployed. (Currently, we use 40-mm Nitinol stents and 20-mm-long Wallstents. The latter in most carotid systems ends up being 40 to 44 mm in length when deployed.)

Wires ranging from soft atraumatic 0.014-inch coronary wires to 0.038-inch stiff Amplatz wires are used during various stages of the procedure. The operator and the assistant must exercise excellent wire control and at all times should be aware of the position of the distal wire tip. This will minimize the risk of wire-induced perforation, spasm, and dissection.

The distal 4-cm Nitinol tip of the 0.018-inch roadrunner wire is conveniently radiopaque. In 7-inch magnification, as long as the operator keeps the radiopaque tip of this wire in constant view, the distal tip will not be way inside the cranium.

If a 0.014-inch coronary wire is used as the initial wire, it is exchanged for the 0.018-inch wire before stent placement. It is easier to advance and accurately place the stent over the stiffer, more robust wire as it straightens the internal carotid artery, facilitating delivery and deployment of the stent.

Currently, almost all self-expanding stents (both Nitinol and Wallstent) are 0.014-inch compatible, rendering use of 0.018-inch wires obsolete.

Stent Deployment

Between September 1994 and August 1995 we used balloon-expandable stents to treat stenosis at the extracranial carotid bifurcation (Figure 41.6). Following observa-

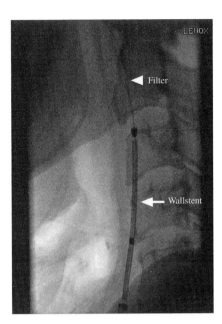

FIGURE 41.6. Following predilatation, a 10- × 20-mm monorail Wallstent (0.014-inch compatible) is advanced and positioned using bony landmarks.

tions of stent deformation/stent crushing (3,6,11), we switched to self-expanding stents (Elgiloy tracheobronchial Wallstent) (Figure 41.6). Currently, with the introduction of Nitinol stents, we use both stent types. At the present time, the only indications for using balloon-expandable stents in the carotid circulation are

1. When stenosis at the *ostium of the common carotid artery* has to be treated.
2. When the *most distal cervical portion* (prepetrous segment) of the internal carotid artery is being treated. [Delivery systems of self-expanding stents can cause dissections in the petrous portion of the internal carotid artery (i.e., within sharp bends of the internal carotid artery).]
3. When the self-expandable stent cannot be smoothly (without resistance) advanced through the stenosis despite adequate balloon predilatation (usually in *heavily calcified rigid stenoses and/or stenosis that have a high tendency to recoil*). In this case, a 4- to 6-mm balloon-expandable stent is first deployed at the bifurcation to prevent recoil at the lesion site and to permit the passage of a self-expanding stent that functions as the definitive stent. Further, collapse of the balloon-expandable stent is prevented by the constant outward force exerted by the self-expanding stent. The self-expanding stent is deployed using the vertebral bodies as landmarks.

Stent Diameter

The unconstrained diameter of the self-expanding stent to be deployed should be at least 1 or 2 mm larger than the largest vessel segment to be covered by the stent, almost always the common carotid artery. In the past we used 8- and 10-mm-diameter stents. Lately, we have used, almost exclusively, 10-mm-diameter stents based on the fact that the stent mesh covering the diseased vessel is tighter, which reduces the possibility of emboli during postdilatation.

Stent Length

In the case of the Wallstent, a 20-mm-long stent is chosen. If the Wallstent were to expand to 10 mm, then the length would be 20 mm. Since there is a size differential between the internal and the common, the former being 5 to 6 mm and the latter being 7 to 9 mm, the Wallstent does not expand to the full 10 mm and hence does not shorten to 20 mm. Instead, in most cases, it ends up being 40 to 44 mm in length. In the case of Nitinol stents, we currently use either a 30- or 40-mm-long (10 mm in diameter) stent. This stent is 30 or 40 mm when deployed (i.e., minimal foreshortening) despite the size differential between the internal and the common.

Other Considerations

The distal end of the stent should not be placed into kinks and tortuosities of the internal carotid artery. These cannot be eliminated and are only displaced distally and become more exaggerated.

The Nitinol stents are less rigid, conform to the "curve" of the vessel, and do not straighten the internal carotid artery as much as the Wallstent.

Since there is no appreciable foreshortening with Nitinol stents, they can be more precisely placed using the distal and proximal markers. An important technical point is to release 3 to 5 mm of the stent distally and wait for the stent to expand fully and stabilize against the vessel wall before releasing the reminder of the stent. These stents have a tendency to "jump" distally if released too fast.

Nitinol stents that are compatible with 0.014-inch and 0.018-inch wires loaded on 5- and 6F delivery systems in both over-the-wire and monorail configurations are in clinical trials.

In our technique, the caudal end of the stent rests in the common carotid artery. Hence a stent with a diameter of 10 mm is preferred. On rare occasion, the stent is placed exclusively in the internal carotid artery; in this case a 6- or 8-mm-diameter stent is selected.

In almost all cases, the stent is placed across the bifurcation into the common carotid artery, crossing the origin of the external carotid artery (Figure 41.7). Covering the origin of the external carotid artery with the stent is not a problem. Follow-up arteriograms show the external carotid artery to be patent with rare exceptions (6).

If the external carotid artery becomes significantly stenosed or occluded after postdilatation of the stent or the patient is symptomatic (jaw, facial pain), this vessel can be approached through the stent mesh and recanalized using

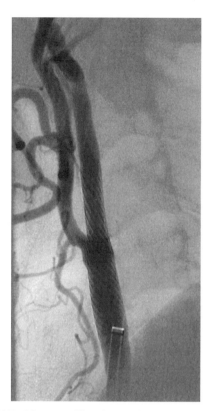

FIGURE 41.7. After postdilatation with a 5.5- × 20-mm balloon and retrieval of the filter (not shown), final angiograms of the carotid bifurcation show excellent resolution of the stenosis.

coronary balloon techniques. A 0.014-inch wire is used to enter the external carotid artery, predilated with a 2-mm balloon, and a 4-mm balloon is used for final dilatation. The goal is not to obliterate the external carotid stenosis completely, but to establish normal flow in the vessel (6).

Postdilatation

The size of the postdilatation balloon is matched to the diameter of the internal carotid artery at the site of the stenosis. Typically, the self-expanding stent is postdilated with a 5- or 5.5-mm (rarely, 6.0 mm diameter, never larger) balloon (0.018-inch Savvy, Cordis, Inc., Miami, FL; 0.014-inch gazelle or Speedy Bypass, BSC, Natick, MA). *The balloon is deflated slowly.* In heavily calcified stenosis, we postdilate using high-pressure balloons (e.g., Titan, Cordis, Inc., Miami, FL). *Postdilatation of the stent is a critical step.* Postdilatation phase is perhaps the time when the most emboli are released and consequently the patient is at greatest risk of a stroke. To minimize the embolic load we recommend (a) using balloons that are no larger than 5.5 mm in diameter; (b) inflating to nominal, not very high, pressures; (c) accepting a 10% to 20% residual stenosis. This does not cause hemodynamic problems. The self-expanding stents have a tendency for late, progressive expansion, especially if oversized (12); (d) restricting to a *single* postdilatation effort; and (e) gradual deflation of the balloon—more than 30 or 45 seconds.

It is safer to underdilate than to overdilate the self-expanding stent. Overdilatation with a high-pressure balloon squeezes the atherosclerotic material through the stent mesh, causing emboli.

In some cases, continued flow via the stent struts into an ulcer occurs. No attempt should be made to obliterate this communication by using larger balloons or higher pressures, as this communication will seal off in the ensuing few days and is of no consequence.

Removal of the Neuroprotective Device

Percusurge Distal Occlusion Balloon

Aspiration

Before deflation of the occlusion balloon, a long, beveled monorail aspiration catheter, *the export catheter,* is introduced over the wire. The distal end of the aspiration catheter has a radiopaque marker and the catheter is advanced until this marker is just below the inflated occlusion balloon. While maintaining constant suction with a 20- or 30-mL syringe, the export catheter is slowly pulled back to the carotid bifurcation and then advanced forward to the occlusion balloon. This back-and-forth maneuver is repeated until approximately 50 to 60 mL of blood is aspirated. The aim is to aspirate the emboli-containing column of blood caudad to the occlusion balloon and any "loose" emboli in the carotid wall, thereby preventing these emboli from traveling intracranially once the occlusion balloon is deflated.

Deflation

While the aspiration of blood is in progress, the assistant reassembles the end of the Percusurge deflation apparatus (the microseal adaptor). As soon as aspiration is completed, the balloon is deflated and final angiograms are acquired. The segment of the ICA that contained the occlusion balloon is carefully evaluated.

Filters

The filters are removed using a retrieval catheter. Either the entire filter (e.g., Accunet, Neuroshield) or part of the filter (Angioguard) is withdrawn into the retrieval catheter, which is then removed as one unit.

Arteria

Following postdilatation, the external carotid and the common carotid balloons are deflated and the system is removed from the artery.

Final Angiographic Assessment

Lesion Site and Cervical ICA

Following stent postdilatation, final angiograms are acquired in the same projection(s) that demonstrated the maximum

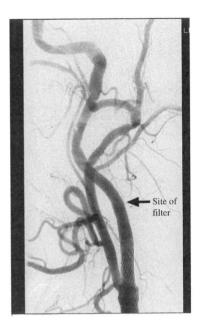

FIGURE 41.8. Angiogram of the segment of the internal carotid artery that housed the filter shows no obvious angiographic abnormality. (The postprocedure course was uneventful and the patient was discharged next morning.)

severity of the lesion in both digitally subtracted and regular formats (Figure 41.7). If a distal neuroprotective device has been used, attention must be directed to the segment of the ICA that contained the protection device (Figure 41.8). It is not unusual to encounter spasm in this segment, particularly if the ICA is tortuous. A small dose of intraarterial nitroglycerine (as a consequence of stretch of the carotid baroreceptors most of the patients will be relatively hypotensive limiting the use of nitroglycerine), and pulling back the Shuttle sheath to the carotid origin aids in relieving the spasm, relaxes the artery, and helps the operator get a better idea of the status of the stented vessel. Distal stent-related linear edge dissections are unusual and when present are short and for the most part inconsequential. Occasionally, such dissections may need treatment, and an additional stent may be needed. On occasion we have noticed linear dissections related to the use of the Percusurge Occlusion balloon. These were more common with the first-generation device when the balloon could be inflated to only two sizes (5.5 and 6.0 mm). Since the second-generation device (the guard wire plus) can be inflated to a range of sizes (3 to 6.0 mm in 0.5-mm increments), the balloon can be more accurately matched to the size of the distal vessel, reducing the risk of dissections related to an oversized balloon. In any event, these small linear dissections did not compromise flow and did not require additional stents.

Intracranial Angiograms

We do not routinely acquire intracranial angiograms, reserving them for those patients who experience intraprocedural neurologic deficits. Several operators will do this as a routine, and almost all the current carotid stent investiga-

TABLE 41.4. DISCHARGE PROTOCOL

1. Ambulate next day
2. NIH stroke scale before discharge
3. Carotid ultrasound
4. ASA 325 mg po qd indefinitely
5. Clopidogrel 75 mg po qd × 1 month
6. Clinical F/U: 1 mo, 6 mo, yearly
7. Ultrasound F/U: 6 mo, yearly
8. Meticulous follow-up records

ASA, aspirin; F/U, follow up; NIH, National Institute of Health.

tional protocols call for repeat intracranial views, which are acquired in the same projections as baseline.

Sheath Removal and Access Site Hemostasis

The Shuttle sheath is pulled back (over a wire) into the iliac artery and exchanged for a short sheath of appropriate size (usually 7F, sometimes 8F) that is removed when the ACT is less than 150 seconds. This takes usually 3 to 4 hours. It is important to inform the person pulling the sheath whether atropine and vasopressors were used intraprocedurally. The effect of these medications wears off in a few hours and typically coincides with the timing of sheath removal. This and the exaggerated vagal response that is not unusual in these patients can lead to profound hemodynamic perturbation for which anticipation and treatment preparation (e.g., ensuring good peripheral venous access, providing adequate hydration, holding antihypertensives prophylactic dosing with atropine, etc.) are extremely helpful.

Although "low blood pressure" is not unusual in the immediate postprocedure phase, it is worth emphasizing that other causes (e.g., retroperitoneal bleed related to access site problems) should be excluded as a cause of any unexplained persistent, disproportionate hypotension.

At the present time, access site hemostasis is achieved at the end of the procedure using a suture closure device (Perclose, Perclose, Inc., Redwood City, CA). We prefer the 6F Perclose device. Following diagnostic angiography, the 5F arterial sheath is exchanged for the 6F Perclose device. The sutures are brought out and left untied, at which point the Perclose device is exchanged for the Shuttle sheath. At the end of the procedure, the Shuttle sheath is removed and the sutures are knotted. This approach is particularly valuable for those patients who are to be discharged the same day (day case carotid stenting). Table 41.4 lists the discharge protocol.

RESULTS

Carotid artery stenting is an alternative revascularization technique for extracranial carotid stenotic disease. In September 1994 while at the University of Alabama at Birmingham, we initiated the program of elective carotid angioplasty with stenting. The team consisted of a multidisciplinary group of physicians and included an interventional neuroradiologist (JV) and interventional cardiologists (SI, GR). From the outset, the group based its technique on the premise that combining angioplasty with elective intravascular stent placement will increase the reliability and safety of the method. The first series of stented patients was reported in 1995 (3).

All patients were treated under a prospectively defined protocol and all gave written informed consent for the procedure. Data were collected prospectively. Neurologic outcome was based on pre- and postprocedural (24 hours) examination by a board-certified neurologist. Follow-up information was obtained by scheduled telephone contact with patients and referring physicians. Events occurring during follow-up were documented by obtaining hospital records and death certificates where appropriate.

Definitions

The following are some important definitions:

1. *Technical success* was defined as the ability to access the carotid artery and successfully stent the lesion.
2. *Complications* include all strokes and deaths occurring within 30 days regardless of their relation to the procedure.
3. *Major stroke* was defined as an increase in the NIH scale of >4 and functionally disabling deficit at 30 days.
4. *Minor stroke* was defined as an increase in the NIH stroke scale of ≤3 or functionally nondisabling at 30 days

Demographics

Between September 1994 and September 2000, we performed carotid artery stenting (CAS) on 712 patients and 805 carotid arteries (hemisph*eres) (Table 41.5). The pati*ents' ages ranged between 35 and 89 years (mean ± SD 69 ± 10); 97 (14%) were older than 80 years. A third of the patients [N = 238 (33%)] were females. Seventy-seven percent (550/712) were hypertensive, 67% (475/712) had hypercholesterolemia, 31% (222/712) were diabetic, and 69% (490/712) had coronary artery disease. A little more than half the patients [N = 427 hemispheres (53%)] were referred for stenting because of an asymptomatic stenosis. Of the remaining 47% (symptomatic), 25% presented with transient ischemic attacks, 20% had had prior stroke, and 2% presented with amaurosis fugax (Table 41.6). A variety of cardiac and noncardiac comorbid conditions and/or unfavorable surgical anatomy (high lesion, above C2; prior neck radiation; radical neck surgery; etc.) would have rendered 88% of symptom-related lesions ineligible for inclusion in the North American carotid endarterectomy trial (NASCET) study (13).

Angiographic Details

To be considered for treatment, symptomatic patients required more than 50% diameter stenosis (14,15). Asymptomatic patients required a ≥70% diameter narrowing (16) by angiography employing NASCET criteria (13). One hundred fifteen of 805 vessels treated (14%) had restenosis

following prior carotid endarterectomy and 9% (72/805) of the patients had occlusion of the contralateral carotid artery. Ninety-three patients with bilateral disease underwent treatment (Table 41.7). Thirty patients underwent treatment during the same procedure. The remaining 63 patients underwent treatment in a staged fashion.

Technical success (Table 41.8) was achieved in 98% of the procedures. Inability to access the carotid artery from the femoral approach was the chief reason for technical failure (9/14). Close to 900 stents have been deployed, 83% of these have been self-expanding stents, the large majority being Wallstents (Table 41.9).

30-Day Outcomes

Overall, the 30-day stroke and death rate was 7.3% (Table 41.10). There were nine deaths [1.3% (9/712)]. Of these, four were neurologic (i.e., stroke related [0.6% (4/712)] and five [0.7% (5/712)] were nonneurologic. Of the four neurologic deaths, one patient expired as a result of multiorgan failure after CVA following carotid artery rupture (7.0-mm postdilatation balloon), one patient died as a result of rupture of a previously unknown ipsilateral internal carotid artery aneurysm after recanalization of an occluded internal carotid artery, one died as a result of intracerebral hemorrhage after an occluded internal carotid artery had been recanalized, and one died from a reperfusion hemorrhage. Of the five nonneurologic deaths, two were from myocardial infarctions (both 3 weeks after the procedure), two from pulmonary embolism (second and third week after the procedure) and one from a large retroperitoneal bleed (related to the procedure).

Major Strokes

There were eight major strokes (1.0%). The first major stroke occurred 3 days after carotid stenting due to an embolus (presumed cardiogenic; prosthetic mitral valve and atrial fibrillation) to the *contralateral* middle cerebral artery. The second major stroke was related to acute stent thrombosis. The third occurred 4 days after successful carotid stenting and followed a period of prolonged hypotension related to cardiac arrest from high-risk elective coronary intervention. The remaining 5 major strokes were periprocedural.

Minor Strokes

In the entire series, there were 35 minor strokes. On an annualized basis, the incidence of minor embolic stroke has declined over the years from 7.1% (1994–1995) to 5.8% (1995–1996), 5.3% (1996–1997) to 3.2% (1997–1998), and 3.1% (1998–1999) to 3.0% (1999–2000).

Late Clinical Outcome

We prospectively evaluated a consecutive series of 703 patients who survived the 30-day periprocedural period (Figure 41.9) (Table 41.11). On late follow-up (21 ± 19

TABLE 41.5. BASELINE VARIABLES

Period:	Sept. 1994–Sept. 2000
Patients:	712
Arteries/hemispheres:	805
Males:	474 (541 arteries)
Females:	238 (264 arteries)
Age range (yr):	35–89
Age (mean ± SD):	69 ± 10
Hypertension:	550
Hypercholesterolemia:	475
Diabetes:	222
CAD:	490

CAD, coronary artery disease.

TABLE 41.6. SYMPTOM STATUS (712 PATIENTS, 805 HEMISPHERES)

Asymptomatic:	427 (53%)
Symptomatic:	378 (47%)
TIA:	258
Stroke:	158
Amaurosis:	22

TIA, transient ischemic attacks.

TABLE 41.7. BASELINE VARIABLES (712 PATIENTS, 805 HEMISPHERES)

Prior CEA:	115
Contralateral occlusion:	72
Bilateral stenosis:	93
Same procedure	30
Staged	63

CEA, carotoid endarterectomy.

TABLE 41.8. PROCEDURAL DETAILS (PART I)

N = patients/artery:	712/805
Procedural success:	791/805 (98%)
Stenosis pre (mean ± sd):	77 ± 14%
Stenosis post (mean ± sd):	3 ± 8%

TABLE 41.9. PROCEDURAL DETAILS (PART II)

Stents	
N = patients/artery:	712/805
Wallstent:	594 (67%)
Smart:	59 (7%)
Memotherm:	85 (10%)
Palmaz:	120 (14%)
Other:	30 (3%)

TABLE 41.10. 30-DAY OUTCOMES

	Males	Females	Totals
N = patients/artery	474/541	238/264	
Minor stroke	26 (4.8%)	9 (3.4%)	35 (6.5%)
Major stroke	5 (0.9%)	3 (1%)	8 (4%)
Fatal stroke	3 (0.6%)	1 (0.4%)	4 (0.6%)
Non–stroke-related death	5 (1.1%)	0	5 (0.7%)
All strokes and deaths	39 (7.4%)	13 (4.8%)	52 (7.3%)

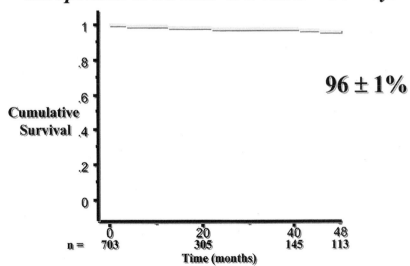

FIGURE 41.9. Incidence of late outcomes after 30 days. There was a 96% freedom from ipsilateral stroke and death.

TABLE 41.11. LATE OUTCOMES

	Males	Females
N = patients/arteries	466/531	237/263
Minor ipsilateral stroke	1 (0.2%)	0
Major ipsilateral stroke	5 (0.9%)	2 (0.8%)
Deaths	3 (0.6%)	2 (0.8%)
All ipsilateral and stroke deaths	9 (1.7%)	4 (1.6%)

months) there were seven major ipsilateral strokes, one minor ipsilateral stroke, and five deaths. Ten patients [6.7% (10/150)] stented with Palmaz biliary balloon-expandable stents were found to have stent deformity (6,11). Eight of these 150 patients (5.3%) had restenosis at the stent site (restenosis = stenosis ≥ 50%), four significant enough to warrant new intervention—PTA of the stent (successful without complications). None of the patients treated with self-expandable stent (Wallstent) had stent deformation.

DISCUSSION

Making Carotid Stenting Safer

Although carotid stenting has been performed since the early 1980s, two important and potentially disastrous complications limited the rapid growth of the technique and procedure—acute closure of the stented vessel and distal embolization. With the introduction in the late 1980s and the subsequent rapid maturation of stent technology the problem of acute closure was effectively resolved. Currently, the major reason for complications during carotid stenting is related to the problem of distal embolization. Hence *increasing safety of carotid stenting is tied in with the issue of reducing embolization during the procedure.* Judicious patient and lesion selection, and refinements in interventional technique (12) have all contributed to reducing the incidence of embolization and hence neurologic complications. From a 7.1% complication rate in 1994–1995 we have reduced the complication rate to 3.0% in the 1999–2000 period.

Patient and lesion selection was modified based on analysis of complications related to different groups of patients (12). Advanced age was the most important predictor of procedural neurologic complications, especially in patients older than 80 years of age (12). Patients with comorbidities, especially those with severe untreated hypertension and patients with recent stroke, are also more prone to neurologic complications. Patients with brain atrophy/dementia and those with extensive lacunar state do not tolerate carotid stenting and should be excluded. We do not accept patients with severe renal impairment (creatinine > 3 to 3.5 mg%), precluding safe use of iodinated contrast agent, and patients unable to tolerate appropriate doses of antiplatelet agents. On the other hand, our analysis showed that a number of higher-risk situations for CEA represent

ideal indications for stenting. These include restenosis after prior CEA, stenosis in patients with prior neck radiation and radical neck surgery and lesions in the distal internal carotid artery or involving high, retromandibular bifurcation. Female gender, presence or absence of neurologic symptoms, presence of coronary artery disease, diabetes mellitus, hypercholesterolemia, smoking, presence of bilateral carotid lesions, ulcerated lesions, or contralateral carotid occlusion do not significantly influence the incidence of neurologic complications.

In general, it should be noted that more systemic factors and comorbidities increase the risk of CEA, whereas local anatomic and lesion factors increase the risk of stenting. At the beginning of our experience, the only contraindication for stenting was pedunculated thrombus at the lesion site. (Thrombi are more easily seen on 7.5 or 15F/sec cineangiography than on DSA.) By analyzing our complications it also became apparent that lesion severity (90% or more diameter stenoses), as well as the length and multiplicity of the stenoses were associated with more embolic complications. We have abandoned recanalization of occluded internal carotid arteries, not only because they were associated with more embolic complications, but also because of an increased risk of intracerebral hemorrhage. The patients at higher risk of neurologic complications are those with severely tortuous, calcified, and atherosclerotic carotid vessels and carotid stenosis with severe concentric calcification. Significant kink, tortuosity, and angulated take-off of the internal carotid artery increase the technical difficulty of stenting and increase the risk of complications.

For stenting we use self-expanding stents. Balloon-expandable stents have several disadvantages when deployed within the carotid bifurcation or its vicinity. Frequently, more then one stent is needed. The stent has to be expanded differentially to conform to the size differential of the internal carotid artery, bifurcation, and common carotid artery. Thus more then one balloon is needed for appropriate dilatation. The balloon can rupture while deploying the stent; there may be difficulties in advancing the balloon–stent assembly (especially 20-mm stent) through the guiding sheath if the aortic arch is significantly distended or the proximal common carotid artery is tortuous. The balloon-expandable stents have a higher tendency to occlude the external carotid artery.

TABLE 41.12. EXPERIENCE WITH NEUROPROTECTION

Period:	February 2000–February 2001
Patients:	102
Minor stroke:	2 (2%)
Major stroke:	0
Deaths:	1 (1%)
Retinal emboli:	1 (1%)
Hyperperfusion:	2 (2%)

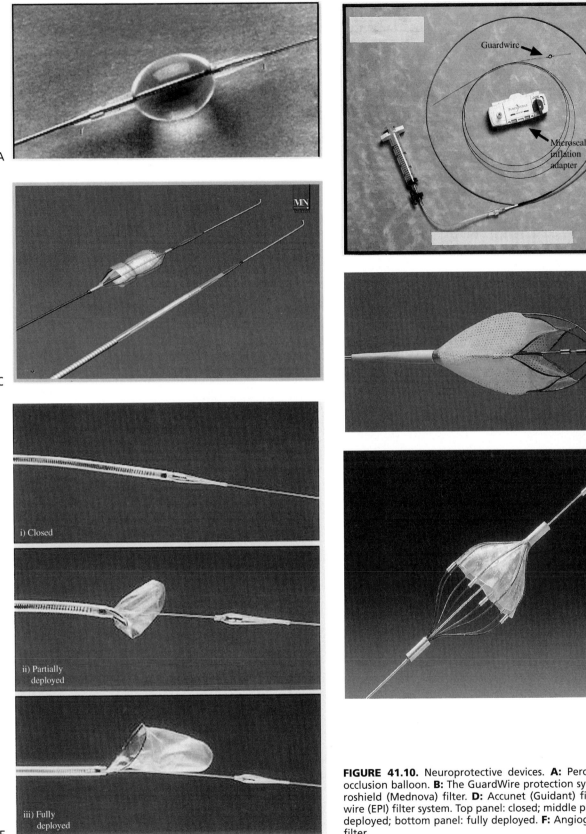

FIGURE 41.10. Neuroprotective devices. **A:** Percusurge distal occlusion balloon. **B:** The GuardWire protection system. **C:** Neuroshield (Mednova) filter. **D:** Accunet (Guidant) filter. **E:** Filterwire (EPI) filter system. Top panel: closed; middle panel: partially deployed; bottom panel: fully deployed. **F:** Angioguard (Cordis) filter.

TABLE 41.13. OVERVIEW OF NEUROPROTECTION DEVICES

Name	GuardWire	Accunet	Angioguard	Neuroshield	FilterWire	ArteriA
Vendor	Percusurge	Guidant	Cordis	Mednova	EPI	ArteriA
Mechanism of neuroprotection	Distal occlusion	Filter	Filter	Filter	Filter	Proximal occlusion
Wire (inch)	0.014	0.014	0.014	0.014	0.014	Not applicable
Crossing profile	0.036	*	*	*	*	Not applicable
CE Mark for carotid use	Yes	No	Yes	Yes	No	Yes
US safety and feasibility study	CAFÉ (n = 220)	Yes (n = 50)	Yes	Picasso (n = 50)	No	No
Current studies	SHELTER		SAPPHIRE			
Comments	†					‡

*Currently all filters are 3F or bigger.
†Largest experience to date in carotids.
‡Only system to confer protection without internal carotid artery instrumentation.
CAFÉ, carotid angioplasty free of emboli; PICASSO, protected internal carotid artery stenting safety observation study; SAPPHIRE, stenting and angioplasty with protection in patients at high risk for endarterectomy; SHELTER, stenting of high risk patients: external cranial lesions trial with emboli removal.

They may also undergo deformation (11) with concomitant restenosis. Exceptions when we use balloon-expandable stents have been mentioned. In heavily calcified stenosis, postdilatation recoil is common (despite predilatation with a 5-mm balloon), and forcing the current, relatively high-profile stent delivery systems may break off plaque and cause embolization. In this situation a short 4- to 6-mm balloon-expandable stent is placed to "hold the stenosis" open before passing a definitive self-expanding stent.

Self-expanding stents have several advantages:

- With exceptions, only one stent is needed.
- They are easily deployed using bony landmarks.
- The distal end is deployed in angiographically normal-appearing internal carotid artery.
- The proximal end of the stent rests in the proximal common carotid.

Significant bradyarrhythmias are not uncommon during predilatation and stent postdilatation, especially when the stenosis is ostial or within the bulb of the internal carotid artery. Bradycardia and asystole usually recover spontaneously after balloon deflation. Premedication with atropine (1.0 mg) is routinely used. (Cardiac pacing has to be available if needed.) Modest fall in blood pressure requires no specific intervention. Occasionally, spasm can develop in the internal carotid artery, especially after placement of the 0.018-inch wire with straightening of the artery or after stent placement. This condition can be treated with intraarterial nitroglycerine (100 to 200 mg) and usually regresses with time. Loss of consciousness can occur with balloon inflation, especially if the ipsilateral hemispheric blood supply is isolated or if the contralateral carotid artery is occluded. This phenomenon recovers spontaneously after balloon deflation (17). Hemodynamic perturbations can be minimized by making sure patients are well hydrated and the procedure is performed earlier during the day. Knowledge of the cardiac status in general and the left ventricular function in particular is therefore important.

Neuroprotection

Why Neuroprotection?

Data from intraprocedural transcranial Doppler monitoring studies have shown us that high-intensity transients (HITS) (presumably representing emboli) are seen in *all* cases of carotid stenting. Although embolization is universal, its clinical expression is random. Periprocedural embolization is not unique to carotid stenting. Muller and colleagues (18) compared TCD and diffusion-weighted magnetic resonance (MR) imaging in patients undergoing CEA for symptomatic stenosis. TCD detected embolic signals in 96% of the patients, and a third of the patients had new defects on diffusion-weighted MR. Five percent of the patients undergoing CEA for symptomatic stenosis had a stroke. The rationale behind the use of neuroprotective devices is to reduce the number of embolic hits and consequently reduce the chance of a clinically relevant neuroembolic event. The effectiveness of one of these devices (Percusurge Guard Wire) to reduce the consequences of particulate distal embolization has been conclusively shown in the context of a randomized trial involving saphenous vein graft angioplasty. Since the distal embolization problem in saphenous vein graft angioplasty and carotid angioplasty appear to be similar, a device that has proven efficacy in reducing distal embolization in vein grafts should also be effective in reducing the distal embolization in the carotid circulation during carotid stenting. Table 41.12 summarizes our experience using two different kinds of neuroprotective devices: the Percusurge occlusion balloon and filters. The overall complication rate using protection devices during

TABLE 41.14. SELF-EXPANDING STENTS AND DELIVERY SYSTEMS (CAROTID USE)

Name	Vendor	Stent Material	Wire Compatibility (in.)	Delivery System (Fr)	Type of Delivery
Tracheobronchial Wallstent	Boston Scientific	Elgiloy	0.035	7 (up to 10-mm diameter)	OTW
Wallstent RP	Boston Scientific	Elgiloy	0.035	6	OTW
Wallstent Monorail	Boston Scientific	Elgiloy	0.014	5.5–6	Monorail
Smart	Cordis	Nitinol	0.035	7 (up to 14-mm diameter)	OTW
Smart 0.018	Cordis	Nitinol	0.018	7	OTW
Smart Precise	Cordis	Nitinol	0.014	6	OTW
Acculink	Guidant	Nitinol	0.014	6	OTW
NEX Stent	Endotex	Nitinol	0.014	5	OTW
X-ACT	Mednova	Nitinol	0.035	7	OTW

OTW, over the wire.

carotid stenting is around 3%. A number of these devices are available and are illustrated in Figures 41.10a through 41.10f and Table 41.13 and were briefly discussed in the preceding section.

CONCLUSION AND FUTURE DIRECTIONS

Carotid artery stenting has rapidly evolved into a less invasive procedure for treating patients with symptomatic and significant asymptomatic carotid stenosis. With today's equipment and technique (Table 41.14), stenting mortality and morbidity from stroke-related complications is in the range of 3%, similar to or lower than comparable patient populations treated with traditional carotid endarterectomy (19–21), and there are no cranial nerve palsies. Rigorous follow-up studies have confirmed low restenosis rates after carotid stenting and a low incidence of late cerebrovascular events (7). In both percutaneous stenting and endarterectomy, stroke related to embolization can occur. In each technique, the incidence of embolic stroke depends on meticulous procedural technique and expertise, and is markedly dependent on the volume of cases performed. The availability of carotid neuroprotective devices such as occlusion balloons (4,22) and filters to reduce the potential for cerebral emboli will further enhance current results of carotid stenting.

REFERENCES

1. Mathias K. Stent placement in supra-aortic artery disease. In: Liermann DD, ed. *State of the art and future developments.* Morin Heights, Quebec, Canada: Polyscience Publication, Inc., 1995: 87–92.
2. Diethrich EB, Ndiaye M, Reid DB. Stenting in the carotid artery: initial experience in 110 patients. *J Endovasc Surg* 1996; 3: 42–62.
3. Roubin GS, Yadav S, Iyer SS, et al. Carotid stent-supported angioplasty: a neurovascular intervention to prevent stroke. *Am J Cardiol* 1996;78:8–12.
4. Theron JG, Payelle GG, Coskun O, et al. Carotid artery stenosis: treatment with protected balloon angioplasty and stent placement. *Radiology* 1996;201:627–636.
5. Wholey MH, Wholey M, Mathias K, et al. Global experience in cervical carotid artery stent placement. *Catheter Cardiovasc Interv* 2000;50:160–167.
6. Vitek JJ, Iyer SS, Roubin GS. Carotid stenting in 350 vessels: problems faced and solved. *J Invasive Cardiol* 1998;10:311–314.
7. Roubin GS, New G, Iyer SS, et al. Immediate and late clinical outcomes of carotid artery stenting in patients with symptomatic and asymptomatic carotid artery stenosis: a 5-year prospective analysis. *Circulation* 2001;103:532–537.
8. Gomez CR, Roubin GS, Dean LS, et al. Neurological monitoring during carotid artery stenting: the duck squeezing test. *J Endovasc Surg* 1999;6:332–336.
9. New G, Roubin GS, Oetgen ME, et al. Validity of duplex ultrasound as a diagnostic modality for internal carotid artery disease. *Catheter Cardiovasc Interv* 2001;52:9–15.
10. Ohki T, Marin ML, Lyon RT, et al. *Ex vivo* human carotid artery bifurcation stenting: correlation of lesion characteristics with embolic potential. *J Vasc Surg* 1998;27:463–471.
11. Mathur A, Dorros G, Iyer SS, et al. Palmaz stent compression in patients following carotid artery stenting. *Catheter Cardiovasc Diagn* 1997;41:137–140.
12. Mathur A, Roubin GS, Iyer SS, et al. Predictors of stroke complicating carotid artery stenting. *Circulation* 1998;97:1239-1245.
13. Beneficial effect of carotid endarterectomy in symptomatic patients with high-grade carotid stenosis. North American Symptomatic Carotid Endarterectomy Trial Collaborators. *N Engl J Med* 1991;325:445–453.
14. Barnett HJ, Taylor DW, Eliasziw M, et al. Benefit of carotid endarterectomy in patients with symptomatic moderate or severe stenosis. *N Engl J Med* 1998;339:1415–1425.
15. North American Symptomatic Carotid Endarterectomy Trial. Methods, patient characteristics, and progress. *Stroke* 1991;22: 711–720.
16. Endarterectomy for asymptomatic carotid artery stenosis. Executive Committee for the Asymptomatic Carotid Atherosclerosis Study. *JAMA* 1995;273:1421–1428.
17. Mathur A, Roubin GS, Gomez CR, et al. Elective carotid artery stenting in the presence of contralateral occlusion. *Am J Cardiol* 1998;81:1315–1317.

18. Müller M, Reiche W, Langenscheidt P, et al. Ischemia after carotid endarterectomy: comparison between transcranial Doppler sonography and diffusion-weighted MR imaging. *Am J Neuroradiol* 2000;21:47–54.

19. McCrory DC, Goldstein LB, Samsa GP, et al. Predicting complications of carotid endarterectomy. *Stroke* 1993;24:1285–1291.

20. Rothwell PM, Slattery J, Warlow CP. A systematic review of the risks of stroke and death due to endarterectomy for symptomatic carotid stenosis. *Stroke* 1996;27:260–265.

21. Wennberg DE, Lucas FL, Birkmeyer JD, Bredenberg CE, Fisher ES. Variation in and patient characteristics [see comments]. *JAMA* 1998;279:1278–1281.

22. Henry M, Amor M, Masson I, et al. Angioplasty and stenting of the extracranial carotid arteries. *J Endovasc Surg* 1998;5:293–304.

42

COVERED STENTS IN THE MANAGEMENT OF INFRARENAL AORTIC ANEURYSMS

GEOFFREY H. WHITE
ANDREW F. LENNOX
JAMES MAY

In the 46 years since the first successful replacement of an abdominal aortic aneurysm (AAA) with a homograft in 1951 (1), the technique of open surgical repair of AAA has been refined to the extent that the elective operative mortality is around 5% (2,3) whereas the mortality rate from surgically repairing ruptured AAA remains around 50% (2). These figures apply only to selected patients, however, and the risks of surgical repair are greater in patients with significant comorbidity (4). As many patients with abdominal aortic aneurysm have coexistent conditions that significantly increase the risk of elective and emergent surgery (4), less invasive techniques of AAA repair that reduce these risks offer a means of reducing morbidity and mortality following AAA repair.

Percutaneous treatment of occlusive arterial disease has become an accepted part of vascular surgical practice since Dotter first reported the percutaneous placement of stainless steel coils within the arterial lumen (5). Percutaneous angioplasty and arterial stenting are now part of routine vascular surgical practice. These endovascular techniques are believed to offer advantages in terms of reduced morbidity and mortality, reduced hospital stay, and shorter convalescence, with results comparable to surgical treatment in appropriately selected patients (6).

At the forefront of this evolution is endovascular aortic aneurysm repair. The minimally traumatic nature of this new technique results in less pain and fewer complications for a cohort of patients who have significant medical comorbidity. Additionally, the procedure may lead to health care cost savings, through reduced lengths of hospital stay and lower utilization of intensive care resources. This chapter reviews the current status of endovascular aneurysm repair of the infrarenal aorta.

DEVICES USED

The technique of endovascular aneurysm repair features a vascular graft affixed to metallic stent or wireform supports, compressed along its long axis and delivered to an aneurysm, usually by a transfemoral, transluminal route. This may be achieved via a small cutdown incision to the artery, or in some cases percutaneously. Once positioned inside the aneurysm, the graft is expanded to bridge the diseased aortic segment, with the aim of unloading it of hemodynamic stress and eliminating the risk of future rupture. In comparison with conventional "open" aneurysm surgery, the principal advantages of endovascular repair include (a) avoidance of a painful, long abdominal or chest incision; (b) avoidance of aortic cross-clamping, with attendant swings in blood pressure and cardiac afterload; and (c) avoidance of blood loss associated with aortotomy.

The first successful use of this technique for human aneurysm repair is attributed to Parodi, who reported results in 1991 (7). Since that date, the technology has matured from initial, homemade devices (fabricated from conventional vascular grafts and vascular stent equipment), to purpose-engineered components, manufactured by cardiovascular and angiography device companies (Table 42.1). The development of the technology has been rapid, so that in some centers endovascular AAA repair has already become the routine rather than the exception.

Geoffrey H. White: Associate Professor of Surgery, Department of Vascular Surgery, University of Sydney, Sydney, New South Wales, Australia

Andrew F. Lennox: Vascular Fellow, Department of Vascular Surgery, Royal Prince Alfred Hospital, Sydney, New South Wales, Australia

James May: Bosch Professor of Surgery, Department of Vascular Surgery, University of Sydney, Sydney, New South Wales, Australia

TABLE 42.1. COMMERCIALLY AVAILABLE ENDOVASCULAR GRAFTS FOR THE TREATMENT OF INFRARENAL AORTIC ANEURYSMS

Manufacturer (Device)	Device Characteristics			Delivery System		
	Graft Material	Stent Material	Stent Pattern	Size (Outside Diameter)	Method of Expansion	Method of Fixation
Guidant/EVT (Ancure)	Polyester	Elgiloy	Proximal and distal stents	27F	Self-expanding + balloon	Hooks
Medtronic (AneuRx)	Polyester (thin-walled)	Nitinol	Continuous mesh (external)	22F	Self-expanding	Friction + compression fit
World Medical (Talent)	Polyester	Nitinol	Intermittent	24F	Self-expanding	Friction + compression fit
Cook (Zenith)	Polyester	Stainless steel (Gianturco type)	Repetitive (total cover)	22F	Self-expanding	Friction + hooks
Edwards LifeSciences (Lifepath)	Polyester	Elgiloy	Intermittent	22F	Balloon expandable	Friction + crimps
Gore (Excluder)	Polytetrofluoroethylene	Nitinol	Continuous (external)	22F	Self-expanding	Friction + small hooks
Bard (Endologix)	Polytetrofluoroethylene	Nitinol	Continous mesh (internal)	22F	Self-expanding	Friction + compression fit

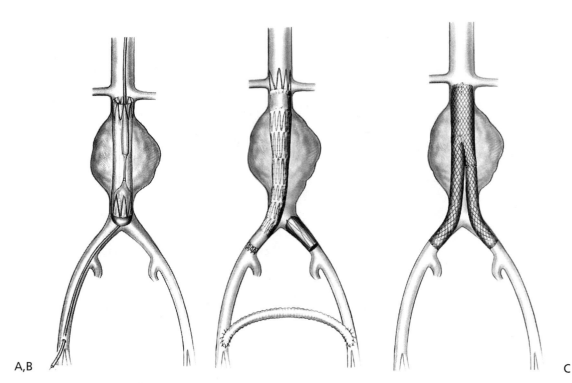

A,B   C

FIGURE 42.1. The different configurations of endoluminal aortic grafts. **A:** Tube graft. **B:** Aorto-uniiliac graft with a contralateral common iliac occluding plug and a femoro-femoral crossover graft. **C:** Bifurcated modular graft. (From Chafour X, May J, White GH, et al. Chirurgie endovasculaire des aneurismes de l'aorte. *Encyclopédie Medico Chirurgicale* 2001;43:155B, with permission.)

Device Configuration and Placement

All present devices for endovascular aneurysm repair consist of two core components: a metal-supported fabric graft ("stent-graft") and a delivery sheath. The latter is always passed over a guide wire. Grafts are available in tube, bifurcated, and aorto-uniiliac (AUI) versions (Figure 42.1) for placement in the abdominal or thoracic aorta. It is possible to repair aneurysms confined only to the aorta, or combined AAA and iliac aneurysms.

Bifurcated grafts are the most common variant employed. Early attempts to treat most patients with tube grafts led to a high incidence of intermediate-term failure due to poor attachment of the distal aspect of the straight graft within the distal aspects of the aneurysmal abdominal aorta. The challenge of placing a bifurcated graft configuration into the aorta by remote access has been met with two designs:

1. *Single-piece bifurcated grafts,* such as the Guidant/EVT Ancure graft (Menlo Park, CA) and the Bard Endologix device (Irvine, CA). This design introduces the entire graft (aortic component and both iliac limbs) into the arterial system via one femoral artery. The contralateral iliac graft limb must be manipulated into position by guide wires and pull-wires directed across the aortic bifurcation by interventional techniques. This design has an inherent advantage of avoiding displacement or leakage between separate segments of a multipiece (modular) graft, but may be prone to twisting or poor positioning during deployment.

2. *Modular bifurcated grafts,* including designs by Boston Scientific (Natick, MA), Cook (Indianapolis, IN), Cordis (Warren, NJ), Edwards LifeSciences (Irvine, CA), Gore (Sunnyvale, CA), and Medtronic (Cupertino, CA). These incorporate two or three components that are assembled intravascularly, to completely form the graft and exclude an aneurysm. The aortic component and one iliac limb are first inserted from one femoral artery and then mated to the opposite iliac limb, inserted by contralateral femoral artery access. The advantage of this modular design is that smaller segments permit smaller-caliber delivery sheaths. The overlap of successive graft segments within one another (the "trombone technique") permits mixing components of different diameters or lengths to complete an entire graft. By this means, a wide variety of aneurysm lengths and disparate proximal and distal neck diameters may be accommodated using a standardized selection of components as demonstrated in Figure 42.2.

PATIENT SELECTION

Patient selection in the management of infrarenal aortic aneurysms has become a controversial issue in recent years with more advanced graft design and the availability of custom-made grafts in addition to smaller delivery sheaths. Suitability for endovascular aneurysm repair is limited by specific anatomic criteria. Table 42.2 lists the most important of these (8). Foremost among qualifying features is the need for an adequate length of normal artery proximal and distal to an aneurysm, for secure graft attachment. Since most abdominal aneurysms extend almost to the aortic bifurcation (without any length of distal cuff or neck), most

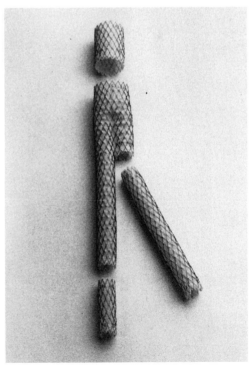

FIGURE 42.2. Modular aortic endoluminal graft demonstrating external metallic stents with multiple components that can be placed either proximally in the aorta or distally in the iliac arteries.

TABLE 42.2. ANATOMIC CRITERIA FOR ENDOVASCULAR REPAIR (GENERAL GUIDELINES)

1. Proximal segment of thrombus-free normal caliber aorta ε 15-mm length
2. Distal segment of thrombus-free normal-caliber aorta (for tube graft) or iliac artery (for aortoiliac or aortobiiliac graft) ε 15-mm length
3. At least one patent external/common iliac artery with diameter ε 7 mm
4. Angulation of proximal aortic neck of less than 60 degrees*
5. Angulation of iliac arteries of less than 90 degrees*
6. Aneurysm does not traverse aortic arch, celiac, superior mesenteric, or renal arteries
7. Reconstruction will preserve patency of at least one internal iliac artery, or inferior mesenteric artery

*As defined by Ad Hoc Committee for Standardized Reporting Practices in Vascular Surgery SVS/ISCVS (8).

patients brought to endovascular repair will require a bifurcated (aorto-biiliac) device. This contrasts with conventional repair, where most patients receive a tube graft, since it is usually possible to suture directly to a rim of aortic wall adjacent to the orifices of the common iliac arteries.

The length of an aneurysm neck and its angulation and geometry determine the ability to attach a stent-graft with long-term security. Other factors, such as calcification, thrombus, and wall strength, may also play a role. With conventional surgery, aneurysms that traverse tributaries (renal and iliac arteries, arch vessels, etc.) can be repaired with reimplantation of tributaries into interposing graft. In general, this is impossible with endovascular repair (except when experimental fenestrated endovascular devices are employed), precluding use of this technique within the aortic arch, or suprarenally around visceral vessels. For infrarenal aneurysms with an inadequate length of infrarenal neck, it is possible to cross the renal orifices with an uncovered portion of stent, achieving anchorage to suprarenal segments. Veith and colleagues have extensive experience with a custom-fabricated, in-house device that frequently covers one or more renal orifices with bare stent, with a low incidence of long-term compromise of renal artery patency (9).

AUI grafts are uniquely suited to two scenarios: (a) when an AAA tapers to a normal caliber above the aortic bifurcation but the segment is too short to anchor a tube graft and too narrow to accommodate both the limbs of an AUI graft, and (b) in combined aneurysmal and atherosclerotic disease (with one iliac artery severely stenosed or chronically occluded) or when there is severe tortuosity of an iliac artery that renders it unsuitable for bifurcated graft. These grafts may also be used to "rescue" failed attempts at placement of an aorto-biiliac device, when the contralateral iliac limb sheath cannot be passed or that graft section is misdeployed. In such cases, an AUI graft may be placed inside the bifurcated graft trunk, occluding the graft contralateral iliac stump. In all cases except contralateral iliac occlusion, placement of an AUI graft must be accompanied by the implantation of an occluding device in the contralateral iliac artery (typically a short, blind-ending stent-graft "sock"), to prevent retrograde AAA filling. Additionally, a femoral-femoral bypass procedure must be performed to revascularize the contralateral leg.

STENT IMPLANTATION

Periprocedural Imaging

Accurate graft sizing is crucial to success after endovascular repair. Correct measurements for device size selection require higher-quality imaging than has routinely been employed for open repair. Contrast-enhanced spiral computerized tomography (CT) scan is the modality of choice, with sections maximally spaced at 5-mm and preferably 2- to 3-mm intervals. Three-dimensional reproduction of the CT images is being used with increasing frequency (Figure 42.3). The scans should include the entire span of the abdominal and pelvic vasculature, with particular views of the infrarenal aortic, and are ideally printed with an enlarged periaortic view (20-cm periaortic field). Thin sections are necessary to gauge length and quality of proximal and distal graft attachment or fixation zones, in segments of nonaneurysmal aorta. Magnetic resonance imaging has also

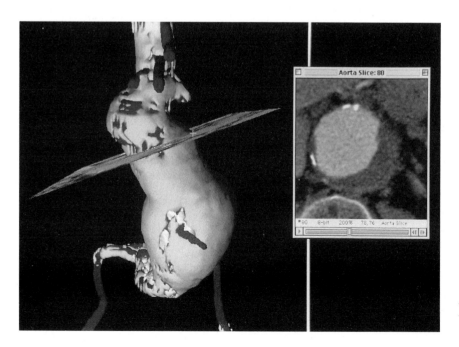

FIGURE 42.3. 3-Dimensional reconstruction of a preoperative aortic computerized tomography (CT) scan. (Image courtesy of Medical Media Systems, Hanover, NH.)

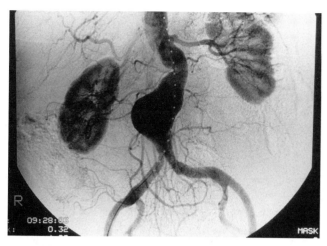

FIGURE 42.4. Calibrated digital subtraction aortogram used to calculate the aortic luminal diameter and length in order to estimate accurately the size of graft required.

been used but rarely provides more information than the CT scan. Many centers also perform aortography, obtained with a calibrated catheter, marked with radiopaque bands at 1-cm intervals (Figure 42.4). This allows measurement of aneurysm length along the flow channel and provides information about patency and caliber of iliac vessels along the pathway to graft insertion, as well as the collateral arteries (lumbar or thoracic intercostal) or a patent inferior mesenteric artery, which may lead to retrograde perfusion of an aneurysm sac after graft placement.

Implantation Technique

High-resolution intraoperative angiographic equipment is essential in managing patients suitable for endovascular AAA repair. Either a mobile C-arm or fixed fluoroscopic system with 12-inch field and digital subtraction facilities is required. An ideal situation is a specifically designed and fully equipped endovascular theater or angiographic suite with dual high-resolution monitors, power injectors, and staff trained in catheter-based techniques.

Delivery sheaths for all devices are relatively large, typically 20 to 22F outside diameter for aortic grafts and 14 to 16F for iliac components. Sheath placement thus usually requires surgical cut-down to the insertion vessel and arteriotomy. Procedures can be done either in an angiography suite equipped for surgery or in an operating room with portable imaging capable of variable field size (from 15- to 30-cm diameter) and digital subtraction. The possibility of urgent conversion to open repair must be considered when choosing a method of anesthesia. Although regional anesthesia is possible, general anesthesia is more commonly employed. This facilitates emergent conversion (however unlikely) and is more comfortable for patients, who must lie supine and still for an extended period.

The procedure employed will vary, depending on the individual graft to be deployed; however, there are basic principles. Following exposure of the femoral artery, the first step is to gain access for an initial angiogram to delineate the position of the renal arteries, aortic bifurcation, and exact location of the proximal and distal deployment sites. This is performed with a 7- to 8F sheath and a pigtail calibrated catheter usually inserted via the contralateral side to the proposed main graft body deployment. Some centers prefer to position an angiographic catheter at the suprarenal level via the left brachial artery, thereby avoiding potential catching on the hooks and metallic stents. This technique, however, does have the risk of distal embolization from a diseased aortic arch.

The angiogram initially confirms the position of the renal arteries and the planned deployment site at the proximal neck. These sites can be referenced by the use of either a vertical marker ruler placed under the x-ray table or an anatomic bony landmark such as the lumbar vertebra. Predilatation of an iliac stenosis is also performed when the angiogram indicates passage of the graft or delivery of the sheath will be difficult. If there is aneurysmal dilatation of the distal common iliac artery, intraoperative coil embolization of the internal iliac arteries can be performed before deployment of the iliac limb of the graft in the external iliac artery. Choice of the ipsilateral access site depends on the degree of both tortuosity and calcification of the iliac vessels. The imaging equipment must be able to outline the passage of the graft through the aortoiliac segment up to the infrarenal position. Once it is in the desired position, the graft is deployed while injecting small boluses of contrast and continuous screening to ensure patency of the renal arteries. After full deployment, the access sheath is withdrawn over the stiff guide wire, which is maintained in the suprarenal aorta. If a modular bifurcated graft is being used, the contralateral limb of the main graft body is cannulated and the second iliac graft is deployed, preferably into the common iliac artery with the internal iliac artery patency maintained. With some grafts routine balloon dilatation is performed at the proximal, junctional, and distal deployment sites to mould the graft against the surrounding arterial wall. With an AUI graft, an occluding plug is deployed into the contralateral common iliac artery before femoro-femoral crossover grafting.

The final task is to perform a completion angiogram to assess the adequacy of the seal between the graft and native vessel both at the proximal and distal deployment sites, as seen in Figure 42.5. Digital subtraction and ceasing ventilation (to remove movement artifacts) improves the quality of the imaging. Should a proximal, distal, or junctional leak of contrast into the aneurysm sac (endoleak) be detected, further balloon dilatation of the graft or the addition of an extension limbs can be used to correct the situation. Only minor fabric "blushes" and lumbar-related leaks should be monitored conservatively.

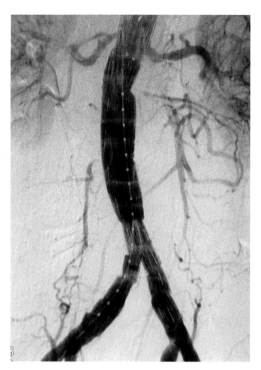

FIGURE 42.5. Completion angiogram following deployment of an endoluminal graft, with suprarenal stents visible and an adequate proximal and distal seal.

The femoral arteries are repaired with direct suturing and the distal circulation is examined for signs of distal embolization before completing the procedure. A postoperative contrast CT scan or duplex is performed to assess for endoleak and graft migration before discharge from the hospital. Currently, the follow-up protocol involves plain x-ray and either CT or duplex imaging to exclude these complications in addition to assessing reduction in the size of the aneurysm sac over time and disruption of the metallic stents. Although different centers vary, most institutions perform these investigations at 3, 6, and 12 months after the procedure, and annually after this if there have been no complications.

RESULTS

Early Results

Experienced centers performing endoluminal AAA repair have initial reported success rates of greater than 90% (10–12) where the aneurysm sac is completely excluded from the circulation without the need for open conversion. These figures appear to be improving. As new technology has developed better stent and material design, including suprarenal stent fixation, stricter criteria for patient selection are being advised and the initial learning curves are being completed. Most published reports have shown that perioperative mortality after endovascular aneurysm repair is similar to that reported for open repair (10–12). In our experience, overall mortality averages approximately 4% (Table 42.3), comparing favorably to large studies of elective conventional repair, including the Canadian Aneurysm Study (4.7%), the UK Small Aneurysm Trial (5.8%), and Michigan statewide mortality (5.6% in 1990) (13–15). The present inability of any large endovascular series to demonstrate an early survival benefit is likely a result of a selection bias for high-risk patients who are offered the procedure on a compassionate basis. In the experience of the UK Registry for Endovascular Treatment of Aneurysms it was reported that 35% of all patients were "unfit" for open surgery (16). At times, our cohort has comprised up to 44% of patients referred for endovascular repair by outside vascular surgeons who had deemed them at excessive risk for conventional repair (11). The impact of comorbidity in this group is best illustrated by the finding in one study that among the first 113 endovascular repairs, all deaths after intraoperative conversion (to open repair) occurred in high-risk patients (17). There was 43% mortality among "unfit" patients requiring conversion, as opposed to no mortality among fit patients requiring conversion. In contrast to these results, more recent results from the US AneuRx Multicenter Trial have demonstrated low mortality (2.6%, Table 42.3), despite 26% of patients being classified as American Society of Anesthesiologists (ASA) Class IV (12). These substantially better results may reflect current improvements in

TABLE 42.3. ENDOVASCULAR VS. OPEN AAA REPAIR: LARGE SERIES RESULTS

	Endovascular			Open
	Sydney (9,23) (*n* = 190)	AneuRx (20) (*n* = 190)	Blum (18) (*n* = 154)	Canadian Aneurysm Study (10,13) (*n* = 680)
30-day mortality	8(4.2%)	5 (2.6%)	1(0.6%)	4.7%
Renal failure*	7(3.6%)	0	2 (1.3%)	0.6%
Wound complication†	1(0.5%)	1 (0.5%)	3(2%)	2%
Embolization†	0	0	4(2.6%)	3.3%
Femoral/iliac/distal limb ischemia	24 (12.6%)	10 (5.2%)	4(2.6%)	3.5%

*Requiring temporary or permanent dialysis.
†Requiring concurrent or subsequent intervention.

endovascular technique and graft design, or may result from patient selection criteria used in the FDA-monitored study.

Technical Complications

A number of technical complications are related specifically to the endovascular method of repair. There has been a greater incidence of postoperative limb ischemia in endovascular-treated patients than in conventional repairs (Table 42.3). Initially, these were attributed to the learning curve for a new technique. However, they may be unavoidable risks of passing firm sheaths through diseased arteries and administering greater x-ray contrast volumes than for open repair. When our collective endovascular experience was analyzed according to date of implant (initial 3 years versus last 2.5 years), we found no significant reduction in adverse events between early and late time periods [49% versus 44% "device adverse events," as defined by the US Food and Drug Administration (FDA)] (18). This was despite the fact that our late experience was heavily weighted with second-generation, purpose-designed prostheses, while most early cases used first-generation or "home-made" devices.

Renal failure after AAA repair is a serious systemic complication. Patients requiring postoperative dialysis in our series experienced a 43% rate of mortality (18). This finding mirrors the experience reported for conventional repair, where postoperative renal failure has been associated with ninefold greater mortality (19). Although most endovascular series report a low incidence of this complication, the incidence remains greater than that reported for open repair (10–12). Renal failure after endovascular grafting may be secondary to the administration of large quantities of intravenous contrast, embolization of thrombus, or atheroma during instrumentation, or inadvertent occlusion of the renal ostia by endografts. Renal artery coverage by graft is rare, but causes the most serious morbidity (11,18).

Repeated instrumentation of the iliac arteries and aneurysm sac may increase the risk of peripheral embolization during endovascular repair. However, this also has not been proven by experience. Embolic events requiring reoperation are reported by the three largest endovascular series to be nearly equal to the 3.3% incidence noted in the Canadian Aneurysm Study (Table 42.3) (10–12,20).

Endoleak

The most common technical complication after endovascular repair is endoleak. This is defined as persistent perfusion of an aneurysm sac, with blood flow outside the graft. Diagnosis can be made on angiography at the time of implantation of the endoluminal graft or on follow-up CT scanning (Figure 42.6). Endoleak has been classified into four subtypes (types I through IV, Figure 42.7) (21–24). Endoleak

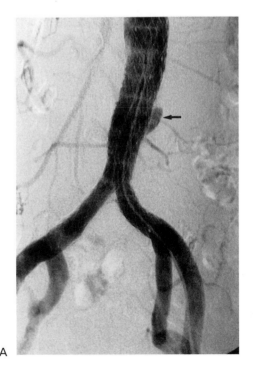
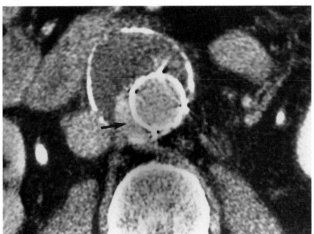

A   B

FIGURE 42.6. Detection of an endoleak. **A:** At completion angiogram, contrast flow outside the graft is indicated with an *arrow.* **B:** Postoperative CT scan again shows contrast within the AAA sac.

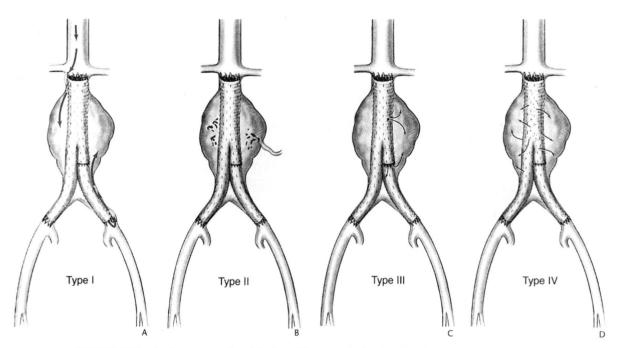

FIGURE 42.7. The four types of endoleaks, with *arrows* indicating the direction of flow into the AAA sac. **A:** Type I endoleak (periprosthetic) occurs at the proximal and/or distal attachment zones. **B:** Type II endoleak is caused by retrograde flow from patent lumbar or inferior mesenteric arteries. **C:** Type III endoleak arises from a defect in the graft fabric, inadequate seal, or disconnection of modular graft components. **D:** Type IV endoleak is due to graft fabric porosity, often resulting in a generalized mild blush of contrast within the aneurysm sac.

is described as "primary" if it arises at the time of graft implant or "secondary" if it occurs later. Primary endoleak results from errors in device sizing, device complications, or errors of technique (although certain grafts, such as the Medtronic AneuRx, have fabric porosity that can cause transient transfabric endoleak). Secondary endoleak results from device failure or a loss of fixation within the proximal or distal attachment zones. In clinical practice, endoleak is the predominant determinant of short- and intermediate-term procedural success. Endoleaks can be associated with aneurysm enlargement and eventual rupture (25–30). This has been most frequently reported with those that directly communicate with aortic lumen (types I and III). The natural history of most successfully excluded AAAs is shrinkage around an endovascular graft. In some cases the aneurysm may completely disappear (31–34). Postoperative aneurysm enlargement is commonly associated with endoleak and mandates selective aortic and iliac angiography to localize its source. Secondary treatment is required for any endoleak of type I or II and for any late endoleak. This may require placement of additional endovascular graft(s), coil embolization of collateral arteries, or conversion to open repair.

Type II endoleaks are those that arise through retrograde perfusion of lumbar arteries or a patent inferior mesenteric artery. These appear to have a more benign natural history.

Some investigators have suggested that most of these are not associated with aneurysm enlargement (35). Conservative management is considered appropriate unless the aneurysm enlarges.

Recently, it has been appreciated that there may be persistent high pressure maintained within the AAA sac, without endoleak. This phenomenon is now referred to as "endotension" (36,37). Possible mechanisms include seal of the aneurysm by a layer of thrombus (which deflects blood flow from the sac but transmits pressure), pressure transmission through the fabric of a highly porous graft, or retrograde perfusion by collateral branches. Pressure measurements obtained during open surgery have shown that thrombus within an aortic sac does not reduce pressure transmission to the aortic wall (38).

CHANGES IN AAA MORPHOLOGY

The changes in morphology that accompany successful endoluminal repair have been recognized since 1995 and reported by a number of groups (39–42). These include a reduction in the maximum transverse diameter of the aneurysm and an increase in diameter of the proximal neck of the order of 10%. In addition to contrast-enhanced, computed tomography demonstrating exclusion of the aneurysm sac from the general circulation, one of the important criteria of successful endoluminal repair is a reduction in maximum transverse diameter (or volume) of the aneurysm.

DURABILITY OF ENDOVASCULAR REPAIR

The most appropriate gauge of success after endovascular aneurysm repair is the percentage of patients who survive with continued aneurysm exclusion (i.e., without endoleak) and endovascular graft patency and without conversion to open repair. Such an endpoint can be compared with the best measure of success after open repair: the percentage of survivors without graft-related complication (pseudoaneurysm at an anastomotic suture line, graft thrombosis, graft-enteric fistula). For open aneurysm repair, an estimate of success can be made by combining results from different studies (realizing the possibility of error inherent in doing so). In a review of more than 300 cases, Hallett reported that the probability of suffering any major graft-related complication (thrombosis, pseudoaneurysm, graft-enteric fistula, graft infection) was 5%, for patients surviving 3 years after open aneurysm repair, and a 3-year survival rate without these complications of 77% (43). In early reports of endovascular repair, survival with successful aneurysm repair at 3 years was 71% (11). Thus a successful outcome is slightly more likely for conventional surgery than for endovascular repair (77% versus 71%) in the intermediate term (3 years post-op). This finding was reproduced for short-term outcomes (30 days) in the US AneuRx trial, which followed concurrent performed endovascular and open aneurysm repairs (12). Success rates for conventional surgery at 30 days were 95%, compared with 89% for endovascular AAA repair. Thus at both early and intermediate-term follow-up, conventional surgery provides an outcome advantage (survival with functioning graft). However, the absolute advantage over endovascular techniques is quite small.

It is important to clarify that the preceding graft success analysis does not consider the important outcome measures of nongraft morbidity (nonfatal myocardial infarction, respiratory failure, etc.) after conventional versus endovascular repair. The US AneuRx trial demonstrated that major morbidity was reduced from 23% after conventional surgery to 12% after stent graft treatment (12). Stent-graft-treated patients demonstrated significant reductions in operative blood loss, time to extubation, ICU stay, and total hospital stay. These findings suggest that endovascular aneurysm repair may be an ideal treatment for patients with significant medical morbidity who are expected to survive at least 4 to 5 years but would be unlikely to survive conventional repair or aneurysm rupture.

DEVICE FAILURE

In addition to specific complications such as endoleak, it is now recognized that the prosthesis may become distorted following endoluminal AAA repair (44–46). This may involve changes in shape and position, and occurs most commonly in the form of kinking in the limbs of bifurcated prostheses at their junction with the trunk, but it may also occur in tube endografts. These structural changes may lead to thrombosis of graft limbs, or result in either dislocation of component parts of a modular prosthesis or dislocation of the limbs of an endograft from the native common iliac arteries. Both forms of dislocation, of course, result inevitably in endoleak, and in some cases have resulted in aneurysm rupture (29,30). Distal migration of the device may also be a significant cause of late complications (47). There is also accumulating evidence that sudden aneurysm rupture may occur in patients who have had apparently successful endovascular treatment, with no evidence of endoleak (28,30). This may be associated with fabric tears or other structural defects, as well as acute dislocation of the segments of a modular device.

Further technologic advances will occur to overcome some of the limitations of the present first- and second-generation devices. Device durability, at the expense of low profile, will be important in improving the long-term results. In the meantime, continued detailed imaging is required in all patients after endovascular graft placement to document changes in AAA size, absence of endoleak, and structural changes in the device.

CONVERSION TO OPEN REPAIR

Conversion to open repair may be required as an acute event due to severe complications during the implant procedure, or as a late event used in management of late failure (48). Endoleak continues to be an important indication for open operative correction if it is not amenable to endoluminal intervention. In general, conversion to open repair will be indicated under the following circumstances:

1. Aortic rupture occurring during the procedure of endoluminal repair or subsequently during observation of an endoleak awaiting spontaneous thrombosis.
2. After implantation of an endograft into a position that obstructs the flow of blood into the renal arteries.
3. In the presence of a persistent endoleak where supplementary attempts at endoluminal repair have been unsuccessful.
4. In the presence of an infected endograft.

Conversion to conventional open repair in the course of an endoluminal repair will undoubtedly become less common as patient selection improves and intraoperative complications are more widely managed by endovascular methods. Infection in the graft is rare, and should be managed by removal of the graft with extraanatomic or in-line restoration of flow.

CURRENT STATUS AND FUTURE PERSPECTIVES

Controversial Issues

Many controversies remain with respect to the use of this new technology. These include the following:

1. Should endovascular grafts be used only for the treatment of patients with high operative risk, because of advanced cardiac disease or other comorbidities?
2. Are the current grafts constructed of materials adequate to withstand device failure, or is further device durability required?
3. Does the advent of endovascular grafts justify the treatment of AAA at an earlier stage (small aneurysms with a maximum diameter of 4 to 5 cm)?
4. Are randomized trials required? Currently, only two major international trials are assessing safety, efficacy, and appropriate patient selection (the EVAR Trial in Great Britain and DREAM Trial in the Netherlands).
5. Should all endoleaks be treated or can type II endoleaks be managed conservatively?
6. Which imaging techniques are best for postoperative surveillance, and how often should follow-up studies be obtained?
7. Are endovascular grafts and their follow-up cost-effective (49,50)?
8. Will the reduced morbidity and early recovery be offset by a lifelong obligation for frequent follow-up investigations?

Current Status

As of 1999, two grafts had been approved by the FDA for general use in the United States. The Guidant Ancure device and Medtronic AneuRx device (Table 42.1) have been used for one year, but the FDA has issued device alerts about their use. With regard to the Ancure device, manufacturing and adverse-event reporting problems have led to a recall of the grafts and suspension of further manufacturing. The manufacturer of the AneuRx graft suspended production after a number of patients presented with aneurysm rupture thought to be associated with

- Suboptimal placement of the graft.
- Endoleak (inadequate proximal seal, collateral vessel retrograde flow, persistent perigraft flow).
- Migration of the main body of the device as well as any attachment cuffs, possibly associated with continuing aortic dilatation.

- Problems with device integrity, due to metal frame fractures, suture breaks, or fabric tears.
- Complex aneurysm anatomy.

The Cook Zenith graft, Gore Excluder, and Bard Endologix graft are currently undergoing further clinical trials and are awaiting FDA approval. All these grafts have a CE mark and can be used in Europe and Britain; they are also used in various centers in Australia. It is uncertain which graft may be superior in the long term, particularly with respect to durability and long-term protection from aneurysm rupture, although it does appear that suprarenal fixation may prevent graft migration and lower the risk of developing late endoleaks. Follow-up data of at least 5 years will be required to provide support for their ongoing and widespread use. Currently, each center performing these procedures will select an appropriate graft, depending on their individual experience and based on the patient's aortic anatomy.

CONCLUSION

Endovascular aortic aneurysm repair is a procedure under trial. Only intermediate-term follow-up is available to date. As with most unproved technologies, there has been an early selection bias to offer this treatment to high-risk patients. Despite this apparent disadvantage, procedural success (patient survival with a patent graft and continued aneurysm exclusion) is equivalent to or slightly less than the gold standard treatment of "open" surgery. Current limitations of the technology preclude its use for patients without an adequate length of proximal and distal aneurysm neck or patients with an aneurysm that traverses a major visceral artery. However, most other aneurysm configurations can be considered for endovascular repair, and the procedure may be preferable in cases of complicated aortic dissection. As the worldwide volume of endovascular repairs increases, its role will become better defined by studies that assess cost efficacy and quality of life, compared with open surgery. Present data suggest an endovascular advantage. Late-term data on device durability are now required, since the long-term performance of an unsutured graft in aneurysmal aorta is not known.

REFERENCES

1. Dubost C, Allary M, Oeconomos N. Resection of an aneurysm of the abdominal aorta: re-establishment of the continuity by a preserved human arterial graft, with results after 5 months. *Arch Surg* 1952;64:405–408.
2. Katz DJ, Stanley JC, Zeloneck GB. Operative mortality rates for intact and ruptured abdominal aortic aneurysms in Michigan: an eleven-year statewide experience. *J Vasc Surg* 1994;19: 804–817.
3. Ernst CB. Abdominal aortic aneurysm. *N Engl J Med* 1993;328: 1167–1172.
4. Katz DJ, Stanley JC, Zelenock GB. Abdominal aortic aneurysm

surgery: statewide variations in prevalence and operative mortality. In: Veith FJ, ed. *Current critical problems in vascular surgery,* vol 7. St. Louis: Quality Medical Publishing, 1996:150–159.

5. Dotter CT. Transluminally placed coil spring endarterial tube grafts: long term patency in canine popliteal artery. *Invest Radiol* 1969;4:329–332.

6. Ferguson JM, Stonebridge PA. Endovascular surgery. *J R Coll Surg Edinb* 1996;41:223–231.

7. Parodi JC, Palmaz JC, Barone HD. Transfemoral intraluminal graft implantation for abdominal aortic aneurysm. *Ann Vasc Surg* 1991;5:491–499.

8. Ad Hoc Committee for Standardized Reporting Practices in Vascular Surgery of the Society for Vascular Surgery/International Society for Cardiovascular Surgery. Reporting standards for infrarenal endovascular abdominal aortic aneurysm repair. *J Vasc Surg* 1997;25:405–410.

9. Ohki T, Veith FJ, Sanchez LA, et al. Varying strategies and devices for endovascular repair of abdominal aortic aneurysms. *Semin Vasc Surg* 1997;10:242–256.

10. Blum U, Voshage G, Lammer J, et al. Endoluminal stent-grafts for infrarenal abdominal aortic aneurysms. *N Engl J Med* 1997; 336:13–20.

11. May J, White GH, Yu W, et al. Concurrent comparison of endoluminal versus open repair in the treatment of abdominal aortic aneurysms: analysis of 303 patients by life table method. *J Vasc Surg* 1998;27:213–221.

12. Zarins CK, White RA, Schwarten D, et. al. AneuRx stent graft versus open surgical repair of abdominal aortic aneurysms: multicenter prospective clinical trial. *J Vasc Surg* 1999;29:292–308.

13. Johnston KW. Ruptured abdominal aortic aneurysm: six-year follow-up results of a multicenter prospective study. *J Vasc Surg* 1994;19:888–900.

14. UK Small Aneurysm Trial participants. Mortality results for randomized controlled trial of early elective surgery or ultrasonographic surveillance for small abdominal aortic aneurysms. *Lancet* 1998;352:1649–1655.

15. Katz DJ, Stanley JC, Zelenock JB. et al. Operative mortality rates for intact and ruptured abdominal aortic aneurysms in Michigan: an eleven-year statewide experience. *J Vasc Surg* 1994;19:804–817.

16. First report on the registry for endovascular treatment of aneurysms (RETA), prepared by the Joint Working Party of the Vascular Surgical Society of Great Britain and Ireland and the British Society of Interventional Radiologists.

17. May J, White GH, Yu W, et al. Conversion from endoluminal to open repair of abdominal aortic aneurysms: a hazardous procedure. *Eur J Vasc Endovasc Surg* 1997;14:4–11.

18. May J, White GH, Waugh R, et al. Adverse effects after endoluminal repair of abdominal aortic aneurysms: a comparison during two successive periods of time. *J Vasc Surg* 1999;29:32–39.

19. Johnston KW. Multicenter prospective study of nonruptured abdominal aortic aneurysm. Part II. Variables predicting morbidity and mortality. *J Vasc Surg* 1989;9:437–447.

20. Johnston KW. Life expectancy after surgical repair of nonruptured abdominal aortic aneurysm. In: Greenhalgh RM, ed. *The durability of vascular and endovascular surgery.* Philadelphia: WB Saunders, 1999:135–147.

21. White GH, Yu W, May J. "Endoleak:" a proposed new terminology to describe incomplete aneurysm exclusion by an endoluminal graft. *J Endovasc Surg* 1996;3:124–125.

22. White GH, Yu W, May J, et al. Endoleak as a complication of endoluminal grafting of abdominal aortic aneurysms: classification, incidence, diagnosis and management. *J Endovasc Surg* 1997;4:152–168.

23. White GH, May J, Waugh RC, et al. Type I and type II endoleaks: a more useful classification for reporting results of endoluminal AAA repair. *J Endovasc Surg* 1998;5:189–191.

24. White GH, May J, Petrasek P, et al. Type III and type IV endoleak: toward a complete definition of blood flow in the sac after endoluminal repair of AAA. *J Endovasc Surg* 1998;5: 305–309.

25. Raithel D, Heilberger P, Ritter W, et al. Secondary endoleaks after endovascular aortic reconstruction. *J Endovasc Surg* 1998;5: 126–127.

26. Lumsden AB, Allen RC, Chaikof EL, et al. Delayed rupture of aortic aneurysms following endovascular stent grafting. *Am J Surg* 1995;170;174–178.

27. White GH, Yu W, May J, et al. Three-year experience with the White-Yu endovascular GAD graft for transluminal repair of aortic and iliac aneurysms. *J Endovasc Surg* 1997;4:124–136.

28. Alimi YS, Chakfe N, Rivoal E, et al. Rupture of an abdominal aortic aneurysm after endovascular graft placement and aneurysm size reduction. *J Vasc Surg* 1998;28:178–183.

29. Zarins CK, White RA, Fogarty TJ. Aneurysm rupture after endovascular repair using the AneuRx stent graft. *J Vasc Surg* 2000;31:960–970.

30. Politz JK, Newman VS, Stewart MT. Late abdominal aortic aneurysm rupture after AneuRx repair: a report of three cases. *J Vasc Surg* 2000;31:599–606.

31. Malina M, Lanne T, Ivancev K, et al. Reduced pulsatile wall motion of abdominal aortic aneurysms after endovascular repair. *J Vasc Surg* 1998;27:624–631.

32. Broeders IA, Blankensteijn JD, Gvakharia A, et al. The efficacy of transfemoral endovascular aneurysm management: a study on size changes of the abdominal aorta during mid-term follow-up. *Eur J Vasc Endovasc Surg* 1997;14:84–90.

33. Matsumara JS, Pearce WH, McCarthy WJ, et al. Reduction in aortic aneurysm size: early results after endovascular graft placement. *J Vasc Surg* 1997;25:113–123.

34. May J, White GH, Yu W, et al. A prospective study of anatomico-pathological changes in abdominal aortic aneurysms following endoluminal repair: Is the aneurysmal process reversed? *Eur J Vasc Endovasc Surg* 1996;12:11–17.

35. Resch T, Ivancev K, Lindh M, et al. Persistent collateral perfusion of abdominal aortic aneurysm after endovascular repair does not lead to progressive change in aneurysm diameter. *J Vasc Surg* 1998;28:242–249.

36. Gilling-Smith G, Brennan J, Harris PL, et al. Endotension after endovascular aneurysm repair: definition, classification and implications for surveillance and intervention. *J Endovasc Surg* 1999;6:305–307.

37. White GH, May J, Waugh RC, et al. Endotension: an explanation for continued aneurysm growth after successful endoluminal repair. *J Endovasc Surg* 1999;6:308–315.

38. Schurink GWH, van Baalen JM, Visser MJT, et al. Thrombus within an aortic aneurysm does not reduce pressure on the aneurysmal wall. *J Vasc Surg* 2000;31:501–506.

39. Broeders IAMJ, Blankensteijn JD, Gvakharia A, et al. The efficacy of transfemoral endovascular aneurysm management: a study on size changes of the abdominal aorta during mid-term follow-up. *Eur J Vasc Endovasc Surg* 1997;14:84–90.

40. Matsumara JS, Pearce WH, McCarthy WJ, et al. Reduction in aortic aneurysm size: early results after endovascular graft placement. *J Vasc Surg* 1997;25:113–123.

41. May J, White GH, Yu W, et al. A prospective study of anatomico-pathological changes in abdominal aortic aneurysms following endoluminal repair: Is the aneurysmal process reversed? *Eur J Vasc Endovasc Surg* 1996;12:11–17.

42. Malina M, Ivancev K, Chuter TAM, et al. Changing aneurysmal morphology after endovascular grafting: relation to leakage or persistent perfusion. *J Endovasc Surg* 1997;4:23–30.

43. Hallett JW, Marshall DM, Petterson RM, et al. Graft-related complications after abdominal aortic aneurysm repair: reassur-

ance from a 36-year population-based experience. *J Vasc Surg* 1997;25:277–286.

44. Harris P, Brennan J, Martin J, et al. Longitudinal aneurysm shrinkage following endovascular aortic aneurysm repair is a source of intermediate and late complications. *J Endovasc Surg* 1999;6:11–16.

45. White GH, May J, Waugh R, et al. Shortening of endografts during the deployment phase in endovascular repair of AAA. *J Endovasc Surg* 1999;6:4–10.

46. Umscheid T, Stelter WJ. Time related alterations of shape, position and structure in self-expanding modular stent grafts for treatment of AAA. *J Endovasc Surg* 1999;6:17–32.

47. Resch T, Ivancev K, Brunkwall J, et al. Distal migration of stent-grafts after endovascular repair of abdominal aortic aneurysms. *J Vasc Intervent Radiol* 1999;10:257–264.

48. May J, White GH, Yu W, et al. Conversion from endoluminal to open repair of abdominal aortic aneurysms: a hazardous procedure. *Eur J Vasc Endovasc Surg* 1997;14:4–11.

49. Holzenbein J, Kretschmer G, Glanzl R, et al. Endovascular AAA treatment: expensive prestige or economic alternative? *Eur J Vasc Endovasc Surg* 1997;14:265–272.

50. Quinones-Baldrich WJ. Achieving cost-effective endoluminal aneurysm repair. *Semin Vasc Surg* 1999;12:220–225.

Catheter Based Devices: For the Treatment of Non-coronary Cardiovascular Diseases in Adults and Children. Edited by P. Syamasundar Rao and Morton J. Kern, Lippincott Williams & Wilkins, Philadelphia © 2003.

43

BIODEGRADABLE STENTS: PROSPECTS FOR THE FUTURE

TAKAFUMI TSUJI
KEIJI IGAKI
HIDEO TAMAI

Coronary stenting has become an established mode of treatment in percutaneous transluminal coronary angioplasty (PTCA), having been shown to reduce late restenosis relative to conventional balloon angioplasty (1,2). Nevertheless, many concerns about stents must be addressed regarding long-term safety. Because all the currently available stents are metallic, they induce varying degrees of thrombogenesis and intimal hyperplasia. Moreover, the long-term effects of metallic stents in human coronary arteries are still unknown.

The important roles of stents are to stabilize the intimal dissections that might be induced by PTCA and to inhibit late restenosis. Intimal dissections that are tacked back in place are likely to heal rapidly, and restenosis commonly occurs within several months of coronary intervention, but only rarely thereafter (3,4). Therefore the clinical need for stents is limited to the first 12 months following angioplasty (5). Consequently, stents made of biodegradable materials may be an ideal alternative to metallic stents, fulfilling the short-term function and avoiding the potential for long-term complications.

In the early 1980s, Stack, Clark and their associates at Duke University developed the first biodegradable stent (5,6). They investigated a number of biodegradable polymers and selected poly-L-lactic acid (PLLA) as the stent material. The stent was constructed of a specialized PLLA polymer woven into a diamond-braided pattern from eight polymeric strands. Eleven PLLA stents sterilized with ethylene oxide were deployed in the canine femoral artery. Animals were sacrificed at intervals ranging from 2 hours to 18

months following deployment, and the femoral arteries were examined histologically. Each vessel was patent at follow-up, except for one that occluded at 48 hours following a traumatic implantation. Little thrombotic and minimal neointimal responses were observed, both in the short term and at 18 months after stent deployment. Bier et al. also developed a biodegradable self-expanding tubular stent constructed of type I collagen (7). Examination *in vitro* revealed the morphometric and hemodynamic compatibility of these stents in porcine arteries. Landau and his group investigated microporous biodegradable polymer stents constructed of PLLA and poly-epsilon-caprolactone (PCL) (8). They loaded recombinant adenovirus vectors into the stents and deployed them in the rabbit carotid artery. Gene transfer and expression were successfully demonstrated. Tamai et al. developed a biodegradable PLLA knitted-type stent in 1994 that was first implanted in canine femoral arteries in 1995 and in porcine coronary arteries in 1996. In 1997 the PLLA stent was modified from a knitted design to a coil design. From our animal study the PLLA coil stent reduced the percent diameter stenosis at 2 weeks from 64% to 19%, in the porcine coronary artery, compared with the PLLA knitted-type stent (9). Histologic examination at 6 weeks revealed that minimal neointimal hyperplasia was found in the PLLA coil stents with minimal vessel wall injury, whereas moderate to severe neointimal hyperplasia was observed in knitted PLLA stents because of deeper vessel wall injury on implantation due to the uneven thickness of the stent struts.

The performance of the PLLA coil stent in the porcine coronary artery was compared with that of the metallic stent (10). Of 15 normocholesterolemic juvenile domestic farm pigs, six received 14 PLLA coil stents, and nine received nine Palmaz-Schatz (P-S) half-stents (Cordis, Warren, NJ). Stents were mounted on delivery catheters of 3.0 mm diameter and were implanted percutaneously into the coronary arteries. Coronary angiography was performed before and immedi-

Takafumi Tsuji: Interventional Cardiologist, Department of Cardiology, Shiga Medical Center for Adults, Moriyama, Shiga, Japan

Keiji Igaki: President, Igaki Medical Planning Company, Limited, Yamashina-ku, Kyoto, Japan

Hideo Tamai: Managing Director, Department of Cardiology, Shiga Medical Center for Adults, Moriyama, Shiga, Japan

ately after stenting and at 2 and 6 weeks in five PLLA pigs and nine P-S pigs. Histologic studies were performed with haematoxylin-eosin and van Gieson's staining in the PLLA pigs: two pigs at 2 weeks (five stents), three pigs at 6 weeks (seven stents), and one pig at 16 weeks (two stents). Sections at the center of each stent were examined for vessel injury and neointimal hyperplasia. The vessel injury score, neointimal thickness, and neointimal area were assessed according to the method of Schwartz et al. (11). Delivery and positioning of the stents were successfully performed in all cases. No acute or subacute thrombotic occlusion was detected in any cases. There was neither coronary obstruction nor restenosis during the follow-up period. Although the percent diameter stenosis tended to be higher in the PLLA group than in the P-S group (23.8 ± 14.4 versus 13.7 ± 6.3%, respectively; $p = .065$) at 2 weeks, there was no significant difference in minimal lumen diameter (MLD) between the two groups at 2 weeks (2.19 ± 0.51 versus 2.27 ± 0.31 mm; $p = .68$) or at 6 weeks (2.18 ± 0.84 versus 2.30 ± 0.58 mm; $p = .82$). The neointimal hyperplasia progressed over 6 weeks and no further proliferation was observed thereafter. Histologic findings with haematoxylin-eosin staining revealed no severe inflammation, foreign-body response, or thrombus formation surrounding the stent struts. Minimal neointima formation and complete coverage of the PLLA stent struts were noted. A tendency to proportionality between the mean neointimal thickness and the mean injury score was observed. This tendency seemed to be comparable to that seen in the scatter plot of mean neointimal thickness versus mean injury score for 26 coronary artery segments injured by tantalum coils presented by Schwartz and colleagues.

DEVICE

The Igaki-Tamai stent (Igaki Medical Planning Co. Ltd., Kyoto, Japan) is made of PLLA monofilament (molecular mass 183 kD) with a zigzag helical coil design (Figure 43.1). The stent is designed to be self-expandable and to reduce vessel wall injury in comparison with the previous model. The thickness of the stent strut is 0.017 mm (0.007 inch), and the stent surface area is 24% of the vessel area. The stent is 12 mm in length with two radiopaque gold markers at each end and is mounted on a correspondingly sized, manufacturer-specified angioplasty balloon of 3.0, 3.5, or 4.0 mm in diameter. This stent is inserted into a covered-sheath system because of its self-expanding capability and requires at least an 8F guiding catheter for delivery.

PATIENT SELECTION

Clinical application commenced in September 1998 in the Shiga Medical Center for Adults. The hospital ethics committee approved the protocol for the Igaki-Tamai stent implantation in humans, and written informed consent, according to the Helsinki Declaration, was obtained from all patients before stent implantation.

STENT IMPLANTATION TECHNIQUE

Eighty-four stents were implanted in 63 lesions in 50 patients. All stent implantations were for elective indications. All patients received 10,000 U of intravenous heparin at the beginning of the procedure. Before stent implantation, the lesions were dilated by optimally sized balloons, or debulked by directional coronary atherectomy (DCA) ($N = 14$) or rotational atherectomy (ROTA) ($N = 2$), as needed. After the pretreatment, the balloon catheter was exchanged for the stent delivery system over a 0.014-inch (0.036-cm) guide wire. The diameter of the stent was chosen, visually, to be 10% to 20% greater than the reference vessel diameter. Multiple stenting was performed, depending on the lesion length, so as to cover the entire lesion. Although this stent is self-expanding, its implantation requires balloon expansion with a heated dye because the PLLA stent requires 13 seconds to

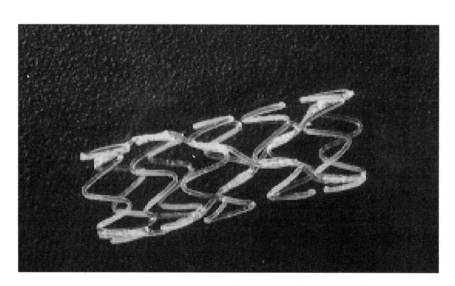

FIGURE 43.1. The Igaki-Tamai stent is a self-expanding biodegradable stent made of PLLA monopolymer.

expand by itself at 50°C, but 20 minutes at 37°C. While the duration of balloon inflation is kept to less than 30 seconds, in order to minimize vessel injury by heating, inflation is repeated until equilibrium is attained between the circumferential elastic resistance of the arterial wall and the dilating force of the PLLA stent. The maximal inflation pressure used was 11.2 ± 1.4 atm. According to local practice, intravenous heparin (15,000 U/day) was continued postoperatively for 3 days. In addition, oral aspirin (81 mg/day) and ticlopidine (200 mg/day) were administered for more than 1 month after implantation. Coronary angiography and intracoronary ultrasound (IVUS) were performed before and immediately after the procedure. Additional assessment by quantitative coronary angiography (QCA) (CMS; Medical Imaging Systems, Nuenen, The Netherlands) and intracoronary ultrasound was performed 1 day, 3 months, and 6 months after the procedure. Continuous variables are expressed as the mean $\pm$ standard deviation. Univariate analysis was performed using the paired t-test for continuous variables. A p value of less than .05 was considered significant.

RESULTS

Baseline clinical characteristics of the 50 patients are shown in Table 43.1. The mean age of the patients was 61 ± 11 years; 44 patients (88%) were men. Twenty-two patients (22%) had a previous myocardial infarction. Nineteen patients (38%) had Canadian Cardiovascular Society class 3 or 4 angina. Table 43.2 shows baseline angiographic characteristics of lesions and procedural variables. The treated vessel was the left anterior descending artery in 28 cases (44%), the left circumflex in 19 cases (30%), and the right coronary artery in 16 cases (25%). All target lesions were American Heart Association/American College of Cardiology type B or C. The mean lesion length was 13.5 ± 5.7 mm. A single stent was implanted in 45 lesions (71%); double stents, in 15 lesions (24%); and triple stents, in three lesions (5%). Debulking before stenting was performed in

TABLE 43.1. BASELINE CLINICAL CHARACTERISTICS OF THE 50 PATIENTS

Variables	No. (%)
Age (years)	61 ± 11
Males	44 (88%)
Previous infarction	22 (44%)
Diabetes	16 (32%)
Hyperlipidemia	18 (36%)
Hypertension	24 (48%)
Current smoker	27 (54%)
Angina	
CCS I	17 (34%)
CCS II	14 (28%)
CCS III	12 (24%)
CCS IV	7 (14%)

Data presented are the mean value ± SD or the number (%) of patients.
CCS, Canadian Cardiovascular Society.

TABLE 43.2. BASELINE ANGIOGRAPHIC CHARACTERISTICS AND PROCEDURAL VARIABLES OF THE 63 LESIONS

Variables	No. (%)
Lesion site	
LAD	28 (44%)
LCX	19 (30%)
RCA	16 (25%)
AHA/ACC lesion type	
A	0
B1	16 (25%)
B2	36 (57%)
C	11 (17%)
Lesion length (mm)	13.5 ± 5.7
No. of stents/lesion	
1 stent	45 (71%)
2 stents	15 (24%)
3 stents	3 (5%)
Stent size (mm)	
3.0	10 (12%)
3.5	52 (62%)
4.0	22 (26%)
Maximal inflation pressure (atm)	11.2 ± 1.4
Debulking prior stenting	
DCA	14 (22%)
Rotablater (Heart Technology, Bellevue, WA)	2 (3%)

Data presented are the mean value ± SD or the number (%) of lesions.
AHA/ACC, American Heart Association/American College of Cardiology; DCA, directional coronary athelectomy; LAD, left anterior descending coronary artery; LCX, left circumflex coronary artery; RCA, right coronary artery.

14 lesions (22%) with DCA and two lesions (3%) with ROTA. All stents were successfully delivered, and angiographic success was achieved in all procedures. Table 43.3 lists the in-hospital complications. There were no deaths, nor were any emergency coronary arterial grafting surgical procedures required during hospitalization. One patient with inadequate anticoagulation and antiplatelet therapy because of gastrorrhagia after the procedure had subacute stent thrombosis with Q-wave myocardial infarction at day 5 and underwent successful emergency PTCA.

Table 43.4 shows the results of QCA. The mean reference vessel diameter was 2.95 ± 0.34 mm before procedure.

TABLE 43.3. IN-HOSPITAL COMPLICATIONS OF THE 50 PATIENTS

Variables	No. (%)
Death	0
Q-wave myocardial infarction	1 (2%)*
Emergency CABG	0
Emergency PTCA	1 (2%)*
Subacute stent thrombosis	1 (2%)*
Bleeding	0

Data presented are the number (%) of patients.
*Same patient.
CABG, coronary artery bypass graft surgery; PTCA, percutaneous transluminal coronary angioplasty.

TABLE 43.4. INTERIM QUANTITATIVE CORONARY ANGIOGRAPHIC DATA

	Before Procedure	After Procedure	1 Day	3 Months	6 Months
No.	63	63	63	19	18
RD (mm)	2.95 ± 0.46	3.04 ± 0.44	3.09 ± 0.48	2.75 ± 0.49	2.69 ± 0.49
MLD (mm)	0.91 ± 0.39	2.68 ± 0.43	2.70 ± 0.46	1.88 ± 0.59	1.84 ± 0.66
DS (%)	69 ± 13	12 ± 8	12 ± 10	33 ± 14	33 ± 18
Loss index				0.44 ± 0.30	0.48 ± 0.32

Data presented are mean value ± SD.
DS, diameter stenosis; MLD, minimal lumen diameter; RD, reference diameter.
The data at 3 months and 6 months are reprinted from Tamai H, Igaki K, Kyo E, et al. Initial and 6-month results of biodegradable poly-L-lactic acid coronary stents in humans. *Circulation* 2000;102:399–404, with permission.

TABLE 43.5. RESULTS OF QUANTITATIVE INTRAVASCULAR ULTRASOUND ANALYSIS

	After Stenting	1 Day After Stenting	3-Month Follow-Up	6-Month Follow-Up
Number	19	19	18	18
Stent cross-section area (mm^2)	7.42 ± 1.51	7.37 ± 1.44	8.18 ± 2.42*	8.13 ± 2.52*
Neointimal area (mm^2)			2.51 ± 0.94	2.50 ± 0.65
Lumen cross-section area (mm^2)	7.42 ± 1.51	7.37 ± 1.44	5.67 ± 2.42†	5.63 ± 2.70‡

*$p < 0.1$ vs after stenting.
†$p < 0.005$ vs after stenting.
‡$p < 0.001$ after stenting.
From Tamai H, Igaki K, Kyo E, et al. Initial and 6-month results of biodegradable poly-L-lactic acid coronary stents in humans. *Circulation* 2000;102:399–404, with permission.

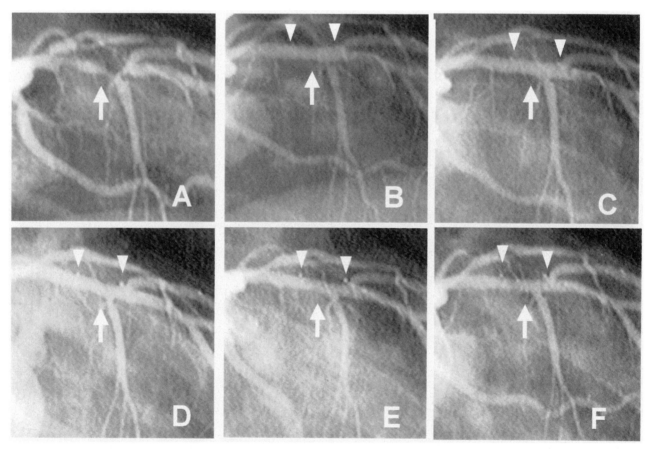

FIGURE 43.2. Serial coronary angiograms of a representative case are shown. The *arrow* shows the stented lesion and *triangles* show the gold-markers at either end of the stent. The percent diameter stenosis was 90% before the procedure (**A**), 7% after the procedure (**B**), 6% at 1 day (**C**), 12% at 3 months (**D**), 13% at 6 months (**E**), and 16% at 12 months (**F**).

The percent diameter stenosis decreased from 69% before stenting to 12% after stenting. The MLD increased from 0.91 mm before stenting to 2.68 mm after stenting. At 1-day angiographic follow-up, the percent diameter stenosis was 12% and the minimal lumen diameter was 2.70 mm. One-day angiographic follow-up revealed no further recoil of the stented segment immediately after stenting.

At present, 6-month follow-up angiography and IVUS have been performed in 15 patients with a total of 19 lesions (12). Only one patient underwent repeat PTCA (two lesions successfully dilated). Follow-up coronary angiograms suitable for QCA were obtained in all 15 patients within 6 months. The mean MLD at 3 months was 1.88 mm and the mean percent diameter stenosis was 33%. At 6 months, the mean MLD was 1.84 mm and the mean percent diameter stenosis was 33%. The angiographic restenosis rate per lesion was 10.5% (two of 19) and that per patient was 6.7% (one of 15) at 3 months. The 3-month target lesion revascularization (TLR) rate per lesion was 5.3% (one of 19), and the individual patient rate was 6.7% (one of 15). At 6 months, both angiographic restenosis rate and TLR rate per lesion were 10.5% (two of 19) and those per patient were 6.7% (one of 15). Finally, the loss index (defined as late loss divided by initial gain) was 0.44 at 3 months and 0.48 at 6 months.

The 3-month IVUS record of one nonrestenotic lesion was missing. One restenotic lesion was treated by repeat angioplasty at 3 months and was unavailable for the analysis at 6 months. Therefore IVUS imaging was analyzed in 18 lesions at 3 months and in 18 lesions at 6 months. IVUS showed the presence of stent struts at 6 months. The mean stent cross-sectional area (CSA) tended to be larger both at 3 months and at 6 months than after stenting (8.18 mm^2 and 8.13 mm^2 versus 7.42 mm^2, $p = .086$ and $.091$) with mild neointimal hyperplasia. The mean stent CSA was similar at 3 months and 6 months (8.18 mm^2 versus 8.13 mm^2, $p = .30$). This difference suggests that the Igaki-Tamai stent continues to expand for at least 3 months. Lumen CSA was similar at 3 months and 6 months (5.67 mm^2 versus 5.63 mm^2, $p = .15$), and the neointimal area was also similar (2.51 mm^2 versus 2.50 mm^2, $p = .65$) (Table 43.5). This result may imply that the Igaki-Tamai stent does not significantly stimulate intimal hyperplasia within the stent between 3 months and 6 months after the procedure.

Figure 43.2 shows the serial coronary angiograms of a representative case. The percent diameter stenosis was 7% immediately after stenting, 6% 1 day after stenting, 12% at 3 months, 13% at 6 months, and 16% at 12 months. Figure 43.3 shows serial IVUS findings of the same case. The stent

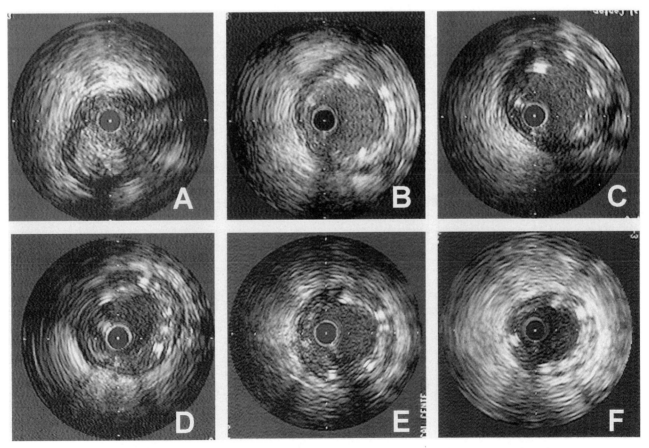

FIGURE 43.3. Serial IVUS findings of the same case are shown. Severe plaque exists before the procedure (**A**). Stent cross-sectional area is 9.40 mm^2 immediately after stenting (**B**), 8.71 mm^2 at 1 day (**C**), 8.04 mm^2 at 3 months (**D**), 8.59 mm^2 at 6 months (**E**), and 8.04 mm^2 at 12 months (**F**).

cross-sectional area was 9.40 mm² immediately after stenting, 8.71 mm² 1 day after stenting, 8.04 mm² at 3 months, 8.59 mm² at 6 months, and 8.19 mm² at 12 months.

DISCUSSION

The biocompatibility of the polymer stent has been controversial. Zidar et al. reported minimal inflammatory reaction and minimal neointimal hyperplasia with the use of PLLA stents in canine femoral arteries (5). However, van der Giessen et al. reported a marked inflammatory response associated with a thick layer containing a fibrocellular component, following polymer stent implantation in a porcine coronary model (13). Lincoff et al. suggested the biocompatibility of high-molecular-weight PLLA in the porcine coronary model (14). Although thrombotic occlusion of polymeric stents has been reported in animal experiments (13,14), Zidar et al. reported reduced platelet adherence and reduced thrombogenicity of the PLLA stent compared with slotted-tube stainless steel metallic stents *in vitro* (5). This property may be one advantage of PLLA stents for clinical usage. PLLA has been used for orthopedic applications in humans and has generally been found to be biocompatible for at least the first few weeks or months after implantation (15–17).

Vessel wall injury caused by neointimal proliferation (18) and the severity of vessel injury are strongly correlated with neointimal thickness and percent diameter stenosis after either balloon angioplasty (19) or stenting (20). No significant difference in neointimal hyperplasia was found between the PLLA coil stents and nine P-S half-stents in nine pigs. PLLA coil stents also demonstrated admirable biocompatibility, with minimal inflammatory response in porcine coronary arteries after 16 weeks (10).

The degradation time of stents is also important. Many factors may affect the biodegradation period, including the type of biodegradable material and its molecular weight, and perhaps biologic conditions, including body temperature and the water content of the tissue and enzymes of the coronary artery. The scaffolding strength of biodegradable stents is reduced as the degradation proceeds. To reduce restenosis in humans, stents must maintain their scaffolding strength for longer than 6 months to overcome late vessel remodeling (21–23). According to the IVUS analysis at follow-up, the PLLA stents used in the present study appeared to maintain their scaffolding property at 6 months. It was impossible to identify signs of biodegradation, but in the IVUS analysis of our human study some of the stent struts appeared to be degraded after 12 months. Long-term follow-up using IVUS is scheduled to clarify the lifetime of the Igaki-Tamai stent in human coronary arteries.

Biodegradable stents can also be useful for the local administration of pharmacologic agents directly to the site of PTCA to prevent late restenosis. Yamawaki et al. loaded a specific tyrosine kinase inhibitor (ST638) into knitted-type Igaki-Tamai stents and implanted them in porcine coronary arteries (24). Drug-loaded PLLA stents gradually released ST638 until day 21 in the porcine coronary artery and significantly reduced neointimal hyperplasia. This study demonstrates the effectiveness of PLLA stents as a local drug delivery system.

CURRENT STATUS

The 12-month clinical and angiographic follow-up of 50 patients enrolled in Igaki-Tamai stent implantation is ongoing. Currently, the Igaki-Tamai stent is available in a few hospitals where the hospital ethics committee approved this stent. In future, a multicenter registry and randomized trial will be undertaken to evaluate the efficacy of the Igaki-Tamai stent.

THE FUTURE: POTENTIAL APPLICATIONS IN PEDIATRIC CARDIOLOGY

Stents are also used in the treatment of peripheral vascular disease and are proving to be ideal endoprostheses in adults. As the transcatheter interventions have been extended for the treatment of congenital and acquired stenotic lesions in children, the clinical needs for stents in pediatric cardiology are increased because of elastic recoil and dissections of the vessel following balloon angioplasty (25,26). However, the most important problem of stent implantation in the growing child is that the stents do not grow with the vessel growth. The Igaki-Tamai stent may overcome such problems because it is self-expanding and biodegradable. The Igaki-Tamai stent can expand as the vessel grows and can be biodegraded within 18 to 24 months. The larger stent can be implanted thereafter, if necessary.

CONCLUSION

This biodegradable, self-expanding stent, made of high-molecular-weight PLLA monopolymer, has been studied in human coronary arteries, yielding promising initial and 6-month results. If the restenosis rate is found to be comparable with metallic stents, PLLA stents will be an attractive alternative to the former and may serve as a vehicle for local drug administration. Long-term follow-up with larger numbers of patients will be required to validate the long-term efficacy of the PLLA stent, and a randomized, comparative study including metallic stents may highlight the advantages of PLLA stents.

REFERENCES

1. Fischman DL, Leon MB, Baim DS, et al. A randomized comparison of coronary-stent placement and balloon angioplasty in the treatment of coronary artery disease. *N Engl J Med* 1994;331:496–501.
2. Serruys PW, de Jaegere P, Kiemeneij F, et al. A comparison of balloon-expandable stent implantation with balloon angioplasty in patients with coronary artery disease. *N Engl J Med* 1994;331:489–495.
3. McBride W, Lange RA, Hills DL. Restenosis after successful coronary angioplasty: pathology and prevention. *N Engl J Med* 1988;318:1734.
4. Holmes DR Jr, Vliestra RE, Smith HC, et al. Restenosis after percutaneous transluminal coronary angioplasty (PTCA): a report from the PTCA registry of National Heart, Lung, and Blood Institute. *Am J Cardiol* 1984;53:77C.
5. Zidar J, Lincoff A, Stack R. Biodegradable stents. In: Topol EJ, ed. *Textbook of interventional cardiology,* 2nd ed. Philadelphia: WB Saunders, 1994:787–802.
6. Stack RS, Califf RM, Phillips HR III, et al. Interventional cardiac catheterization at Duke Medical Center: new interventional technology. *Am J Cardiol* 1988;2(Suppl F):3F–24F.
7. Bier JD, Zalesky P, Li ST, et al. A new bioabsorbable intravascular stent: *in vitro* assessment of hemodynamic and morphometric characteristics. *J Interv Cardiol* 1992;5:187–194.
8. Ye YW, Landau C, Willard JE, et al. Bioresorbable microporous stents deliver recombinant adenovirus gene transfer vectors to the arterial wall. *Ann Biomed Eng* 1998;26:398–408.
9. Tsuji T, Tamai H, Kyo E, et al. The effect of PLLA stent design on neointimal hyperplasia (in Japanese). *J Cardiol* 1998;32:235A (abst).
10. Tamai H, Igaki K, Tsuji T, et al. A biodegradable poly-L-lactic acid coronary stent in porcine coronary artery. *J Interv Cardiol* 1999;12:443–450.
11. Schwartz RS, Huber KC, Murphy JG, et al. Restenosis and the proportional response to coronary artery injury: results in a porcine model. *J Am Coll Cardiol* 1992;19:267–274.
12. Tamai H, Igaki K, Kyo E, et al. Initial and 6-month results of biodegradable poly-L-lactic acid coronary stents in humans. *Circulation* 2000;102:399–404.
13. Van der Giessen WJ, Lincoff AM, Schwartz RS, et al. Marked inflammatory sequelae to implantation of biodegradable and nonbiodegradable polymers in porcine coronary artery. *Circulation* 1996;94:1690–1697.
14. Lincoff AM, Furst JG, Ellis SG, et al. Sustained local delivery of dexamethasone by a novel intravascular eluting stent to prevent restenosis in the porcine coronary injury model. *J Am Coll Cardiol* 1997;29:808–816.
15. Schkenraad JM, Oosterbaan P, Nieuwenhuis P. Biodegradable hollow fibers for the controlled release of drugs. *Biomaterials* 1988;9:116–120.
16. Bos RRM, Boering G, Rozema FR, et al. Resorbable poly (L-lactide) plates and screws for the fixation of zygomatic fractures. *J Oral Maxillofac Surg* 1987;45:751–753.
17. Suganuma J, Alexander H. Biological response of intramedullary bone to poly-L-lactic acid. *J Appl Biomat* 1993;4:13–27.
18. Schwartz RS, Huber KC, Murphy JG, et al. Restenosis and the proportional response to coronary artery injury: Results in a porcine model. *J Am Coll Cardiol* 1992;19:267–274.
19. Karas SP, Gravanis MB, Santoian EC, et al. Coronary intimal proliferation after balloon injury and stenting in swine: an animal model of restenosis. *J Am Coll Cardiol* 1992;20:467–474.
20. Kornowski R, Hong MK, Tio FO, et al. In-stent restenosis: contributions of inflammatory responses and arterial injury to neointimal hyperplasia. *J Am Coll Cardiol* 1998;31:224–230.
21. Currier JW, Faxon DP. Restenosis after percutaneous transluminal coronary angioplasty: Have we been aiming at the wrong target? *J Am Coll Cardiol* 1995;25:516–520.
22. Minz GS, Popma JJ, Pichard AD, et al. Arterial remodeling after coronary angioplasty: a serial intravascular ultrasound study. *Circulation* 1996;94:35–43.
23. Lansky AJ, Mintz GS, Pompa JJ, et al. Remodeling after directional coronary atherectomy (with and without adjunct percutaneous transluminal coronary angioplasty): a serial angiographic and intravascular ultrasound analysis from the Optimal Atherectomy Restenosis Study. *J Am Coll Cardiol* 1998;32:329–337.
24. Yamawaki T, Shimokawa H, Kozai T, et al. Intramural delivery of a specific tyrosine kinase inhibitor with biodegradable stent suppresses the restenotic changes of the coronary artery in pigs *in vivo. J Am Coll Cardiol* 1998;32:780–786.
25. Rao PS. Interventional pediatric cardiology: state of the art and future directions. *Pediatr Cardiol* 1998;19:107–124.
26. Benson L, Nykanen D. Interventional pediatric cardiology: an overview. In: Beyar R, Keren G, Leon MB, et al., eds. *Frontiers in interventional cardiology.* London: Martin Dunitz Ltd, 1997:409–432.

Catheter Based Devices: For the Treatment of Non-coronary Cardiovascular Diseases in Adults and Children. Edited by P. Syamasundar Rao and Morton J. Kern, Lippincott Williams & Wilkins, Philadelphia © 2003.

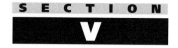

MISCELLANEOUS

44

COIL EMBOLIZATION THERAPY IN THE ADULT PATIENT

VENERANDO S. SEGURITAN[1]
ROBERT N. WOOD-MORRIS
MICHAEL D. EISENHAUER

In the last decade there has been much renewed interest in transcatheter vascular embolization, or embolotherapy. Nonetheless, it should be recognized that much of the current published literature consists only of anecdotal or individual case reports. There are almost no longitudinal follow-up studies, or randomized clinical trials comparing the different types of embolotherapy. Because of this, it remains difficult to identify the single most effective therapy for any individual patient. Certainly, in most cases multiple therapeutic options exist, whether with conventional surgery, radiotherapy, sclerotherapy, pharmacotherapy, or embolotherapy. All these techniques have proven safe in individual patients, but care must be taken to recognize operator skill and anticipate potential complications when planning these procedures.

The principle of embolotherapy dates back to 1904, when Dawbain described preoperative injection of melted paraffin-petrolatum into the external carotid arteries of patients suffering from head and neck tumors (1). In 1963, Baum and Nusbaum, in a landmark paper, demonstrated that bleeding at rates as low as 0.5 mL/min could be detected angiographically (2). This finding led directly to the increasing practice of transcatheter management of hemorrhage, which was first achieved with selective infusions of vasopressin. The explosion of interest in embolization therapy seen in the 1970s was fueled by parallel developments in catheter technology and embolic agents. The practice of embolizing autologous clot, skin, or muscle fragments quickly gave way to synthetic agents such as detachable balloons, gel foam particulates, silicone or stainless steel microspheres, methylmethacrylate, gelatinates, polyvinyl alcohol (Ivalon), and even direct tissue and vascular

ablation using transcatheter absolute alcohol injections or electrocoagulation.

COIL EMBOLIZATION

Coils are the most widely used mechanical agents for percutaneous transcatheter embolotherapy. Coil embolization has been described in almost every blood vessel and organ system (3). Although an in-depth discussion of coil embolotherapy for each and every indication is beyond the scope of this chapter; some general categories of use are presented and discussed.

In 1975, Gianturco and colleagues developed the steel coil, and demonstrated its utility in arterial occlusion (4). The coils are not intended to completely occlude the vessel primarily; instead, they are meant to induce thrombosis. To increase thrombogenicity, early coil designs were feathered with wool strands ("tails") to promote a local inflammatory response. Unfortunately, the wool proved to be too inflammatory, with the brisk host immune response resulting in severe arteritis and granulomatous intimal erosion in animal studies (5). As a result, wool strands were subsequently replaced by synthetic Dacron strands. Several modifications of this original coil design remain in use today.

The end result of coil embolization is similar to surgical ligation. However, if complete control of hemorrhage or complete organ infarction is desired, the combination of coil embolization with another, more peripherally occluding agent (such as gel foam) is recommended, as coiling alone does not impede distal flow resulting from collateral supply or venoarterial flow reversal. Alternatively, coil embolization should be performed on both sides of the bleeding site.

Venerando S. Seguritan: Director, Interventional Radiology, Department of Radiology, William Beaumont Army Medical Center, El Paso, Texas

Robert N. Wood-Morris: Resident, Internal Medicine, Department of Medicine, William Beaumont Army Medical Center, El Paso, Texas

Michael D. Eisenhauer: Assistant Professor of Medicine, Uniformed Services, Health Sciences University, Bethesda, Maryland; Chief, Cardiology Service, Department of Medicine, William Beaumont Army Medical Center, El Paso, Texas

[1]**Disclaimer:** The opinions or assertions contained herein reflect the views of the authors, and are not to be construed as official, or as representing the position of the United States Army Medical Department, the Department of Defense, or the United States Federal Government.

The principal indications for coil embolotherapy in the adult are obliteration of large arteriovenous fistulae or malformations, vessel occlusion after trauma, preoperative embolization of renal or other solid-organ tumors, obliteration of esophageal varices, or occlusion of systemic-pulmonary shunts (6).

TECHNIQUES FOR COIL DEPLOYMENT

Most coil designs are passive, in that they are merely "pushed" out of the guide catheter lumen by the use of any straight-tipped guide wire. Once deployed (even partially), these coils cannot be retrieved or repositioned reliably without the use of a snare or similar extraction device. Fortunately, newer detachable occlusion coils are available that have a controlled-release mechanism allowing for complete control and accurate positioning of the occlusive coil before release (7–12). Furthermore, these devices are completely removable and retractable, even after coil deployment or advancement beyond the end of the delivery catheter, providing for a margin of safety should imprecise positioning occur (Figure 44.1).

Although generally safe, several potential complications are noteworthy and have been reported (6,13). Many of these complications can be categorized as follows:

Coil deployment through a noncustomized or inappropriately sized delivery catheter. Minicoils are designed for insertion through a 5F polyethylene nontorquable catheter using a 0.035-inch guide wire as a pusher. If larger 6- or 7F catheters are used, the coils tend to buckle inside the larger lumen, allowing the pushing wire to prolapse past the coil, potentially wedging and locking the coil inside the delivery catheter. This can be particularly problematic if part of the coil is already extended beyond the distal tip of the delivery catheter, as dislodgment and imprecise embolization can occur with catheter withdrawal. Similarly, if the delivery catheter lumen is too small or has a tapered tip that encroaches on the minimal luminal dimensions required, the coil may become lodged within the catheter tip, preventing deployment. There is no substitute for an *in vitro* "dry run" of equipment before attempting this procedure.

Improper selection of coil size. A coil with an intrinsic diameter too small for the arterial lumen will not wedge into position effectively and could either migrate distally or be washed back with aggressive catheter flushes or catheter withdrawal from the target site. In general, the coil helical diameter should be at least one and a half to two times larger than the diameter of the target vessel to allow for appropriate folding and buckling of the deployed coil into a wedged position. A coil that is too large in diameter for the target vessel will remain elongated and not fold back on itself during deployment, and may be less effective in promoting a permanent vascular occlusion. Although immediate thrombosis commonly occurs, the relative degree of

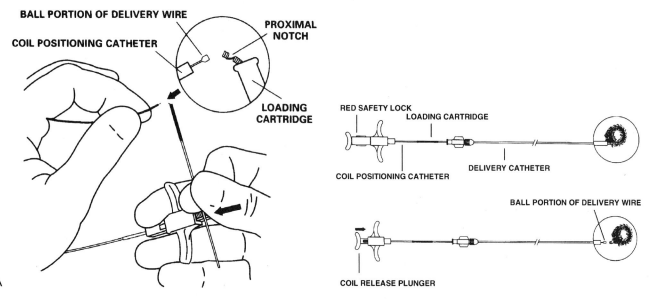

A   B

FIGURE 44.1. A: One example of several available detachable coils. Optimal positioning is easily obtained with the operator-controlled, safety-release mechanism of this device. After removing a safety lock, the coil release plunger must be depressed to expose the ball portion of the delivery wire for loading. After aligning the ball with the proximal notch in the coil, the plunger is released. The proximal coil segment is thereby retracted within the coil positioning catheter, and the safety lock is replaced. The loading cartridge is retained and guided into the proximal end of the delivery catheter. The coil is then advanced through the loading cartridge and delivery catheter by pushing the coil-positioning catheter forward. **B:** Coil deployment. Following definitive coil positioning, and after manually removing the safety lock, the coil release plunger is depressed. The action advances the ball portion of the delivery wire from the distal end of the coil positioning catheter, releasing the coil.

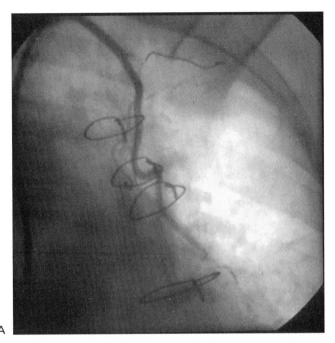

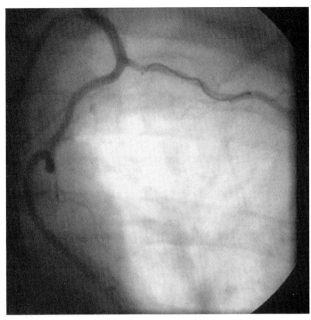

A

B

FIGURE 44.2. A: Angiogram demonstrating successful deployment of a 3-cm by 5-mm helical diameter coil in the side-branch of an internal mammary artery bypass graft to the left anterior descending coronary artery. The helical diameter of this coil was oversized, which prevented the desirable effect of coil folding or prolapse, resulting in an "elongated" coil position within the side branch. Thromboocclusion was immediate. **B:** Angiogram performed 6 months later, demonstrating partial recanalization of the side-branch despite the presence of the embolization coil, although the luminal diameter and contrast opacity are decreased. In this case, the deployment of multiple coils may have provided an additional "bulk effect" that may have promoted permanent vascular occlusion.

mechanical obstruction to flow remains minimal. With time, the extended coil may become endothelialized and vessel flow restored (Figure 44.2).

Inadequate number of coils deployed. Although thrombus formation may be rapid and vascular occlusion initially may appear complete, the principle of "bulk" in the obstructing coil entanglement remains important. The decision regarding the number of coils to be deployed at the target site remains with the operator and may be quite subjective. It seems intuitive that "more is better," in that the more mechanically complete the obstruction with a steel "plug," the less likely that any subsequent intrinsic fibrinolysis (that inevitably occurs as the vascular system attempts to remove thrombus and recanalize the vessel) will be successful at restoring distal flow (Figure 44.3).

Excessive number of coils deployed. Sometimes too many coils are inserted, resulting in "that last coil" that will not fully deploy within the target site, which extrudes back into the parent vessel. This may be particularly problematic if a bifurcation is present, as an unintended branch vessel may be unavoidably occluded. If the coil extrudes proximally into the aorta, it may become a recurrent nidus for thrombus formation that can embolize.

Improper coil placement. If the target vessel is tortuous, the delivery catheter must have enough support to prevent sudden delivery catheter recoil as the coil is expelled from

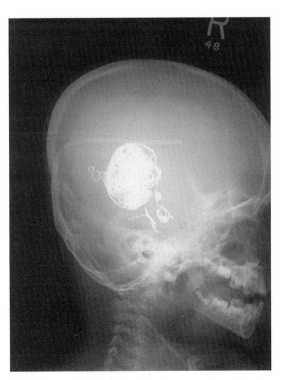

FIGURE 44.3. Vein of Galen aneurysm in a child. Approximately 260 coils were required to adequately block flow. Mechanical obstruction with coiling is preferred in this setting compared with injectable sclerosing agents, microspheres, gelatinates, or gelfoam because of the risk of iatrogenic cerebrovascular accident without controlled embolization.

the catheter. Should this occur, the coil might be errantly deposited in an unsatisfactory location, making it only more difficult to get the next coil beyond the "new" obstacle in its pathway. If the delivery catheter retracts or prolapses during a trial run (advancing the "pusher" wire only, without a coil in front of it), either a stiffer delivery catheter or a less rigid pusher wire may be necessary.

Failure of vessel occlusion. As previously alluded to, the occlusive action of coils depends on the patients' ability to form and organize a thrombus. In patients receiving anticoagulants, the use of cast-forming embolic agents (silicone, isobutyl a-cyanoacrylate [IBCA]) may be preferable (14) either alone or in combination with coil embolization. If target vessel occlusion is not observed during the procedure, the operator should not assume that "delayed thrombosis" will occur. The opposite, in fact, is truer, in that immediate thrombosis does not ensure permanent vascular occlusion.

CARDIAC AND CORONARY ARTERY COIL EMBOLIZATION

Abnormal communications of the coronary arteries with venous structures of the heart and cardiac chambers are well described. The first pathologic report was published in 1865 (15). Coronary artery fistulas may be congenital or may occur following surgical or accidental cardiac trauma. Although coronary artery malformations or fistulas are rare (0.2% to 0.25% of patients referred for coronary angiography), they account for the most common hemodynamically significant congenital defect of the coronary vascular system, and usually occur in isolation (16–20). These malformations commonly bridge the myocardial bed, shunting a significant amount of coronary arterial flow to the coronary veins or coronary sinus, pulmonary vein, superior vena cava, or right or left heart chambers (arteriocameral fistulas). In 1983, Reidy et al. reported the first transcatheter embolization of a coronary artery fistula (21,22).

Most patients with these coronary anomalies are asymptomatic, but late complications can occur, and include congestive heart failure due to a large left-to-right shunt, myocardial ischemia, arrhythmias, endocarditis, pulmonary hypertension, venous rupture or thrombosis, and venous obstruction (20). Consequently, surgical ligation of the anomalous connection has been recommended in most series, with open perioperative mortality ranging from 2% to 4% (16,23–26). Although still uncommon, numerous case reports and small trials have demonstrated the utility and safety of transcatheter coronary embolization (12).

Coronary arteries involved in the anomalous connection are typically dilated and ectatic, elongated and extremely tortuous, and are readily apparent on angiography. Subselective cannulation of these arteries may be required to fully opacify the vessel and identify the anomalous connection, as well as any important side branches that may affect the treatment plan. The aim of coronary artery embolization is complete occlusion of all involved vessels, while sparing the normal adjacent vessels. In general, mechanical devices such as balloons, umbrellas, or coils are used to obstruct flow, as opposed to injectable polymers or sclerosing agents. This is because of the need to absolutely avoid unwanted or accidental obstruction of adjacent normal coronary artery segments.

The risks associated with transcatheter embolization of coronary artery fistulas include coronary artery disruption with the guiding catheter or guide wire, and distal systemic or pulmonary embolization from debris or occluder materials, as well as the inherent risk of myocardial ischemia or infarction.

The techniques and indications for transcatheter intervention of other congenital or acquired cardiac defects, such as atrial or ventricular septal defect and patent ductus arteriosus, are discussed in detail elsewhere in this text.

NONCARDIAC COIL EMBOLIZATION

Arteriovenous Malformations and Arteriovenous Fistulas

Congenital or acquired arteriovenous malformations and arteriovenous fistulas are abnormal vascular connections that bypass the capillary bed, with a marked decrease of peripheral resistance. Blood flows preferentially into this low-resistance system, resulting in a steal phenomenon and decreased pressure in the adjacent normal circulation. These lesions are occasionally significant because of possible complications, such as paradoxical embolization, hemorrhage, mass effect, and ischemia. The most commonly affected vascular beds supply the lungs and the brain.

Pulmonary arteriovenous malformations may become large enough to cause a right-to-left shunting of blood flow (with subsequent poor arterial oxygen saturation or paradoxical emboli) and are amenable to coil embolization (27). Patients with Osler-Weber-Rendu syndrome may have multiple malformations, which are usually located in the lungs but also may affect the cerebrovascular system.

For embolization to be successful, both the draining vein and the feeding artery of the arteriovenous malformation or fistula need to be embolized. The lesion is usually embolized with multiple coils. Initially, multiple large coils are deployed followed by smaller coils to occlude any gaps the large coils may leave behind. Long-term angiographic follow-up is required (usually at 6- to 12-month intervals) because successful complete obliteration of the arteriovenous malformation has been shown to occur in only about 25% of lesions with initial therapy (27). Despite the occasional need for repeated embolotherapy, the procedure is extremely well tolerated, and clinical symptoms often improve.

Hemorrhage

The utility of coil embolotherapy depends upon the location, etiology, and severity of bleeding. Although

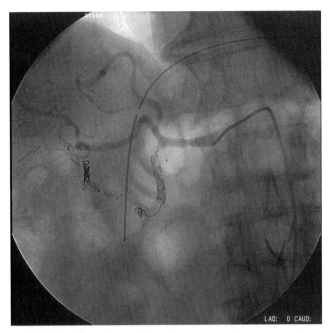

FIGURE 44.4. Gastroduodenal artery hemorrhage. This patient had an actively bleeding duodenal ulcer that was not amenable to endoscopic sclerotherapy. The entire gastroduodenal artery is embolized with coils, with subsequent angiography demonstrating adequate embolization with stasis of blood flow.

embolization to control hemorrhage is nearly always possible, it will result in permanent vascular occlusion, and care must be taken to preserve as much normal tissue as possible.

One of the most common applications for coil embolotherapy is gastrointestinal hemorrhage (28), which can be further classified as either upper or lower gastrointestinal bleeding, with the ligament of Treitz as the anatomic divider. Classifying the source of hemorrhage is important because of the different therapeutic options. In general, coil embolization is performed after transcatheter intraarterial vasopressin infusion fails to control the hemorrhage, but primary coil embolization is occasionally performed. The upper gastrointestinal system is more amenable to coil embolization because of the rich collateral vascular supply to the visceral organs. Common vessels that can be embolized without significant adverse sequelae include the gastroduodenal artery and the left gastric artery (Figure 44.4). The pancreaticoduodenal and gastroepiploic arcades more than adequately give good collateral blood supply to the duodenum and stomach, respectively. Although not historically promoted, more recently lower gastrointestinal bleeding is believed amenable to coil embolotherapy with superselective catheterization and targeted embolization (29). Potential complications include the possibility of intestinal ischemia or subsequent infarction, or procedural failure to control the hemorrhage.

Hemorrhage caused by trauma is also amenable to coil embolotherapy (Figure 44.5) (30). Hemorrhage due to

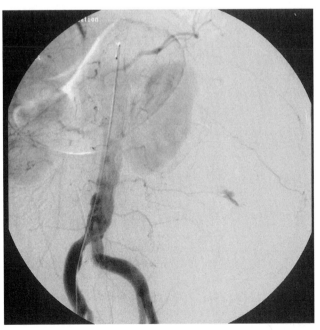

A

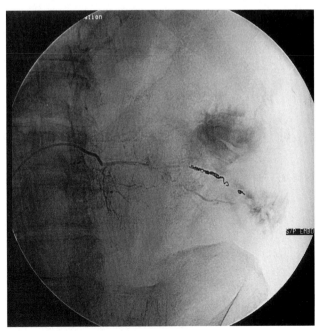

B

FIGURE 44.5. A: Iatrogenic injury to left lumbar artery following a biopsy procedure. Bolus contrast aortography demonstrates active extravasation of contrast. **B:** Successful embolization of the bleeding lumbar artery with multiple coils, demonstrating hemostasis.

pelvic trauma can be life-threatening, often requiring prompt evaluation with rapid angiography looking for active extravasation of flow. Arterial injuries most commonly involve the internal iliac arteries, either unilaterally or bilaterally. The bleeding internal iliac artery is often initially embolized with gel foam. However, if the bleeding is not controlled, then coils are added. If needed, both internal iliac arteries can be occluded simultaneously without significant sequelae, because of good collateral blood supply in the pelvis. In trauma to the extremities, both coils and gel foam are used to embolize actively bleeding vessels. However, the target vessel must be able to be sacrificed without leaving a significant ischemic burden to the extremity.

ANEURYSMS AND PSEUDOANEURYSMS

Aneurysms and pseudoaneurysms occur throughout the body. Most true aneurysms are idiopathic, whereas pseudoaneurysms are usually secondary to traumatic or iatrogenic injury. Aneurysms or pseudoaneurysms can rupture, causing hemorrhage and other complications particular to the anatomic location.

The cerebral arterial system is one anatomic area that has benefited greatly with an improved ability to treat both aneurysms and pseudoaneurysms with embolization coils (31). Advances in coil and microcatheter technology enable the interventionalist to exclude the aneurysm by packing it with coils, thereby preserving parent vessel patency (Figure 44.3). Success is more likely achieved in saccular aneurysms with a narrow neck, and with the use of Guglielmi detachable coils (31).

Depending on their location, saccular aneurysms elsewhere in the body can also be packed with coils in an effort to preserve parent vessel patency. However, the vessel feeding the aneurysm is more commonly embolized with coils both distal and proximal to the aneurysm itself. Frequent applications of this technique include splenic artery pseudoaneurysms caused by pancreatitis, hepatic artery pseudoaneurysms, and renal artery pseudoaneurysms caused by iatrogenic trauma (Figure 44.6).

Endovascular stent-grafts for the treatment of abdominal aortoiliac aneurysms are increasingly used in an effort to avoid an open abdominal aortic aneurysm repair. Occasionally, one of the limbs of these stent-grafts may need to be placed across the internal iliac artery bifurcation. To prevent the occurrence of endoleaks (reversed or forward blood flow that remains intraluminal but outside the aortic stent-graft that pressurizes the aortic wall), the internal iliac artery may need to be preoperatively embolized (32). For this relatively specific indication, embolization with coils has been shown to be effective.

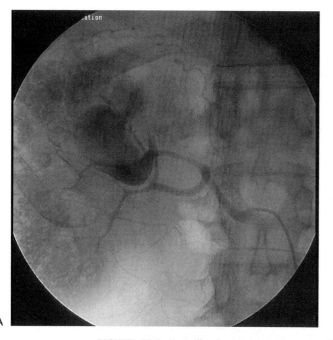
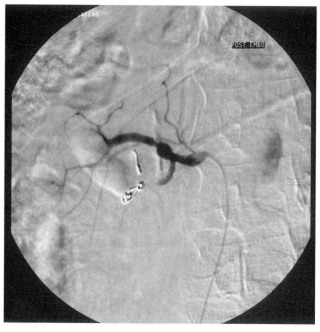

A   B

FIGURE 44.6. A: Following right pyeloureterolithotomy, the patient suffered from persistent hematuria requiring blood transfusions. Right renal angiography demonstrates a pseudoaneurysm arising from one of the lesser branches of the renal artery. **B:** Successful coil embolization of the feeding renal artery segment. Delayed angiography confirms hemostasis. The patient's hematuria resolved shortly thereafter.

ORGAN AND TUMOR ABLATION

Therapeutic embolization is performed on both solid organs and tumors for both definitive and preoperative reasons. Preoperative tumor embolization decreases operative blood loss during resection. Indications for primary embolotherapy include palliation for unresectable malignant lesions, or reduction of the size of a tumor or organ. Coils are often deployed in conjunction with other embolic material, such as polyvinyl alcohol or gel foam.

Splenic partial embolization can be performed with selective coil embolization for the treatment of idiopathic thrombocytopenia (33) as well as for blunt trauma (34). Embolization is helpful during the resection of renal carcinomas, in an effort to decrease the intraoperative blood loss. The liver is also amenable to partial embolization with coils following blunt trauma (35). Recognizing that the liver has a dual blood supply (the portal venous system and the hepatic arterial system), the hepatic arteries can be embolized safely without adversely affecting liver function.

VENOUS EMBOLIZATION

The most common application of coil embolization in the venous system is the treatment of varicoceles (and its female counterpart, pelvic congestion syndrome) (36). Incompetent venous valves allow reflux of blood with distention of the gonadal veins. In men this may cause infertility, whereas in women this frequently causes chronic pelvic pain. Although varicoceles are often surgically ligated during an open procedure, percutaneous transcatheter embolization with coils remains minimally invasive. During the procedure the entire length of the gonadal vein is laced with multiple coils, in conjunction with either gel foam or sodium tetradecyl sulfate (Figure 44.7). In men, only the symptomatic gonadal vein is treated, but women usually require treatment of both gonadal veins.

QUALITY IMPROVEMENT GUIDELINES

The Society of Cardiovascular and Interventional Radiology has published a set of Quality Improvement Guidelines for Percutaneous Transcatheter Embolization that briefly describe the importance of patient selection, procedural technique, and periprocedural patient monitoring (37). The document also includes composite success and complication rates for general categories of percutaneous embolization procedures.

SUMMARY AND CONCLUSION

Coils can be safely and effectively deployed (embolized) in almost every location and in almost every clinical situation,

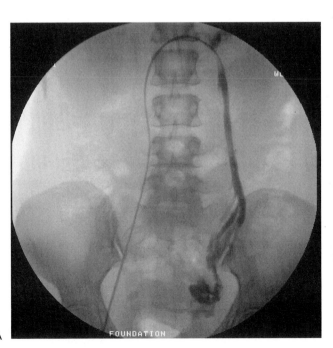
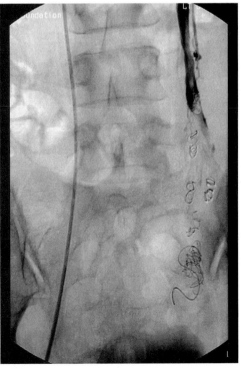

A   B

FIGURE 44.7. A: Pelvic congestion syndrome. Left ovarian venography demonstrates a distended ovarian vein with pelvic varicoceles. **B:** Successful coil embolization of the entire length of the left ovarian vein, resulting in varicocele obliteration.

limited only by the judgment and experience of the operator. Some of the more general and common uses of coil embolotherapy have been described in this chapter, although clearly this discussion is not all-inclusive. The clinical indications for coil embolotherapy will only increase in the future, as this therapeutic modality often avoids significant mortality and morbidity associated with more invasive surgical options that are usually available to the patient with vascular compromise.

REFERENCES

1. Dawbain G. In Lussenhop AJ, Spence WT. Artificial embolization of cerebral arteries: report of use in a case of aterioyenous malformation. *JAMA* 1960;172:1153–1155.
2. Baum S, Nusbaum M. The control of gastrointestinal hemorrhage by selective mesenteric arterial infusion of vasopressin. *Radiology* 1971;98:497–505.
3. Coldwell DM, Stokes KR, Yakes WF. Embolotherapy: agents, clinical applications, and techniques. *Radiographics* 1994;14:623–643.
4. Gianturco C, Anderson JH, Wallace S. Mechanical devices for arterial occlusion. *Am J Roentgenol* 1975;124:428–435.
5. White RI, Strandberg JV. Therapeutic embolization with long-term occluding agents and their effects on embolized tissues. *Radiology* 1977;125:677–687.
6. Young A, Tadavarthy SM, Coleman CC, et al. Embolotherapy: agents, equipment, and techniques. In: Castaneda-Zuniga WR, Tadavarthy SM, eds. *Interventional radiology.* Baltimore: Williams & Wilkins, 1988:13–76.
7. Eisenhauer MA, Mego DM, Cambier PA. Coronary steal by IMA bypass graft side-branches: a novel therapeutic use of a new detachable embolization coil. *Catheter Cardiovasc Diagn* 1998;45:301–306.
8. Ogoh Y, Akago T, Abe T, et al. Successful embolization of coronary arteriovenous fistula using an interlocking detachable coil. *Pediatr Cardiol* 1997;18:152–155.
9. Hazama K, Nakanishi T, Tsuji T, et al. Transcatheter occlusion of arterial duct with new detachable coils. *Cardiol Young* 1996;6:332–336.
10. DeWolf D, Terriere M, DeWilde P, et al. Embolization of a coronary fistula with a controlled delivery platinum coil in a 2 year-old. *Pediatr Cardiol* 1994;15:308–310.
11. Quek SC, Wong J, Tay JSH, et al. Transcatheter embolization of coronary artery fistula with controlled release coils. *J Paediatr Child Health* 1996;32:542–544.
12. Qureshi SA, Reidy JF, Alwi MB, et al. Use of interlocking detachable coils in embolization of coronary arteriovenous fistulas. *Am J Cardiol* 1996;78:110–113.
13. Mazer MJ, Baltaxe HA, Wolf GL. Therapeutic embolization of the renal artery with Gianturco coils: limitations and technical pitfalls. *Radiology* 1981;138:37–46.
14. Freeny PC, Bush WH, Kidd R. Transcatheter occlusive therapy of genitourinary abnormalities using isobutyl 2-cyanoacrylate (Bucrylate). *Am J Radiol* 1979;133:647–656.
15. Krause W. Über den Ursprung einer akzessorischen A. coronaria aus der A. pulmonalis. *Z Ration Med* 1865;24:225.
16. Wilde P, Watt I. Congenital coronary artery fistulae: six new cases with a collective review. *Clin Radiol* 1980;31:301–311.
17. Levin DC, Fellows KE, Abrams HL. Hemodynamically significant primary anomalies of the coronary arteries. *Circulation* 1978;58:25–34.
18. Effler DB, Sheldon WC, Turner JJ, et al. Coronary arteriovenous fistulas: diagnosis and surgical management: report of fifteen cases. *Surgery* 1967;61:41–50.
19. Baltaxe AH, Wixson D. The incidence of congenital anomalies of the coronary arteries in the adult population. *Radiology* 1977;122:47–52.
20. Harris WO, Andrews JC, Nichols DA, et al. Percutaneous transcatheter embolization of coronary arteriovenous fistulas. *Mayo Clin Proc* 1996;71:37–42.
21. Reidy JF, Anjos RT, Qureshi SA, et al. Transcatheter embolization in the treatment of coronary artery fistulas. *J Am Coll Cardiol* 1991;18:187–192.
22. Reidy JF, Sowton E, Ross DN. Transcatheter occlusion of coronary to bronchial anastomosis by detachable balloon combined with coronary angioplasty at same procedure. *Br Heart J* 1983;49:284–287.
23. Haberman JH, Howard JL, Johnson ES. Rupture of the coronary sinus with hemopericardium. *Circulation* 1963;28:1143–1144.
24. Blanche C, Chaux A. Long-term results of surgery for coronary artery fistulas. *Int Surg* 1990;75:238–239.
25. Kirklin JW, Barratt-Boyes BG. *Cardiac surgery.* New York: John Wiley, 1986:945–955.
26. Perry SB, Keane JF, Lock JE. Pediatric intervention. In: Grossman W, Baim DS, eds. *Cardiac catheterization, angiography, and intervention.* Philadelphia: Lea & Febiger, 1991:543–544.
27. Dutton JAE, Jackson JE, Hughes JMB, et al. Pulmonary arteriovenous malformations: results of treatment with coil embolization in 53 patients. *Am J Roentgenol* 1995;165:1119–1125.
28. Ledermann HP, Schoch E, Jost R, et al. Superselective coil embolization in acute gastrointestinal hemorrhage: personal experience in 10 patients and review of the literature. *J Vasc Int Radiol* 1998;9:753–760.
29. Evangelista PT, Hallisey MJ. Transcatheter embolization for acute lower gastrointestinal hemorrhage. *J Vasc Int Radiol* 2000;11:601–606.
30. Selby JB. Interventional radiology of trauma. *Radiol Clin North Am* 1992;30:427–439.
31. Murayama Y, Vinuela F, Duckwiler GR, et al. Embolization of incidental cerebral aneurysms by using the Guglielmi detachable coil system. *J Neurosurg* 1999;90:207–214.
32. Razavi MK, DeGroot M, Olcott C III, et al. Internal iliac artery embolization in the stent-graft treatment of aortoiliac aneurysms: analysis of outcomes and complications. *J Vasc Int Radiol* 2000;11:561–566.
33. Miyazaki M, Ito H, Kaiho T, et al. Partial splenic embolization for the treatment of chronic idiopathic thrombocytopenic purpura. *Am J Roentgenol* 1994;163:123–126.
34. Hagiwara A, Yukioka T, Ohta S, et al. Nonsurgical management of patients with blunt splenic injury: efficacy of transcatheter arterial embolization. *Am J Roentgenol* 1996;167:159–166.
35. Hagiwara A, Yukioka T, Ohta S, et al. Nonsurgical management of patients with blunt hepatic injury: efficacy of transcatheter arterial embolization. *Am J Roentgenol* 1997;169:1151–1156.
36. Maelux G, Stockx L, Wilms G, et al. Ovarian vein embolization for the treatment of pelvic congestion syndrome: long-term technical and clinical results. *J Vasc Int Radiol* 2000;11:859–864.
37. Drooz AT, Lewis CA, Allen TE, et al. Quality improvement guidelines for percutaneous transcatheter embolization. *J Vasc Int Radiol* 1997;8:889–895.

45

TRANSCATHETER EMBOLIZATION OF UNWANTED BLOOD VESSELS IN CHILDREN

P. SYAMASUNDAR RAO

A number of congenital and/or acquired anomalous vascular connections may produce significant hemodynamic burden or may bypass the natural or artificially created vascular pathways causing hypoxemia. Whereas some of these superfluous vascular connections can be surgically closed, the extra time and effort required to identify and surgically close are generally thought to be detrimental to the patients. Consequently, most cardiologists/surgeons prefer transcatheter occlusion. Selective occlusion of such vessels by embolization has been extensively undertaken in adult patients, and Berenstein and Kricheff (1,2) reviewed the technical considerations a little more than two decades ago. Subsequently, a number of reviews addressing pediatric and congenital heart disease applications have been published (3–8). Transcatheter embolization may serve as an adjunct to surgery or may be the sole procedure. The preceding chapter discussed embolization therapy in adults. This chapter reviews pediatric applications of embolotherapy. Transcatheter occlusion of patent ductus arteriosus (PDA) was reviewed in detail in Section II of this book and will not be dealt with in this chapter.

EMBOLIC MATERIALS

A variety of embolic materials have been used that are either absorbable biodegradable materials or nonabsorbable particulate materials. The nonabsorbable particulate materials are more commonly utilized and include silicone spheres, Ivalon, isobutyl-2-cyanoacrylate (IBCA), silicone fluid mixtures, tantalum powder, Gianturco coils (Cook, Bloomington, IN), and silicone balloons (1,2,9,10). The Gianturco-Grifka vascular occlusion device (11) and PDA occlusion

devices (12–14) have also been used as embolic materials. Embolization with Gianturco coils, initially developed for renal vessel occlusion (15), has been the most commonly used method in children.

Described initially in 1975 (15), the coils have undergone considerable changes. The coils are made up of stainless steel (or platinum) wire embedded with thrombogenic synthetic (Dacron) fibers. The wire diameter varies from 0.018 to 0.052 inch. The coil may have a single curl (loop) or multiple curls. Straight coils are also available: Hilal embolization microcoils (Cook, Bloomington, IN) or platinum microcoils (Target, Meditech, Natick, MA) are used for occlusion of small vessels. The helical diameter of the coil loop varies from 2 through 3, 5, 8, 10, 15, and 20 mm. Other coils with different-sized diameters could also be custom-made by the manufacturer. The length of the coil varies from 1.0 to 15 cm. The manufacturer's description of the coil includes wire diameter, length of the coil, and helical diameter of the coil loop, in that order. The number of coil loops in the embolus is not given but can be calculated as follows: number of loops = length of the coil in mm/πD, where D is the diameter of the coil loop in millimeters.

Whereas the free coils are most commonly used for occlusion of superfluous vessels, detachable coils that provide controlled release and allow repositioning, if necessary (16), have been introduced. Other modifications include staking of one or more coils in a plastic sac (11).

The devices (Chapters 22 through 24, 26) (11–14) and detachable balloons (10,17–22) have been described elsewhere and will not be detailed in this chapter.

TECHNIQUE

Safety, superselectivity, occlusion of the nidus of the lesion, rather than of just the feeding vessel, and prevention of distal migration of the embolus should be considered before embarking on the embolization procedure (1,2). The pro-

---

P. Syamasundar Rao: Professor of Pediatrics, Medicine, and Cardiology, Department of Pediatrics, University of Texas-Houston Medical School; Director, Division of Pediatric Cardiology, Memorial Hermann Children's Hospital, Houston, Texas

cedure is usually performed under conscious sedation. Informed consent is obtained from parents or the patient as appropriate. Percutaneous cannulation of the femoral vein and artery is undertaken, and a 4 or 5F sheath is inserted to allow exchange of multiple catheters, which may be required. Larger sheaths may be required if devices or detachable balloons are used (Chapters 22 through 24, 26) (10–14,17–22). Heparin 100 U/kg is given intravenously and activated clotting times (ACTs) are monitored. Additional doses of heparin are given to maintain ACTs between 200 and 250 seconds. Systemic heparinization does not seem to prevent clot formation in the implanted coils (23). Therefore we do not hesitate to anticoagulate during the procedure.

Angiography from the blood vessel giving origin to the target vessel to be occluded, and selective angiography of the target vessel itself are obtained to measure the diameter of the vessel, define any constrictions in the vessel, and discern the extent of target vessel distribution. An understanding of the local vascular anatomy, natural history of the lesion to be occluded, physiologic results of occlusion, and potential complications of occluding such a vessel is important before embarking on the occlusion procedure. Test occlusion with a balloon-tipped catheter for 5 to 10 minutes, while monitoring for potential adverse effects, usually arterial oxygen saturation and electrocardiogram, may be necessary in some of the lesions.

After identifying the target vessel to be occluded, an end-hole catheter is introduced into it. Most commonly we use a 4 or 5F Judkins right coronary artery catheter (Cordis, Miami, FL), although other catheters (e.g., internal mammary artery, Cobra, Head Hunter, and Glidecath) are used on occasion. For occlusion of very small and tortuous vessels, we use a 3F (Target-18) catheter (24), which can be advanced through a large-bore 4 or 5F right coronary artery catheter. Larger, specifically designed catheters may be necessary to deliver detachable balloons (10,17–22) or devices (Chapters 22 through 24 and 26) (11–14). The remaining part of this section will discuss only deployment of Gianturco coils (Cook, Bloomington, IN).

Coils for embolization are chosen on the basis of diameter of target vessel and presence of a constrictive lesion in the target vessel. In the presence of the latter, coil diameter should be approximately double the diameter of the constrictive lesion so that the coil is entrapped proximal to the constriction. Otherwise, the diameter of the coils should be 20% to 30% larger than the diameter of the target vessel. The target vessel may stretch (dilate) following occlusion, and this should be considered in the selection of coil diameter. If the coil is too small, it may completely curl in the vessel and may not cause complete occlusion. Too large a coil may not curl at all and remains straight, and again may not produce effective thrombosis of the vessel. We prefer 0.038-inch wire diameter coils in preference to small wire diameter coils because of their greater thrombogenic effect.

The tip of the delivery catheter is positioned at the desired location, and a test angiogram is made to confirm the catheter position. The selected coil is loaded into the catheter with the stiff end of a 0.038-inch guide wire. However, the soft end of the catheter is used to advance and deliver the coil. This is to prevent any change in the position of the tip of the delivery catheter. If in doubt or if a new type of catheter is being used to deliver the coil, an *in vitro* trial of coil delivery should be performed. During deployment of the coil, either advancement of the coil alone, withdrawal of the catheter while holding the guide wire firmly in position, or a combination of the two may be utilized, depending upon the delivery site, curvature and/or tortuosity of the catheter, and fluoroscopic appearance during coil delivery. Occasionally, detachable coils (16) or coils grasped with bioptome (25,26) are used if greater control than is provided by free Gianturco coils is deemed important.

Selective angiography is performed 5 to 10 minutes after coil placement to document effectiveness of occlusion. If there is residual flow, a second coil may be necessary. Temporary balloon occlusion of the vessel for a 5-minute period, tamponading the flow, may be beneficial in producing complete occlusion and is worth a trial. More than one coil is needed in large vessels. Initially, we deploy a larger coil, then implant additional smaller coils to produce complete occlusion.

Three doses of cefazolin 25 mg/kg/dose are given at 6-hour intervals. The first dose is started in the catheterization laboratory. Heparin is not continued, nor is the effect of already administered heparin reversed.

Follow-up chest roentgenograms on the morning after the procedure and at the 1-month follow-up visit are performed to ensure that the coil(s) has (have) not moved. Follow-up angiography is not performed unless other clinical indications suggest the need for repeat catheterization and angiography.

MECHANISM OF OCCLUSION

Occlusion of the target blood vessel occurs by thrombosis secondary to mechanical effect of synthetic (Dacron) fibers attached to the coils. Heparin does not seem to prevent thrombosis of the embolized vessels (23). Therefore, as mentioned in the preceding section, we use heparin in all our cases (8). Some workers advocate presoaking of the coils in thrombin (4) before implantation, but the rate of vessel occlusion is not altered by it (6). For this reason we do not advocate presoaking coils in thrombin before their implantation.

COMPLICATIONS

A number of complications have been reported. These include embolization into the pulmonary or systemic circuit, inability to implant the coil, transbronchial migration, segmental infarction, infection, and hemolysis (4–6, 27–30). Complications may be avoided or their rate decreased by meticulous attention to the technique and detailed understanding of the local vascular anatomy. *In vitro* testing of coil delivery via the catheters, particularly if that type of catheter has not been used by the operator previously, is helpful. Using a shorter-length coil will avoid protrusion into the blood vessel giving origin to the target vessel. Securing the catheter well into the target vessel will also prevent inadvertent catheter recoil or coil misplacement. If the coil embolizes, transcatheter retrieval with a snare or a variety of other retrieval devices (31) is possible and should be attempted. Gooseneck snares (Microvena, White Bear Lake, MN) have been most useful in our own experience (8,31). If retrieval is impossible, repositioning the coil into the vessel that is least likely to cause physiologic abnormality should be attempted. Hemolysis is usually related to residual shunt through the partially occluded vessels. If the hemolysis does not decrease or disappear, reocclusion of the vessel to abolish residual shunt is recommended.

SPECIFIC CLINICAL APPLICATIONS

Embolization of the superfluous vessels is useful in a number of clinical situations in pediatric cardiac patients. These clinical scenarios will be described separately in the ensuing sections. Central nervous system and visceral (hepatic, renal, and gastrointestinal) applications will not be discussed.

PULMONARY ARTERIOVENOUS FISTULA

The first known report of pulmonary arteriovenous fistula (PAVF) dates back to the late nineteenth century (32). PAVFs are rare pulmonary vascular anomalies in which a direct communication between the pulmonary arteries and veins exists, producing intrapulmonary right-to-left shunt. Systemic arterial desaturation, cyanosis, polycythemia, and digital clubbing will follow (33). Exercise intolerance is usually present. Serious complications such as stroke, brain abscess, and hemoptysis may develop with resultant fatality in nearly 10% patients (34). Most cases are due to hereditary hemorrhagic telangiectasia or Osler-Rendu-Weber syndrome (33). PAVF may also occur in patients with schistosomiasis (35) hepatic fibrosis (36,37) and classic Glenn anastomosis (38,39). Most patients with PAVF present after the second decade of life, and 25% of the cases may be seen during childhood (40). However, the clinical presentation may be seen as early as in the neonatal period (41–45) and infancy (46).

A high index of suspicion is necessary to diagnose PAVF. Cyanosis without any major cardiac findings is most usual. Radiopaque density may be seen on chest roentgenograms in some patients. Conventional two-dimensional and color Doppler echocardiography do not show major cardiac abnormalities. However, contrast echocardiography shows rapid and early contrast bubble appearance in the left atrium following peripheral intravenous injection of agitated saline solution or other contrast material. Computed tomography of the chest or gadolinium-enhanced MRI (14) may be helpful in the diagnosis. Selective pulmonary arteriography is confirmatory.

Since the early reports in the 1970s of therapeutic embolization (47,48), detachable balloons (10,21,22,39,49) and Gianturco coils (3,42,45,46,48,50–54) have been extensively used in successfully occluding the PAVFs. More recently, the Amplatzer Duct Occluder (14) and the Gianturco-Grifka vascular occlusion device (55) have also been used in occluding large PAVFs.

The technique of coil occlusion is as described in the preceding section. Selective pulmonary artery branch angiography is performed first to identify the feeding vessel supplying the fistula. Then the delivery catheter is positioned in the target vessel, and a test injection is made. A coil 20% to 30% larger than the target vessel is delivered. In large vessels, several coils may have to be implanted to achieve successful occlusion. Selective angiography is repeated 10 to 15 minutes after coil deployment in order to assess effectiveness of occlusion. Additional coils may be delivered if there is residual shunt. Figures 45.1 and 45.2 show a few examples from our own experience. An increase in arterial oxygen saturation is also suggestive of a successful procedure. When multiple vessels are involved, embolization procedures may have to be performed in more than one session (51,52).

The results of PAVFs are generally good, with increase in arterial oxygen saturation and improvement of other ventilation/perfusion abnormalities (22,51,52). Angiography several weeks after coil deployment demonstrated continued occlusion of the embolized vessels (51). However, some follow-up studies demonstrate a high incidence [eight of 14 (57%)] of recanalization (53). Difficulty in occluding all involved vessels at the same sitting, development or opening up of new fistulae, and recanalization may necessitate repeating the embolization procedure. Because of the observation that recanalized PAVFs are fed by bronchial artery branches, coil placement should be as close to PAVFs as possible (53). Transcatheter embolization appears to be a safe and effective alternative to surgical resection of the lung in the management of PAVFs (21,40,46,49–55). Because of its simplicity and accessibility, coil embolization is becoming a preferred method of transcatheter occlusion, although devices may be particularly useful in very large PAVFs.

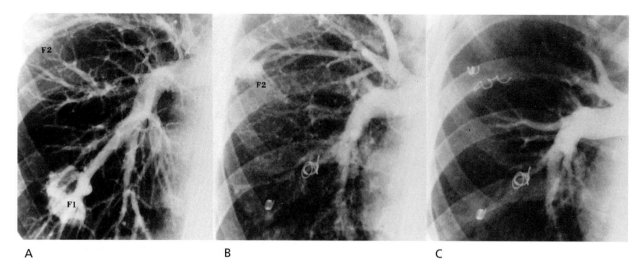

A   B   C

FIGURE 45.1. Selective pulmonary arteriographic frames in posteroanterior view showing two pulmonary arteriovenous fistulae, F1 and F2 (**A**). Following coil occlusion (**B**) the larger fistula F1 is no longer opacified. After implantation of additional coils (**C**), the smaller fistula F2 is also occluded. (From Siblini G, Rao PS. Coil embolization in the management of cardiac problems in children. *J Invasive Cardiol* 1996;8:332–340, with permission.)

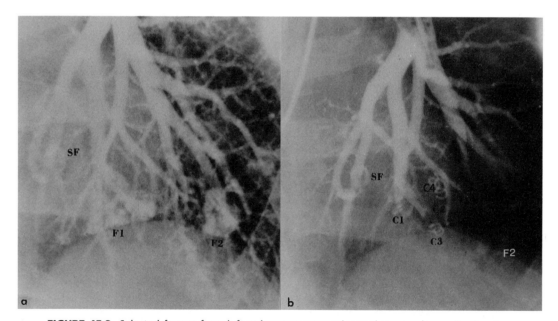

FIGURE 45.2. Selected frames from left pulmonary artery cineangiograms demonstrating two large (F1 and F2) and one small (SF) pulmonary arteriovenous fistulae before (**a**) and following (**b**) occlusion with four Gianturco coils (C1, C2, C3, and C4). The coils C1, C2, and C3 appear to have completely occluded F1. Coil C4 seems to have almost completely occluded F2. No attempt was made to occlude the SF.

AORTOPULMONARY COLLATERAL VESSELS

In patients with pulmonary atresia or tetralogy of Fallot, persistent embryonic collateral (PEC) vessels, erroneously called *bronchial collateral vessels,* arise most commonly from the descending aorta or from brachiocephalic vessels. Such blood vessels may also arise from celiac, renal, and visceral arteries (5). Whereas the pulmonary blood flow through these vessels is useful in maintaining good systemic arterial oxygen saturation, such vascular connections may become problematic and require attention in certain clinical situations:

1. Excessive pulmonary blood flow through these vessels may precipitate congestive heart failure. This is much more true if a surgical systemic arterial-to-pulmonary shunt had been performed previously.
2. Excessive hemodynamic burden in the immediate post-operative period following surgical correction.
3. Contemplated surgical unifocalization in patients with pulmonary atresia.

Issues related to venous and arterial collateral vessels associated with bidirectional Glenn and Fontan procedures will be discussed later.

A number of embolic materials have been used to occlude PECs and include tissue adhesives (9), detachable silicone balloons (3,7,17), and Gianturco coils (4–6, 56–60). At the present time coils are most commonly used for this purpose.

The technique of coil embolization is similar to that described in the preceding section. However, the operator must ensure that an alternative source of blood supply to the lung segment supplied by the target vessel exists before occluding the PEC. Test occlusion with a balloon-tipped catheter may be necessary to verify that the systemic arterial oxygen saturation does not decrease to levels below 80%. Peculiar origin and tortuosity of the collateral vessels may cause difficulty in proper positioning of the tip of the catheter, but various guide wires and catheters (5,8), including the 3F Target catheters, are available and may help achieve an ideal position of the catheter to ensure safe implantation of the embolic material (Figure 45.3). A coil that is 30% to 50% larger than the diameter of the target vessel is recommended because of likely distention of the vessel following coil placement.

The results of occlusion PECs are generally good and have high effective occlusion rates. In one study (4), complete occlusion was demonstrated in 42 (72%) of 58 vessels. In 14 (24%) there was trivial residual shunt. Failure to implant or partial occlusion was observed in only two (3%) patients. Similar results were observed by other workers (6); 14 (82%) of 17 vessels were completely occluded. In another study involving 67 aortopulmonary collateral vessels, complete occlusion in 51 (76%), subtotal obstruction in seven (10%), and partial obstruction in four (6%) was noted (60). In five (8%) the procedure could not be accomplished. Figures 45.4 and 45.5 demonstrate a few examples from our experience.

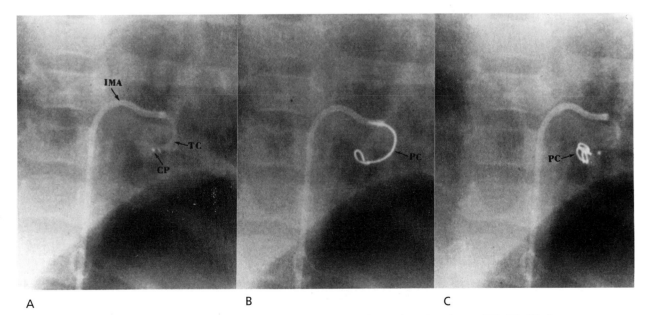

A   B   C

FIGURE 45.3. Cineradiographic frames showing a TurboTracker-18 catheter (TC) (MediTech–Boston Scientific, Natick, MA) passing through a 4F internal mammary artery (IMA) catheter (Cook, Inc., Bloomington, IN) through which a Coil Pusher-16 (CP) (MediTech–Boston Scientific) has been advanced (**A**). The tip of the IMA catheter is in the mouth of the collateral vessel, but could not be advanced further. **B,C:** Delivery of a platinum coil (CP) through the Turbo Tracker. (From Rao PS. Tricuspid atresia. *Curr Treat Options Cardiovasc Med* 2000;2:507–570, with permission.)

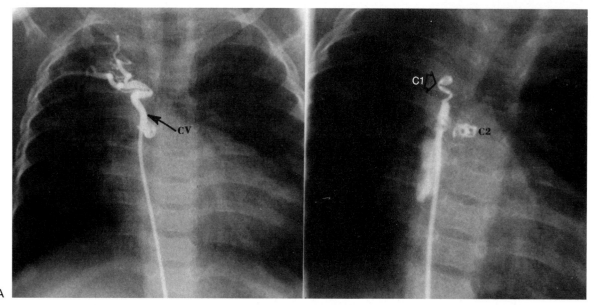

FIGURE 45.4. Selected cine frames from angiograms obtained in a 2-year-old child with pulmonary atresia and a large ventricular septal defect (tetralogy of Fallot) who underwent a Blalock-Taussig shunt several months previously. To manage congestive heart failure uncontrolled by conventional anticongestive measures, two collateral vessels were coil-embolized. **A:** One such collateral vessel (CV) which was occluded with a Gianturco coil (C1) with resultant complete occlusion (**B**). **B** also shows the second coil (C2), which also completely occluded the second CV (not shown).

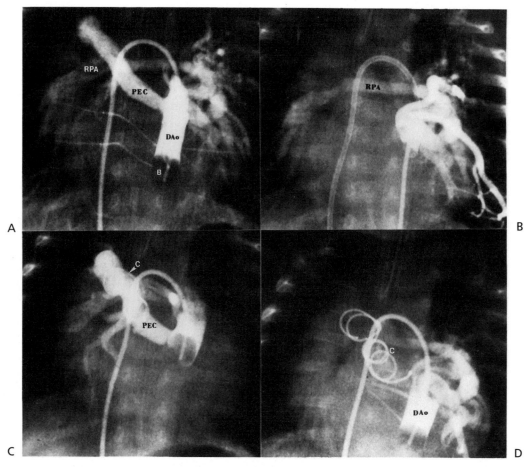

FIGURE 45.5. Selected cineangiographic frame from balloon (B) occlusion aortography in a neonate with severe congestive heart failure demonstrating a large persistent embryonic collateral (PEC) vessel connecting the descending aorta (DAo) to the right pulmonary artery (RPA) (**A**). Alternative blood supply to RPA is demonstrated from a PEC on the left side (**B**). Occlusion with an 8-mm-diameter Gianturco coil (C) did not result in complete occlusion of the PEC (**C**). A second overlapping coil was placed, which resulted in complete occlusion of the PEC (**D**). The infant improved remarkably from congestive heart failure and eventually underwent unifocalization and complete correction.

Follow-up studies (58) revealed complete occlusion in 31 (89%) of 35 PECs. This study also demonstrates endothelialization of coils protruding into the aortic lumen. Furthermore, no episodes of stroke, embolic events, endarteritis, or coil migration were observed in this study (58).

In conclusion, transcatheter coil embolization of the PECs is feasible, safe, and effective, and is helpful in the overall management of this patient subset.

COLLATERAL VESSELS AFTER BIDIRECTIONAL GLENN AND FONTAN PROCEDURES

Development of veno-venous (61–65) and arteriovenous (66–70) collateral vessels following bidirectional Glenn operation has been well documented. Such collateral vessels may cause hypoxemia (61–65,71,72) or left ventricular volume overload (66–70) and need attention. Such collateral vessels may also develop following Fontan operation (66,68,73–77).

Venovenous Collateral Vessels

Detailed studies by two groups of workers (64,65) revealed development of collateral channels between the superior and inferior vena caval system following bidirectional cavopulmonary anastomosis. Nearly one-third of the patients were shown to develop such collateral vessels, causing arterial hypoxemia secondary to "steal" from the pulmonary circulation (72,78). Various venous channels were identified and include azygos or hemiazygos veins; persistent left or right superior vena cavae; pericardiophrenic, pericardial, internal thoracic, intercostal, or paravertebral veins; and others. Most vessels seem to represent reopening of vessels present during embryonic development. These collateral vessels are more common in the presence of abnormal superior vena caval connections, pulmonary artery distortion, high superior vena caval or pulmonary artery pressure, and absent upper lobe pulmonary blood flow. A large difference between superior vena caval and right (or left) atrial pressures appears to be a common denominator. Although most of these vessels may have been dormant and not demonstrable at the time of preoperative catheterization, careful scrutiny for the presence of such vessels (e.g., by left innominate vein angiography) and, if present (Figure 45.6), their occlusion in the catheterization laboratory or during bidirectional Glenn surgery may be appropriate and beneficial in the overall management of these babies.

Significant systemic arterial desaturation is an indication to occlude abnormal channels connecting the superior and inferior vena caval systems unless immediate Fontan conversion is contemplated. Occlusion of such vessels demonstrated increase in median oxygen saturation from 65 to 84% (64). Systemic venous to pulmonary venous connections should, however, be occluded irrespective of planned Fontan. Most workers used Gianturco coils to occlude these vessels (6,65,71,72). Figure 45.7 shows one such example from our case series.

Development of collateral vessels bypassing the lung following Fontan (4,66,68,73,77), both early (76) and late (77), has been reported. Occlusion of such vessels with conventional Gianturco coil (Cook, Bloomington, IN) is feasi-

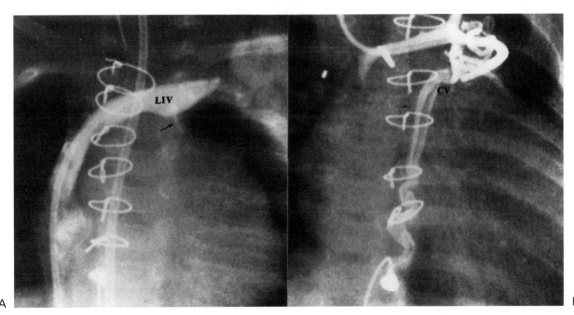

FIGURE 45.6. Left innominate vein (LIV) cineangiographic frame (**A**) showing a tiny twig, presumably representing persistent left superior vena cava *(arrow)*. Following a bidirectional Glenn procedure, a large collateral vessel (CV) developed, causing hypoxemia (**B**).

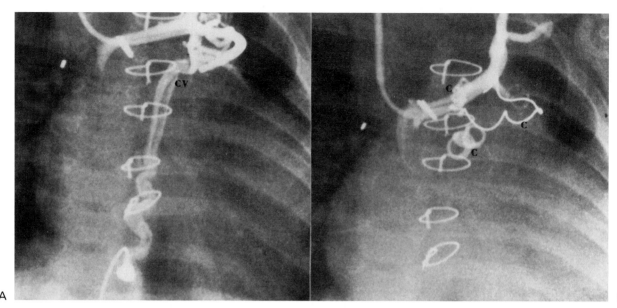

FIGURE 45.7. The left panel (**A**) is from the same patient demonstrated in FIGURE 45.6. Following occlusion with several coils (C), there is complete occlusion (**B**) with resultant improvement in systemic arterial oxygen saturation.

ble. However, when these vessels are large, 0.052-inch coils (77), devices, or innovative solutions (79) should be sought to occlude them.

Systemic Artery to Pulmonary Collaterals

Systemic artery to pulmonary collaterals cause excessive pulmonary blood flow and left ventricular volume overload, and

may be problematic, causing increased mortality and morbidity in the immediate postoperative period after Fontan operation. Between 59% and 84% of children catheterized before Fontan procedure were found to have aortopulmonary collateral vessels (66,68,69). In one large study (70) nearly one-third of the patients required occlusion of one to 11 vessels (mean, 3.6 vessels) preoperatively. An additional 20% of patients required occlusion in the immediate postoperative

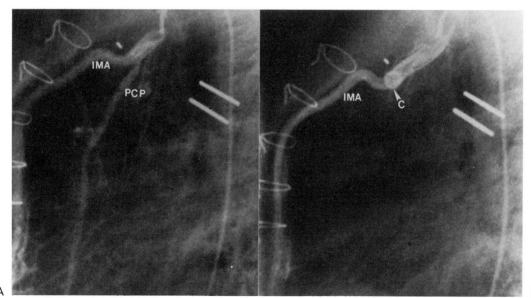

FIGURE 45.8. Selective internal mammary artery (IMA) cineangiograms in the lateral view demonstrating multiple, small collateral vessels arising from the pericardiophrenic (PCP) branch (**A**) which resulted in a significant levophase (not shown). **B:** Following occlusion with a Gianturco coil (C), there is complete occlusion of this vessel.

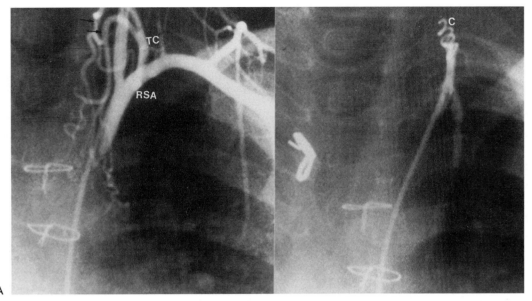

FIGURE 45.9. A: Right subclavian artery (RSA) cineangiogram showing branches *(arrows)* of the thyrocervical (TC) trunk that supplied a number of small vessels, giving a good degree of levophase. Complete occlusion occurred following implantation of a coil (C) **(B).**

period because of elevated pulmonary artery pressure, heart failure, or prolonged chest tube drainage. Morbidity and mortality appear to be higher in patients who had significant aortopulmonary collateral vessels. It is for this reason that these collateral vessels should be sought during preoperative catheterization. We routinely perform descending aortography and left and right subclavian arteriography. Most of these vessels can be occluded with Gianturco coils (Cook, Bloomington, IN) (Figures 45.8 and 45.9). Sometimes use of the 3F Target catheter may facilitate entry into these vessels and they can be embolized with 0.018-inch wire coils (Figure 45.3).

AORTOPULMONARY SURGICAL SHUNTS

Palliation by a variety of shunts, including classical or modified (Gore-Tex) Blalock-Taussig (BT) shunt, is undertaken if the patients with complex pulmonary atresia/stenosis cannot be totally corrected at the time of presentation. Such shunts may also be necessary to treat hypoxemia (secondary to decreased right ventricular compliance and right-to-left shunting across the patent foramen ovale) following transcatheter therapy of critical pulmonary stenosis or atresia with intact ventricular septum. However, these shunts may require occlusion at a later date for a number of reasons:

1. Excessive pulmonary blood flow (e.g., multiple shunts).
2. Resolution of the original cardiac defect (e.g., critical pulmonary stenosis or atresia managed by balloon or surgical valvotomy).
3. Residual shunts following ligation during total surgical repair.

4. Elective preoperative occlusion to avoid surgical exploration.
5. Shunts created at the time of bidirectional Glenn procedure to augment arterial saturation.

Blalock-Taussig Shunts

Detachable balloons (3,18–20,80,81), Gianturco coils (4–6,8,60,81–85), Rashkind PDA devices (12,81), Duct-Occlude pfm (13), detachable coils (85), and Gianturco-Grifka vascular occlusion devices (85,86) have been used to occlude BT shunts.

Effective occlusion of both classic and modified BT shunts is feasible, but the procedure is more challenging because of high-velocity flow, lack of distal stenosis (in some cases), high prevalence of embolization into the pulmonary arteries (4,81,85), residual shunts (4,85), and difficult access. Each of the preceding issues can be adequately addressed. Temporary balloon occlusion of the shunt during coil delivery (4,5,84), appropriate choice of coil diameter (1 mm larger than BT shunt diameter), meticulous attention to the technique, use of multiple coils, and use of a variety of available catheter/guide wire systems, respectively, may circumvent these difficulties.

Several large series of BT shunt occlusion have been reported to date (4,81,85). Perry et al. (4) utilized Gianturco coils in 14 patients. In one (7%) patient, the coil could not be implanted because of technical difficulties. Complete closure was demonstrated in six (43%), subtotal occlusion was found in five (36%), and partial closure occurred in two (14%). Coils embolized into the pul-

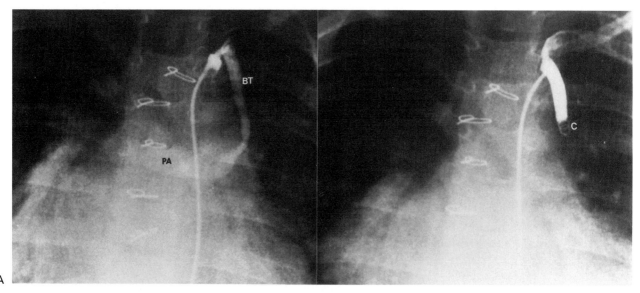

FIGURE 45.10. Selective cineangiogram demonstrating a patent modified Blalock-Tausig (BT) shunt opacifying the pulmonary artery (PA) (**A**). Following coil (C) implantation, complete occlusion was demonstrated (**B**).

monary artery in three (12%) patients. Burrows et al. (81) utilized Gianturco coils, detachable balloons, and Rashkind devices; occlusion was eventually successful in 14 (82%) of 17 patients. Device embolization into the pulmonary artery occurred in five (29%) patients. Moore and his associates (85) attempted 19 BT shunt occlusions in 18 patients. Seventeen were modified and two were classical BT shunts. Detachable coils and/or Gianturco coils were used in 16 patients and the Gianturco-Grifka occlusion device was used in two patients. In several patients, stents were implanted in the narrowed branch pulmonary artery, thus essentially preventing coil embolization into the pulmonary artery. Complete closure was achieved in all but one patient. In the lone exception, there was a small residual leak. Embolization of coils or devices into the pulmonary artery did not occur. Based on these data, the authors concluded that transcatheter occlusion of BT shunt is safe and effective. Our own experience with BT shunt occlusion was with Gianturco coils in eight patients. In one patient the coil migrated into the pulmonary artery, requiring removal by a snare. Complete occlusion (Figures 45.10 and 45.11) was demonstrated in seven patients; trivial residual shunt

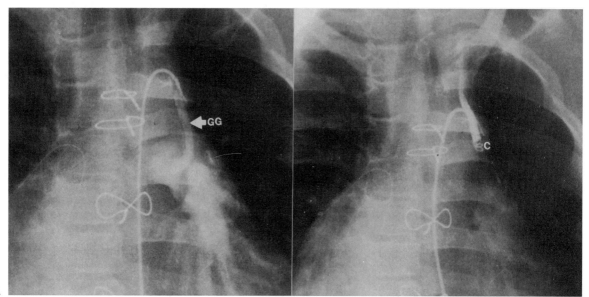

FIGURE 45.11. Angiographic frame in posteroanterior view demonstrating a patent Goretex graft (GG) from a previous modified Blalock-Taussig shunt (**A**). Note complete occlusion (**B**) following coil (C) occlusion. (From Siblini G, Rao PS. Coil embolization in the management of cardiac problems in children. *J Invasive Cardiol* 1996;8:332–340, with permission.)

was present in one. Based on the data presented earlier, we can conclude that Gianturco coil occlusion is commonly used and that transcatheter occlusion of BT shunts with a number of devices is feasible, safe, and effective.

Other Surgical Shunts

Occlusion of other surgical shunts such as Pott's (descending aorta-to-left pulmonary artery anastomosis) (87) or ascending aorto-to-right pulmonary artery Gortex graft (88) and other types of shunts is also feasible, and special techniques may be required (87), depending upon the type of the communication. However, surgical shunts other than BT shunts are not frequently performed at the present time; therefore the need for occlusion of such shunts becomes less.

CORONARY ARTERIOVENOUS FISTULAE

Coronary arteriovenous fistula (AVF) is a rare anomaly comprising 0.2% of all cases undergoing cardiac catheterization (89) or selective coronary angiography (90). Nearly half of the fistulae arise from the branches of the right coronary artery. The other half come from the left coronary artery (91). However, the vast majority (90%) of them empty into the right atrium, right ventricle, or pulmonary artery (91). The remaining few enter the left heart structures, coronary sinus, or a bronchial artery (91,92). The usual mode of presentation is a murmur on auscultation, which is continuous in nature. More than half of the patients, especially in childhood, are otherwise asymptomatic. However, complications during follow-up, namely, aneurismal dilatation (92,93), rupture (94), myocardial ischemia, and/or infarction (91,92,95–100) presumably related to coronary steal, congestive heart failure (89,97,101,102), endocarditis (89,103), arrhythmia (103), and pulmonary hypertension (101,102) may be seen. Therefore closure of these fistulae is recommended even in asymptomatic patients. However, it should be noted that clinically silent coronary AVF that are incidentally diagnosed on routine two-dimensional and color Doppler echocardiographic studies tend to regress with time and remain asymptomatic (104), and that, consequently, no treatment is indicated.

A number of embolic materials have been used to transcatheter-occlude coronary AVF. These include Ivalon foam (105,106), ductal closure devices (107,108), coils (8,92,93, 107,109-127), and silicone- or contrast-filled detachable balloons (92,128–131). Coils appear to be the most commonly used embolus. Regular Gianturco coils, detachable coils (117,119,120,123,127), and platinum microcoils (115,116,118,122,124) have been used in occluding coronary fistulae.

The method of coil delivery for occlusion of coronary AVF is similar to that described earlier. Embolization into the pulmonary circuit and inadvertent blockage of branch vessels supplying the myocardium can occur. Therefore careful study of morphology and distribution of anomalous coronary circulation should be undertaken to ensure suitability for transcatheter occlusion. Stenotic segment distal to the site of coil embolus (or any other type of device) and absence of coronary artery branches supplying the myocardium beyond the proposed site of coil placement are important prerequisites for successful embolization. Skimming et al. (131) retrospectively reviewed their case material and came to the conclusion that 15 (88%) of their 17 patients had suitable features for effective occlusion of coronary AVF. A similar review by another group of workers (132) indicated that only six (38%) of 16 are suitable for transcatheter embolization. This review appears to be from a surgical perspective.

Initially, selective coronary angiography to discern the anatomy of the coronary AVF and visualize coronary artery branches should be performed. However, coronary steal may not result in adequate visualization of all branches. Test occlusion may reveal these vessels. Whenever possible, test occlusion should be performed not only to visualize these vessels, but also to uncover any myocardial ischemia. Then coil occlusion should follow. Most workers use transcoronary artery embolization of AVF (Figure 45.12). Rarely, it may be possible to embolize it antegradely (i.e., via the pulmonary artery) (119,121). However, in most cases it is difficult to cannulate the fistula from this end. Following coil implantation, coronary arteriography should be repeated to evaluate for residual shunt; if present, it should be occluded by placement of additional coils.

By and large, most of the reported experiences are based on one or two case reports. To have a greater understanding of the utility of transcatheter occlusion, the data from five case series (92,107,119,125,131), each containing three to 13 patients, were combined. Thirty-six patients underwent transcatheter occlusion of coronary AVF. Gianturco coils, detachable balloons, and a combination of the two were used to close the fistulae. Complete occlusion was demonstrated in 32 (89%) of the 36 patients. Clinical evaluation several months to 4 years following the procedure did not reveal any evidence for recanalization; however, the patients have not been systematically studied by repeat coronary angiography. Although the procedure has been most commonly performed in children, it is also feasible to perform it in infants (124), if clinically indicated.

Surgical correction is safe with low, 0 to 4% mortality rates (89,132,133). However, morbidity is universal and the potential for myocardial infarction (133) exists. Furthermore, the recurrence rate associated with surgery is unknown. Given these considerations, transcatheter closure is an excellent initial treatment option in patients with coronary AVF. Based on the published reports, as reviewed and our own, although limited, experience, the transcatheter treatment option is feasible, safe, and effective. Coils, particularly microcoils introduced through Target

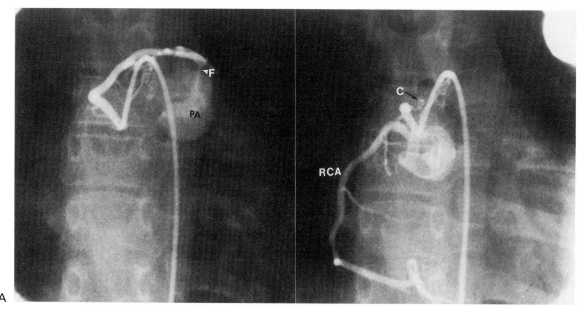

FIGURE 45.12. Selective right coronary angiography with the catheter tip in the feeding vessel shows a coronary arteriovenous fistula (F) opacifying the pulmonary artery (PA) **(A)** which after coil (C) occlusion **(B)** is no longer visualized. RCA, right coronary artery.

catheters, are useful in avoiding occlusion of normal coronary branches.

PULMONARY SEQUESTRATION

Pulmonary sequestration may either be intralobar or extralobar (134) and may be associated with scimitar syndrome (135,136). The sequestered lung, however, receives blood supply from an anomalous systemic artery, usually arising from the abdominal or thoracic aorta. The pulmonary venous drainage may be normal or may drain anomalously into the azygos system, portal vein, or inferior vena cava. Atrial septal defect may also be present. The large intrapulmonary shunt may result in congestive heart failure in infancy. Whereas surgical resection of the sequestered lung along with ligation of the vessel supplying the sequestered lung segment has been the conventional

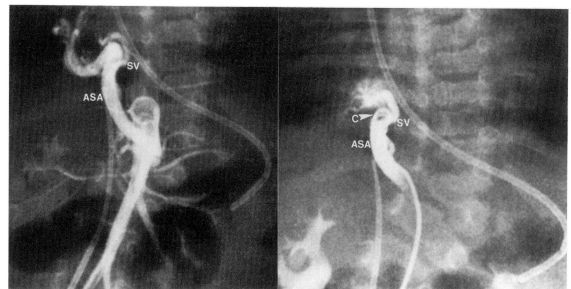

FIGURE 45.13. Abdominal aortogram demonstrating a large anomalous systemic artery (ASA) opacifying a sequestered lung **(A)** in an infant with severe congestive heart failure. The ASA was occluded with a coil (C) resulting in complete occlusion of the ASA **(B)**. A small vessel (SV) was not occluded. The infant also had a patent ductus arteriosus that was also coil-occluded (not shown). Following the procedure the infant improved dramatically.

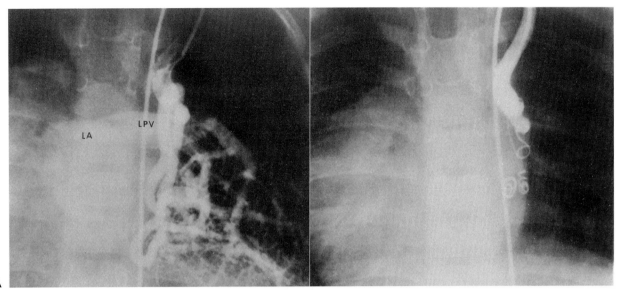

FIGURE 45.14. Systemic arteriovenous fistula (**A**) arising from the internal mammary artery shown on posteroanterior view in a patient with dextrocardia, but without any intracardiac anomalies. Note opacification of the left pulmonary vein (LPV) and left atrium (LA) during the levoangiographic phase. Following implantation of multiple coils (**B**), arteriovenous fistulas are no longer visualized. A continuous murmur heard on auscultation is no longer heard following occlusion.

approach, several workers over the years (4,6,137–139) employed transcatheter embolization and found successful results! Gelfoam fragments and Gianturco coils have been used successfully (4,6,137–139). Severe or difficult-to-treat heart failure constitutes an indication for transcatheter intervention in infants. Transcatheter coil occlusion (Figure 45.13) is safe, feasible, and effective.

OTHER LESIONS

A number of other congenital or acquired anomalous connections would benefit from transcatheter occlusion. These include anomalous systemic arteriovenous (Figures 45.14 and 45.15) or veno-venous connections (5,6,140–143) and bleeding vessels causing hemoptysis (144–147).

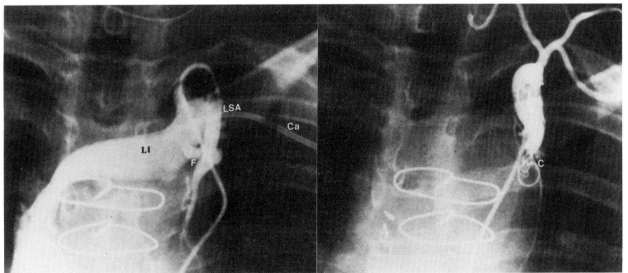

FIGURE 45.15. Selective cineangiogram from the left subclavian artery (LSA) revealed dense opacification of the left innominate (LI) vein (**A**). This fistula (F) was presumed to be secondary to prior subclavian vein punctures related to her care for cardiac transplantation. Following coil (C) occlusion (**B**), the fistulous connection and LI vein are no longer opacified. The catheter (Ca) is in the LI vein beyond the level of the fistula.

CURRENT STATUS

The Gianturco coil, currently the most commonly used embolus, is available for general clinical use. The PDA occluding devices and balloons are available for investigational use at the participating institutions. The Gianturco-Grifka vascular occlusion device is approved by the FDA for general clinical use.

CONCLUSION

Occlusion of unwanted, superfluous vascular connections is feasible with a number of embolic materials. Whereas a combination of several methods of occlusion appears logical, experience with embolization of the target vessel with Gianturco coils is simple and effective in the vast majority of clinical scenarios and can be accomplished via small-diameter catheters. The devices may be necessary when occluding large vascular connections. Knowledge of the vascular anatomy, pathophysiologic effects of embolic occlusion of the target vessel, and potential complications, and availability of appropriate catheter/guide wire systems and embolic material are essential before embarking on transcatheter occlusion. Transcatheter methods have advantages over conventional surgery and should be the first-choice treatment option in the management of these abnormal vascular connections.

REFERENCES

1. Berenstein A, Kricheff II. Catheter and material selection for transcatheter embolization: technical considerations. I. Catheters. *Radiology* 1979;132:616–630.
2. Berenstein A, Kricheff II. Catheter and material selection for transcatheter embolization: technical consideration. II. Materials. *Radiology* 1979;132:631–642.
3. Reidy JF, Jones ODH, Tynan MJ, et al. Embolization procedures in congenital heart disease. *Br Heart J* 1985;54:184–192.
4. Perry SB, Radtke W, Fellows KE, et al. Coil embolization to occlude aortopulmonary collateral vessels and shunts in patients with congenital heart disease. *J Am Coll Cardiol* 1989;13:104–108.
5. Orsmond G. Coil embolization in congenital heart disease. *Prog Pediatr Cardiol* 1992;1:44–54.
6. Rothman A, Tong AD. Percutaneous coil embolization of superfluous connections in patients with congenital heart disease. *Am Heart J* 1993;126:206–213.
7. Kan JS. Role of embolization therapy in the treatment of infants and children. In: Rao PS, ed. *Transcatheter therapy in pediatric cardiology.* New York: Wiley-Liss, 1993:371–376.
8. Siblini G, Rao PS. Coil embolization in the management of cardiac problems in children. *J Invasive Cardiol* 1996;8:332–340.
9. Zuberbuhler JR, Danker E, Zoltun R, et al. Tissue adhesive closure of aortic-pulmonary communications. *Am Heart J* 1974;88:41–46.
10. White RI Jr., Kaufman SL, Barth KH, et al. Embolotherapy with detachable silicone balloons: technique and clinical results. *Radiology* 1979;131:619–627.
11. Grifka RG, Mullins CE, Gianturco C, et al. New Gianturco-Grifka vascular occlusion device: initial studies in canine model. *Circulation* 1995;91:1840–1846.
12. Houde C, Zahn EM, Benson LN. Transcatheter closure of Blalock-Taussig shunts with a modified Rashkind umbrella delivery system. *Br Heart J* 1993;69:56–58.
13. Tometzki AJP, Houston AB, Redington AN, et al. Closure of Blalock-Taussig shunts using a new detachable coil device. *Br Heart J* 1995;73:383–384.
14. Waight DJ, Hijazi ZM. Pulmonary arteriovenous malformations: transcatheter embolization options (Editorial). *Catheter Cardiovasc Intervent* 2000;50:52–53.
15. Gianturco C, Andersen JH, Wallace S. Mechanical devices for arterial occlusion. *Am J Roentgenol* 1975;124:428–435.
16. Uzun O, Hancock S, Parsons JM, et al. Transcatheter occlusion of arterial duct with Cook detachable coils: early experience. *Heart* 1996;76:269–273.
17. Grinnel VS, Mehringer CM, Hieshima GB, et al. Transaortic occlusion of collateral arteries to the lung by detachable valved balloons in a patient with tetralogy of Fallot. *Circulation* 1982;65:1276–1278.
18. Reidy JF, Baker E, Tynan M. Transcatheter occlusion of a Blalock-Taussig shunt with a detachable balloon in a child. *Br Heart J* 1983;50:101–103.
19. Florentine M, Wolfe RR, White RI Jr. Balloon embolization to occlude Blalock-Taussig shunt. *J Am Coll Cardiol* 1984;3:200–202.
20. Gewilling M, Van der Hauwaert L, Daenen W. Transcatheter occlusion of high flow Blalock-Taussig shunts with a detachable balloon. *Am J Cardiol* 1990;65:1518–1519.
21. Barth KH, White RJ, Kaufman SL, et al. Embolotherapy of pulmonary arteriovenous malformations with detachable balloons. *Radiology* 1982;142:599–606.
22. Terry PB, White RI Jr., Barth KH, et al. Pulmonary arteriovenous malformations: physiologic observations and results of therapeutic balloon embolization. *N Engl J Med* 1983;308:1197–1200.
23. Johnson WH, Peterson RK, Howland DF, et al. Systemic heparinization does not prevent clot formation in coil embolization. *Catheter Cardiovasc Diagn* 1990;20:267–270.
24. Rao PS. Tricuspid atresia. *Curr Treat Options Cardiovasc Med* 2000;2:507–570.
25. Hayes MD, Hoyer NH, Glasgow PF. New forceps delivery technique for coil delivery of patent ductus arteriosus. *Am J Cardiol* 1997;39:209–211.
26. Grifka RG, Jones TK. Transcatheter closure of large PDA using 0.052-inch Gianturco coils: controlled delivery using a bioptome catheter through a 4F sheath. *Catheter Cardiovasc Intervent* 2000;49:301–306.
27. Chang VP, Wallace S, Gianturco C, et al. Complications of coil embolization: prevention and management. *Am J Roentgenol* 1981;131:809–813.
28. McCarthy P, Kennedy A, Dawson P, et al. Pulmonary embolus as a complication of therapeutic peripheral arteriovenous malformation embolization. *Br J Radiol* 1991;64:177–178.
29. Abad J, Villar R, Parga G, et al. Bronchial migration of pulmonary arterial coil. *Cardiovasc Intervent Radiol* 1990;13:345–346.
30. Remy-Jardin M, Wattinne L, Remy J. Transcatheter occlusion of pulmonary arterial circulation and collateral supply: failures, incidents and complications. *Radiology* 1991;180:699–705.
31. Rao PS. Transcatheter retrieval of intravascular/intracardiac foreign bodies. In: Rao PS, ed. *Transcatheter therapy in pediatric cardiology.* New York: Wiley-Liss, 1993:377–392.
32. Churtor T. Multiple aneurysm of pulmonary artery. *Br Med J* 1897;1:1223–1225.

33. Dines DE, Arms RA, Bernatz PE, et al. Pulmonary arteriovenous fistulas. *Mayo Clin Proc* 1974;49:460–465.

34. Lindskog GE, Liebow AA, Kausel H, et al. Pulmonary arteriovenous aneurysm. *Ann Surg* 1950;132:591–606.

35. Lopes de Faria J. Pulmonary arteriovenous fistulas and arterial distribution of eggs of *Schistosoma mansoni. Am J Trop Med Hyg* 1956;5:860–862.

36. Karlish AJ, Marshall R, Reid L, et al. Cyanosis with hepatic cirrhosis: a case with pulmonary arteriovenous shunting. *Thorax* 1967;22:555–561.

37. Maggiore G, Borgna-Pignatti C, Marni F, et al. Pulmonary arteriovenous fistulas: an unusual complication of congenital hepatic fibrosis. *J Pediatr Gastroenterol Nutr* 1983;2:183–186.

38. Gomes AS, Benson L, George B, et al. Management of pulmonary arteriovenous fistulas after superior vena cava–right pulmonary artery (Glenn) anastomosis. *J Thorac Cardiovasc Surg* 1984;87:636–639.

39. Von Scheidt W, Von Arnium T, Schneider B, et al. Balloon embolization of a pulmonary arteriovenous fistula after cavopulmonary anastomosis in tricuspid atresia. *Am Heart J* 1988;116:182–185.

40. Gasul B, Arcilla R, Lev M. *Heart disease in children: diagnosis and treatment.* Philadelphia: JB Lippincott, 1966:459–468.

41. Hall RJ, Nelson WP, Blake HA, et al. Massive pulmonary arteriovenous fistula in the newborn: a correctable form of cyanotic heart disease; an additional cause of cyanosis with left axis deviation. *Circulation* 1965;31:762–767.

42. Grady RM, Sharky AM, Bridges ND. Transcatheter coil embolization of a pulmonary arteriovenous malformation in a neonate. *Br Heart J* 1994;71:370–371.

43. Amarall FV, Felix PR, Grannzotti JA, et al. Massive pulmonary arteriovenous fistula: a rare potentially curable cause of hypoxia in the newborn. *Arq Bras Cardiol* 1996;66:353–355.

44. Von-Segesser L. Pulmonary arteriovenous fistula: a rare cause of progressive asymptomatic cyanosis in neonates. *Arch Mal Coeur Vaiss* 1997;90:713–717.

45. Fletcher SE, Cheatham JP, Bolam D. Primary transcatheter treatment of congenital pulmonary arteriovenous malformation causing cyanosis of the newborn. *Catheter Cardiovasc Intervent* 2000;50:48–51.

46. Marin-Garcia J, Lock JE. Catheter embolization of pulmonary arteriovenous fistulas in an infant. *Pediatr Cardiol* 1992;13:41–43.

47. Porstmann W. Therapeutic embolization of arteriovenous pulmonary fistula by catheter technique. In: Kelop O, ed. *Current concept in pediatric cardiology.* Berlin: Springer, 1977:23–71.

48. Taylor BG, Cockerill EM, Manfredi F, et al. Therapeutic embolization of the pulmonary artery in pulmonary arteriovenous fistula. *Am J Med* 1978;64:360–365.

49. White RJ Jr, Lynch-Nyhan A, Terry P, et al. Pulmonary arteriovenous malformations: techniques and long-term outcome of embolotherapy. *Radiology* 1988;169:663–669.

50. Keller FS, Rosch J, Baker AF, et al. Pulmonary arteriovenous fistulas occluded by percutaneous introduction of spring coils. *Radiology* 1984;152:373–375.

51. Hartnell GG, Jackson JE, Allison DJ. Coil embolization of pulmonary arteriovenous malformations. *Cardiovasc Intervent Radiol* 1990;13:347–350.

52. Kirsh LR, Sos TA, Engle MA. Successful coil embolization for diffuse, multiple pulmonary arteriovenous fistulas. *Am Heart J* 1991;122:245–247.

53. Sagara K, Miyazono N, Inoue H, et al. Recanalization after coil embolotherapy of pulmonary arteriovenous malformations: study of long-term outcome and mechanism of recanalization. *Am J Roentgenol* 1998;170:727–730.

54. Ghani M, Yusuf M, Sdringola S, et al. Percutaneous coil embolization of multiple arteriovenous malformation in the left lung causing persistent hypoxemia. *Circulation* 2000;102:E-118.

55. Ebeid MR, Braden DS, Gaymes CH, et al. Closure of a large pulmonary arteriovenous malformation using multiple Gianturco-Grifka vascular occlusion devices. *Catheter Cardiovasc Intervent* 2000;49:426–429.

56. Szarnicki R, Krebber HJ, Wack J. Wire coil embolization of systemic-pulmonary artery collaterals following surgical correction of pulmonary atresia. *J Thorac Cardiovasc Surg* 1981;81:124–126.

57. Fuhrman BP, Bass JL, Castenada-Zuniga W, et al. Coil embolization of congenital thoracic vascular anomalies in infants and children. *Circulation* 1984;70:285–289.

58. Verma R, Lock BG, Perry SB, et al. Intra-aortic spring coil loops: early and late results. *J Am Coll Cardiol* 1995;25:1416–1419.

59. Louis JF, Gomes AS, Smith DC, et al. Systemic-to-pulmonary collateral vessels and shunts: treatment with embolization. *Radiology* 1988;169:671–676.

60. Sharma S, Kothari SS, Krishnakumar R, et al. Systemic-to-pulmonary artery collateral vessels and surgical shunts in patients with cyanotic congenital heart disease: perioperative treatment by transcatheter embolization. *Am J Roentgenol* 1995;164:1505–1510.

61. Gross GJ, Jonas RA, Castaneda AR, et al. Maturational and hemodynamic factors predictive of increased cyanosis following bidirectional cavopulmonary anastomosis. *Am J Cardiol* 1994;74:705–709.

62. Webber SA, Horvath P, LeBlanc JG, et al. Influence of competitive pulmonary blood flow on the bidirectional superior cavopulmonary shunt: a multi-institutional study. *Circulation* 1995;92:II-279–II-286.

63. Gatzoulis MA, Shinebourne EA, Redington AN, et al. Increasing cyanosis early after cavopulmonary connection caused by abnormal systemic venous channels. *Br Heart J* 1995;73:182–186.

64. McElhiney DB, Reddy VM, Hanley FL, et al. Systemic venous collateral channels causing desaturation after bi-directional cavopulmonary anastomosis: evaluation and management. *J Am Coll Cardiol* 1997;30:817–824.

65. Magee AG, McCrindle BW, Mawson J, et al. Systemic venous collateral development after bi-directional cavopulmonary anastomosis: prevalence and predictions. *J Am Coll Cardiol* 1998;32:502–508.

66. Triedman JK, Bridges ND, Mayer JE, et al. Prevalence and risk factors for aortopulmonary collateral vessels after Fontan and bidirectional Glenn procedures. *J Am Coll Cardiol* 1993;28:207–215.

67. Ichikawa H, Yagihara T, Kishimoto H, et al. Extent of aortopulmonary collateral blood flow as a risk factor for Fontan operation. *Ann Thorac Surg* 1995;59:433–437.

68. Salim MA, Case CL, Sade RM, et al. Pulmonary to systemic flow ratio in children after cavopulmonary anastomosis. *J Am Coll Cardiol* 1995;25:735–738.

69. Spicer RL, Uzark KC, Moore JW, et al. Aortopulmonary collateral vessels and prolonged pleural effusions after modified Fontan procedures. *Am Heart J* 1996;131:1164–1168.

70. Kantor KR, Vincent RN, Raviele AA. Importance of acquired systemic-to-pulmonary collateral vessels in the Fontan operation. *Ann Thorac Surg* 1999;68:974–975.

71. Michel-Behnke J, Akinturk H, Schranz D. Reopening of a persistent left superior vena cava in early postoperative period following bi-directional cavopulmonary anastomosis: treatment by coil embolization. *Z Kardiol* 1999;88:555–558.

72. Vance MS, Cohen MH. Management of azygos vein "steal" fol-

lowing hemi-Fontan by transcatheter coil embolization. *Catheter Cardiovasc Diagn* 1996;39:403–406.

73. Hayes AJ, Burrows PE, Benson LN. An unusual cause of cyanosis after the modified Fontan procedure: closure of venous communications between the coronary sinus and left atrium by transcatheter techniques. *Cardiol Young* 1994;4:172–174.

74. Stamper O, Wright JGC, Sadiq M, et al. Late systemic desaturation after total cavopulmonary shunt operation. *Br Heart J* 1995;74:282–286.

75. Bernstein HS, Ursell PC, Hanley F, et al. Fulminant development of pulmonary arteriovenous fistulae in an infant following total cavopulmonary shunt. *Pediatr Cardiol* 1996;17:46–50.

76. Clapp S, Morrow WR. Development of superior vena cava to pulmonary vein fistulae following modified Fontan operation: case report of a rare anomaly and embolization therapy. *Pediatr Cardiol* 1998;19:363–365.

77. Tomita H, Ishikawa Y, Hasegawa S, et al. Use of 0.052-inch Gianturco coil to embolize a persistent right superior vena cava following extracardiac cavopulmonary connection. *Catheter Cardiovasc Intervent* 2000;52:481–483.

78. Robicsek F, Sanger PW, Taylor FH, et al. The azygos "steel" syndrome in cavo-pulmonary anastomosis. *Ann Surg* 1963;158:1007–1011.

79. Moore JW, Murphy JD. Use of a bow tie stent occluder for transcatheter closure of a large anomalous vein. *Catheter Cardiovasc Intervent* 2000;49:437–440.

80. Dubois J, Cohen L, Brunell F, et al. Modified Blalock-Taussig shunt anastomosis in a three-month-old child with pulmonary stenosis: embolization therapy. *Pediatr Radiol* 1991;21:198–199.

81. Burrows PE, Edwards TC, Benson LN. Transcatheter occlusion of Blalock-Taussig shunts: technical options. *J Vasc Intervent Radiol* 1993;4:673–680.

82. Culham JAG, Izukawa T, Burns JE, et al. Embolization of a Blalock-Taussig shunt in a child. *Am J Roentgenol* 1981;137:413–415.

83. Shrivastava S, Sharma S, Sanghri S, et al. Coil embolization of a Blalock-Taussig shunt. *Indian Heart J* 1993;45:219–220.

84. Limsuwan A, Sklansky MS, Kashani IA, et al. Wire-snare technique with distal flow control for coil occlusion of a modified Blalock-Taussig shunt. *Catheter Cardiovasc Intervent* 2000;49:51–54.

85. Moore JM, Ing FF, Drummond D, et al. Transcatheter closure of surgical shunts in patient with congenital heart disease. *Am J Cardiol* 2000;85:636–640.

86. Hoyer MH, Leon RA, Fricker FJ. Transcatheter closure of modified Blalock-Taussig shunt with the Gianturco-Grifka vascular occlusion device. *Catheter Cardiovasc Intervent* 1999;48:365–367.

87. Ing FF, Recto MR, Saidi A, et al. A method providing bi-directional control of coil delivery in occlusion of patent ductus arteriosus with shallow ampulla and Pott's shunt. *Am J Cardiol* 1997;79:1561–1563.

88. Lane GK, Lucas VW, et al. Percutaneous coil occlusion of ascending aorta to pulmonary artery shunts. *Am J Cardiol* 1998;81:1389–1391.

89. Wilde RPA, Walt I. Congenital coronary artery fistulae: six new cases with a collective review. *Clin Radiol* 1980;31:301–311.

90. Baltaxe HA, Wixson D. The incidence of congenital anomalies of the coronary arteries in the adult population. *Radiology* 1977;122:47–52.

91. Levin DC, Fellows KE, Abrahams HL. Hemodynamically significant primary anomalies of the coronary arteries. *Circulation* 1978;58:25–34.

92. Reidy JF, Anjos RT, Qureshi SA, et al. Transcatheter embolization in the treatment of coronary artery fistulas. *J Am Coll Cardiol* 1991;18:187–192.

93. Meyer MH, Stephenson HE, Keats TE, et al. Coronary artery resection for giant aneurismal enlargement and arteriovenous fistula. *Am Heart J* 1967;74:603–613.

94. Haberman JH, Howard ML, Johnson ES. Rupture of the coronary sinus with hemopericardium. *Circulation* 1963;28:1143–1144.

95. Morgan JR, Forker AD, O'Sullivan MJ Jr, et al. Coronary arterial fistulas. *Am J Cardiol* 1972;30:432–436.

96. Bishop JO, Mathur VS, Guinn GA. Congenital coronary artery fistula with infarction. *Chest* 1974;65:233–234.

97. Liberthson RR, Sagar K, Berkoben JP, et al. Congenital coronary arteriovenous fistula. *Circulation* 1979;59:849–854.

98. Velvis H, Schmidt KG, Silverman NH, et al. Diagnosis of coronary artery fistula by two-dimensional echocardiography, pulsed Doppler ultrasound and color flow imaging. *J Am Coll Cardiol* 1989;14:968–976.

99. Kimball TR, Daniels SR, Meyer RA, et al. Color-flow mapping in the diagnosis of coronary artery fistula in the neonates: benefits and limitations. *Am Heart J* 1989;117:968–971.

100. St. John Sutton MG, Miller GAH, Kerr IH, et al. Coronary artery steal via large coronary artery to bronchial artery anastomosis successfully treated by operation. *Br Heart J* 1980;44:460–463.

101. Davidson PH, McKracken BH, McIlveen DJS. Congenital coronary arteriovenous aneurysm. *Br Heart J* 1965;17:569–572.

102. Neill C, Mounsey P. Auscultation in patent ductus arteriosus with a description of two fistulae simulating patent ductus. *Br Heart J* 1958;20:61–75.

103. McNamara JJ, Gross RE. Congenital coronary artery fistula. *Surgery* 1969;65:59–69.

104. Sherwood MC, Rockenhacher S, Colan SD, et al. Prognostic significance of clinically silent coronary artery fistulas. *Am J Cardiol* 1999;83:407–411.

105. Bennett JM, Marie E. Successful embolization of a coronary arterial fistula. *Int J Cardiol* 1989;23:405–406.

106. Strunk BL, Hieshema GB, Shafton EP. Percutaneous treatment of a congenital coronary arteriovenous malformation with micro-particle embolization. *Catheter Cardiovasc Diagn* 1991;22:133–136.

107. Perry SB, Rome J, Keane JF, et al. Transcatheter closure of coronary artery fistulas. *J Am Coll Cardiol* 1992;20:205–209.

108. Hakim F, Madani A, Goussous Y, et al. Transcatheter closure of a large coronary arteriovenous fistula using new Amplatzer Duct Occluder. *Catheter Cardiovasc Intervent* 1998;45:155–157.

109. Fuhrman BP, Bass JL, Castaneda-Zuniga W, et al. Coil embolization of congenital thoracic vascular anomalies in infants and children. *Circulation* 1984;70:285–289.

110. Petrosjan JS. Der transluminale verscheuss angeborener koronarer fistein. *Radiol Diagn* 1987;28:489–470.

111. Nguyen K, Myler RK, Hieshima G, et al. Treatment of coronary artery stenosis and coronary arteriovenous fistula by interventional cardiology techniques. *Catheter Cardiovasc Diagn* 1989;18:240–243.

112. Issenberg HJ. Transcatheter closure of coronary arterial fistula. *Am Heart J* 1990;120:1441–1443.

113. Moskowitz WB, Newkumet KM, Albrecht GT, et al. Case of steel versus steal: coil embolization of coronary arteriovenous fistula. *Am Heart J* 1991;121:909–911.

114. Latson LA, Forbes TJ, Cheatham JP. Transcatheter coil embolization of a fistula from the posterior descending coronary artery to the right ventricle in a two-year-old child. *Am Heart J* 1992;124:1624–1626.

115. Kienast W, Emmich K, Schultz J, et al. Coronary artery fistula. surgical or percutaneous embolization treatment? *Z Kardiol* 1993;82:436–442.

116. DeWolf D, Terriere M, DeWilde R, et al. Embolization of coronary fistula with controlled delivery platinum coil in a 2-year-old. *Pediatr Cardiol* 1994;15:308–310.

117. Quek SG, Wong J, Tay JSH, et al. Transcatheter embolization of coronary artery fistula with controlled release coils. *J Paediatr Child Health* 1996;32:542–544.

118. Harris WO, Andrews JC, Nichols DA, et al. Percutaneous transcatheter embolization of coronary arteriovenous fistulas. *Mayo Clin Proc* 1996;71:37–42.

119. Qureshi SA, Reidy JF, Alwi MB, et al. Use of interlocking detachable coil in embolization of coronary arteriovenous fistulas. *Am J Cardiol* 1996;78:110–113.

120. Ogoh Y, Akagi T, Abe T, et al. Successful embolization of coronary arteriovenous fistula using an interlocking detachable coil. *Pediatr Cardiol* 1997;18:152–155.

121. Wax DF, MaGee AG, Nykanen D, et al. Coil embolization of a coronary artery to pulmonary artery fistula from an antegrade approach. *Catheter Cardiovasc Diagn* 1997;42:68–69.

122. Vance MS. Use of platinum microcoils to embolized vascular abnormalities in children with congenital heart disease. *Pediatr Cardiol* 1998;19:145–149.

123. Descalzo Senorans S, Santos de Soto J, Gonzalez Garcia A, et al. Congenital coronary fistula to right ventricle: treatment with transcatheter coil embolization. *Rev Esp Cardiol* 1999;52:526–528.

124. Lee ML, Chaou WT. Successful transcatheter coil embolization of coronary artery fistula in an infant. *J Thorac Imaging* 2000;15:153–156.

125. McElhinney DB, Burch GH, Kung GC, et al. Echocardiographic guidance for transcatheter coil embolization of congenital coronary arterial fistulas in children. *Pediatr Cardiol* 2000;21:253–258.

126. Chopra V, Saxena A, Kothari SS, et al. Isolated coronary arteriovenous fistula. *Indian J Pediatr* 2000;67:661–664.

127. Haneda N, Miura T, Taketani T. Transcatheter coil closure of a coronary artery fistula in a 2-year-old child. *Pediatr Int* 2000;42:570–572.

128. Hartnell GG, Jordon SC. Balloon embolization of a coronary arterial fistula. *Int J Cardiol* 1990;29:381–383.

129. Doorey AJ, Sullivan KL, Levin DC. Successful percutaneous closure of a complex coronary-to-pulmonary artery fistula using a detachable balloon: benefits of intraprocedural physiologic and angiographic assessment. *Catheter Cardiovasc Diagn* 1991;23:23–27.

130. Krabill KA, Hunter DW. Transcatheter closure of congenital coronary arterial fistula with a detachable balloon. *Pediatr Cardiol* 1993;14:176–178.

131. Skimming JW, Gessner IH, Victorica BE, et al. Percutaneous transcatheter occlusion of coronary artery fistula using detachable balloon. *Pediatr Cardiol* 1995;16:38–41.

132. Mavroudis C, Backer CL, Rocchini AP, et al. Coronary fistulas in infants and children: a surgical review and discussion of coil embolization. *Ann Thorac Surg* 1997;63:1235–1242.

133. Kirklin JW, Barrat-Boyes BG. *Cardiac surgery*. New York: John Wiley, 1987:945–955.

134. DeParades CG, Pierce WS, Johnson DG, et al. Pulmonary sequestration in infants and children: a 20-year experience and review of the literature. *J Pediatr Surg* 1970;5:136–147.

135. Neill CA, Ferencz C, Sabisten DC, et al. The familial occurrence of hypoplastic right lung with systemic arterial supply and venous drainage "Scimitar syndrome." *Bull Johns Hopkins Hosp* 1960;167:1–21.

136. Mardini MK, Rao PS. Scimitar syndrome: experience with four patients and review of literature. *Arab J Med* 1984;3:13–23.

137. Dickinson DF, Galloway RW, Massey R, et al. Scimitar syndrome in infancy: role of embolization of systemic arterial supply to right lung. *Br Heart J* 1982;47:468–472.

138. Park ST, Yoon CH, Sung K, et al. Pulmonary sequestration in a newborn infant: treatment with arterial embolization. *J Vasc Intervent Radiol* 1998;9:668–670.

139. Tokel K, Boyvat F, Varan B. Coil embolization of pulmonary sequestration in two infants: a safe alternative to surgery. *Am J Radiol* 2000;175:993–995.

140. Cobby MJD, Culling W, Jordan SC, et al. Balloon embolization of a congenital arterio-venous fistula between the internal mammary artery and a portal vein radicle. *Br J Radiol* 1989;62:371–373.

141. Gerson LP. Arteriovenous fistulae. In: Garson A, Jr, Bricker JT, Fisher DJ, et al., eds. *The science and practice of pediatric cardiology*. Philadelphia: Lea Febiger, 1990:1471–1481.

142. Miranda AA, Hill JA, Mickle JP, et al. Balloon occlusion of an internal mammary artery to anterior interventricular vein fistula. *Am J Cardiol* 1990;65:257–258.

143. Slack MC, Jedeikin R, Jones JS. Transcatheter coil closure of right pulmonary artery to left atrial fistula in an ill neonate. *Catheter Cardiovasc Intervent* 2000;50:330–333.

144. Fellows KE, Khaw KT, Schuster S, et al. Bronchial artery embolization in cystic fibrosis: technique and long-term results. *J Pediatr* 1979;95:959–963.

145. Kaufman S, Kan JS, Mitchell SE, et al. Embolization of systemic to pulmonary artery collaterals in the management of hemoptysis in pulmonary atresia. *Am J Cardiol* 1988;58:1130–1132.

146. Hofbeck M, Wild F, Singer H. Successful termination of acute pulmonary hemorrhage in a patient with pulmonary atresia and ventricular septal defect by coil embolization of a systemic-to-pulmonary collateral artery. *Z Kardiol* 1993;82:384–387.

147. Golej J, Trittenwein G, Marx M, et al. Aortopulmonary collateral artery embolization during postoperative extracorporal membrane oxygenation after arterial switch procedure. *Artif Organs* 1999;23:1038–1040

Catheter Based Devices: For the Treatment of Non-coronary Cardiovascular Diseases in Adults and Children. Edited by P. Syamasundar Rao and Morton J. Kern, Lippincott Williams & Wilkins, Philadelphia © 2003.

46

DEVICES IN THE MANAGEMENT OF ARRHYTHMIAS

PREBEN BJERREGAARD

Electrical stimulation on a chronic basis as treatment of a cardiac disorder is best known from pacemaker therapy of patients with various forms of bradycardia and heart block, and is well known to all physicians. Therefore this chapter will not discuss it. Instead, the focus will be on more advanced applications of devices using permanent transvenous implantation of intracardiac electrode-catheters for treatment of not only ventricular tachyarrhythmias but also congestive heart failure and atrial tachyarrhythmias. The goal for many companies making these devices is to incorporate all these applications of electrical stimulation into a single integrated cardiac rhythm management system, which would create a unique opportunity to tailor therapy to individual patients simply by programming the device after implantation. The following discussion focuses on various forms of electrical stimulation therapy, which currently are separate entities but could be part of a single unit.

IMPLANTABLE DEFIBRILLATOR

The use of the implantable cardioverter defibrillator (ICD) in preventing sudden cardiac death from ventricular tachyarrhythmias has produced dramatic improvement in the prognosis for patients at high risk for sudden cardiac death (SCD), which claims between 400,000 and 600,000 lives annually in the United States alone.

The inventor of the ICD, Michel Mirowski, died in 1990 at the age of 65 years. In 1968 he presented his first data and vision for the future with a "standby automatic defibrillator" (1). The first human implantation took place in 1980, and FDA approval was obtained in 1985. Since 1996, dual-chamber ICDs with the capability of atrio-ventricular (AV) synchronized pacing have been available (2).

Preben Bjerregaard: Professor of Medicine, Director, Section of Electrophysiology and Arrhythmia Division of Cardiology, Saint Louis University School of Medicine, Saint Louis University Hospital, Saint Louis, Missouri

The first approved device was nonprogrammable. Its volume was 150 cm^3 and it weighed 240 g. It had an expected longevity of 18 months. Today's single-chamber devices are approximately 40 cm^3, weigh 90 g, and are highly programmable while supporting a wide range of testing and diagnostic features (3). Some have an expected longevity of 6 to 8 years. The smaller size has led to almost 100% infraclavicular (pectoral) subcutaneous implantation (4). The case material is hermetically sealed titanium, and the power derives from lithium-silver vanadium oxide. The basic single-chamber ICD uses a single right ventricular (RV) endocardial electrode with a biphasic shock delivered between a coil electrode in the RV and the active "can" of the ICD. If needed, a second coil electrode can be placed in the superior vena cava either as a second coil on a single lead or as a single coil on a second lead. Dual-chamber devices require in addition an atrial pacing/sensing lead. (See a bi-ventricular pacemaker in Figure 46.1.) When an arrhythmia, which requires treatment, is detected, a 30- to 40-J shock is delivered within 10 seconds. The shock size is programmable and can be tailored to the individual patient according to the defibrillatory threshold (DFT), which is the smallest amount of energy necessary to defibrillate induced ventricular fibrillation during implantation. It is usually recommended that the output be programmed at least 10 J above the DFT.

Sensing

Separate sensing amplifiers are used for the atria and the ventricles, which is important to the proper device function as both a pacemaker and a defibrillator. Some systems have an automatic gain-controlled sensing system; others have a manually programmed sensing range. An Achilles heal of many systems is how to approach the use of blanking periods and refractory periods, which are used to minimize undersensing and oversensing, without adversely affecting the device's ability to classify certain types of arrhythmias and thereby resulting in inappropriate therapy.

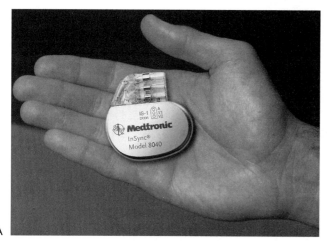

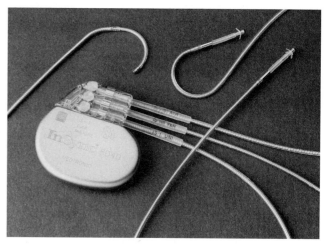

A   B

FIGURE 46.1. Bi-ventricular pacemaker. **A:** Showing the size of the device compared to an adult human hand. **B:** Showing the device connected to the 3 leads: (from left to right) the coronary sinus (left ventricular) lead, the right atrial lead, and the right ventricular lead.

Arrhythmia Detection

Bradycardia detection is based upon a beat-by-beat analysis of the timing relationship between the ventricular events, atrial events, and escape time-outs for each chamber. Tachyarrhythmia detection is based upon analysis of the incoming signals over a specified number of beats or a period of time. First of all, a percentage of ventricular intervals needs to be faster than a specified rate limit. Then a variety of detection enhancements—including abrupt or slow onset of the tachycardia, stability of the rhythm, and some type of morphology assessment—comes into play. Dual-chamber devices offer a great advantage in differentiating between atrial and ventricular tachyarrhythmias using atrial rate to ventricular rate comparisons (5). If the ventricular rate is faster than the atrial rate, it is assumed that the ventricular rhythm is ventricular in origin and should be treated. Sustained rate duration is a safety enhancement that will override other detection enhancements that can withhold therapy. After a programmable period of time, this feature will allow the device to override all other detection enhancements and deliver therapy.

Bradycardia Therapy

ICDs also function as common pacemakers. Gradually, most of the features seen in pacemakers, such as rate responsiveness, rate smoothing, and mode switching, have been incorporated (6).

Ventricular Tachytherapy

In addition to programmable shocks, the ICD can deliver programmable antitachycardia pacing (ATP). This is mainly used to treat hemodynamically stable monomorphic ventricular tachycardia (VT). A sequence of fast ventricular stimuli ("burst") is delivered during tachycardia and often can terminate VT before the patient even realizes there is a problem. In this setting, low-energy shocks (3 to 5 J) may also be effective and prevent the patient from getting painful high-energy shocks.

Diagnostic Storage Capabilities

Current ICDs not only offer an array of diagnostic storage features that have proven very valuable in patient management, but also provide new insight into the mechanism of how ventricular tachyarrhythmias are initiated. Real-time recording of the intracardiac electrogram is available with signal interpretation channels, which will show how the ICD interprets the electrical activity of the heart during its normal rhythm, and similar recordings are stored of arrhythmic events leading to ICD therapy. R-R intervals (distance between two heart beats) are available from immediately before, during and after an arrhythmic event with a graphical display of R-R cycle length over time for each arrhythmic episode (Figure 46.2).

Additionally, ICDs contain information about battery status, lead integrity, and need for bradycardia pacing. An ICD usually needs to be replaced whenever the battery voltage gets below a certain level or the time it takes for the battery's to form the capacitors to full capacity (charge time) exceeds a certain number of seconds specific for each type of device. Some devices have audible tones that will alert the patient in case of system malfunction detected by the device itself.

Implantation Technique

With the advent of transvenous ICD lead systems, the non-thoracotomy approach with a significantly lower periopera-

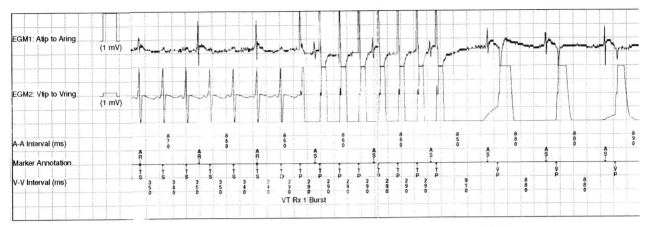

FIGURE 46.2. Antitachycardia pacing (ATP) for episode of ventricular tachycardia followed by AV synchronous pacing. EGM1 is the atrial electrogram showing an atrial rate of 72 beats/min. EGM2 is the ventricular electrogram showing a ventricular rate before ATP of 175 beats/min. The marker channel underneath the electrograms gives the AA and VV intervals along with annotations to each beat.

tive mortality has been established as the preferred technique in ICD implantation (4). Initially, the large size of the ICD devices required that the pulse generator be implanted in an abdominal site, which entailed subcutaneous lead tunneling from the infraclavicular area. However, with the availability of smaller devices it is feasible to implant the ICDs safely in the thorax. The endocardial lead(s) is/are inserted preferably via a cephalic vein cutdown or by subclavian puncture with the pocket for the subcutaneously placed ICD. In patients with a thin layer of subcutaneous tissue the pocket may be placed prepectorally (7). Most implantations are performed by electrophysiologists in the electrophysiology laboratory under conscious sedation. VF is induced at least twice by either low-energy shock on a T-wave or burst-pacing and in order to make sure that the device is sensing appropriately and can defibrillate with a shock at least 10 J below the maximum output for the device.

CLINICAL TRIALS INVOLVING ICDS

In the 1980s the use of ICDs was based on clinical experience from large centers and the benefit of therapy was so obvious that many electrophysiologists considered it unethical to even consider a randomized trial against other effective therapies. Others felt, however, that such trials would be necessary to define the role of the ICD in the treatment of patients at high risk of sudden cardiac death. In the 1990s several such studies were performed (8–14) using the ICD both as secondary and as primary prophylaxis against SCD (Tables 46.1 and 46.2). In all of these trials except the coronary artery bypass graft (CABG)-Patch trial, ICD therapy showed significant benefit compared with conventional therapy. The reason for the negative result in CABG-Patch may have been the low mortality (18%) in the control group and the possibility that CABG by eliminating ischemia greatly reduced the risk for SCD. In the Multicenter unsus-

TABLE 46.1. ICD THERAPY IN SECONDARY PROPHYLAXIS AGAINST SCD

	AVID	CASH	CIDS
Patient population	Primary VF; or VT with syncope; or VT with symptoms + EF <41%; or VT with BP <80 mm Hg and EF <41%	Sudden cardiac death survivors with documented ventricular tachyarrythmias	Documented VF: or cardiac arrest or sustained VT with hemodynamic collapse
Randomization	ICD or Class III antiarrhythmic drugs (primarily amiodarone)	ICD or treatment with amiodarone, propafenone, or metoprolol	ICD or treatment with amiodarone
Primary end point	Total (all-cause) mortality	Total (all-cause) mortality	Total (all-cause) mortality
Result	39% reduction in mortality for ICD patients compared with patients managed with Class III antiarrhythmic drugs	38% reduction in mortality for ICD patients compared with patients receiving amiodarone or metoprolol	20% reduction in mortality for ICD patients compared with patients receiving amiodarone

AVID, antiarrhythmia versus implantable defibrillators; CASH, cardiac arrest study, Hamburg; CIDS, Canadian implantable defibrillator study; EF, ejection fraction; ICD, implantable cardioverter defibrillators; SCD, sudden cardiac death; VF, ventricular fibrillation; VT, ventricular tachycardia.

TABLE 46.2. ICD THERAPY IN PRIMARY PROPHYLAXIS AGAINST SCD

	MADIT	CABG-PATCH	MUSTT
Patient population	Prior MI and EF <86%, NYHA Class I–III and nonsustained VT	Coronary bypass surgery, EF <86%, positive signal-averaged ECG	Coronary artery disease, EF <41%, asymptomatic nonsustained VT
Randomization	ICD or conventional medical therapy	ICD or no ICD	After positive EP study: EP-guided therapy, including ICD or no Rx
Primary end point	Total (all-cause) mortality	Total (all-cause) mortality	Cardiac arrest or death from arrhythmia
Result	54% reduction in mortality for ICD patients compared with conventionally managed patients	No statistically significant difference in mortality between the two groups	27% reduction in cardiac arrest or death from arrhythmia in EP-guided therapy group compared with no Rx

CABG-PATCH, Coronary Artery Bypass Graft Patch Trial; ECG, electrocardiogram; EP, electrophysiology; ICD, implantable cardioverter defibrillator; MI, myocardial infarction; MADIT, Multicenter Automatic Defibrillator Implantation Trial; MUSTT, Multicenter Unsustained Tachycardia Trial; NYHA, New York Heart Association; Rx, treatment; SCD, sudden cardiac death; VT, ventricular tachycardia.

tained tachycardia trial (MUSTT) it is important to emphasize that the 5-year rate of cardiac arrest or death from arrhythmia was only 9% among patients assigned to EP-guided therapy that received an ICD. This contrasted with 37% among those who did not receive an ICD ($p < .001$) and constituted a reduction in mortality of 75%. Results from most of these trials have been incorporated in current guidelines for ICD therapy. On an average, the reduction in 2-year mortality by ICD therapy in primary prevention trials (efficacy of ICD therapy) has been 51% and in secondary prevention trials, 29% with an efficiency of ICD therapy as primary prevention of 14% and as secondary prevention of 6% over a 2-year period. In this high-risk population on an average one in every ten implantations will be lifesaving within the first 2 years of implantation.

GUIDELINES AND RECOMMENDATIONS FOR ICD THERAPY

As a general rule ICD therapy should be restricted to those well-defined categories of high-risk patients who are most likely to benefit from ICD implantation in terms of a significant survival benefit (14). Looking at it from an economic perspective, based on current trial-based evidence the cost-effectiveness of ICD therapy varies between $115,000 and $145,000 per life-year gained when used for secondary prevention and approximately $27,000 per life-year gained when used for primary prevention (15). Unfortunately, there is a great difference in access to the device in different countries, with approximately 80% of the estimated 65,000 ICDs implanted worldwide being implanted in the United States, where the implantation rate is 120 per million population compared with 10 per million in the United Kingdom and France. The ACC/AHA guidelines for implantation of ICDs from 1998 specifically mention

four categories of patients where there is evidence and/or general agreement that implantation of an ICD is beneficial, useful, and effective:

1. Cardiac arrest due to VF or VT not due to a transient or reversible cause.
2. Spontaneous sustained VT.
3. Syncope of undetermined origin with clinically relevant hemodynamically significant sustained VT of VF induced at electrophysiologic study when drug therapy is ineffective, not tolerated, or not preferred.
4. Nonsustained VT with coronary disease, prior MI, LV dysfunction, and inducible VF or sustained VT at electrophysiologic study that is not suppressible by a class I antiarrhythmic drug.

In addition, ICDs are used in some specific categories of patients with diseases known to have a high incidence of SCD, such as arrhythmogenic right ventricular dysplasia, Brugadas syndrome, hypertrophic obstructive cardiomyopathy, and Long QT syndrome.

Studies in progress are looking at populations at high risk for SCD based more upon LV dysfunction than on the presence of arrhythmias, since a low EF in most studies has been the strongest predictor of SCD (16).

ATRIAL DEFIBRILLATION

Atrial fibrillation is the most common arrhythmia resulting in hospital admission and often treated by 200-360 J external DC-shocks in order to restore normal sinus rhythm. It has been shown, however, that internal DC shocks delivered through electrode catheters placed in the right atrium and the coronary sinus are more successful at much lower energy levels (1 to 6 J) (17). This has led to the introduction of implantable atrial defibrillators either as stand-alone device (METRIX Atrioverter system (InControl, Inc.) or as part of a combined dual-chamber system (Jewel AF 7250, Medtronic, Inc.). The METRIX system consists of a low-output (6 J) atrial defibrillator with a volume of 53 cm³ and weight of 79 g, and three leads (a pair of defibrillation leads in the right atrium and the coronary sinus and a separate right ventricular lead for ventricular pacing and sensing). The device can operate in automatic and patient-activated mode. It detects atrial fibrillation and delivers R-wave synchronized shocks. In clinical trials AF was detected with 100% specificity and 96% sensitivity. No ventricular proarrhythmia has been observed, and therapy has been successful in approximately 90% of patients. Initially, this device was used only in hospital settings, but recently the first report of ambulatory use was published (18). In 48 patients the atrial defibrillator restored sinus rhythm in 368 of 388 episodes of atrial fibrillation (95%) with no ventricular proarrhythmia. A questionnaire evaluating the impact of ambulatory therapy showed high patient satisfaction with only moderate discomfort. The Jewel AF is an atrioventricular pacemaker defibrillator with a volume of 55 cm³ and a weight of 93 g that may use up to three transvenous leads: ventricular, right atrial, coronary sinus, and/or subcutaneous patch in any desired combination (19). In addition to DC shock therapy that is programmable from 0.4 to 27 J, treatments available for atrial arrhythmias include the following (5):

1. Preventive therapies: antibradycardia pacing (AAI, DDI, DDD with mode switch), atrial rate stabilization, and temporary high-rate post-AF atrial overdrive pacing.
2. Pacing therapies of atrial tachycardia/atrial flutter (burst, ramp, and high-frequency 50 Hz).

Also this device can be programmed to automatic or patient-activated modes. Automatic therapies have programmable options of day, time to start therapy, and a limit of the number of shocks per day. The device has the ability to store 60 pre- and posttherapy events, and this feature has already been able to provide a lot of new information about the natural history of atrial tachyarrhythmias, which cannot be based on symptoms alone, because many events are asymptomatic.

Patients with symptomatic recurrences of long-lasting episodes of AF, despite the use of antiarrhythmic drug therapy, represent potential candidates for atrial defibrillator therapy. The optimum frequency of recurrence is probably between weekly and every 2 or 3 months. To date it is unclear whether AF patients provided with such a device will be of lower risk for stroke. In addition, cost-effectiveness and improvement in quality of life must be demonstrated before automatic atrial defibrillation by an implantable device will be an acceptable form of therapy for paroxysmal AF.

BI-VENTRICULAR PACING FOR HEART FAILURE

Emerging data support the novel use of pacemakers as therapy for patients with symptomatic congestive heart failure (CHF) in the setting of dilated cardiomyopathy and intraventricular conduction delay (IVCD), especially LBBB (20). IVCD can cause an inefficient pattern of contraction in which segments of the ventricles contract at different times, leading to diminished contractile performance, mitral valve regurgitation, and a shortened diastole. In addition, IVCD identifies a heart failure patient at increased mortality risk and is observed in up to 30% of patients with dilated cardiomyopathy. Pacemakers capable of simultaneous stimulation of both ventricles may improve ventricular performance by a variety of mechanisms, including the following:

1. Restoration of ventricular contractile synchrony.
2. Resynchronization of ventricular septal motion.
3. Pacing-induced decrease in atrioventricular valve regurgitation.
4. Pacing-related increase in ventricular diastolic filling time.

The greatest benefit has been observed in patients with LBBB, and the most important technical component is placement of the left ventricular pacing electrode. In the earliest studies left ventricular epicardial stimulation was accomplished via a small thoracotomy, but lately specially designed coronary sinus electrode catheters (EASYTRAK; Guidant, Inc.) have been used and placed with good success in a coronary sinus branch, preferably at the lateral wall of the left ventricle. In their chronic implant position, leads implanted in this way can stimulate the myocardium through the coronary vein wall. The obvious advantage of this technique is the reduction in surgical risk, procedure complexity, and elimination of the need for general anesthesia. Bi-ventricular pacemakers (Figure 46.1) are now available and at least two manufacturers have obtained FDA approval for a combined ICD and bi-ventricular pacing device. In patients with LBBB and normal AV conduction ventricular synchronization can be accomplished without a right ventricular lead (atrial synchronous LV pacing) (21).

The impression from a growing number of clinical trials conducted so far is that bi-or left ventricular pacing can ameliorate symptoms and improve quality of life in approximately two-thirds of patients with dilated cardiomyopathy, NYHA functional class III and IV, and QRS greater than 120 msec, but it is still unknown whether it will improve long-term prognosis for these patients, unless combined with ICD capabilities.

COMPLICATIONS

Complications seen with ICD implantation are no different from those seen with pacemaker implantation, where the acute complication rate clearly is related to the introducer method of vein access and operator activity and experience. In the AVID trial (8), where 507 patients received an ICD (93% nonthoracotomy lead system), the 30-day mortality was 2.4%, which was less than in the medically treated group (3.5%). The rate of nonfatal complications of implantation was 5.7%. Bleeding requiring reoperation or transfusion occurred in six patients (1%), and serious hematomas occurred in 13 (2.5%). Infections were seen in ten patients (2%); pneumothorax, in eight (1.6%); and cardiac perforation, in one (0.2%). Early dislodgment or migration of leads occurred in three patients. The first attempt at implantation of the ICD without thoracotomy was unsuccessful in five patients—in four because of excessive high DFT and in one because of cardiac perforation. Three of these five patients subsequently underwent a successful implantation procedure. Late complications are mainly skin erosion, infection, conductor fracture, and insulation failure, which all may require lead extraction. In a French study (22) 15 ICD leads were removed in 11 patients with only one complication in terms of subclavian vein thrombosis, but the experience from larger studies involving pacing electrodes found life-threatening complications to extraction in 2.5% and a mortality of 0.6%. In 8% the lead was only partially removed, and in 6% extraction failed (23).

DISCUSSION AND CONCLUSION

Electrical stimulation techniques for management of cardiac disorders have undergone significant developments since implantation of the first pacemaker in 1958, and new indications are constantly emerging. Future devices are likely to be hybrids of current brady and tachy devices with the ability to provide very comprehensive treatment of both rhythm disorders and heart failure. Cardiac contractility and ventricular filling time can be monitored by impedance measurement technique and heart rate and pacing modality automatically adjusted for optimization of cardiac output. Calculations of heart rate variability (HRV) are readily available and when monitored over a prolonged period of time would afford the clinician data to assess the effect of both device and pharmacologic therapy. Certain changes in HR, HRV, and frequency of ectopic beats have been seen before episodes of VT and VF and could form the basis for preventive measures such as fast pacing to avert the onset of an arrhythmia. Finally, a pacing-lead might contain drug ports through which a variety of agents (e.g., antiarrhythmics, diuretics, or inotropic drugs) could be delivered in response to information collected by the ICD. Diuretics may be administered according to hemodynamic parameters and an antiarrhythmic drug given when certain tachyarrhythmias would develop. The result should be optimization of overall cardiac care for patients. It would seem just as important, however, to make the industry interested in making available an ICD for prophylactic use and able to provide basic defibrillator therapy in a cost-effective way.

REFERENCES

1. Mirowski M, Mover MM, Staewen WS, et al. Standby automatic defibrillator: an approach to prevention of sudden coronary death. *Arch Intern Med* 1970;126:158–161.
2. Higgens SL, Pak JP, Barone J, et al. The first year experience with the dual chamber ICD's. *Pacing Clin Electrophysiol* 2000;23:18–25.
3. Sarter BH, Callans DJ, Gottlied CD, et al. Implantable defibrillator storage capabilities: evolution, current status and future utilization. *Pacing Clin Electrophysiol* 1998;21:1287–1298.
4. Bollmann A, Marx A, Sathavorn C, et al. Patient discomfort following pectoral defibrillator implantation using conscious sedation. *Pacing Clin Electrophysiol* 1999;22:212–215.
5. Dijkman B, Wellens HJJ. Diagnosis and therapy of atrial tachyarrhythmias in the dual chamber implantable cardioverter defibrillator. *J Cardiovasc Electrophysiol* 2000;11:1196–1205.
6. Elliot L, Gilkerson J. Advances in dual chamber implantable cardioverter-defibrillators. *J Interven Cardiol* 1998;11:187–196.
7. Manolis AS, Chiladakis J, Vassilikos V, et al. Pectoral cardioverter defibrillators: comparison of pectoral and submuscular implantation techniques. *Pacing Clin Electrophysiol* 1999;22:469–478.
8. The Antiarrhythmics Versus Implantable Defibrillators (AVID) Investigators. A comparison of antiarrhythmic-drug therapy with implantable defibrillators in patients resuscitated from near-fatal ventricular arrhythmias. *N Engl J Med* 1997;337:1576–1583.
9. Siebels J, Kuck K-H, CASH Investigators. Implantable cardioverter defibrillator compared with antiarrhythmic drug treatment in cardiac arrest survivors (the Cardiac Arrest Study Hamburg). *Am Heart J* 1994;127:1139–1144.
10. Sheldon R, Connolly S, Krahn A, et al. Identification of patients most likely to benefit from implantable cardioverter-defibrillator therapy. The Canadian Implantable Defibrillator Study. *Circulation* 2000;101:1660–1664.
11. Moss AJ, Hall WJ, Cannom DS, et al. Improved survival with an implanted defibrillator in patients with coronary disease at high risk for ventricular arrhythmia. *N Engl J Med* 1996;335:1933–1940.
12. Bigger JT Jr, for the Coronary Artery Bypass Graft (CABG) Patch Trial Investigators. Prophylactic use of implanted cardiac defibrillators in patients at high risk for ventricular arrhythmias after coronary-artery bypass graft surgery. *N Engl J Med* 1997;337:1569–1575.
13. Buxton AE, Lee KL, Fisher JD, et al. A randomized study of the prevention of sudden death in patients with coronary artery disease. *N Engl J Med* 1999;341:1882–1890.
14. Gregoratos G, Cheitlin MD, Conill A, et al. ACC/AHA Guidelines for Implantation of Cardiac Pacemakers and Arrhythmia Devices. A Report of the American College of Cardiology/American Heart Association Task Force on Practice Guidelines (Committee on Pacemaker Implantation). *J Am Coll Cardiol* 1998;31:1175–1209.
15. Noorani HZ, Connolly SJ, Talajic M, et al. Canadian Coordinating Office for Health Technology Assessment. Implantable cardioverter defibrillator (ICD) therapy for sudden cardiac death. *Can J Cardiol* 2000;16:1293–1324.
16. Moss AJ. Implantable cardioverter defibrillator therapy: the sickest patients benefit the most. *Circulation* 2000;101:1638–1649.
17. Levy S, Richard P, Gueunoun M, et al. Low energy cardioversion of spontaneous atrial fibrillation. Immediate and long term results. *Circulation* 1997;96:253–259.
18. Daoud EG, Timmermans C, Fellows C, et al. Initial clinical experience with ambulatory use of an implantable atrial defibrillator for conversion of atrial fibrillation. *Circulation* 2000;102:1407–1413.

19. Jung W, Luderitz B. Implantation of an arrhythmic management system for ventricular and supraventricular tachyarrhythmias. *Lancet* 1997;349:853–854.

20. Breithardt OA, Stellbrink C, Franke A, et al. Echocardiographic evidence of hemodynamic and clinical improvement in patients paced for heart failure. *Am J Cardiol* 2000;86(Suppl): 133K–137K.

21. Auricchio A, Klein H, Tackman B, et al. Transvenous biventricular pacing for heart failure: can the obstacles be overcome? *Am J Cardiol* 1999;83:136D–142D.

22. Le Franc P, Klug D, Jarwe M, et al. Extraction of endocardial implantable cardioverter-defibrillator leads. *Am J Cardiol* 1999; 84:187–191.

23. Sellers TD, Smith HJ, Fearnot NE. Intravascular lead extraction: technique, tips and U.S. database results. *Pacing Clin Electrophysiol* 1993;16:1538–1548.

Catheter Based Devices: For the Treatment of Non-coronary Cardiovascular Diseases in Adults and Children. Edited by P. Syamasundar Rao and Morton J. Kern, Lippincott Williams & Wilkins, Philadelphia © 2003.

47

VENA CAVAL FILTERS IN THE PREVENTIVE MANAGEMENT OF PULMONARY EMBOLISM: CURRENT STATE OF THE ART

S. WILLIAM STAVROPOULOS

Pulmonary embolism (PE) is a major source of morbidity and mortality in the United States, accounting for approximately 140,000 deaths per year (1). Lower-extremity deep vein thrombosis (DVT) occurs in up to 5 million patients per year, and there are nearly 750,000 cases of nonlethal pulmonary embolus annually (2–5).

Standard therapy for PE and some forms of DVT remains anticoagulation with heparin followed by warfarin. This therapy can decrease the mortality of untreated PE from 30% to 2.5% (6). Iliofemoral DVT is more effectively treated with catheter-directed thrombolysis. There is a subset of patients for whom anticoagulation is either contraindicated or ineffective. These patients require mechanical interruption of the inferior vena cava (IVC).

IVC ligation was one of the initial surgical approaches to mechanical interruption of the IVC. This approach requires an extensive retroperitoneal dissection and general anesthesia. In addition, patients undergoing IVC ligation have problems associated with lower-extremity venous stasis and clinical failures ranging from 4% to 50% (7). Ligation of both common femoral veins is another surgical approach that resulted in recurrent PE in 10% to 26% of patients (8). This high incidence of recurrent PE is due to the development of collateral vessels following occlusion of the IVC or common femoral veins. IVC fenestration has been attempted, using suture or surgical clips. This maintained flow through the IVC and decreased the recurrent PE rate to 4%. However, this technique still requires major surgery, and problems with venous stasis continue to occur at unacceptably high rates (9).

Less invasive procedures have been developed to provide PE prophylaxis. Temporary placement of a balloon in the IVC has been tried. The main disadvantage of this approach is that the clot that has been trapped by the device may embolize to the pulmonary arteries once the balloon is deflated and removed (10). Initial IVC filters were large devices that required a venous cutdown to insert them. As technological advancements enabled these devices to be placed through smaller introducer sheaths, the larger IVC filters have been phased out and all the commonly available IVC filters can now be placed percutaneously. It is important to remember that the only function of IVC filters is to prevent PE. IVC filters do not treat PE or prevent or treat DVT. Filters are placed in the IVC, because 75% to 90% of pulmonary emboli originate from the lower extremities. The remainder of pulmonary emboli come from the right atrium and upper-extremity veins. This probably accounts for some of the cases of recurrent pulmonary emboli seen following IVC filter placement. Placement of superior vena cava (SVC) filters can be performed in the unique setting of symptomatic PE with no lower-extremity DVT and documented upper-extremity DVT.

INFERIOR VENA CAVAL FILTERS

Stainless Steel Greenfield Filter

The Stainless Steel Greenfield filter (SSGF) (Medi-tech, Boston Scientific Corp., Watertown, MA) was originally introduced in 1973 and was designed to be placed via a surgical cutdown. Percutaneous techniques for placement of this 24F device were soon developed (11). This filter forms a conical shape with six legs extending from a central hub. The legs have hooks at the base that allow for stabilization in the IVC. This filter is designed to be placed in a vena cava that measures up to 28 mm in diameter.

Thrombus is captured by the central portion of the cone, which allows flow of blood around the periphery of the filter. When the filter is 70% filled with clot, 50% of the cross-sectional diameter is preserved (12,13). The rates of recurrent PE following placement of this filter range between 2% and 5%. IVC patency rates have ranged

S. William Stavropoulos: Assistant Professor, Department of Radiology, University of Pennsylvania School of Medicine, Philadelphia, Pennsylvania

between 92% and 98% (14–16). The SSGF resists migration during MRI, however there is significant artifact. Because of the large 24F sheath needed to introduce the filter and the development of smaller-profile systems, few interventionalists currently use this filter.

Titanium Greenfield Filter

The titanium Greenfield Filter (TGF) (Medi-tech, Boston Scientific Corp., Watertown, MA) can be placed through a 12F sheath and was initially designed in 1987 to be placed percutaneously. This filter has a conical shape similar to that of its predecessor, the SSGF, and has similar properties with respect to recurrent PE and caval patency. The TGF is primarily placed through the right common femoral vein or right internal jugular vein. However, placement via the left internal jugular vein and left common femoral vein has been reported. This filter can be placed in a vena cava with up to a 28-mm diameter.

The initial version of this filter reported unacceptably high rates of filter migration and caval perforation. This was due to the anchoring hooks at the bottom of the legs. These hooks have been modified, and the incidence of filter migration and caval perforation has decreased (17,18). The TGF is MRI compatible and exhibits little artifact on MR images (19). Asymmetry of the legs of the TGF continues to be noticed following deployment. Whether leg asymmetry affects the clinical efficacy of this filter is debatable. The legs can be repositioned by gentle manipulation with an angled catheter; however, this increases the risk for migration and is not recommended by the manufacturer.

Stainless Steel Over-the-Wire Greenfield Filter

The stainless steel over-the-wire Greenfield filter (OTWG) (Medi-tech, Boston Scientific Corp., Watertown, MA) (Figure 47.1) was recently introduced with a 12F delivery sheath. This filter maintains the conical shape of the SSGF and may be used in vena caval sizes up to 28 mm. The OTWG is meant to be placed over a stiff guide wire that is included in the set. This stiff wire helps stabilize the filter during deployment and can help in navigating tortuous venous anatomy. With the over-the-wire design, the incidence of leg asymmetry has decreased compared with the other Greenfield filter designs. This filter is MRI compatible; however, because it is stainless steel, MR artifact does occur.

LGM Vena Tech Filter

The LGM Vena Tech Filter (LGM) (B Braun/Vena Tech, Evanston, IL) was designed in France and initially released in the United States in 1989, with a modified version released in 1991. This filter has a conical design similar to that of the Greenfield filter. However, side rails are attached to the filter, which contact the walls of the IVC and help center the

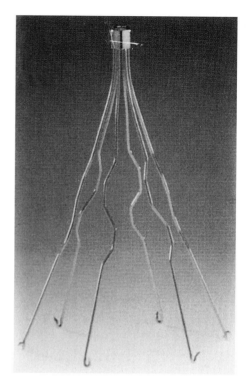

FIGURE 47.1. The stainless steel over-the-wire Greenfield filter (OTWG) (Medi-Tech, Boston Scientific Corp., Watertown, MA).

device. These side rails have small hooks that slightly penetrate the IVC wall and fix the filter in place. The filter is designed to be placed in caval sizes up to 28 mm.

The Vena Tech filter is made of a nonferromagnetic alloy called Phynox. It is MRI compatible and creates minimal artifact on MR images (20). This filter is deployed through a 10F sheath and is quite easy to use. Although it is preferred to use the right internal jugular or right common femoral vein for placement, the Vena Tech filter has been placed from the left side. The modified version of this filter released in 1991 decreased the incidence of filter migration and incomplete opening noted with the initial model (21). The Vena Tech filter is packaged so it can be placed from either a jugular or femoral approach using the same kit. A study by Crochet et al. described recurrent PE in 3.5% of patients and a caval patency rate of 92% at 2 years, 80% at 4 years, and 70% at 6 years (21).

Bird's Nest Filter

The Gianturco Bird's Nest Filter (BNF) (Cook, Inc., Bloomington, IN) was the first filter designed specifically for percutaneous placement. It was released in 1982 and was modified in 1986 to correct problems causing proximal migration and prolapse. The BNF is deployed through a 12F delivery system and has two struts made of stainless steel, which fix to the caval wall via hooks. These struts are connected with four wires, which form a random wire mesh when finally deployed. This filter is MRI compatible, but it does create significant local artifact on MR images (22).

The unique design of the BNF provides an advantage in that this filter can be placed in patients with a caval diameter of up to 40 mm. In addition, each BNF kit can be placed from either the jugular or femoral approach. A disadvantage of the design is the length of the filter, which is 7 cm. This can limit the use of the BNF if a patient has a short segment of usable IVC. Also, placing the BNF requires more steps than are required by all the available filters, and its proper placement is the most operator dependent. Wires from the mesh can occasionally prolapse past the struts. This is cosmetically unappealing; however, the BNF retains its ability to capture thrombus in its prolapsed form (23). A multicenter trial consisting of 440 patients reported a caval occlusion rate of 2.9% and recurrent PE rate of 2.7% (24). The caval occlusion rates are suspected to be higher than this because most of the data from this study were obtained from clinical follow-up and questionnaires rather than from direct imaging of the IVC.

Simon Nitinol Filter

The Simon Nitinol IVC filter (SNF) (Nitinol Medical Technologies, Woburn, MA) has a 7F sheath introducer and is made of a nickel–titanium alloy. This nonferromagnetic alloy gives the filter a property of thermal memory that allows the filter to attain its preformed shape when it reaches body temperature. The SNF is MRI compatible and creates minimal artifact on MR images. The filter has an upper domelike structure made of seven petals. Six wires extend from the dome and embed into the caval wall with terminal hooks. The filter is 3.8 cm long and can be placed in patients with caval diameters up to 28 mm. The manufacturer suggests placing the SNF in a maximal caval diameter of 24 mm in patients who have surgery with general anesthesia planned within 2 weeks of placement.

Because of the small sheath size, this filter can be placed via an antecubital approach. Placing this filter from a left internal jugular or left common femoral approach is also easier than with some of the other filters. The SNF can tilt when placed in the IVC. This does not appear to decrease the clinical effectiveness of the filter (25). When placing the SNF from the transfemoral approach, it can jump caudally 1 to 2 cm. This usually is not clinically significant. However, it can be important when precise filter placement is needed. This jump can be compensated for by gently advancing the filter after the dome has been formed but before deploying the legs, or by slightly advancing the filter pusher, when performing the unsheathing maneuver. The rates of recurrent PE with the SNF are approximately 2%, and the rates of caval occlusion are between 7% and 9% (26–28). The caval occlusion rate is slightly higher than that with other IVC filters.

TrapEase Filter

The TrapEase Filter (Cordis Endovascular, Johnson & Johnson, Warren, NJ) (Figure 47.2) is one of three new IVC filters approved for use in the United States. This filter is also made from a nonferromagnetic nickel–titanium alloy, which gives it thermal memory properties similar to the SNF. The TrapEase has a six-pointed star configuration.

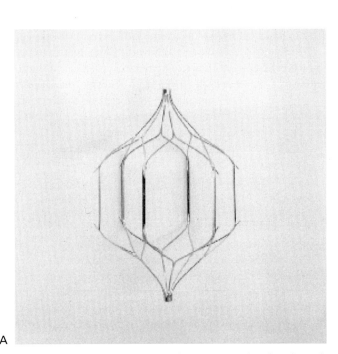

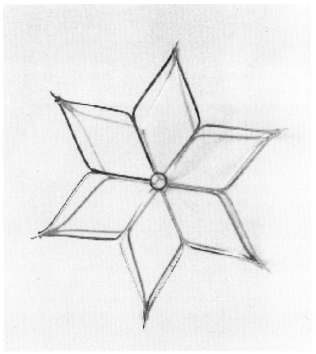

A   B

FIGURE 47.2. The TrapEase Filter (Cordis Endovascular, Johnson & Johnson, Warren, NJ) as seen in an AP view (**A**) and as seen from above (**B**).

A single kit can be used for either jugular or femoral deployment. This filter can be used in patients with caval diameters of up to 30 mm.

This filter is easy to deploy and has a 6F inner diameter introducer sheath, which is the smallest introducer system currently available. This allows the TrapEase to be deployed from the antecubital vein as well as the left internal jugular vein and left common femoral vein with relative ease compared with some of the other IVC filters described. The largest published series using the TrapEase is a multicenter European trial with 65 patients and 6 months' follow-up. No recurrent PE occurred, and only one asymptomatic filter thrombosis was detected at 6-month follow-up (29). Long-term data on recurrent PE rates and caval patency are unavailable with this filter. Those studies are currently ongoing.

Gunther Tulip Filter

Cook, Inc., recently introduced the Gunther Tulip IVC filter to the US market. This filter can be ordered for either femoral or jugular placement through an 8.5F sheath. This filter is FDA approved as a permanent filter; however, it is manufactured with a hook on the tip of it, and trials are currently being performed to evaluate this as a retrievable filter. Currently, it can be used as retrievable in an off-label manner. A snare is used to grab the hook, and a sheath can then be placed over the filter. At our institution, we have done this within 14 days of implantation and only after performing a cavogram to ensure that a large clot is not within the filter.

Vena Tech LP Filter

The Vena Tech LP filter was recently introduced by B Braun, as a low-profile version of the original Vena Tech. It can be placed from either the jugular or the femoral approach. A 7F sheath is used for placement. This filter is currently approved for placement in patients with caval diameters up to 28 mm, but an FDA application is pending for use in caval diameters up to 35 mm.

Temporary/Retrievable IVC Filters

Although the available permanent IVC filters are relatively safe and effective, there are certain patient populations for which a temporary or retrievable filter would be beneficial. Temporary filters are removed when no longer needed. A retrievable filter can be removed within a certain time period or may be left in place as a permanent filter. The patient populations that would benefit from a temporary IVC filter include young trauma patients, perioperative patients, pregnant patients, patients with a temporary contraindication to anticoagulation, and those patients undergoing DVT thrombolysis (30).

Currently, no temporary IVC filters are approved for use in the United States. As discussed earlier, the Gunther Tulip filter can be used as a retrievable filter on an off-label basis.

Outside the United States a variety of temporary and retrievable devices are currently in use. Lorch et al. recently reported results from a multicenter registry for temporary IVC filters. Three different types of filters were used in a total of 188 patients. Four patients died of PE with a filter in place. Filter thrombosis occurred 16% of the time, and filter dislocation occurred in 4.8% of patients (31).

One of the major drawbacks to temporary IVC filters is dealing with filter thrombosis before explantation. When a temporary filter traps thrombus, removing the filter can cause the thrombus to embolize to the pulmonary arteries. To prevent this, physicians can either place a permanent IVC filter above the temporary filter or perform thrombolysis using pharmacologic and mechanical techniques (31). Although there are clear advantages to temporary IVC filters, dealing with thrombus before explantation remains the Achilles heal of temporary IVC filters. New temporary filter designs will have to account for this problem.

PATIENT SELECTION

Indications for IVC Filter Placement

For patients with pulmonary embolus or lower-extremity deep vein thrombosis (DVT), standard therapy remains anticoagulation with intravenous heparin followed by oral warfarin. For patients with contraindications to anticoagulation, placement of IVC filters represents a safe alternative for PE prophylaxis. This would include patients with ongoing bleeding from any organ system, recent central nervous system hemorrhage, or noncompliance with drug therapy or follow-up. In addition, anticoagulation can be risky in patients for whom a small amount of undetected bleeding would cause significant morbidity, such as those with vascular brain metastases. A complication from anticoagulation therapy, such as thrombocytopenia or bleeding while in the therapeutic range, represents another contraindication to anticoagulation. It has been reported that approximately 20% of anticoagulated patients have complications directly related to anticoagulation therapy that requires that it be discontinued (14,32). IVC filters are indicated for patients suffering from recurrent PE or progressive DVT despite adequate anticoagulation. There is an 18% rate of recurrent PE in these patients (33,34). Two other groups in whom IVC filter placement is generally accepted are those with massive PE or limited cardiopulmonary reserve and DVT, as well as those with free-floating iliofemoral or IVC thrombus (Figure 47.3).

Prophylactic IVC filter placement involves placing an IVC filter in patients who are at increased risk for, but do not currently have, DVT or PE. This is a controversial indication but has been advocated by several authors (35,36). This patient population includes trauma patients and preoperative patients with DVT risk factors. When they are approved for use in the United States, temporary IVC filters would seem suited for these patient populations.

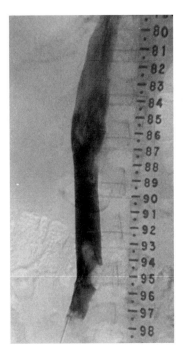

FIGURE 47.3. Floating thrombus extending into the IVC. An infrarenal IVC filter was placed through a right internal jugular vein puncture.

Contraindications to IVC Filter Placement

Few absolute contraindications to IVC filter placement exist. The inability to gain venous access or complete thrombosis of the IVC would preclude placement of an IVC filter. There are numerous relative contraindications to filter placement. Some patients with severe coagulopathy may not be candidates for percutaneous procedures. However, with the development of 6- and 7F delivery systems, we do not require complete reversal of anticoagulation before placing filters. Some interventionalists are resistant to placing IVC filters in patients with septic emboli or positive blood cultures. Because the effects of IVC filters beyond 15 to 20 years have not been completely established, placement of filters in young patients should be avoided if possible. If absolutely needed, it is generally suggested that Greenfield filters be placed in younger patients because the longest follow-up is available with this filter. Similarly, IVC filters should not be placed in pregnant patients, if possible. If a filter is needed in a pregnant patient, it should be placed in a suprarenal location because the expansion of the uterus can deform the filter and cause IVC damage. In addition, there is a slight decrease in radiation exposure to the fetus if a filter is placed at the suprarenal level.

IMPLANTATION TECHNIQUE

Venacavography

Before placing any of the filters, performing a venacavogram is critical. This is done whether the approach is from the jugular, femoral, or antecubital vein. Venacavography is done to evaluate the size and patency of the cava. The position of the renal veins and presence of IVC anomalies is also noted. Clinically relevant information is detected in 26% of venacavograms (37).

Before performing the cavogram, informed consent is obtained and the patient is kept without parental nutrition for at least 4 hours. A platelet count and coagulation profile are obtained. Appropriate conscious sedation and local anesthesia should also be given. The entry site is prepped and draped in the usual sterile fashion. Using a single-wall needle to gain access to the vein will decrease the chance of puncturing the artery. Ultrasound is always used to guide entry into the internal jugular vein and can be used if trouble is encountered during a common femoral vein approach. Once venous access is obtained, a small hand injection of contrast under fluoroscopy through a dilator or catheter should be done to exclude the presence of thrombus in the accessed vein. If significant thrombus is identified, an alternate access site should be selected.

Venacavography can then be performed using a 5F pigtail catheter placed with the side holes at the caval bifurcation. Some interventionalists perform venacavography exclusively from the left common femoral vein approach or place the catheter in the left common iliac vein when using the jugular approach, to decrease the chance of missing a caval anomaly. Use of a sizing catheter with radiopaque markers on the catheter facilitates measuring the cava, which is critical when selecting the proper filter to place. The BNF can be placed in patients with caval diameters up to 40 mm, while the TrapEase can be placed in IVCs with diameters up to 30 mm. The remainder of the filters must be placed in patients with caval diameters no greater than 28 mm. If iodinated contrast cannot be used due to patient allergy or increased creatinine, the venogram can be performed using gadolinium or carbon dioxide.

The renal veins appear as inflow defects on venacavogram (Figure 47.4). Noting the level of the renal veins is important because, if possible, IVC filters should be placed below the renal veins to decrease the incidence of renal vein thrombosis following clot capture or caval thrombosis. If there is any doubt about the location of the renal veins, selective injection of the renal veins should be performed. A suprarenal filter may need to be placed if there is thrombus in the IVC at or above the level of the renal veins (Figure 47.5). Placement of suprarenal filters has been described in pregnant women, as discussed earlier. Patients with an infrarenal IVC filter in place but with recurrent PE and no upper-extremity DVT can also benefit from suprarenal filters. Lastly, suprarenal filters are beneficial in patients with PE known to be originating from thrombus in the left ovarian vein.

Evaluating for IVC anomalies is important during venacavogram. IVC duplication occurs in 0.2% to 0.3% of patients (38). The left IVC typically terminates in the left renal vein. Patients with IVC duplication generally require filters in both the left and right IVCs because placement of a

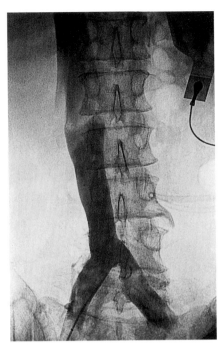

FIGURE 47.4. Normal cavagram showing inflow defects at the level of the renal veins.

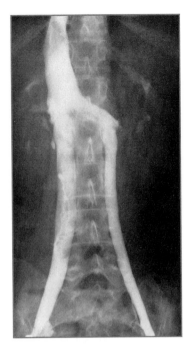

FIGURE 47.6. Cavogram demonstrating a duplicated IVC. Filters were placed in both the right IVC and the left IVC.

right IVC filter only protects the patient from pulmonary emboli originating from the left lower extremity (Figure 47.6).

Left-sided IVCs occur in 0.2% to 0.5% (38) of patients. This vessel usually crosses over to the right side of the abdomen at the level of the left renal vein and continues in the position of the normal right-sided renal and suprarenal segments of the IVC. Because the anatomy from the left

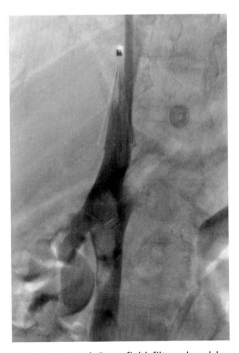

FIGURE 47.5. Suprarenal Greenfield filter placed because IVC thrombus was detected at the level of the renal veins.

side can be tortuous, placement of the more flexible SNF or TrapEase filters may be helpful in these patients.

The circumaortic left renal vein forms a venous ring around the aorta and has a prevalence of between 1.5% and 8.7% (39,40). The anterior segment of the ring connects with the IVC at the expected level of the left renal vein. The posterior segment connects to the IVC below the insertion of the anterior segment. Recognizing this anomaly is important, because the filter must be placed below the level of the lowest renal vein segment because this vein can act as a pathway for emboli to circumvent the IVC filter and pass to the lungs. For a similar reason, IVC filters must be placed below the level of the lowest renal vein in patients with accessory renal veins.

IVC Filter Insertion

Once the venocavagram is performed, the appropriate filter can be chosen and the tract can be dilated to accommodate the delivery sheath. Placing a ruler with radiopaque markings under the patient can facilitate placement of the filter by giving an easy reference point to mark the renal veins. Some operators prefer placement through the femoral vein. Others prefer a jugular approach. Being comfortable with both approaches allows the interventionalist more flexibility in dealing with a variety of patients. The femoral approach is more familiar to many interventionalists and may be better in terms of sterility and patient comfort. The right jugular approach provides a more direct route and allows the operator slightly better control of the filter during release because the delivery sheath is superior to the filter. In addition, a central line can easily be left in place following filter placement from a jugular approach. However, the risk of air embolism increases when using a jugular approach. The incidence of air embolism can be decreased by placing the patient in Trendelenburg position or by having the patient perform a Valsalva maneuver during placement of the delivery sheath and filter. Single kits allow placement of the Vena Tech, BNF, and TrapEase filters from either the jugular or the femoral approach, whereas separate femoral and jugular kits are made for the other filters.

When dilating the tract and placing the delivery sheath, it is important not to retract the wire or advance the introducer sheath when it is not over a guide wire. Doing either of these maneuvers can result in malposition of the filter, possibly in a renal, hepatic, or gonadal vein. Constant fluoroscopic guidance during this procedure is essential.

Although all the approved filters have relatively easy-to-follow instructions for placement, the steps vary between manufacturers. It is essential that the interventionalist have a thorough understanding of the specific instructions needed to place the chosen filter before starting the procedure. Once the filter has been placed, a repeat venacavagram should be performed to confirm proper placement. The sheath can then be removed and hemostasis achieved. A central line or PICC line can be left in place through the puncture site if it is clinically necessary.

After placement of the filter, the patient is kept at bed rest for frequent monitoring of the vital signs. Trained medical staff performs puncture site observation for at least 4 hours. The patient is instructed not to do any heavy lifting or to increase abdominal pressure for 24 hours.

RESULTS

If fluoroscopic guidance is used, a filter can be placed in a patent IVC in almost 100% of cases (41). Failed deployment is usually due to extensive thrombus in the IVC or the inability to access the IVC.

The published long-term results indicate that all the approved IVC filters are quite effective in preventing symptomatic recurrent PE. The rates for recurrent PE range from approximately 3% to 5% in published reports (32,42–45). These rates are based on clinical finding of PE, and objective imaging data in patients to detect symptomatic, as well as asymptomatic, PE is limited. In DVT patients without filters the rates of asymptomatic PE ranges from 35% to 51% (46,47). Although all the approved IVC filters are similarly effective in protecting patients from symptomatic PE, the rates of asymptomatic recurrent PE are largely unknown.

COMPLICATIONS

Complications from filter placement related to access include hematoma, arteriovenous fistula, venous thrombosis, arterial puncture, and IVC perforation. If the jugular vein is used, additional complications include air embolism and pneumothorax. With the 12F delivery systems, occlusive thrombosis has been reported in up to 10% of patients (41,43,48). This rate appears to be significantly less with the smaller 6- and 7F delivery systems.

Complications related to the device include filter migration, malposition, fracture, infection, IVC perforation, and failed deployment (Figure 47.7). The rates of filter malpo-

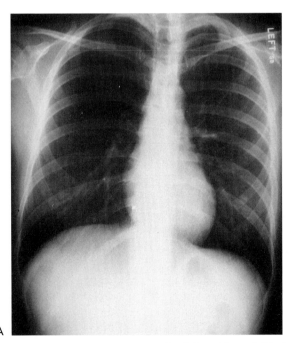
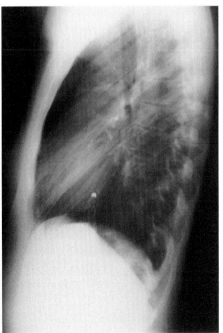

FIGURE 47.7. Posteroanterior (**A**) and lateral (**B**) chest x-ray demonstrating a Greenfield filter which has migrated to the junction of the IVC and right atrium.

sition can be greatly reduced with the use of fluoroscopic guidance for filter placement. A small amount of filter migration is common and is usually not of clinical significance. IVC filter migration into the right atrium and pulmonary artery has been reported and can be fatal (49). Techniques have been described to snare a migrated filter percutaneously and remove it through a large sheath. However, filters that have significantly migrated often need to be removed surgically (50,51). IVC filters can be dislodged by wires or catheters placed during venous access performed at a later time without fluoroscopic guidance. The incidence of this can be decreased by thorough documentation of filter position and good communication with the clinicians.

Caval occlusion following IVC filter placement can occur due to trapped thrombus in the filter or can be due to spontaneous thrombosis of the filter. While caval occlusion may not be clinically apparent because it happens gradually and collaterals have time to form, it can be a serious or life-threatening event. Although reports in the literature place the rate of symptomatic IVC occlusion generally between 2% and 10%, asymptomatic rates of caval occlusion can occur in up to 30% of patients (41,52–54).

DISCUSSION

Because no perfect IVC filter is available, it is important that the interventionalist be comfortable placing more than one filter. The decision on which filter to place is often based on operator preference and design differences between the IVC filters, because there is no significant evidence to suggest one filter has better clinical outcomes when compared with the others. The BNF, Vena Tech, and TrapEase filters can be obtained in a single kit that can be placed from either a jugular or femoral approach. When placing a filter from the left side, or from an antecubital approach, using a SNF or TrapEase filter is preferred because of the small size and relative flexibility of these filters. Because the longest follow-up is available with the Greenfield filter, this filter is often chosen for younger patients. The BNF is needed for patients with a large vena cava. This is the only filter approved for use in patients with IVC diameters as large as 40 mm. The TrapEase is approved for caval diameters of up to 30 mm; the other filters are approved for caval diameters of up to 28 mm. If a BNF is unavailable and the patient has a megacava, then IVC filters can be placed in each of common iliac veins. In such situations as when there is a low insertion of a renal vein, there may be only a short segment of usable IVC to place the filter. In these cases, placing one of the Greenfield filters, which can be secured in a small length of usable cava, may be preferable.

Temporary IVC filters will probably be approved for use in the United States in the near future. This will greatly increase the number of patients in which IVC filters will be placed. Although this may benefit certain patients, prospective studies detailing appropriate indications and clinical effectiveness of permanent versus temporary IVC filters for different patient populations will need to be performed.

REFERENCES

1. Dalen JE, Albert JS. Natural history of pulmonary embolism. *Progr Cardiovasc Dis* 1975;17:259–270.
2. Harmon B. Deep venous thrombosis: a prospective on anatomy and venographic analysis. *J Thoracic Imaging* 1989;4:15–19.
3. Schuman LM. The epidemiology of thromboembolic disorders: a review. *J Chronic Dis* 1965;18:815–845.
4. Dalen JE, Albert JS. Natural history of pulmonary emboli. *Progr Cardiovasc Dis* 1975;17:257–270.
5. Evans AJ, Sostmann HD, Knilson MH, et al. Detection of deep venous thrombosis: prospective comparison of MR imaging with contrast venography. *Am J Roentgenol* 1993;161:131–139.
6. Freiman DG, Suyemoto J, Wessler S. Frequency of pulmonary thromboembolism in man. *N Engl J Med* 1965;290:1278–1286.
7. Carson JL, Kelly MA, Duff A, et al. The clinical course of pulmonary embolism. *N Engl J Med* 1992;326:1240–1245.
8. Schroeder TM, Elkins RC, Greenfield LJ. Entrapment of sized emboli by the KMA-Greenfield intracaval filter. *Surgery* 1978;83:435.
9. Coleman CC. Overview of interruption of the inferior vena cava. *Semin Intervent Radiol* 1986;3:175–187.
10. Greenfield LJ. Current indications for and results of Greenfield filter placement. *J Vasc Surg* 1984;1:502–504.
11. Tadavarthy SM, Castaneda-Zuniga W, Salamonowitz E, et al. Kimray-Greenfield filter: percutaneous introduction. *Radiology* 1984;151:525–526.
12. Thompson BH, Cragg AH, Smith, TP, et at. Thrombus-trapping efficiency of the Greenfield filter *in vivo*. *Radiology* 1989;172:979–981.
13. Elkins RC, McCurdy JR, Brown PP, et al. Clinical results with an extracaval prosthesis and description of a new intracaval filter. *J Okla State Med Assoc* 1973;66:53–59.
14. Golueke PJ, Garrett WV, Thompson JE, et al. Interruption of the inferior vena cava by means of the Greenfield filter: expanding the indications. *Surgery* 1988;103:111–117.
15. Greenfield LJ, Michna BA. Twelve-year clinical experience with the Greenfield vena cava filter. *Surgery* 1988;104:706–712.
16. Greenfield LJ, Peyton R, Crute S, et al. Greenfield vena cava filter experience: late results in 156 patients. *Arch Surg* 1981;116:1451–1456.
17. Greenfield LJ, Cho KJ, Pais SO, et al. Preliminary clinical experience with the titanium Greenfield vena cava filter. *Arch Surg* 1989; 124:657–659.
18. Greenfield LJ, Cho KJ, Proctor M, et al. Results of a multicenter study of the modified hook-titanium Greenfield filter. *J Vasc Surg* 1991;14:253–257.
19. Teitelbaum GP, Ortega HV, Vinitski S, et al. Low artifact intravascular devices: MR imaging evaluation. *Radiology* 1988;168:713–719.
20. Kiproff PM, Deeb ZL, Contractor FM, et al. Magnetic resonance characteristics of the LGM vena cava filter: technical note. *Cardiovasc Intervent Radiol* 1991;14:254–255.
21. Palestrant AM, Prince MR, Simon M. Comparative *in vitro* evaluation of the Nitinol inferior vena cava filter. *Radiology* 1982;145:351–355.
22. Watanabe AT, Teitelbaum GP, Gomes AS, et al. MR imaging of the bird's nest filter. *Radiology* 1990;177:578–579.
23. Katsamouris AA, Waltman AC, Delichatsios MA, et al. Inferior

vena cava filters: *in vitro* comparison of clot trapping and flow dynamics. *Radiology* 1988;166:361–366.

24. Roehm JOF Jr, Johnsrude IS, Barth MH, et al. The bird's nest inferior vena cava filter: progress report. *Radiology* 1988;168:745–749.

25. Simon M, Athanasoulis CA, Kim D, et al. Simon Nitinol inferior vena cava filter: initial clinical experience. Work in progress. *Radiology* 1989;172:99–103.

26. Dorfman GS, Esparza AR, Cronan JJ. Percutaneous large bore venotomy and tract creation: comparison of sequential dilator and angioplasty balloon methods in a porcine model—preliminary report. *Invest Radiol* 1988;23:441–446.

27. Loesberg A, Taylor FC, Awh MH. Dislodgement of inferior vena cava filters during "blind" insertion of central venous catheters. *Am J Roentgenol* 1993;161:637–638.

28. Kaufman JA, Thomas JW, Geller SC, et al. Guide-wire entrapment by inferior vena cava filters: *in vitro* evaluation. *Radiology* 1996;198:71–76.

29. Rousseau HP, Stockx L, Golzarian J, et al. First clinical experience with a new 6F Nitinol inferior vena cava filter: results from a European multicentre trial. *J Vasc Interv Radiol* 2000;11:196.

30. Stoneham GW, Burbridge BE, Millward SF. Temporary inferior vena cava filters: *in vitro* comparison with permanent IVC filters. *J Vasc Interv Radiol* 1995;6:731–736.

31. Lorch H, Welger D, Wagner V, et al. Current practice of temporary vena cava filter insertion: a multicenter registry. *J Vasc Interv Radiol* 2000;11:83–88.

32. Ferris EJ, McCowan TC, Carver DK, et al. Percutaneous inferior vena cava filters: follow-up of seven designs in 320 patients. *Radiology* 1993;188:851–856.

33. Mobin-Uddin K, Utley JR, Bryant LR. The inferior vena cava umbrella filter. *Progr Cardiovasc Dis* 1977;17:391–399.

34. Santos GH, Lansman S. Prevention of pulmonary embolism with use of Mobin-Uddin filter. *NY State J Med* 1982;82:185.

35. Rogers FB, Shackford SR, Wilson J, et al. Prophylactic vena cava filter insertion in severely injured trauma patients: indications and preliminary results. *J Trauma* 1993;35:637.

36. Winchell RJ, Hoyt DB, Walsh JC, et al. Risk factors associated with pulmonary embolism despite routine prophylaxis: implications for improved protection. *J Trauma* 1994;37:600.

37. Martin KD, Kempczinski RF, Fowl RJ, et al. Are routine inferior vena cavograms necessary before Greenfield filter placement. *Surgery* 1989;106:647–651.

38. Ferris EJ. The inferior vena cava. In: Abrahms HL ed. *Abrahms angiography*. Boston: Little, Brown, 1983:939–975.

39. Giordano JM, Trout HH III. Anomalies of the inferior vena cava. *J Vasc Surg* 1986;3:924–928.

40. Kahn PC. Selective venography of the branches. In: Ferris EJ, Hipona FA, Kahn PC, et al., eds. *Venography of the inferior vena cava and its branches.* Huntington, NY: Krieger, 1973:154–224.

41. Cho KJ, Greenfield LJ, Proctor MC, et al. Evaluation of a new percutaneous stainless steel Greenfield filter. *J Vasc Interv Radiol* 1997;8:181.

42. Kinney TB, Rose SC, Weingarten KW, et al. IVC filter tilt and asymmetry: comparison of over-the-wire stainless-steel and titanium Greenfield IVC filters. *J Vasc Interv Radiol* 1997;8:1029.

43. Wojtowycz MM, Stoehr T, Crummy AB, et al. The bird's nest inferior vena cava filter: review of a single-center experience. *J Vasc Interv Radiol* 1997;8:171.

44. Becker DM, Philbrick JT, Selby JB. Inferior vena cava filters: indications, safety, effectiveness. *Arch Intern Med* 1992;152:1985.

45. Bull PG, Mendel H, Schlengl A. Guenther vena caval filter: clinical appraisal. *J Vasc Interv Radiol* 1992;3:395.

46. Dorfman GS, Cronan JJ, Tupper TB, et al. Occult pulmonary embolism: a common occurrence in deep venous thrombosis. *Am J Roentgenol* 1987;148:263–266.

47. Huisman MV, Buller HR, ten Cate JW, et al. Unexpected high prevalence of silent pulmonary embolism in patients with deep venous thrombosis. *Chest* 1989;95:498–502.

48. Molgaard CP, Yucel EK, Geller SC, et al. Access site thrombosis after placement of inferior vena cava filters with 12–14F delivery sheaths. *Radiology* 1992;185:257.

49. Friedell ML, Goldenkranz RJ, Parsonnet V, et al. Migration of a Greenfield filter to the pulmonary artery: a case report. *J Vasc Surg* 1986;3:929.

50. Malden ES, Darcy MD, Hicks ME, et al. Transvenous retrieval of misplaced stainless steel Greenfield filters. *J Vasc Interv Radiol* 1992;3:703.

51. Deutsch LS. Percutaneous removal of intracardiac Greenfield vena caval filter. *Am J Roentgenol* 1988;151:677.

52. Grassi CJ, Matsumoto AH, Teitelbaum GP. Vena caval occlusion after Simon Nitinol filter placement: identification with MR imaging in patients with malignancy. *J Vasc Interv Radiol* 1992;3:535.

53. Millward SF, Marsh JI, Peterson RA, et al. LGM (Vena Tech) vena cava filter: clinical experience in 64 patients. *J Vasc Interv Radiol* 1991;2:429.

54. Engmann E, Asch MR. Clinical experience with the antecubital Simon Nitinol IVC filter. *J Vasc Interv Radiol* 1998;9:774.

48

VASCULAR CLOSURE DEVICES FOR TRANSARTERIAL INTERVENTIONS

TIMOTHY A. SANBORN

Randomized clinical trials have demonstrated that four different vascular closure devices are able to shorten hemostasis time, reduce the discomfort of manual or mechanical compression, and allow for earlier ambulation without increasing peripheral vascular complications after cardiac catheterization and percutaneous coronary interventions (1–4). Whether the mechanism of action of these devices is mechanical suturing or collagen stimulation of hemostasis combined with a "plugging" or "sandwiching" of the arteriotomy, each provides rapid hemostasis at the puncture site until the natural healing process occurs. Table 48.1 summarizes the techniques and material utilized for each of these four FDA-approved sealing or suturing devices.

COMPARATIVE STUDIES

Several reports in the literature have compared these various closure devices (5–7). In a study of more than 1,600 patients in which AngioSeal (Daig, Minnetonka, MN), VasoSeal (Datascope Corp., Mahwah, NJ), Perclose (Abbott, Redwood City, CA), and manual compression were compared after diagnostic catheterization (80%) and coronary interventions (20%), there was a slight but statistically significant variation in the incidence of major complication rates of the four methods of hemostasis (AngioSeal, 3.2%; Perclose, 2.3%; manual compression, 1%; and VasoSeal, 0.6%). However, in two other studies in which these devices were used after percutaneous coronary interventions, there was no significant difference in the incidence of femoral artery complications, even with the use of platelet glycoprotein IIb/IIIa blockade. All these studies were conducted as a prospective series of patients; however, none were randomized trials. In addition, these studies were conducted with first-generation devices, and the results may have been in part related to operator learning curves.

SECOND-GENERATION DEVICES

In an attempt to develop devices that are safer, easier to use, and more "user-friendly," each of these devices has gone through considerable modification and improvement such that second-generation devices have now been released. For example, more precise delivery of a collagen "plug" to the surface of the artery is now possible with the VasoSeal ES device, which utilizes a temporary wire anchor to help place the collagen on top of the artery as compared with the original needle depth measurement technique. Likewise, improvement and downsizing of the AngioSeal device has simplified its ease of use. The Perclose suturing devices are also smaller and easier to use since the release of the Closure system, with its knot-tying apparatus.

The most recently approved device, Duett (Vascular Solutions, Minneapolis, MN), is not simply another collagen sealing device but a device that employs a concept of mixing two biochemicals, collagen and thrombin, in an attempt to create a better "seal" and stimulus for hemostasis than collagen alone. With the introduction of the Duett sealing device, it is clear that emphasis will now be placed on creating a rapid, strong biochemical or hemostatic bond at the arteriotomy site that will form a sufficient temporary seal until healing and fibrosis occur and arteriotomy closure is complete. If the hemostasis process can be stimulated to occur faster or to yield a stronger or more complete seal of the arteriotomy with these new biochemical approaches, then these devices may represent an improvement over the current collagen sealing devices.

Timothy A. Sanborn: Professor of Medicine, Department of Medicine, Division of Cardiology, The Feinberg School of Medicine Northwestern University; Head, Division of Cardiology, Evanston Northwestern Healthcare, Evanston, Illinois

TABLE 48.1. FDA-APPROVED VASCULAR SEALING AND SUTURING DEVICES

	Technique	Material
VasoSeal	Plug	Collagen
AngioSeal	Sandwich	Collagen and anchor
Perclose	Suture	Suture
Duett	Gel	Collagen and thrombus

Several manufacturers are also developing and initiating clinical investigation of other suture-type closure devices (X-Site, Sutura, etc.). Whether these new suturing devices will prove to be safe and reliable awaits randomized clinical trial results. Thus the suture approach to access site closure will also continue to mature in the next few years.

FURTHER CONSIDERATIONS

In view of the additional cost of these devices, there will be a need to justify their use and to determine their appropriate indications for use. For example, ambulatory cases performed late in the day may be able to be discharged earlier in the evening with these devices. In very selected cases, some institutions are performing ambulatory stenting with arterial closure devices. Finally, the relative role of alternative catheterization techniques such as the radial approach will also need to be compared.

CONCLUSION

Each approach for arterial access site closure after cardiac catheterization or percutaneous coronary intervention, whether it be sealing or suturing, will undoubtedly be available in the future. It may be that certain anatomic or clinical situations will favor one device over another. There also may be certain operator preferences. Ultimately, the extent to which vascular closure devices are accepted in clinical practice in the future will depend on which device or devices provide a simple approach with reliable hemostasis.

REFERENCES

1. Sanborn TA, Gibbs HH, Brinker JA, et al. A multicenter randomized trial comparing a percutaneous collagen hemostasis device with conventional manual compression after diagnostic angiography and angioplasty. *J Am Coll Cardiol* 1993;22: 1273–1279.
2. Kussmaul WG, Buchbinder M, Whitlow PL, et al. Rapid arterial hemostasis and decreased access site complications after cardiac catheterization and angioplasty: results of a randomized trial of a novel hemostasis device. *J Am Coll Cardiol* 1995;25:1685–1692.
3. Baim DS, Knopf WD, Hinohara T, et al. Suture-mediated closure of the femoral access site after cardiac catheterization: results of the suture to ambulate and discharge (STAND I and STAND II) trials. *Am J Cardiol* 2000;85:864–869.
4. Ellis SG, Mooney M, Talley JD, et al. DUETT femoral artery closure device vs. manual compression after diagnostic or interventional catheterization: results of the SEAL trial. *Circulation* 1999; 100:I-513.
5. Shrake KL. Comparison of major complication rates associated with four methods of arterial closure. *Am J Cardiol* 2000;85: 1024–1025.
6. Chamberlin JR, Lardi AB, McKeever LS, et al. Use of vascular sealing devices (VasoSeal and Perclose) versus assisted manual compression (Femostop) in transcatheter coronary interventions requiring Abciximab (ReoPro). *Catheter Cardiovasc Interv* 1999; 47:143–147.
7. Cura FA, Kapadia SR, L'Allier PL, et al. Safety of femoral closure devices after percutaneous coronary interventions in the era of glycoprotein IIa/IIIa platelet blockade. *Am J Cardiol* 2000;86: 780–782.

49

TRANSCATHETER IMPLANTATION OF PROSTHETIC VALVES

DUŠAN PAVČNIK

In 1981, Charles Dotter (1) suggested transcatheter valve placement in his review paper on interventional radiology with the following words: "Catheter based devices have met clinical success in the closure of patent ductus arteriosus and atrial septal defects. Why not catheter-placed prosthetic valves? Femoral vein valve incompetence might offer a reasonable initial target. Other, simpler means might pay off in a percutaneous catheter treatment for varicose vein, even hemorrhoids." Since then minimally invasive catheter therapy has progressed at a breathtaking pace, and there does not appear to be an end in sight.

This chapter describes the initial design and experimental evolution of mechanical and biological prosthetic aortic and venous valves for percutaneous placement developed by Pavcnik et al. (2–4), Andersen et al. (5), Moazami et al. (6), Sochman et al. (7), Uflacker et al. (8), Gomez-Jorge et al. (9), Bonhoeffer et al. (10,11), and Osse et al. (12). All current devices for percutaneous transcatheter valve placement rely on some form of a vascular stent for valve attachment (2–10). Self- expandable Gianturco Z-stents served as carriers for most of these devices.

AORTIC VALVE

Square Stent-Based Aortic Valve

The square stent was designed to be an intravascular implant device carrier (3,4,13,14). Compared with other stents, it has a minimal amount of metal and thus requires a smaller-diameter catheter for introduction. Despite the small amount of metal present in this stent, the square stent has adequate expansile force. The square stent becomes a valve when the stent with barbs on all four corners is covered with low porous material such as small intestine submucosa (SIS) (Figure 49.1). SIS provides an acellular framework that becomes remodeled by host tissue, while degrading and reab-

sorbing over time (15). This makes SIS a unique covering for intravascular devices. The square stent's diagonal axis is constrained to the length of πr, forming a diamond to fit in the aortic circumference of $2\pi r$. Two separate triangular pieces of SIS are sutured to the square frame with 7.0 Prolene monofilament running sutures, allowing for the gap between the diagonal axes of the square. The valves ranging from 16 to 32 mm in diameter are front-loaded into a 10F guiding catheter. For deployment a special pusher with a small hook at its end is used. It ensures valve placement in proper position and prevents its dislodgment by blood flow before its barbs engage into the vessel wall. The valve is self-expanding, so that upon insertion it automatically assumes its operational form.

We tested aortic valves *in vitro* in a flow model at a hydrostatic pressure of 100 mm Hg and with continuous or pulsatile antegrade flow at 2.5 L/min. A 100-mL silicone bag attached by a side arm at the lower end of the flow model provided pulsatile flow. Manual bag compression lasting less than 1 second was used to stimulate ventricular contractions during systole. In the resting state without flow, the aortic valve was closed with a hydrostatic pressure of 101 mm Hg below and 100 mm above the valve. With pulsatile flow, immediately after a fast compression rate of the bag the pressure above it increased to 110 mm Hg (5) and decreased to 79 mm Hg (7) below the valve (3).

In vivo acute and short-term experiments up to 4 weeks were conducted in swine and dogs. SIS valves ranging from 16 to 28 mm in diameter were placed into the ascending aorta from common carotid arteries through a 10F sheath, either in the subcoronary or in the supracoronary position (Figure 49.2). With the aortic valve deployed, two valvular sinuses were created between the aortic wall and SIS leaflets. Systolic pressure opened the aortic valve and permitted blood to flow through it. In diastole, the valve closed as its two triangular leaflets sealed against each other preventing blood flow through it. The animals tolerated the procedure well, and no arrhythmia or aortic pressure changes were observed. Valve movements were regular, and there was no gradient across the valve. In animals with subcoronary placed valves, one of the cusps of the native valve was

---

Dušan Pavčnik: Research Professor, Dotter Institute, Oregon Health and Science University; Josef Rosch Chair, Dotter Interventional Institute, Portland, Oregon

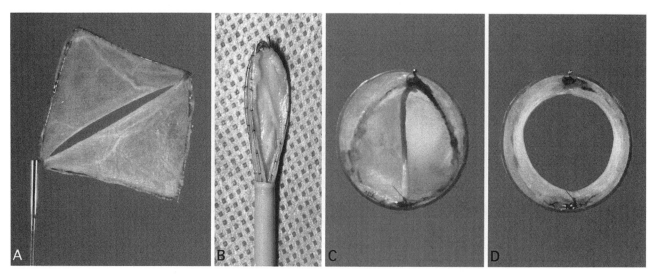

FIGURE 49.1. Small intestine submucosa (SIS) aortic valve model. **A:** Unrestricted valve 30 mm long retained by a wire pusher connected to a barb. **B:** Valve partially front-loaded into a 10F sheath. **C:** Valve deployed in a plastic tube 20 mm in diameter, closed position. **D:** Open position. (See Color Figure 49.1)

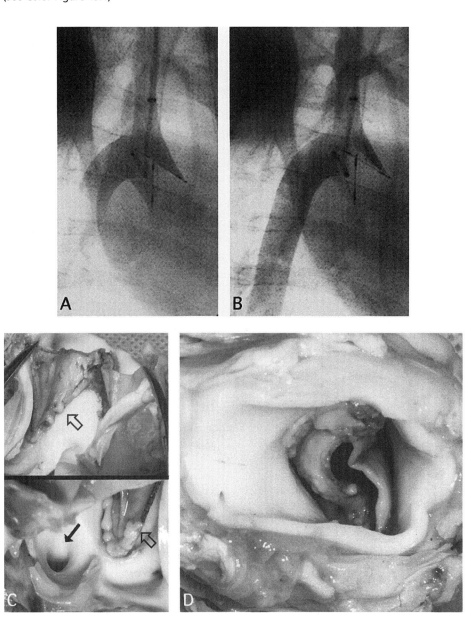

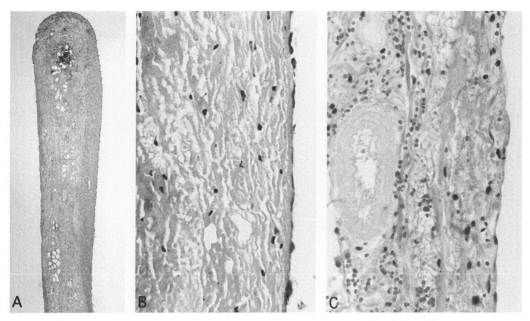

FIGURE 49.3. Photomicrographs of the SIS aortic valve 2 and 4 weeks after implantation into porcine aorta. **A:** A longitudinal cross section of aortic valve at 2 weeks shows early remodeling. **B:** Magnified view of the partially remodeled part of the SIS leaflet at 2 weeks shows collagenous tissue stroma with fibrocytes and endothelial cells covering valve leaflet. (Hematoxylin and eosin stain, original magnification 200×.) **C:** High magnification of the SIS leaflet with endothelial lining at 4 weeks shows remodeling of the SIS by collagenized fibrous tissue and numerous capillaries. (Hematoxylin and eosin stain; original magnification 400×.) (See Color Figure 49.3.)

trapped between the square stent and the aortic wall. This created considerable regurgitation. Such placement is an appropriate model for evaluating SIS-valve efficacy.

Follow-up aortograms revealed minimal regurgitation and no interference with coronary blood flow. All animals survived the initial postimplantation procedure. Rupture of the ascending aorta was seen in one animal after 1 week due to nonoptimal deployment of the square stent. Postmortem examination found all valves to be securely anchored. Histologic evaluation at 2 and 4 weeks revealed early remodeling of the SIS with fibrocytes, fibroblasts, capillaries, endothelial, and some inflammatory cells (Figure 49.3).

Ball-in-Cage Valve

The catheter balloon valve principle was suggested in 1980 with the idea of balloon periodical closures of the insufficient aortic valve orifice using a system attached to an aortic balloon pump control unit (16). A completely revolutionary concept in a catheter-based aortic valve was introduced in 1992 with a percutaneously introduced valve, based on the caged-ball and seat design (Figure 49.4) (2).

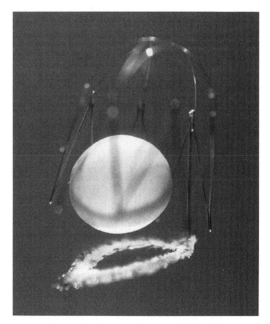

FIGURE 49.4. Caged-ball valve for percutaneous transcatheter placement. The three main components of the prosthesis (cage, ring, and ball) are depicted. (See Color Figure 49.4.)

FIGURE 49.2. SIS aortic valve in supracoronary position in ascending aorta of a swine 2 weeks after placement. **A:** Aortogram shows competency of the prosthetic aortic valve in diastole with closure and (**B**) opening in systole. **C:** Side views of the specimen show incorporation of the bicuspid valve into aortic wall *(open arrows)* and patent coronary arteries *(arrow)*. **D:** View from above shows bicuspid valve. (See Color Figures 49.2 C, D.)

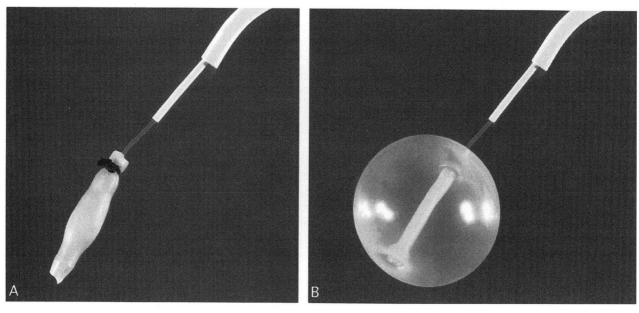

FIGURE 49.5. Detachable latex balloon used as the ball. The balloon is attached to a 5F catheter, which is passed coaxially through the Teflon introducer sheath. **A:** Noninflated latex balloon. **B:** Latex balloon filled with the air. (See Color Figure 49.5.)

- *The cage* was a barbed Gianturco self-expanding stainless steel stent consisting of four to six flat, flexible stainless steel wire 3-cm lengths attached at the cranial end to form the top of the cage.
- *The seat,* or ring, was constructed of two stainless steel wires coiled together in a springlike configuration and covered with an expandable nylon mesh. Barbs were located at various points around the ring for stabilization after placement. The ring was attached to the cage assembly with a length of stainless steel tubing.
- *The ball* was a detachable latex balloon placed at the tip of a 60-cm-long 5F high-flow catheter for delivery and was designed for placement within the cage and ring assembly (Figure 49.5). It was filled with a liquid silicone prepolymer system before detachment. Polymerization of the mixture occurred within 25 minutes after mixing, and when fully cured, the polymer had the consistency of soft rubber.

Whereas in the previous systems the inserted valve remained connected to the introducing catheter, the deployed ball valve stayed in the aorta without any support of the catheter. The cage was deployed first, followed by introduction of the detachable balloon.

Development of the final ring design allowed delivery through an 11- or 12F Teflon sheath (Figure 49.6). In all 12 animals the ring assembly was successfully placed below the ostia of the coronary arteries. The cusps of the aortic valve were trapped between the ring and the aortic wall, resulting in complete incompetence of the natural valve.

The ring and cage assembly consistently self-expanded after being pushed from the sheath, and the unit was easily positioned and securely anchored in place. Once the assembly was in position, the detachable balloon was inserted into the valve and released between the ring and cage. In the first nine dogs the ball was filled with air (three dogs) or

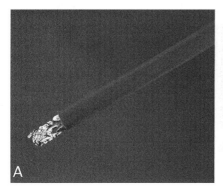
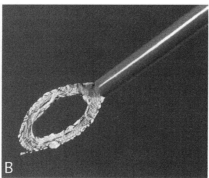
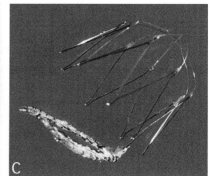

FIGURE 49.6. Collapsed prosthetic valve being pushed out of 12F Teflon sheath. **A:** The ring with anchoring barbs is just beginning to emerge from the sheath. **B:** Self-expanding ring is covered with nylon mesh. **C:** Self-expanding ring and the cage. (See Color Figure 49.6.)

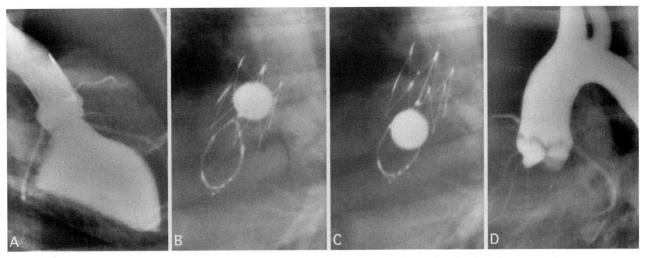

FIGURE 49.7. Ball-in-cage valve function. **A:** Aortogram obtained immediately after placement of the cage and ring assembly in ascending aorta. The animal is in the right anterior oblique position. Note the massive regurgitation resulting from compression of the native cusps by the ring. **B:** Radiographs showing movement of the ball during diastole and **(C)** systole. **D:** Aortogram in left anterior oblique position demonstrates competency of prosthetic valve and patency of coronary arteries. The filling defect seen in the aortic annulus is due to the ring.

contrast medium (six dogs). In the final three animals, the radiopaque silicone prepolymer system was used to fill the latex ball.

The last three valves that were placed showed excellent functional results for up to 3 hours. However, in all three cases, the ball escaped into the aorta through the top of the cage after 1, 2.5, and 3 hours, respectively.

During the time when the valve remained functional, the ring and surrounding structures were sufficiently close together to prevent leakage of blood between them, and the coronary arteries remained patent. A thin layer of clot formed on the nylon mesh immediately after valve placement. This provided a barrier that effectively channeled blood flow through the central opening of the ring during systole and prevented leakage of blood around the ball back into the left ventricle during diastole (Figure 49.7).

This pilot study showed that the development of a mechanical prosthetic aortic valve for transcatheter placement was feasible.

Stent Valve Bioprosthesis

The "stent valve" bioprosthesis was introduced in 1992 (5). The foldable valve was a porcine aortic valve taken from a 90-kg pig. The stent valve was prepared by mounting the cleaned aortic valve inside the homemade stent (Figure 49.8). The aortic annulus, which included three commissural sites, was fixed to the metallic stent by 45 to 50 Prolene 5-0 sutures. The external diameter of the stent valve was approximately 12 mm when collapsed and 32 mm when entirely expanded. After the stent valve was manually compressed on the balloon catheter carrier, the metal stiff-

ness prevented it from uncoiling spontaneously. After expansion, the metal stiffness minimized spontaneous recoil when the balloon was deflated. The carrier balloon catheter used for implantation was a conventional 12F three-foiled aortic valvuloplasty balloon dilatation catheter (Schneider, Zurich, Switzerland). It was mounted in a 41F flexible introducer sheath (external diameter, 13.6 mm; internal diameter, 12.5 mm; length, 75 cm). The stent-valve-loaded carrier balloon catheter was retracted into the introducer sheath during intravascular introduction and advancement to minimize friction against the vessel wall. The biological valve was tested in nine swine, and the valves were introduced surgically by the abdominal aortic route. Implantation was easy in both the ascending and descending aortas, where small movements of the carrier balloon catheter were not critical. However, with subcoronary implantation such movements proved to be problematic (5).

All the animals survived the initial postimplantation period. None of the stent valves caused severe stenoses, and only trivial contrast regurgitation was seen in two pigs. Left ventricular end-diastolic pressures were unchanged after stent-valve implantation in five of seven pigs but increased in two due to left ventricular failure caused by restriction of the coronary blood flow (5).

Another " stent valve" was developed in 2000 in Jena, Germany, using porcine aortic valve and a Nitinol self-expanding stent. At present the Nitinol stent aortic valve has been tested only *in vitro* (Figure 49.9) (*personal communication,* Dr. T. Peschel, 2000). A similar model with a valve made from the porcine pericardium mounted on a stent base was tested successfully in animals. This model required a 24F catheter for introduction (6).

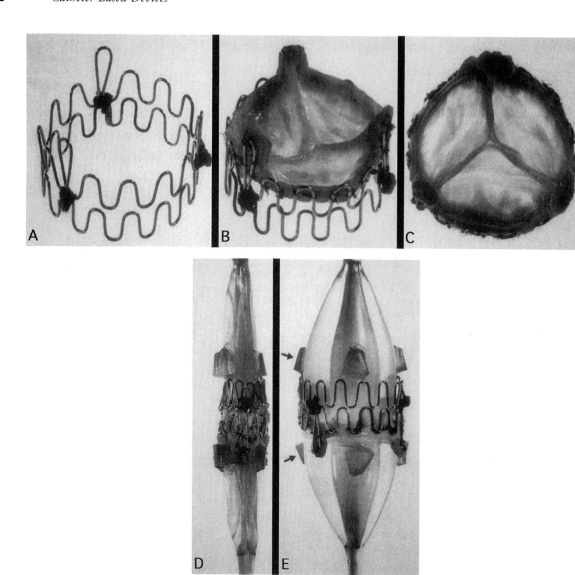

FIGURE 49.8. Stent valve bioprosthesis. **A:** The stent was constructed with two 0.55-mm stainless steel wires folded in 15 loops. **B,C:** A three-leaflet porcine aortic valve was mounted inside the stent and fixed to the metal by sutures to form the stent valve. **D:** Before implantation, the stent valve was mounted on a deflated three-foiled balloon dilatation catheter. **E:** Balloon inflation expanded the stent valve to an external diameter of 32 mm. *Arrows* point to balloon catheter modification. (From Anderson HR, Knudsen LL, Hasenkam JM. Transluminal implantation of artificial heart valves: description of a new expandable aortic valve and initial results with implantation by catheter technique in closed chest pig. *Eur Heart J* 1992;13:704–708, with permission.)

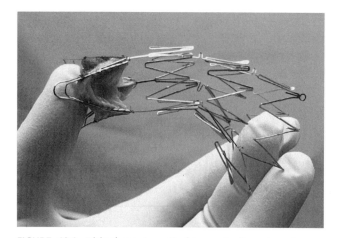

FIGURE 49.9. Nitinol stent aortic bioprosthetic valve. (Reproduced, courtesy of Dr. T Peschel.) (See Color Figure 49.9.)

Disk Valve

A percutaneously introduced disk valve was described in 2000 (7). Like the SIS square stent, the ball-in-cage valve, and stent valve bioprosthesis, the disk valve was delivered with a catheter, but it stayed in place on its own. The disk valve consisted of a Z-stent-based valve cage with locking mechanism and a prosthetic flexible tilting valve disk (Figure 49.10). The valve cage was delivered first followed by deployment and locking the disk. The elliptical tilting valve disk was made of a Nitinol wire .010 inch in size and contained a narrow stainless steel plate with an eyehole for locking into the spring mechanism of the valve cage. The whole disk, except the plate-eye, was covered with polyurethane membrane approximately 0.1 mm thick. A loop forming polytetrafluroethylene (PTFE) ligature 5-0 introduced through the disk plate eye was used for delivering and

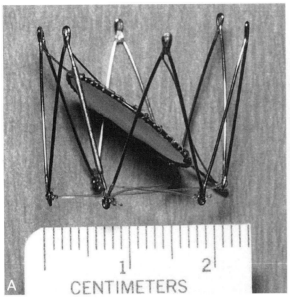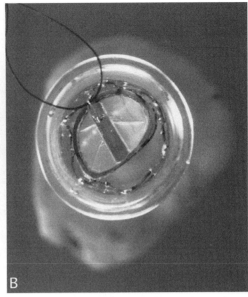

FIGURE 49.10. Expanded valve cage with anchored disk in a plastic tube. **A:** Side view. **B:** Axial view from above. (From Sochman J, Peregrin J, Pavčnik D, et al. Percutaneous transcatheter aortic disc valve prosthesis implantation: a feasibility study. *Cardiovasc Intervent Radiol* 2000;23: 384–388, with permission.) (See Color Figure 49.10.)

locking the valve disk. For delivery, the disk was folded, loaded into a cartridge, and introduced through a 10F catheter.

The size of the delivery catheter for the disk valve was similar to that for delivery of the square stent or the ball-in-cage valve (10 to 12F) and much smaller than the size of the stent valve bioprosthesis delivery catheters (24 to 45F) (2,3,5–7).

In acute experiments, valve implantation was tested in four dogs. The valve implantation was successful in all animals. The implanted valve functioned well for the duration of the experiments, up to 3 hours (Figure 49.11). The study

showed implantation feasibility and short-term function of the tested catheter-based aortic disk valve.

VENOUS VALVE

Venous valves are intended for the extracardiac conduits, pulmonary arteries, and venous system. In 1993 Uflacker (8) reported on an artificial monocusp venous valve consisting of a single-body Z-stent with insertion of the poly-

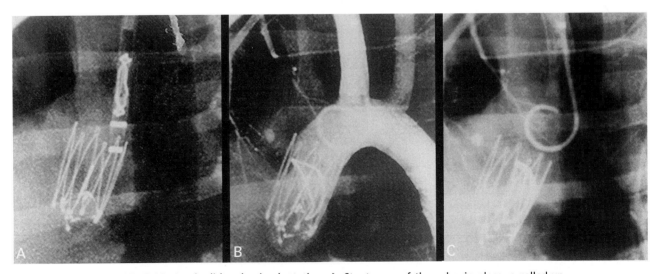

FIGURE 49.11. Aortic disk valve implantation. **A:** Stent cage of the valve in place, a rolled-up disk is being inserted using an introducing catheter. **B:** Aortogram demonstrates blocked flow of contrast medium into the left ventricle by the disk valve (diastole). **C:** Disk is in opening phase of systole. (From Sochman J, Peregrin J, Pavčnik D, et al. Percutaneous transcatheter aortic disc valve prosthesis implantation: a feasibility study. *Cardiovasc Intervent Radiol* 2000;23:384–388, with permission.)

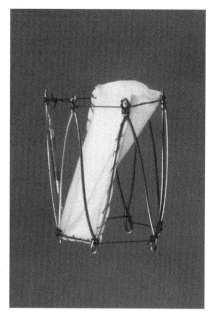

FIGURE 49.12. Monocusp Z-stent valve. (Reproduced, courtesy of Barry Uchida.) (See Color Figure 49.12.)

etherurethane or PTFE membrane into the stent lumen (Figure 49.12). Valve implantation in the inferior vena cava (IVC) of swine through 12F sheath for a week has shown promising results, although the thrombosis was of concern. In 2000, Thorpe, Osse, and Correa (12) reported a bicuspid venous valve made from the porcine small intestinal

submucosa mounted on a single-body Z-stent base. This model required a 16F catheter for introduction. The valve showed promising *in vitro* and short-term results.

The development of extracardiac conduits for the establishment of right ventricular to pulmonary artery continuity has been one of the major advances in pediatric heart surgery. Conduits have permitted repair of previously uncorrectable congenital heart defects. Prosthetic conduits are valveless or use xenograft, pericardial, or homograph valves. Conduit stenting during percutaneous catheterization is an efficient technique to reopen the conduit narrowing, but the valve in conduit has to be sacrificed (11). Bonhoeffer et al. (11) have recently reported successful percutaneous valve replacement in the failed conduit from the right ventricle to the pulmonary artery in a 12-year-old boy. They used a bovine jugular vein valve mounted inside the stent (Figures 49.13 and 49.14).

Bovine Jugular Vein Valve Mounted Inside an Expandable Stent

Gomez-Jorge et al. (9) reported in 2000 the outcome of a 2-week study of the valve-stent device in a swine model. A segment of a gluteraldehyde fixed bovine external jugular vein with valves was trimmed and sutured inside a Nitinol stent (Boston Scientific, Watertown, MA) (Figure 49.15). Valve devices were compressed and loaded into a 12- to 24F introducer sheath and deployed percutaneously into the IVC (*N* = 3) and common iliac veins (*N* = 6). The animals were anti-

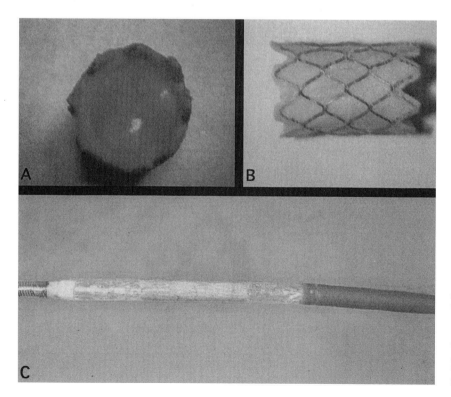

FIGURE 49.13. Valved stent. **A:** Closed jugular valve mounted in the stent. **B:** Profile of the valved stent before compression. **C:** Valved stent in the delivery system. (From Bonhoeffer P, Boudjemline Y, Saliba Z, et al. Percutaneous replacement of pulmonary valve in a right-ventricle to pulmonary-artery prosthetic conduit with valve dysfunction. *Lancet* 2000;356:1403–05, with permission.) (See Color Figure 49.13.)

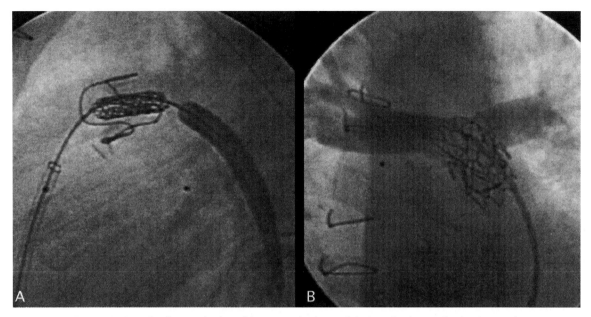

FIGURE 49.14. Valved stent deployed into prosthetic conduit **A:** Valved stent in the Carpentier-Edwards conduit before deployment. **B:** Angiography after expansion of the valved stent demonstrates competence of the valve (From Bonhoeffer P, Boudjemline Y, Saliba Z, et al. Percutaneous replacement of pulmonary valve in a right-ventricle to pulmonary-artery prosthetic conduit with valve dysfunction. *Lancet* 2000;356:1403–05, with permission.)

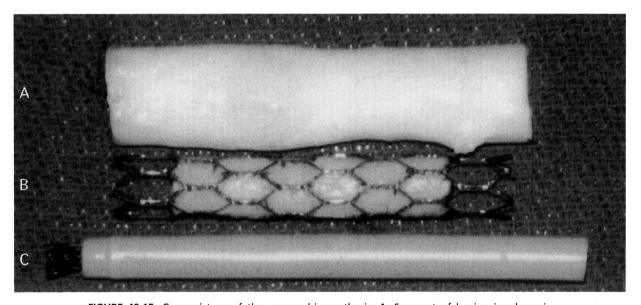

FIGURE 49.15. Gross picture of the venous bioprosthesis. **A:** Segment of bovine jugular vein with leaflets. **B:** Vein segments trimmed and sutured to a Nitinol stent. **C:** Bioprosthesis compressed and loaded within an 18F introducer. (Reproduced, courtesy of Dr. Jackeline Gomez-Jorge.)

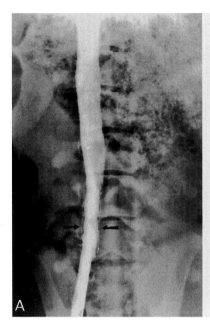

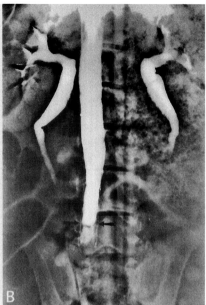

FIGURE 49.16. Function of the venous valve bioprosthesis 2 weeks after placement into a porcine inferior vena cava (IVC) in supine position with injection of contrast medium distal and proximal to the stent. **A:** Ascending venogram demonstrates patency of the valve prosthesis. No thrombus is visualized above and below the bioprosthesis. **B:** Descending venogram demonstrates interrupted column of contrast by competent leaflets *(arrows).* (Reproduced, courtesy of Dr. Jackeline Gomez-Jorge.)

coagulated and euthanized at 2 weeks (*N* = 4). Descending and ascending venograms were performed before sacrifice (Figure 49.16). Their studies have demonstrated that stent-bovine valve can remain patent and competent for up to 2 weeks. This technique has potential application in venous valvular incompetence (Figure 49.17).

Bonhoeffer et al. (10) reported implantation of a similar bovine jugular vein valve device into a lamb's pulmonary artery. A fresh bovine jugular vein containing a native valve was sutured into a platinum balloon-expandable stent and then cross-linked with 0.6% glutaraldehyde solution for 36 hours. The valve device was crimped onto a balloon catheter

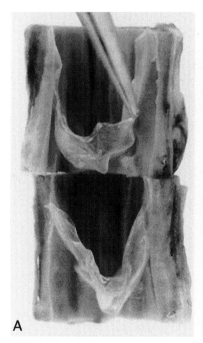

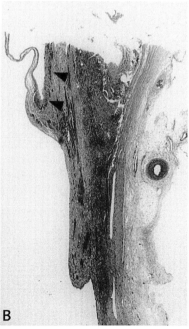

FIGURE 49.17. Histology of the bioprosthesis. **A:** Gross photograph of the venous valve leaflets (longitudinal bisection). **B:** Microscopic view of venous valve segment shows no thrombus in the lumen. More prominent endothelial cells noted at the base of the valve *(arrowheads).* (Reproduced, courtesy of Dr. Jackeline Gomez-Jorge.) (See Color Figure 49.17.)

and deployed through an 18F delivery catheter in the position of the native pulmonary valve in 11 lambs. The pulmonary valve replacement was successful in seven animals and was followed up for 2 months. The valve remained functional after 2 months in five animals. The study showed the implantation feasibility and long-term function of a bovine valve deployed with standard stent implantation technique.

Square-Stent-Based Venous Valve

Venous and aortic valve have the same construction and differ only by the sizes of the square stent and diameter of the wire, from which they are made. The square stent with four barbs becomes a venous valve when two triangular pieces of SIS are sutured to a constrained stent (1,3). SIS pieces are sutured with 7.0 Prolene monofilament in such a way that they allow for the gap between the diagonal axis of the square. Valves ranging from 8 to 20 mm in diameter are folded and front-loaded into a 9F guiding catheter and

delivered coaxially through an 11F sheath (Figure 49.18). For deployment the valve is attached by one barb to a bird's nest retention wire (Cook, Inc.) with a locking mechanism. This ensures valve placement in a proper position and prevents its migration by blood flow before valve barbs engage into the vessel wall. After deployment the valve self-expands automatically and assumes its functional form, creating two valvular sinuses between the vein wall and SIS on the square stent. The valve is open during continuous antegrade flow, permitting fluid flow through it. When retrograde pressure is applied, the valve closes, with the two triangular leaflets sealing against each other and preventing retrograde flow through it (Figure 49.19).

In vitro testing proved that the valve is competent and able to withstand high retrograde hydrostatic pressures in the vertical position in the flow model. A SIS valve 15 mm in diameter was functioning well with antegrade flow of 250 mL/min and with pulsations simulating the exercise pump of the calf.

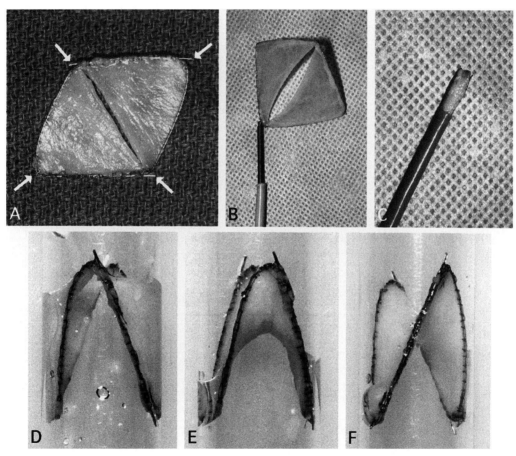

FIGURE 49.18. Venous valve model. **A:** Nonrestricted valve 20 mm long with four barbs *(arrows)*. **B:** Valve retained by a wire pusher connected to one barb. **C:** Valve front-loaded into a 9F guiding catheter. **D:** Deployed valve in a plastic tube, open position. **E:** Deployed valve in a plastic tube, closed position. **F:** Deployed valve in a plastic tube, oblique view, closed position. (See Color Figure 49.18.)

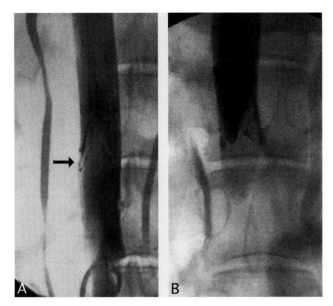

FIGURE 49.19. Function of the SIS venous valve placed into a porcine inferior vena cava (IVC) in supine and upright position with injection of contrast medium distal and proximal to the valve. **A:** Cavogram in supine position and injection below valve shows valve patency with unrestricted flow to proximal IVC. *Arrow* shows valve position. **B:** Cavogram in upright position with the high flow injection of contrast medium above the valve demonstrates competent valve with minimal reflux into lower IVC.

In a resting state without flow, the valve closed with a hydrostatic pressure of 61 mm Hg below and 60 mm Hg above the valve. Initiation of continuous nonpulsatile antegrade flow caused the valve to open immediately, and it remained open during continuous flow. Pulsating flow and either a mild or strong pulsation caused the valve to open. However, it closed immediately after flow was discontinued. Exposure to retrograde flow caused the valve to close immediately. It remained closed with increasing pressure up to 300 mm Hg. Valves placed in a reverse position into vessels such as the inferior vena cava are effective enough to become vascular occluders.

Valves ranging from 10 to 18 mm in diameter were percutaneously placed into the IVC from either femoral or jugular approach in our acute experiments conducted on dogs and swine. Function and stability of these valves were studied in the supine and upright positions with both venograms and pressure measurements proximal and distal to the valve. Good valve function was observed with no or only minimal initial leak and no pressure gradient through valve in supine position. Exercising both legs in the upright position caused an immediate pressure gradient of 12 to 15 Hg mm with less pressure below the valves. For short-term

testing valves were placed into the iliac veins of swine. At 6 weeks veins remained patent with smooth incorporation of the SIS valves into the vein mimicking the natural vein valves. Histologic evaluation of the SIS valves demonstrated host tissue replacement and collagen remodeling of the tissue stroma (3).

We are presently performing a long-term study in sheep to evaluate valve patency, competency, stability, durability, and biocompatibility. Of the 26 valves placed into jugular veins, good valve function with minimal or no leak was observed on immediate venograms in 25 valves (96%). The one valve with poor function was due to placement into a curved vein, resulting in the valve tilting with one leaflet unable to function. This valve was partially thrombosed at 1 month. Fifteen valves have been evaluated at present, with animal sacrifice at 1 and 3 months. Gross pathology showed smooth incorporation of 14 SIS valves into the vein wall. Histologic evaluation of the SIS valves demonstrated early SIS remodeling with endothelial cells, variable fibrocytes, capillaries, and some inflammatory cells (Figure 49.20).

Our early observations are very promising. They demonstrate that the SIS valve is nonthrombogenic. This is a great advantage in the venous circulation, where, in contrast to the arterial circulation, hardly any thrombogenic surface is tolerated. Early after implantation venous endothelial cells get attached to SIS. As this process continues, other cells infiltrate and multiply to completely envelop the SIS bioscaffolding in 4 weeks. The SIS is gradually reabsorbed.

The SIS valves are intended to replace venous valves that are destroyed during thrombophlebitis or are incompetent from birth. We expect the SIS valve will be remodeled with the recipient's own cells and will function without need for continuous blood-thinning medications. Experimental studies are warranted to test the valve in the pulmonary position and several other locations.

SUMMARY AND CONCLUSION

The past 25 years have witnessed experimental efforts at catheter-based management of aortic, pulmonary, and venous valve regurgitation. This chapter describes the initial designs and experimental evolution of mechanical and bioprosthetic aortic, pulmonary, and venous valves that can be implanted by using a transcatheter technique. Although a great deal of work remains to be done, these early results indicate that the development of mechanical and biological prosthetic aortic, pulmonary, and venous valves for transcatheter placement is more than feasible.

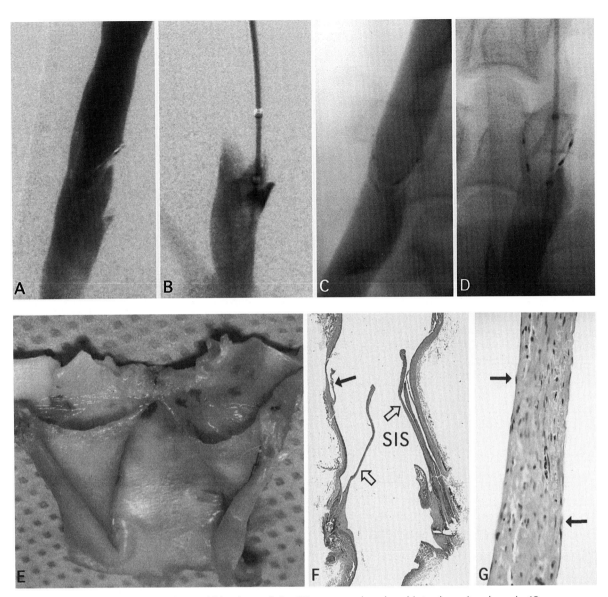

FIGURE 49.20. Function and histology of the SIS venous valve placed into sheep jugular vein 13 mm in diameter. **A:** Jugular venogram immediately after valve placement demonstrates valve patency. **B:** A high-volume injection of contrast medium below the valve immediately after valve placement demonstrates closure of the valve with no leak. **C:** Jugular venogram with injection above the valve 1 month after placement demonstrates valve patency. **D:** A high-volume injection of contrast medium below the valve 1 month after placement does not reveal any reflux and demonstrates closure of the valve. **E:** One-month jugular vein specimen shows smooth incorporation of the valve into the vein wall. **F:** Longitudinal microscopic view of both SIS leaflets *(open arrows)* in original size. Native valve is visible *(arrow)*. **G:** Magnified view of the remodeled SIS leaflet reveals host tissue replacement and collagenous stroma remodeling with fibrocytes, plasma cells, and lymphocytes. Vascular endothelial cells *(arrows)* cover valve leaflet. (Hematoxylin and eosin stain; original magnification, 400×.) (See Color Figures 49.20 E, F, G.)

REFERENCES

1. Dotter CT. Interventional radiology-review of an emerging field. *Semin Radiol* 1981;16:7–12.

2. Pavcnik D, Wright KC, Wallace S. Development and initial experimental evaluation of a prosthetic aortic valve for transcatheter placement. *Radiology* 1992;183:151–154.

3. Pavcnik D, Uchida BT, Keller FS, et al. Aortic and venous valve for percutaneous placement. *Minim Invasive Ther Allied Technol* 2000: 9:287–292.

4. Pavcnik D, Uchida B, Timmermans HA, et al. Square stent: a new self-expandable endoluminal device and its applications. *Cardiovasc Intervent Radiol* 2001;24:207–217.

5. Andersen HR, Knudsen LL, Hasenkam JM. Transluminal implantation of artificial heart valves: description of a new expandable aortic valve and initial results with implantation by catheter technique in closed chest pigs. *Eur Heart J* 1992;13: 704–708.

6. Moazami N, Basller M, Argencia M, et al. Transluminal aortic valve replacement: a feasibility study with a newly designed collapsible aortic valve. *ASAIO J* 1996;42:M381–M385.

7. Sochman J, Peregrin J, Pavcnik D, et al. Percutaneous transcatheter aortic disc valve prosthesis implantation: a feasibility study *Cardiovasc Intervent Radiol* 2000;23:384–388.

8. Uflacker R. Percutaneously introduced artificial venous valve: experimental use in pigs. The 1993 Annual Meeting of the Western Angiographic & Interventional Society, Portland, OR, Abstract book 1993;30.

9. Gomez-Jorge J, Venbrux AC, Magee C. Percutaneous development of a valved bovine jugular vein in the swine venous system: a potential treatment for venous insufficiency. *J Vasc Interv Radiol* 2000;11:931–936.

10. Bonhoeffer P, Boudjemline Y, Saliba Z, et al. Transcatheter implantation of a bovine valve in pulmonary position: a lamb study. *Circulation* 2000;102:813–816.

11. Bonhoeffer P, Boudjemline Y, Saliba Z, et al. Percutaneous replacement of pulmonary valve in a right-ventricle to pulmonary-artery prosthetic conduit with valve dysfunction. *Lancet* 2000;356:1403–1405.

12. Thorpe PE, Osse FJ, Correa LO. The valve-stent: development of a percutaneous prosthesis for treatment of valvular insufficiency. The 12th Annual meeting of the American Venous Forum, Phoenix, Arizona. Abstract book 2000;82.

13. Pavcnik D, Uchida BT, Keller FS, et al. Retrievable IVC square stent filter: experimental study. *Cardiovasc Intervent Radiol* 1999; 22:239–245.

14. Pavcnik D, Uchida B, Timmermans HA, et al. Square stent based large vessel occluder. *J Vasc Interv Radiol* 2000;11: 1227–1234.

15. Hiles MC, Badylak SF, Lantz GC, et al. Mechanical properties of xenogenic small-intestinal submucosa when used as an aortic graft in the dog. *J Biomed Mater Res* 1995;29:883–895.

16. Moulopoulos SD, Anthopoulos LP, Antonatos PG, et al. Intra-aortic balloon pump for relief of aortic regurgitation. Experimental study. *J Thorac Cardiovasc Surg* 1980;80: 38–44.

50

PERCUTANEOUS REPLACEMENT OF THE PULMONARY VALVE

YONES BOUDJEMLINE
PHILIPP BONHOEFFER

Stents have revolutionized the treatment of right heart lesions in the child (1) and are now even utilized in the technology for percutaneous valve implantation (2,3). They have been largely used in the treatment of branch pulmonary artery stenosis (4), but they have also been used in conduit obstruction from the right ventricular to the pulmonary artery (5). Balloon dilatation with isolated stent placement opens the conduit narrowing but creates or aggravates pulmonary regurgitation. Obviously, pulmonary insufficiency also occurs after valveless repair of the right ventricular outflow tract. Pulmonary regurgitation is generally well tolerated for many years when pulmonary vasculature is normal. However, in the long term, it results in progressive right ventricular dilatation and finally in right heart failure (6). Exercise tolerance decreases with an increased risk for arrhythmia and sudden death (7). Preservation of the right ventricular function appears to be important for the long-term survival of patients who underwent cardiac surgery in their infancy.

Thus pulmonary valve replacement is recommended in patients with deterioration of their clinical status and/or objective signs of right ventricular dysfunction (8). Unfortunately, the recovery of a normal right ventricular function after valve replacement cannot be guaranteed. Further, symptoms often occur only when irreversible damage to the right ventricle is already established. There is no consensus on the optimal timing for valve implantation (9). Classically, the surgical approach is the only technique to replace a pulmonary valve. The mortality and the morbidity of the reoperations are low but are not negligible. In addition, the need for re-replacement also exists. Thus a potentially less invasive approach is appealing. We developed an innovating device for percutaneous implantation of a valve in the pul-

monary position. Here we describe our experience with experimental percutaneous valve implantation in animal models and the initial cases of nonsurgical heart valve implantation in the human subjects.

THE VALVE

Many herbivorous animals have native venous valves in their jugular veins that allow avoiding stasis of the blood in the head during feeding. Venous valves are found in different configurations. Most of them are incomplete, but occasionally perfectly formed bi- or tricuspid valves can be found. These valves have already been harvested and used in surgical pulmonary valve replacement. They became popular because their leaflets are extremely thin and mobile and the venous wall is ideal for suturing by the surgeon. The geometrical structure of the valve allows it to function at different diameters and in different geometrical conformations. In surgery, this allows for the implantation of a stentless valved segment of the vein in form of a right-ventricular-to-pulmonary-artery conduit. With the idea of percutaneous implantation, this permits compression of the valve and to reexpand it to the original diameter. In clinical studies the thin leaflets of the valve have been shown to resist to diastolic pulmonary pressures. Our experimental *in vitro* studies at short term have also shown their resistance to pressures above 100 mm Hg. The feasibility of using such a valve in aortic position still needs to be evaluated.

Preparation of the Assembly

The biologic valve is harvested from the jugular vein of a fresh bovine cadaver. The thickness of the bovine jugular vein is too large to permit percutaneous placement in children when attached to the stent. Therefore the external wall is trimmed and tanned to remove unnecessary tissue. The prepared tubular portion (Figure 50.1) is then sutured in a preexpanded vascular platinum stent (Numed, Hopkinton,

Yones Boudjemline: Service de Cardiologic Pédiatrique, Hôpital Necker-Enfants Malades, Paris, France

Philipp Bonhoeffer: Director, Cardiac Catheterization Laboratory, Hospital for Sick Children, London, United Kingdom

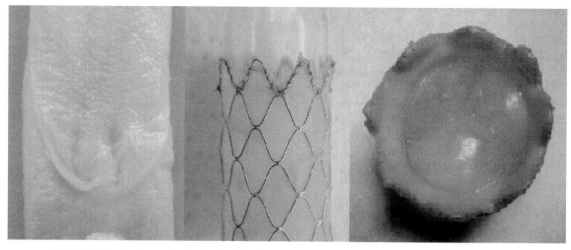

A, B   C

FIGURE 50.1. Photograph of a bovine jugular venous valve **(A)**. The tubular vein graft, trimmed and mounted in a preexpanded stent, is shown in **(B)**. **C:** Shows *en face* view of the closed venous valve.

NY). This stent is made of a platinum iridium wire that is interconnected by welds. This structure allows compression and reexpansion that is an essential characteristic. After crimping, the overall diameter of the valve assembly when fitted on the balloon catheter does not exceed 18F.

Sterilization protocols in the animal experience were by simple use of glutaraldehyde. For the human application, they were prepared according to industrial standards.

THE ANIMAL EXPERIENCE

Eleven lambs 2 months old and weighing 16 to 18 kg underwent catheterization for percutaneous pulmonary valve implantation under general anesthesia. All lambs were treated according to European regulations for animal experimentation (10).

The device was hand-crimped just before its implantation onto the inflatable portion of a balloon catheter. After positioning a guide wire in the pulmonary artery through the internal jugular vein, the device was front-loaded in a Mullins long sheath and the whole system was loaded and advanced onto the previously positioned guide wire. The valve assembly was finally inserted in the desired position according to standard stent placement technique.

Hemodynamic evaluation was performed before and after the implantation and at the end of the protocol to measure the right ventricular and pulmonary arterial pressures. Angiography was performed before the implantation to precisely locate the position of the native pulmonary valve. This was repeated after the procedure and at the end of the protocol to confirm the good function of the implanted valve.

Grafts were retrieved after 2 months (60 to 74 days), and explanted valved stents were macroscopically

inspected, tested *in vitro,* and finally fixed in 10% formaldehyde and individually stored for histologic examination. Specimens were embedded in paraffin. Serial sections were cut at 10-μm thickness and stained with hematoxylin, eosin, and a histologic method for calcium deposit. The morphologic examination protocol consisted of multiple microphotographs, histology, and transmission electron microscopy of the venous wall and valve leaflets.

Results in the Animal Model

Seven (64%) of 11 lambs had a pulmonary valve implanted through the internal jugular approach. Technical failure occurred in the four remaining lambs. Stent implantation failure was due to the narrow angle between the tricuspid valve and the right ventricular outflow in lambs. Indeed, the femoral vein used in humans allows a straight course of the catheter. This approach is impossible in the lamb because of the small size of this vein.

In the successful seven implantations, five valved stents were implanted in good position impinging on the function of the native valve. Two stents were implanted in unsatisfactory position adjacent to the native valve.

There were no significant complications during the procedure and in the early follow-up. No early or late stent migration was noted. Somatic growth was normal in all implanted lambs.

Pulmonary artery pressures showed unchanged diastolic pressures in all lambs during the entire study. One stent was mildly stenotic, with a pressure gradient between the right ventricle and the pulmonary artery of 15 mm Hg. Six of these seven valved stents were angiographically competent at the early evaluation. The evaluation of the seventh showed a mild insufficiency aggravated by the position of the catheter in the pulmonary valve during the angiography.

Macroscopic findings at autopsy revealed that four of the five valves implanted in precise position were competent with no sign of valvar calcification. The remaining graft was moderately stenotic with macroscopic calcification at examination. Two of the three cusps were immobilized and retracted. Partial fusion of the commissures was also found in this particular case. We attributed this early degeneration to the suboptimal sterilization process used in our early experience. The wall of all stents showed diffuse fibrous tissue ingrowth predominantly in the extremities of the stents. Removal of the grafts was always possible without major damage to the pulmonary trunk.

The two stents implanted in incorrect position adjacent to the native pulmonary valve were not totally functioning. The normal hemodynamics of these animals were due to the residual function of the native pulmonary valve. The first stent showed a valve totally covered by a fibrous tissue. The function was restored *in vitro* after the removal of this tissue. The covered leaflets were thin, transparent, and not calcified. The other valved stent impinged the function of only one leaflet of the native valve. Only one leaflet of the implanted stent was functional, the other being embedded in fibrous tissue. There were no macroscopic evidence surface thrombi and infected vegetations in any of the explanted valves.

Multiple longitudinal sections of the grafts were then inspected under light microscopy. Neointimal formation with endothelium-like cell was observed in all luminal portions of the stents. The valves were free of this formation. The extremities and the external wall of the stents were covered by abundant fibrin deposit associated with slight calcification. No thrombus formation and no fibroblast migration were observed.

The explanted stenotic valve had major microscopic alteration, including calcific deposits, endocarditis, neovascularization, and collagen degeneration. Calcific deposits formed oval-shaped nodules and were mainly localized in the middle of the cuspal fibrosa. Multiple calcific nodules protruded through the cuspal tissue into the outflow surface deforming the structure of this valve. Morphologic examination also disclosed that endocarditis had occurred. Indeed, inflammatory infiltrates composed by lymphocytes and giant cells were found in cusp sections. The presence of these early degenerative processes in this valve strengthened our hypothesis of a suboptimal sterilization process used in the protocol.

This animal experimentation confirmed that biologic valves could be implanted with good functional results. Once implanted, there is no difference between surgical and percutaneous placement in term of lifespan. Technical implantation difficulties were related to the animal model. Stent experience exists already in the right ventricular outflow tract in the human. Therefore human application was the next step.

THE HUMAN EXPERIENCE

Patient Selection

Children with a failing prosthetic conduit connected between the right ventricle and the pulmonary arteries were selected for a preliminary study. Characteristics of the patients are reported in Table 50.1. The patients had congenital heart defects (namely, tetralogy of Fallot, pulmonary

TABLE 50.1. PATIENT CHARACTERISTICS AND RESULTS

Patients	Age (in years)	Congenital Heart Defect	Conduit Type	Systolic Pressure Ratio Between Right Ventricle and Aorta (%)		Pulmonary Artery Pressures Distal to Conduit (Systolic/Diastolic/Mean)	
				Before	After	Before	After
1	12	Pulmonary atresia with ventricular septal defect	18-mm Carpentier–Edward valved conduit	85	66	30/8/16	30/16/20
2	12	Pulmonary atresia with ventricular septal defect	18-mm Goretex conduit non-valved conduit	71	33	22/6/16	28/14/20
3	10	Pulmonary atresia with ventricular septal defect	18-mm Hancock valved conduit	71	33	25/8/15	30/14/18
4	11	Tetralogy of Fallot	RVOT reconstruction with Dacron patch	70	60	60/10/18	40/10/22
5	11	Absent pulmonary valve syndrome	16-mm Carpentier–Edward valved conduit	50	50	31/8/15	32/14/18
6	18	Tetralogy of Fallot	20-mm Carpentier–Edward valved conduit	60	33	28/12/16	32/16/20

atresia with ventricular septal defect, and absent pulmonary valve syndrome) initially palliated with one or more modified Blalock-Taussig shunts. Subsequently, total repair with closure of the ventricular septal defect and placement of a conduit from the right ventricle to the pulmonary artery was performed. These children were symptomatic and in need of surgery for conduit replacement because of significant stenosis and insufficiency of the conduit.

Device Implantation Technique

Approval for percutaneous pulmonary valve replacement was given by a certified ethical committee Comité Consultatif pour la Protection des Personnes dans la Recherche Biomédicale (CCPPRB), Cochin, Paris, France). Informed consent was then obtained from the parents.

Angiographic and hemodynamic evaluation were first performed to locate the position of the stenosis, to study the anatomy of the right ventricular outflow tract, and to confirm the need of valved stent implantation. The stenosis was first dilated to ascertain that the obstruction could be sufficiently dilated to place the valved stent inside without creating additional obstruction.

A new delivery system (Numed, Hopkinton, NY) was used for human application (Figure 50.2). The initial delivery system was too stiff to allow a safe course of the system into the pulmonary trunk. Therefore we improved the delivery system to allow a safer procedure and to reduce the failure rate of the technique. This new system is made for front-loading of the valve assembly and has a structure, which avoids kinking. The balloon is based on the BIB (balloon-in-balloon) catheter system.

After positioning a guide wire in the pulmonary artery, the delivery system, containing the hand-crimped valved stent, was advanced into the prosthetic pulmonary trunk. The plastic sheath of the delivery system was then retrieved to uncover the valved stent. First, the inner balloon is inflated to 9 mm to secure the stent to the inflatable portion of the delivery system and to limit the risk of dislodg-

ment during final precise positioning. The outer balloon was then inflated additionally, expanding the stent to the final radial diameter such that the stent fixes the device to the prosthetic pulmonary wall and relieves the stenosis and the insufficiency of the old damaged valve. Each balloon was subsequently deflated and the catheter was removed from the patient, leaving the valve implant in the desired position. Angiographic and hemodynamic evaluation concluded the procedure.

Results

Immediate Results

In three patients, angiography before implantation showed severe calcifications of the conduit. Calcification was seen in the area of the valve contained in the conduit. In two patients, the stenosis was located in the bifurcation of the pulmonary artery. Patients 2 and 4 had a dilatation of pulmonary branch stenosis before valve implantation. Patient 3 had a severe stenosis of the left pulmonary artery with multiple pulmonary stenoses behind.

The results of hemodynamic study are listed in Table 50.1. The valved stent was successfully implanted in all patients. The hemodynamic and angiographic evaluation confirmed good function of the new valve (Figure 50.3) in five patients and the partial relief of the conduit obstruction in patients 1 and 4. In patient 4 an insignificant paraprosthetic insufficiency was observed because of suboptimal positioning of the valved stent. The paraprosthetic insufficiency in patients 4 and 5 could not be detected by echocardiography. There were no significant complications in the early follow-up, and patients were discharged with aspirin at a low dose.

Follow-up

The follow-up ranged from 15 days to 8 months, with a mean at 4 months. Echocardiography showed a perfectly competent pulmonary valve and a normal-sized right ven-

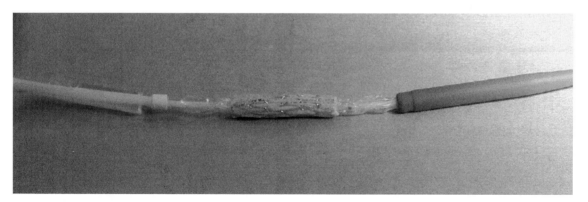

FIGURE 50.2. Photograph of a front-loaded stent valve assembly on a balloon-in- balloon (BIB) catheter ready for implantation.

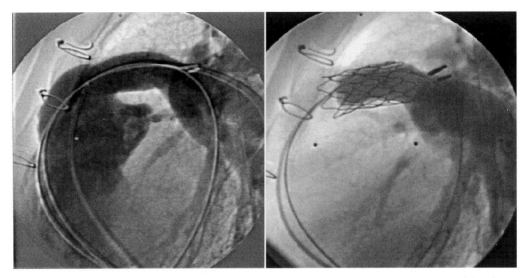

FIGURE 50.3. Selected cineangiographic views of pulmonary arteriograms via a multitrack catheter before **(A)** and after **(B)** percutaneous pulmonary valve implantation. The left panel demonstrates opacification of the right ventricle (pulmonary regurgitation) before valve insertion, which completely disappears **(B)** after placement of the bovine jugular valve.

tricle with normal systolic function in all patients. It also confirmed the partial relief of the conduit obstruction in patients 1 and 4, but the systolic pressure ratio between the right ventricle and aorta tended to be lower during the follow-up. No migration of the valved stent occurred. One stent had a fracture of a weld between the wires due to difficulties at the time of insertion through the skin. That fracture had no influence on valve function. The physical condition of all patients improved after implantation.

DISCUSSION

Percutaneous valve implantation in the right heart is possible. Our early experiments in animals have shown the feasibility of such a technique and the perfect valvular function after implantation. The good results in the animal study allowed us to begin with human application. With a number of technical modifications, it was possible to implant pulmonary valves in children with a conduit from the right ventricle to the pulmonary artery that was obstructed and insufficient. Further technical improvements will allow for a user-friendly implantation of such a valve. The impact of nonsurgical pulmonary valve replacement in the human is obviously manifold. Surgical indication to pulmonary valve replacement has always been difficult. Patients requiring such an operation usually have a long surgical history with numerous operations and reoperations. Their symptoms related to pulmonary insufficiency usually occur late, when right ventricular function has already attained irreversible damage. In addition, the benefit of pulmonary valve replacement is difficult to predict. A less traumatic nonsur-

gical approach for such a patient is therefore obviously beneficial. Furthermore, the technique is less painful, causes less anxiety, and permits an early discharge, without additional sternal scar.

In common with other heterografts, our device can degenerate. The degeneration of the bioprosthetic valves has been studied extensively over the past 10 years (11). Many factors have been reported to influence this progressive failure. In particular, biologic and metabolic factors—including immunologic (foreign-body reaction), fibrin deposition, calcification, and infection—contribute to the failure of bioprostheses. Calcification is the major cause of failure leading to valve replacement. The calcification also depends largely on host factors, mainly on the patient's age and the type of the cross-linking (12).

The type of preparation of our device could theoretically alter the function and the durability of the valve. Anyway, as far as the function of the valve is considered, we verified by multiple *in vitro* testing that this had not led to any side effects, and most of the implanted valves functioned perfectly without any major macroscopic or microscopic alterations.

The initially implanted patients were carrying a failing prosthetic conduit in the right ventricular outflow tract. Clinical results of valve implantation were excellent in the early follow-up stage in all patients. The use of a valved stent was very attractive due to the simple model. We chose this model because of the potential benefit of relieving both stenosis and insufficiency during the same procedure. Indeed, stents are commonly used to reopen obstructed conduits, delaying the need for surgical replacement (13–17), but they may aggravate pulmonary insufficiency.

The long-term function of the right ventricle is impaired by the chronic regurgitation that volume overloads the non-systemic ventricle. The implantation of valved stents preserves the right ventricular function. In all our patients, right ventricular function and size were normal after the valve implantation.

Obviously, one of the major challenges of the future will be to implant such a valve in more variable anatomy. Indeed, pulmonary insufficiency frequently occurs after repair of tetralogy of Fallot (18), and early treatment of this condition might be beneficial. This experience reports the first step in percutaneous implantation of heart valves. The replacement of the aortic and atrioventricular valves still remains a major challenge for the future.

CURRENT STATUS

The device is custom manufactured by Numed (Hopkinton, NY) and Venpro (Irvine, CA). Ethical Committee approval for its use is limited to our institution. Submission for the CE Mark is planned for the European market in 2004.

REFERENCES

1. O'Laughlin MP, Perry SB, Lock JE, et al. Use of endovascular stents in congenital heart disease. *Circulation* 1991;83:1923–1939.
2. Bonhoeffer P, Boudjemline Y, Saliba Z, et al. Transcatheter implantation of a bovine valve in pulmonary position: a lamb study. *Circulation* 2000;102:813–816.
3. Bonhoeffer P, Boudjemline Y, Saliba Z, et al. Percutaneous replacement of pulmonary valve in a right-ventricle to pulmonary-artery prosthetic conduit with valve dysfunction. *Lancet* 2000;356:1403–1405.
4. Fogelman R, Nykanen D, Smallhorn JF, et al. Endovascular stents in the pulmonary circulation: clinical impact on management and medium-term follow-up. *Circulation* 1995;92:881–885.
5. Conte S, Jashari R, Eyskens B, et al. Homograft valve insertion for pulmonary regurgitation late after valveless repair of right ventricular outflow tract obstruction. *Eur J Cardiothorac Surg* 1999;15:143–149.
6. Schamberger MS, Hurwitz RA. Course of right and left ventricular function in patients with pulmonary insufficiency after repair of tetralogy of Fallot. *Pediatr Cardiol* 2000;21:244–248.
7. Bove EL, Byrum CJ, Thomas FD, et al. The influence of pulmonary insufficiency on ventricular function following repair of tetralogy of Fallot: evaluation using radionuclide ventriculography. *J Thorac Cardiovasc Surg* 1983;85:691–696.
8. Connelly MS, Webb GD, Somerville J, et al. Canadian Consensus Conference on Adult Congenital Heart Disease 1996. *Can J Cardiol* 1998;14:395–452.
9. Therrien J, Siu SC, McLaughlin PR, et al. Pulmonary valve replacement in adults late after repair of tetralogy of fallot: are we operating too late? *J Am Coll Cardiol* 2000;36:1670–1675.
10. Convention européenne sur la protection des animaux vertébrés utilisés à des fins expérimentales ou à d'autres fins scientifiques. *Journal Officiel des Communautés Européennes.* L222/29 à L222/37. August 24, 1999.
11. Rao KP, Shanthi C. Reduction of calcification by various treatments in cardiac valves. *J Biomater Appl* 1999;13:238-268.
12. Grabenwoger M, Sider J, Fitzal F, et al. Impact of glutaraldehyde on calcification of pericardial bioprosthetic heart valve material. *Ann Thorac Surg* 1996;62:772–777.
13. Saliba Z, Bonhoeffer P, Aggoun Y, et al. Traitement des obstructions des prothèses tubulaires par implantation percutanée de stents. *Arch Mal Cœur Vaiss* 1999;92:591–596.
14. Ovaert C, Caldarone CA, McCrindle BW, et al. Endovascular stent implantation for the management of postoperative right ventricular outflow tract obstruction: clinical efficacy. *J Thorac Cardiovasc Surg* 1999;118:886–893.
15. O'Laughlin MP, Slack MC, Grifka RG, et al. Implantation and intermediate-term follow-up of stents in congenital heart disease. *Circulation* 1993;88:605–614.
16. Hosking MC, Benson LN, Nakanishi T, et al. Intravascular stent prosthesis for right ventricular outflow obstruction. *J Am Coll Cardiol* 1992;20:373–380.
17. Powell AJ, Lock JE, Keane JF, et al. Prolongation of right ventricular to pulmonary artery conduit life span by percutaneous stent implantation intermediate-term results. *Circulation* 1995;92:3282–388.
18. Murphy JG, Gersh BJ, Mair DD, et al. Long-term outcome in patients undergoing surgical repair of tetralogy of Fallot. *N Engl J Med* 1993;329:593–599.

51

NEW AND MISCELLANEOUS DEVICES

P. SYAMASUNDAR RAO

Although we have allocated 50 chapters to discuss catheter-based devices, some devices still have not been mentioned. In this chapter we review a number of other devices that are beginning to appear as well as those that have not been included in the preceding chapters, because of the format of the book. Also included here is a discussion of devices/device applications that have come to light since the initial preparation of this book.

STAGED FONTAN: NONSURGICAL COMPLETION

The current practice in surgical management of tricuspid atresia and other "single-ventricle" physiology cardiac defects is staged total cavopulmonary connection (1,2). Initially, a bidirectional Glenn procedure is performed, followed later by "Fontan conversion" by an extracardiac conduit diversion of the inferior vena caval flow into the pulmonary artery (3). The latter procedure, seemingly simple, continues to have significant morbidity and some mortality. To avoid this morbidity and to do away with the second-stage surgery, Konert (4), Hausdorf (5), and their associates proposed a staged surgical–catheter approach. The first stage consists of performing a modified hemi-Fontan; the second involves transcatheter completion of Fontan.

The first stage (i.e., modified hemi-Fontan) involves performing the usual bidirectional Glenn shunt, anastomosis of the lower end of the divided superior vena cava to the undersurface of the right pulmonary artery, banding of the superior vena cava slightly above the caval–atrial junction around a 16-gauge catheter with 6-0 prolene, creating a lateral tunnel with a Goretex baffle, diverting the inferior vena caval blood flow toward the superior vena cava and fenestrating the baffle with three to seven 5-mm punch holes (Figure 51.1). As can be seen, the first stage accomplishes a physiologic bidirectional Glenn.

Other problems such as subaortic obstruction, prior aortopulmonary shunt, antegrade flow through the main pulmonary artery, interatrial obstruction, and pulmonary artery distortion, if present, are also addressed during the hemi-Fontan operation.

The second stage (i.e., the transcatheter stage) consists of balloon dilatation of superior vena caval band and closure of the fenestrations. The latter may be achieved by a variety of atrial septal occlusion devices (Chapters 11 and 14) or by implantation of a covered stent (4–7). Incorporation of perforatable membrane within the covered stent may facilitate fenestration should it be necessary during follow-up.

A limited number of procedures utilizing the preceding concepts have been performed (4–7). The preliminary data

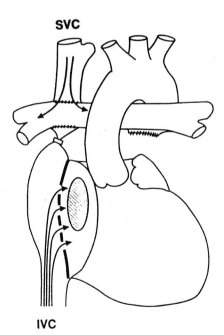

FIGURE 51.1. Artist's representation of a stage 1 surgical procedure. Note the banding of the superior vena cava (SVC) close to cavopulmonary anastomosis and multifenestrated baffle, which allows inferior vena caval (IVC) return to mix with pulmonary venous return. (From Konert W, Schneider M, Herwig V, et al. Modified hemi-Fontan operation and subsequent nonsurgical Fontan completion. *J Thorac Cardiovasc Surg* 1995;110:865–867, with permission.)

P. Syamasundar Rao: Professor of Pediatrics, Medicine, and Cardiology, Department of Pediatrics, University of Texas–Houston Medical School; Director, Division of Pediatric Cardiology, Memorial Hermann Children's Hospital, Houston, Texas

suggest that the usual post-Fontan complications, such as pleural effusion, ascites, and long postoperative stay in the hospital have not occurred with this approach. This ingenious and innovative approach should be seriously considered as an alternative to conventional two-stage Fontan. However, scrutiny of immediate and long-term results in a larger series of patients and ready availability of atrial septal defect closure devices and covered stents for general clinical use are needed before routine use of this method.

COVERED STENTS

Aortic Coarctation

The conventional surgical repair of coarctation of the aorta is being slowly replaced by transcatheter techniques (8–12). Catheter management of neonatal and infant coarctations is controversial (12), but use of balloon angioplasty in children and stents in adolescents and adults appears to be the current trend. Issues related to use of stents (regular, uncovered) have been discussed in Chapter 35. The experience with the use of covered stents in the treatment of aortic coarctation is limited (13), although there is extensive experience in their use in the treatment of infrarenal aortic aneurysms, discussed in detail in Chapter 42. A brief review of the role of covered stents in the management of coarctation will be undertaken in this section.

There is extremely limited experience in the use of covered stents in the management of aortic coarctation (13). De Giovani used Jostent grafts (Jomed International, Helsingborg, Sweden) to treat aortic coarctation. The grafts vary in length from 38 to 58 mm and can be expanded to diameters of 10 to 18 mm. They are covered with PTEE (polyterafluorethylene) and are hand-mounted onto the balloon valvuloplasty catheters. They can be delivered to the implantation site via 9- to 11F sheaths.

The indications for intervention are similar to those used for balloon angioplasty and deployment of a standard stent (Chapter 35) (9). The indications for use of covered stents are postangioplasty aneurysm, tortuous aortic arch and isthmus, associated patent ductus arteriosus, prior surgical conduit, and Takayasu's arteritis (13). When the assessed risk for development of aneurysm or dissection is high, a covered stent was used.

The patients' ages varied between 10 and 43 years (median, 12), and their weights varied between 28 and 96 kg (median, 76) (13). The stents crimped on Crystal valvuloplasty balloons (Merck KGa A, Hampsphire, UK) were delivered to implantation sites via 9- to 11F sheaths. The delivery sheath is 1F larger than that required for the balloon catheters. Expanded stent diameters were 9 to 18 mm (median, 14), whereas the lengths varied between 38 and 58 mm (median, 48). Peak systolic pressure gradients across the aortic obstruction decreased from 32 ± 22 mm Hg to 11 ± 6 mm Hg, and the coarctation segment diameter increased from 10 ± 5 mm to 14 ± 4 mm following stent

deployment. Platelet-inhibiting drugs (mostly aspirin) were administered for 1 to 6 months. No complications were encountered during stent implantation or during a short period of follow-up from 4 to 32 months (13).

A number of other covered stents are detailed in Chapter 42. Both self-expandable and balloon-expandable stents are available. The preference to use Jostent is related to its low profile (13). However, it can be expanded to a diameter of only 18 mm. Also, the stent shortens when expanded to larger diameters. Use of covered stents has another disadvantage in that the vessels arising from the aorta are blocked.

Based on the currently available data, the covered stents may be useful in highly selected patients with aortic coarctation.

Other Uses

The covered stents may also be useful in closing multiple vascular connections, such as pulmonary arteriovenous fistulae, or for Fontan applications, as detailed in a preceding section.

DEVICES TO KEEP ATRIAL FENESTRATIONS OPEN

Interatrial communication with shunting across it is highly beneficial in some congenital heart defects. Most important of these is transposition of the great arteries with intact ventricular septum in which interatrial mixing is essential for survival. Other lesions in which the presence of adequate interatrial communication is important are mitral atresia, hypoplastic left heart syndrome, tricuspid atresia, pulmonary atresia with intact ventricular septum, and total anomalous pulmonary venous connection. Surgical atrial septostomy/septectomy was originally used to relieve interatrial obstruction. In 1966, Rashkind and Miller (14) described a technique of nonsurgical enlargement of the patent foramen ovale in which a balloon filled with diluted radiopaque liquid is rapidly pulled back across the atrial septum, thus rupturing the lower margin of the atrial septum forming the patent foramen ovale. The procedure is now called Rashkind balloon atrial septostomy. The usefulness of balloon atrial septostomy in palliation of transposition of the great arteries (15,16), mitral atresia (17,18), hypoplastic left heart syndrome (19), tricuspid atresia (20,21), pulmonary atresia with intact ventricular septum (22,23), and total anomalous pulmonary venous return (24,25) has been well documented.

The original concept and subsequent success of balloon atrial septostomy are predicated on the fact that the lower margin of the foramen ovale is very thin and membranous, and can be torn by Rashkind balloon septostomy. The lower margin of the foramen ovale, however, becomes thick and muscular beyond the neonatal period (26,27) and cannot be ruptured by balloon septostomy. This appears to be the reason for failure of this procedure in older infants and children (26–28). To address this difficulty, Park and his associates (29,30) developed a catheter with a built-in, retractable blade (knife) to cut the lower margin of the foramen ovale (septum primum of the fossa ovales). This is then followed by balloon septostomy to further enlarge the atrial defect. Following the initial report by Park (30) a number of other studies (31–34) confirmed the efficacy of this procedure, with success rates ranging between 70% and 90% (31–34). Availability of different sizes of blade catheters and long introducer sheaths has improved the success rate. However, adequate septostomy is impossible or difficult in patients with small and hypoplastic left atria.

When balloon angioplasty technique became available, it was applied to address this issue. Mitchell, Sideris, and their colleagues (35,36) were able to produce large atrial septal defects by static balloon dilatation in animal models and suggested that the static balloon dilatation could be performed instead of dynamic Rashkind balloon septostomy. The first human application of static balloon dilatation was successfully undertaken by Shrivastava and her colleagues (37) to improve mixing in an infant with transposition of the great arteries. Subsequently, several reports of its use in treating a number of conditions appeared and were reviewed elsewhere (38).

More recently, the need for creation and maintenance of interatrial communication was recognized in two situations, namely, Fontan patients to relieve systemic venous hypertension (39,40) and pulmonary hypertension (pulmonary vascular obstructive closure) as a bridge to transplantation (41,42). Whereas the atrial defects can be enlarged or produced following Brockenbrough puncture or radiofrequency perforation (43,44), some of these defects tend to close spontaneously, requiring repeat intervention in some patients. Also, the currently available methods are not conducive to control the size of the defect. To circumvent these problems two different types of solutions are envisioned (9,45). Stenting of the atrial septum is one such option (9). Mounting a balloon-expandable stent on a dumbbell-shaped balloon and implanting across the atrial septum may prove useful (9). The waist of the balloon can be selected (4, 5, or 6 mm) and the stent implanted in such a way that the waist is at the level of the atrial septum and the stent is expanded to 10 mm on either side of the atrial septum (Figure 51.2) to ensure the stability of the expanded stent across the atrial septum. Precise positioning of the stent and, more important, assurance that the stent will remain in place are important. Preliminary experience (46,47) appears to be encouraging. The dumbbell shape of the stent was achieved either by using a 2-0 silk suture placed circumferentially around the stent (46) or by limiting the balloon expansion with a loop created from a temporary pacing wire (47). Procedural success in most patients and improvement in hemodynamic parameters along with symptomatic improvement occurred in the majority of patients. An alternative to mounting the stent on dumbbell-shaped balloons is construction of a dumbbell-shaped stent with a shape-memory alloy.

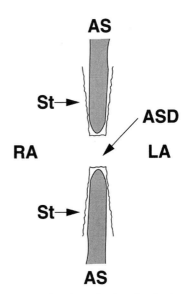

FIGURE 51.2. Artist's drawing of a longitudinal cross section of the atrial septum (AS) and implanted stent (St) to keep open the atrial septal defect (ASD). LA, left atrium; RA, right atrium. (From Rao PS. Interventional pediatric cardiology: state of the art and future directions. *Pediatr Cardiol* 1998;19:107–124, with permission.)

The second option is to create a fenestration in an atrial septal defect occluding device and implant it across the atrial septum. This was undertaken with the Amplatzer Septal Occluder, the fenestrated Amplatzer (45). Preliminary data indicate usefulness of this concept. The Amplatzer Septal Occluder was modified by incorporating a 4-mm tunnel near the center of the device. The method of device implantation is similar to that used for secundum atrial septal defect closure, described in Chapter 6. The modified device was successfully implanted in two patients who had protein-loosing enteropathy or refractory pleural effusions following Fontan (45). Both patients experienced relief of symptoms. Follow-up echocardiography 6 months later revealed functional fenestration. The authors concluded that the fenestrated Amplatzer device is a valuable tool in the overall management of failing Fontan circulation and that it can be performed without surgical intervention. A similar approach may be taken in creating controlled-size atrial defect in patients with pulmonary vascular obstructive disease, as a bridge to transplantation.

DEVICE CLOSURE OF AORTOPULMONARY WINDOW

The aortopulmonary window (APW) is an uncommon congenital cardiac malformation representing no more than 0.1% of all congenital cardiac defects (48). Most APWs require surgical closure. A variety of surgical techniques have been used to repair the defect successfully (49–53). Furthermore, most APWs are large, have little inferior or superior rim, and may not be good candidates for trans-

TABLE 51.1. TRANSCATHETER CLOSURE OF AORTOPULMONARY WINDOW (APW)

Authors	Age (yr)	Weight (kg)	Size of APW (mm)	Qp:Qs	Device Used	Size of Delivery Sheath	Result	Complications
Stamato et al. (55)	3	11	3	—	Rashkind PDA occluder 12 mm	7F	Small residual shunt	None
Tulloh and Rigby (56)	0.8	8	3	—	Rashkind PDA occluder 12 mm	8F	Full occlusion	None
Jureidini et al. (57)	27	—	3.7	>2.1	Buttoned Device 15 mm	8F	Full occlusion	None

catheter device closure. However, a small percentage [three of 25 (12%)] of the defects, intermediate defects, may have well-formed inferior and superior rims (54) and are amenable to the transcatheter approach.

Extensive review of the literature revealed less than a handful of case reports of device closure of APWs (Table 51.1) (55–57). Rashkind patent ductus arteriosus (PDA) occluder devices and buttoned device have been used. Initially, an arteriovenous guide wire "rail" was established by passing a guide wire from the femoral artery (via a catheter) through the APW into the pulmonary artery, with the guide wire snared and brought out through the femoral vein. The delivery sheath was then positioned transvenously over the guide wire. The delivery and implantation of the selected device are similar to the implantation of the PDA devices (58). The results were good with minimal or no residual shunt. Figure 51.3 shows one case from our personal experience (57).

The previously described experience, though limited, suggests feasibility, safety, and effectiveness of device closure of the APWs. However, only a small proportion of APWs

are amenable for transcatheter closure. Accurate assessment of the size, if necessary by balloon sizing, ensuring that adequate superior and inferior margins surround the defect and that there is no interference with critical structures (coronary artery, pulmonary artery), are important for successful use of transcatheter methodology.

PALLIATION OF PULMONARY OLIGEMIA

Patients with large interventricular communication and severe right ventricular outflow obstruction including atresia most commonly require surgical intervention. Corrective surgery, when feasible, is the current choice. When corrective surgery is not feasible, palliation with a variety of aortopulmonary shunts, most commonly modified Blalock-Taussig, shunt is undertaken. In highly selected cases catheter interventional techniques (59–66) may be used either as a primary procedure or as an adjunct to surgery. This section reviews application of stents and devices in the treatment of pulmonary oligemia.

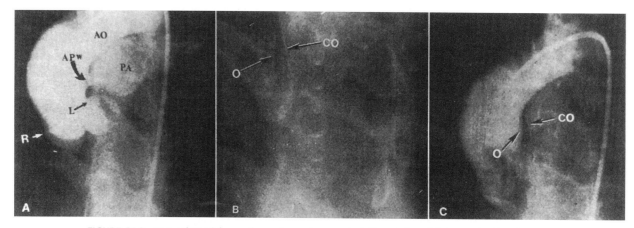

FIGURE 51.3. A: A selected frame from cineaortogram in left anterior oblique projection demonstrating the location, size, and shape of the aortopulmonary window (APW) *(curved arrow)*. There is dense filling of the pulmonary artery (PA). The distance between the defect and left coronary artery (L) *(straight arrow)* is foreshortened in this view but outlined better in the lateral view (not shown). **B:** The occluder (O) and counteroccluder (CO) of the buttoned device are shown *(arrow)* after buttoning across the defect. **C:** Repeat aortogram in left anterior oblique view after implantation of the buttoned device, showing minimal, if any, residual shunt. The *arrows* point to O and CO. (From Jureidini SB, Spadaro JJ, Rao PS. Successful transcatheter closure with the buttoned device of aortopulmonary window in an adult. *Am J Cardiol* 1998;81:371–372, with permission.)

Ductal Stents

The role of stenting the ductus is discussed in Chapter 36 and will not be reviewed except to state that availability of new technology (e.g., flexible stents) may facilitate more frequent use of stents than previously reported (67). In addition, there appears to be progressive, spontaneous closure of the ductal stents following implantation (67). To address some of the problems associated with ductal stents, Amin et al. (66) modified the Amplatzer Septal Occluder (AGA Medical Corp., Golden Valley, MN) by creating a 4- to 6-mm diameter tunnel through the waist of the device and implanted it across the ducti of newborn lambs. They demonstrated feasibility of implantation and short-term patency of such devices. Further studies in animal models, followed by human trials, will be necessary to determine the role of such devices in the management of congenital heart defects.

Stenting of Aortopulmonary Collateral Vessels

The preferred treatment approach for patients with ventricular septal defects, pulmonary atresia, and persistent aortopulmonary collateral arteries (PACAs) is surgical treatment with unifocalization and closure of the ventricular septal defect (68). However, surgical correction may not be feasible in some patients, particularly those with severe pulmonary artery hypoplasia. The condition of some of these patients may be improved by surgical systemic artery to pulmonary artery shunts. In others transcatheter palliation may be feasible (62,64). The embryonic PACAs tend to involute (69) and become stenotic. Stenosis may also

develop because of excessive proliferation of intimal tissue (70,71). Balloon angioplasty may be undertaken to enlarge the stenosed vessels. However, balloon dilatation of stenosed PACAs not only is associated with dissection, occlusion, and rupture (62) but also is ineffective (60,61,64). Therefore stenting the stenosed vessel may be a better option. Zahn et al. (59) were the first to report successful use of a stent in relieving stenosis of PACA. They implanted a 7-mm-diameter, 15-mm-long Palmaz stent into a PACA in a 12-year-old child with pulmonary atresia with ventricular septal defect, with resultant increase in arterial saturation from 60% to 82%. Several other reports of stenting PACAs followed (60–62,64).

The technique involves initially defining the angiographic anatomy of the stenosed vessel followed by access to the vessel beyond the stenotic region using a soft-tipped guide wire and an angled catheter [right coronary artery catheter (Cook, Bloomington, IN) or Glidecath catheter (Meditech, Boston, MA)]. The selected stent is mounted on a delivery balloon, usually 5 or 6 mm in diameter, and the stent is delivered and implanted across the stenotic region. More recently, the availability of premounted stents [Medtronic AVE bridge stents (Santa Rosa, CA) (Chapters 33 and 39) and IntraTherapeutic Paramount IntraStents (St. Paul, MN) (Chapter 33)] may make the procedure simpler. Additional stents in the same vessel or other stenotic PACAs may be necessary (64). Crisscross placement of stents (64,72) may be needed to maintain access and prevent obstruction if two vessels arise in close proximity to each other. Simultaneous stenting of the previously created, stenosed aortopulmonary shunts may also be necessary.

TABLE 51.2. STENTS IN PERSISTENT AORTOPULMONARY COLLATERAL ARTERIES (PACA)

Authors	Age (yr)	Weight (kg)	Vessels Stented	Stent(s) Used	O₂ Saturation Pre (%)	Post (%)	Comment
Zahn et al. (59)	12	—	PACA to left lung	Palmaz shunt*	60	82	—
McLeod et al. (60)	22	—	PACA to right and left lower lobes	Strecker stent†	78	85	—
Redington et al. (61)							
First case	24	56	PACA to right lobe	Self-expanding wall stent‡	67	83	—
Second case	32	63	PACA to right lobe	Self-expanding wall stent‡	66	86	—
Brown et al. (62)	4 patients, 8 Palmaz stents,* 7 collateral vessels—Patients not individually listed						
El-Said et al. (64)							
First case	33	—	PACA to left upper lobe	Two P-204 Palmaz-Statz stents*	70	81	Stenosed right BT shunt was also stented
Second case	6	—	PACA to left lower lobe	Two P-154 Palmaz stent*	68	88§	Pulmonary hemorrhage, dissection of lobar PAs

*Johnson and Johnson, Sommerville, NJ.
†Boston Scientific Ltd., Natick, MA.
‡Schneider, Bülach, Switzerland.
§At 2-month follow-up.
BT, Blalock-Taussig shunt; PAs, pulmonary arteries.

The reported experience (Table 51.2) in stenting stenosed PACAs (60–62,64), though limited, appears feasible and effective. Improvement in oxygen saturation, the primary objective, was achieved in most cases. Reported complications of pulmonary hemorrhage, aneurysm formation, and dissection (62,64) raise questions of safety. Use of soft-tipped guide wires for initial vessel access, careful attention to the details of the technique, and use of more flexible stents than those previously used may improve feasibility, safety, and effectiveness of this procedure.

Stenting of Aortopulmonary Shunts

As mentioned in the preceding section, surgical aortopulmonary shunts are performed if total correction is not feasible. Classic (73) or modified (74) Blalock-Taussig (BT) shunts are most commonly used for this purpose. Obstruction of such surgical stents can also occur, causing hypoxemia. If stenosis of the shunt develops before planned surgical correction, additional palliative surgery may be necessary. In such situations, transcatheter intervention to relieve the obstruction should be considered.

Balloon angioplasty of the narrowed BT shunts was first described by Fisher et al. (75), who reported improvement in oxygen saturation for 68% to 80% following balloon dilatation in a 4-year-old child. Subsequently, a number of interventionalists have reported on their experience with balloon angioplasty of both classic and modified BT shunts, reviewed elsewhere (76–79). However, balloon angioplasty is not uniformly effective (79,80), and some develop restenosis with time. Deployment of stents across the stenosed BT shunts to ensure their patency appears to be an attractive option.

Stent placement for treating obstruction that developed immediately after surgical creation of shunt (63,65) and during follow-up (64) appears possible. Both modified BT shunts (64,65) and central aortopulmonary Goretex grafts (63) were effectively stented. Obstructions at proximal (64) or distal (63) anastomotic sites as well as those in the middle portion of the graft secondary to intimal proliferation (64) could be treated successfully.

The procedure is similar to that described for stenting PACAs stenotic lesions. In the limited number of cases reported thus far (63–65) the procedure was successful in increasing arterial oxygen saturation.

Much wider experience than reported thus far, further miniaturization of stent delivery systems, and greater flexibility of the stents to pass through tortuous courses are necessary before routinely using this method of treatment.

LEFT ATRIAL APPENDAGE OCCLUSION TO PREVENT STROKES

It is estimated that 500,000 new strokes occur annually in the United States. Of these, 15% to 20% are accounted for by atrial fibrillation (AF). The AF-related strokes have high mortality. Annual health care costs run into $30 billion per year in the United States alone. The source of the emboli appears to be the left atrial appendage (LAA). Anticoagulation with warfarin has been the strategy used thus far to prevent strokes. Randomized clinical trials with warfarin suggest 60% to 70% reduction in strokes. However, anticoagulation is underutilized, is sometimes difficult to use, and does not have 100% efficacy. Therefore alternative approaches to prevent/reduce strokes in AF patients are worthy of further study. One such approach is occlusion or elimination of LAA from circulation. When other types of cardiac surgery (e.g., mitral valve repair/replacement) are performed, the obliteration of LAA is an established practice for stroke prophylaxis. Percutaneous device occlusion of LAA would therefore seem attractive.

A self-expandable Nitinol cage covered with e-PTFE has recently been developed, which can be implanted percutaneously (81). The device is named PLAATO (Appriva Medical, Sunnyvale, CA) and stands for "percutaneous left atrial appendage transcatheter occlusion." Preliminary experience in 31 patients demonstrated feasibility of successful implantation without major adverse events. Longer-term follow-up and randomized clinical trials comparing with the warfarin group may be necessary before widespread use of this device.

OTHER USES OF ATRIAL SEPTAL DEFECT CLOSURE DEVICES

Section I of this book discussed the usefulness of atrial septal defect (ASD) closure devices in occluding ostium secundum ASDs, ASDs/patent foramen ovalia (PFOs) presumed to be the sites of paradoxical embolism causing cerbrovascular accidents and transient ischemic attacks, ASDs/PFOs causing cyanosis and hypoxemia in partially corrected congenital heart defects or fenestrated Fontan patients, and atrial defects related to platypnea-orthodeoxia syndrome. Recently, some interest has been expressed in closure of the ASDs/PFOs in the management of decompression illness and migraine.

Decompression Illness

Decompression illness in divers appears to be caused by gas nucleation or gas embolism into the systemic arterial circulation. The potential for paradoxical embolism of venous gas bubbles via the PFO exists (82–85). Indeed, a higher frequency of decompression illness and of ischemic brain lesions in divers with PFO than in those without PFO was demonstrated (86). Some workers have used device closure of PFO to prevent ischemic brain lesions (87,88). However, at the present time abstaining from diving is recommended (89). The role of either surgical or device closure of PFO in the management of decompression illness should be investigated in future studies.

Migraine

An association between migraine with aura and right-to-left shunt has been suggested (90–92). In some of these subjects, shunting across PFO may have a causal association with migraine. The logical extension of such observations is to close PFO to prevent such migraine attacks. Indeed, device closure for such purposes has been undertaken (92). A more definitive establishment of a causal relationship between migraine with aura and right-to-left shunt through PFO should first be established in large cohorts of patients, followed by clinical studies to investigate the role of device closure in such defects.

AMPLATZER DEVICE MODIFICATIONS

Following the initial description of the Amplatzer device for closure of atrial septal defects (93), it has been clinically used in closure of atrial septal defects (Chapter 6). The device was subsequently modified/redesigned to close patent ductus arteriosus (Chapter 24) and muscular ventricular septal defects (Chapter 28).

The ASD closure device, because of the method of its construction, may not adapt to the septum when used for occlusion of patent foramen ovalia. Furthermore, the short and wide waist may not produce effective apposition of the device components against the atrial septum and, consequently, occlusion of the defect. Therefore the device was modified (94); there is now a larger right atrial disk and the connecting waist is thin and flexible. The new design is expected to be useful in closing PFOs with floppy atrial septum and channel-type defects. Clinical trials are under way with this modified device.

Additional modifications of the ASD device, by creation of a fenestration (45), and of the PDA device to stent the ductus open (66) have been undertaken and were discussed in preceding sections of this chapter.

The Amplatzer ventricular septal defect (VSD) occluder designed to close muscular VSDs (Chapter 28) may not be useful for closing the more common perimembranous VSDs because the left ventricular disk may interfere with the aortic valve function. To circumvent this problem, the device was redesigned (95) so that the aortic end of the left ventricular disk is short (0.5 mm) while the opposite end is longer (5.5 mm). A platinum marker, to indicate the lower pole of the left ventricular disc, is built into the system and should be appropriately positioned during the device delivery and implantation. This modified device was used in six children, aged 3.5 to 19 years, with small VSDs (95), and the results were good. Other anecdotal and abstracted (96) reports also suggest good results. Further experience with this device is necessary before its widespread use.

The Amplatzer Duct Occluder has been used in closing moderate to large PDAs (discussed in Chapter 24).

Although it has been generally effective, its use in infants and young children has been reported to produce aortic obstruction (97,98). To circumvent this problem, the device was modified (99): the retention disk was made thinner and concave and was built at a 32-degree angulation with the cylindrical long axis of the device so that the device conforms to the descending thoracic aorta. A platinum marker was placed in the downstream rim of the retention disc. Experimental evaluation (99) suggested that the objective of preventing aortic obstruction was achieved. Further modifications using finer wire mesh and without polyester disk was undertaken and was used successfully in a single case (100). Additional experience with this and other modified (swivel disk or diskless) (101–103) devices appears to address the aortic obstruction in infants associated with the use of the conventional Amplatzer Duct Occluder. Greater experience with longer duration of follow-up is indicated.

PERCUTANEOUS VALVE IMPLANTATION

The historical aspects and experimental work in relation to percutaneous valve implantation were discussed in Chapter 49. Human experience with pulmonary valve implantation was detailed in Chapter 50. Such implantations are feasible in patients with prior conduits across the right ventricular outflow tract (RVOT) for seating the valve implant. In the absence of a prior conduit, the RVOT is large and may not hold the valve implant in place. To circumvent this problem, an Amplatzer type of cage may be delivered initially into which the pulmonary valve may be implanted. Feasibility and efficacy studies to test this approach are needed in the future.

More recently, Eltchaninoff and Cribier in Rouen, France, implanted an aortic valve percutaneously (104) to treat a 57-year-old patient with severe aortic stenosis with poor left ventricular function and cardiogenic shock, resistant to balloon aortic valvuloplasty. This was a bovine pericardial valve mounted in a stent. There was immediate improvement. At 2-month follow-up, the valve function remained good with only mild aortic regurgitation. Further experience with this technique is awaited.

MISCELLANEOUS

Since the initial writing of several preceding chapters, there has been some progress in availability and approval of devices. The Amplatzer Septal Occluder for closure of ASDs is now approved by the FDA and is available for use by all cardiologists following appropriate training required by the FDA. Additional flexible stents have since been released and include Palmaz Genesis (Cordis Endovascular), Mega LD, and Max LD (Sulzer IntraTherapeutics, St. Paul, MN).

CURRENT STATUS

The devices described in this chapter fall into three major categories, namely, stents, covered stents, and occluding devices. Most stents are used on an off-label basis and are generally available at most institutions. Covered stents and devices (except the Amplatzer ASD occluder) are available only at institutions participating in FDA-approved clinical trials with investigation device exemption (IDE) and with local IRB (Institutional Review Board) approval.

SUMMARY AND CONCLUSION

The devices that have not been included in the preceding chapters are briefly discussed in this chapter. Surgical management of functionally single-ventricle-physiology patients by Fontan operation may be simplified and a second surgery avoided by appropriate surgical preparation during the initial bidirectional Glenn by a modified hemi-Fontan followed by catheter completion of Fontan. A larger experience with this approach and ready availability of covered stents and/or ASD closure devices are prerequisites for routine adaptation of this approach.

Although creating or enlarging an ASD appears not too difficult, maintenance of patency in the long run appears problematic. Innovative use of stent and fenestrated ASD closure devices may have a role in the management of certain cardiac/pulmonary problems.

A small percentage of aortopulmonary windows is suitable for transcatheter occlusion. Limited experience thus far is encouraging.

Transcatheter management of pulmonary oligemia associated with complex congenital heart defects is feasible in a number of clinical scenarios. Placement of endoluminal stents or modified PDA closure devices, stenting narrowed aortopulmonary collateral arteries, and implantation of stents in the narrowed surgical aortopulmonary shunts appear to improve systemic arterial oxygen saturation and may serve as simpler alternatives to repeat surgical intervention.

Percutaneous occlusion of LAA by PLAATO implant appears to be an attractive alternative to long-term anticoagulation in prevention of strokes in patients with atrial fibrillation. Feasibility of the procedure has been demonstrated in a limited number of patients. Long-term follow-up and comparative studies with the warfarin group are needed in the future.

Percutaneous closure of ASDs/PFOs in the management of decompression illness and migraine has recently been suggested. Although this less invasive approach appears attractive, establishment of a causal relationship between the atrial defects and the diseases in question is needed. Following such confirmation, clinical trials on large cohorts to confirm the effectiveness and safety of device closure of the defects should be undertaken.

A number of modifications of the Amplatzer device have been undertaken to extend its use to close other cardiac defects and to address the identified problems. Larger clinical experience and evaluation of follow-up data are in order.

Limited clinical experience with percutaneous aortic valve implantation was briefly reviewed.

Many of the preceding procedures have been tried in only a limited number of patients. Larger experience, longer follow-up, and ready availability of stents/devices are necessary for routine use of this technology.

REFERENCES

1. Rao PS. Tricuspid atresia. In: Moller JH, Hoffman JIE , eds. *Pediatric cardiovascular medicine.* New York: Churchill Livingstone, 2000:421–441.
2. Rao PS. Tricuspid atresia. In: e-medicine-Pediatrics: *http:www. emedicine.com.*
3. Marcelleti C, Corno A, Giannico S, et al. Inferior vena cava-pulmonary artery extra cardiac conduit: a new form of right heart bypass. *J Thorac Cardiovasc Surg* 1990;100:228–232.
4. Konert W, Schneider M, Herwig V, et al. Modified hemi-Fontan operation and subsequent nonsurgical Fontan completion. *J Thorac Cardiovasc Surg* 1995;110:865–867.
5. Hausdorf G, Schneider M, Konertz W. Surgical pre-conditioning and completion of total cavopulmonary connection by interventional cardiac catheterization: a new concept. *Heart* 1996;75:403–409.
6. Hijazi ZM, Ruiz CE, Patel H, et al. Catheter therapy for Fontan baffle obstruction and leak, using an endovascular covered stent. *Catheter Cardiovasc Diagn* 1998;45:158–161.
7. Ruiz CE. Personal Communication, 2001.
8. Rao PS. Should balloon angioplasty be used instead of surgery for native aortic coarctation? (Editorial) *Br Heart J* 1995;74:578–579.
9. Rao PS. Interventional pediatric cardiology: state of the art and future directions. *Pediatr Cardiol* 1998;19:107–124.
10. Rao PS. Aortic coarctation: who should be dilated or operated. *First Virtual Congress on Cardiology,* 1999. *http:pcvc.sminter. com.arcvirtual.*
11. Rao PS. Stents in treatment of aortic coarctation (Editorial). *J Am Coll Cardiol* 1997;30:1853–1855.
12. Rao PS. Current status of balloon angioplasty for neonatal and infant aortic coarctation. *Prog Pediatr Cardiol* 2001;14:35–44.
13. De Giovanni JV. Covered stents in the treatment of aortic coarctation. *J Intervent Cardiol* 2001;14:187–190.
14. Rashkind WJ, Miller WW. Creation of an atrial septal defect without thoracotomy. *JAMA* 1966;196:991–992.
15. Baker F, Baker L, Zoltun R, et al. Effectiveness of Rashkind procedure in transposition of the great arteries in infants. *Circulation* 1971;43:II-6.
16. Kidd L. Balloon atrial septostomy: current perspective. In: Rao PS, ed. *Transcatheter therapy in pediatric cardiology,* New York: Wiley-Liss, 1993:7–15.
17. Mickell JJ, Mathews RA, Park SC, et al. Left atrioventricular valve atresia: clinical management. *Circulation* 1980;61: 123–127.
18. Rao PS, Kulungara RJ, Moore HV, et al. Syndrome of single

ventricle without pulmonary stenosis but with left atrioventricular valve atresia and interatrial obstruction: palliative management with simultaneous atrial septostomy and pulmonary artery banding. *J Thorac Cardiovasc Surg* 1981;81:127–130.

19. Sinha SM, Rusnak SL, Sommers HM, et al. Hypoplastic left heart syndrome: analysis of thirty autopsy cases in infants with surgical considerations. *Am J Cardiol* 1968;21:166–173.

20. Rashkind WJ, Waldhausen JA, Miller WW, et al. Palliative treatment in tricuspid atresia: combined balloon atrial septostomy and surgical alteration of pulmonary blood flow. *J Thorac Cardiovasc Surg* 1969;57:812–818.

21. Rao PS, Covitz W, Moore HV. Principles of palliative management of patients with tricuspid atresia. In: Rao PS, ed. *Tricuspid atresia,* 2nd ed. Mt. Kisco, NY: Futura Publishing Co., 1992: 297–320.

22. Shams A, Fowler RS, Trusler GA, et al. Pulmonary atresia with intact ventricular septum: report of 50 cases. *Pediatrics* 1971;47: 370–377.

23. Rao PS. Comprehensive management of pulmonary atresia with intact ventricular septum. *Ann Thorac Surg* 1985;40: 409–413.

24. Serrato M, Bucheleres HG, Bicoff P, et al. Palliative balloon atrial septostomy for total anomalous pulmonary venous connection in infancy. *J Pediatr* 1968;73:734–739.

25. Mullins CE, El-Said GM, Neches WH, et al. Balloon atrial septostomy for total anomalous pulmonary venous return. *Br Heart J* 1973;35:752–757.

26. Korns ME, Garabedian HA, Lauer RM. Anatomic limitation of balloon atrial septostomy. *Hum Pathol* 1972;3:345–349.

27. Meng CCL, Wells CR, Valdes-Dapnena M, et al. The anatomy of the foramen ovale in relation to balloon atrial septostomy. *Pediatr Res* 1973;7:304(abst).

28. Leanage R, Agnetti A, Graham G, et al. Factors influencing survival after balloon atrial septostomy for complete transposition of the great arteries. *Br Heart J* 1981;45:559–572.

29. Park SC, Zuberbuhler JR, Neches WH, et al. A new atrial septostomy technique. *Catheter Cardiovasc Diagn* 1975;1: 195–201.

30. Park SC, Neches WH, Zuberbuhler JR, et al. Clinical use of blade septostomy. *Circulation* 1978;58:600–606.

31. Park SC, Neches WH, Mullins CE, et al. Blade atrial septostomy: collaborative study. *Circulation* 1982;66:258–266.

32. Rao PS. Transcatheter blade atrial septostomy. *Catheter Cardiovasc Diagn* 1984;10:335–342.

33. Ali Khan MA, Bricker JT, Mullins CE, et al. Blade atrial septostomy: experience with first 50 procedures. *Catheter Cardiovasc Diagn* 1991;23:257–262.

34. Park SC, Neches WH. Blade atrial septostomy. In: Rao PS, ed. *Transcatheter therapy in pediatric cardiology.* New York: Wiley-Liss, 1993:17–27.

35. Mitchell SE, Kan JS, Anderson JH, et al. Atrial septostomy: stationary angioplasty balloon technique. *Pediatr Res* 1986;20: 173A(abst).

36. Sideris EB, Fowlkes JP, Smith JE, et al. Why atrial septostomy and not foramen ovale angioplasty? *Abstracts of cardiology and cardiovascular surgery: interventions.* 18th Annual Symposium of the Texas Heart Institute, Sept 28–Oct 1, 1988:36.

37. Shrivastava S, Radhakrishnan S, Dev V, et al. Balloon dilatation of atrial septum in complete transposition of great artery: a new technique. *Indian Heart J* 1987;39:298–300.

38. Rao PS. Static balloon dilatation of the atrial septum (Editorial). *Am Heart J* 1993;125:1824–1827.

39. Feldt RH, Driscoll DJ, Offord KP, et al. Protein-losing enteropathy after Fontan operation. *J Thorac Cardiovasc Surg* 1996;112:672–680.

40. Rychick J, Rome JJ, Jacobs ML. Late surgical fenestration after the Fontan operation. *Circulation* 1997;96:33–36.

41. Hausknecht MJ, Sims RE, Nihill MR, et al. Successful palliation of primary pulmonary hypertension by atrial septostomy. *Am J Cardiol* 1990;65:1045–1046.

42. Nihill MR, O'Laughlin MP, Mullins CE. Effect of atrial septostomy in patients with terminal cor pulmonale due to pulmonary vascular disease. *Catheter Cardiovasc Diagn* 1991;24: 166–172.

43. Coe JY, Timinsky JJ, Villnave DJ, et al. Transcatheter puncture of the atrial septum using a new radiofrequency catheter. *Catheter Cardiovasc Interv* 1998;44:116.

44. Justino H, Benson LN, Nykanen DG. Catheter creation of an atrial septal defect using radiofrequency perforation. *Catheter Cardiovasc Interv* 2001;54:83–87.

45. Amin Z, Danford D. Initial experience with a new Amplatzer device to maintain patency of Fontan fenestration. *Cardiol Young* 2001;11(Suppl 1):71(abst).

46. Sommer RJ, Rhodes JF, Kamenir SA, et al. Transcatheter creation of atrial septal defect and Fontan fenestration with butterfly stent technique. *J Am Coll Cardiol* 1999;33:529A(abst).

47. Stumper O, Vettukattil J, Chessa M, et al. Modified technique of stenting the atrial septum after Fontan operation. *Cardiol Young* 2001;11(Suppl 1):70(abst).

48. Tiraboschi R, Salmone D, Crupi G, et al. Aortopulmonary window in the first year of life: report on 11 surgical cases. *Ann Thorac Surg* 1988;46:438–441.

49. Mori K, Ando M, Takao A, et al. Distal type of aortopulmonary window: report of 4 cases. *Br Heart J* 1978;40:681–689.

50. Gross RE. Surgical closure of an aortic septal defect. *Circulation* 1952;5:858–863.

51. Cooley DA, McNamara DG, Latson JR. Aortopulmonary septal defect: diagnosis and surgical treatment. *Surgery* 1957;42: 101–120.

52. Johansson L, Michaelsson M, Westerholm CJ, et al. Aortopulmonary window: a new operative approach. *Ann Thorac Surg* 1978;25:564–567.

53. Schmid FX, Hake U, Iversen S, et al. Surgical closure of aortopulmonary window without cardiopulmonary bypass. *Pediatr Cardiol* 1989;10:166–169.

54. Ho SY, Gerlis LM, Anderson C, et al. The morphology of aortopulmonary window with regard to their classification and morphogenesis. *Cardiol Young* 1994;4:146–155.

55. Stamato T, Benson LN, Smallhorn JF, et al. Transcatheter closure of an aortopulmonary window with a modified double umbrella occluder system. *Catheter Cardiovasc Diagn* 1995;35: 165–167.

56. Tulloh RM, Rigby ML. Transcatheter umbrella closure of aortopulmonary window. *Heart* 1997;77:479–480.

57. Jureidini SB, Spadaro JJ, Rao PS. Successful transcatheter closure with the buttoned device of aortopulmonary window in an adult. *Am J Cardiol* 1998;81:371–372.

58. Rao PS, Kim SH, Choi J, et al. Follow-up results of transvenous occlusion of patent ductus arteriosus with buttoned device. *J Am Coll Cardiol* 1999;33:820–826.

59. Zahn EM, Lima VC, Benson LN, et al. Use of endovascular stents to increase pulmonary blood flow in pulmonary atresia with ventricular septal defect. *Am J Cardiol* 1992;70:411–412.

60. McLeod KA, Blackburn ME, Gibbs JL. Stenting of stenosed aortopulmonary collaterals: a new approach to palliation in pulmonary atresia with multifocal aortopulmonary blood supply. *Br Heart J* 1994;71:487–489.

61. Ridington AN, Well J, Somerville J. Self-expending stents in congenital heart disease. *Br Heart J* 1994;72:378–333.

62. Brown SC, Eysken B, Mertens L, et al. Percutaneous treatment

of stenosed major aortopulmonary collaterals with balloon dilatation and stenting: what can be achieved? *Heart* 1998;79:24–28.

63. Alcibar J, Cabrera A, Martinez P, et al. Stent implantation in a central aortopulmonary shunt. *J Invasive Cardiol* 1999;11: 506–509.

64. El-Said HG, Clap S, Fagan TE, et al. Stenting of stenosed aortopulmonary collaterals and shunts for palliation of pulmonary atresia/ventricular septal defect. *Catheter Cardiovasc Interv* 2000;49:430–436.

65. Zahn EM, Chang AC, Aldousany A, et al. Emergent stent placement for acute Blalock-Taussig shunt obstruction after stage I Norwood surgery. *Catheter Cardiovasc Diagn* 1997;42: 191–194.

66. Amin Z, Radio S, Danford, et al. A new Amplatzer device to maintain ductus arteriosus patency: preliminary results in lambs. *Cardiol Young* 2001;11(Suppl):61(abst).

67. Gibbs J, Orhan U, Blackburn MEC, et al. Fate of the stented arterial duct. *Circulation* 1999;99:2621–2625.

68. Reddy VM, Liddicoat JR, Hanley FL. Midline one-stage complete unifocalization and repair of pulmonary atresia with ventricular septal defect and major aortopulmonary collaterals. *J Thorac Cardiovasc Surg* 1996;109:832–844.

69. Haworth SG. Collateral arteries in pulmonary atresia with ventricular septal defect: a precarious blood supply. *Br Heart J* 1980;44:5–13.

70. Haworth SG, Macartny FJ. Growth and development of pulmonary circulation in pulmonary atresia with ventricular septal defect and major aortopulmonary arteries. *Br Heart J* 1980;44: 14–24.

71. Freedom RM, Rabinovitch M. Pulmonary atresia with ventricular septal defect. In: Freedom RM, Benson LN, Smallhorn JF, eds. *Neonatal heart disease.* London: Springer-Verlag, 1992: 229–256.

72. Zeller TM, Mullins CE, Nihill MR, et al. Simultaneously implanted "cross crossing" stents provide excellent relief for postoperative bilateral proximal pulmonary artery stenosis with closely related ostia. *J Am Coll Cardiol* 1998;31:57A.

73. Blalock A, Taussig HB. The surgical treatment of malformations of the heart in which there is pulmonary stenosis or atresia. *JAMA* 1945;128:189–202.

74. DeLeval M, McKay R, Jones M, et al. Modified Blalock-Taussig shunt: use of subclavian orifice as a flow regulator in prosthetic systemic-pulmonary artery shunts. *J Thorac Cardiovasc Surg* 1981;18:112–119.

75. Fischer DR, Park SC, Neches WH, et al. Successful dilatation of stenotic Blalock-Taussig anastomosis by percutaneous transluminal balloon angioplasty. *Am J Cardiol* 1985;55:861–862.

76. Rao PS, Levy J, Chopra PS. Balloon angioplasty of stenosed Blalock-Taussig anastomosis: role of balloon-on-wire in dilating occluded shunts. *Am Heart J* 1990;120:1173–1178.

77. Rao PS. Transcatheter management of cyanotic congenital heart defects: a review. *Clin Cardiol* 1992;15:483–496.

78. Rao PS. Transcatheter treatment of pulmonary outflow tract obstruction: a review. *Prog Cardiovasc Dis* 1992;35:119–158.

79. Wang J, Wu M, Chang C, et al. Balloon angioplasty of obstructed modified systemic pulmonary artery shunts and pulmonary artery stenosis. *J Am Coll Cardiol* 2001;37: 940–947.

80. Rao PS. Concurrent balloon dilatation of stenosed aortopulmonary Gore-Tex shunts and branch pulmonary arteries (Editorial). *J Am Coll Cardiol* 2001;37:948–950.

81. Sievert H, Lesh MD, Trepels T, et al. Percutaneous left atrial appendage transcatheter occlusion (PLAATO) to prevent stroke in patients with atrial fibrillation: first human experience. *J Am Coll Cardiol* 2002;39:6A(abst).

82. Wilmshurst PT, Ellis BG, Jenkins BS. Paradoxical gas embolism in a scuba diver with atrial septal defect. *Br Med J* 1986;293: 1277.

83. Moon RE, Camporesi EM, Kisslo JA. Patent foramen ovale and decompression sickness in divers. *Lancet* 1989;1:513–514.

84. Wilmshurst P. Right-to-left shunt and neurologic decompression sickness in divers (Letter). *Lancet* 1990; 336:1071–1072.

85. Knauth M, Ries S, Pohimann S, et al. Cohort study of multiple brain lesions in sport divers: role of a patent foramen ovale. *Br Med J* 1997;314:701–705.

86. Schwerzmann M, Seller C, Lipp E, et al. Relation between directly detected patent foramen ovale and ischemic brain lesions in sports divers. *Ann Intern Med* 2001;134:21–24.

87. Wilmshurst P, Walsh K, Morrison L. Transcatheter occlusion of foramen ovale with a buttoned device after neurological decompression illness in professional divers. *Lancet* 1996;348: 752–753.

88. Walsh K, Wilmshurst PT, Morrison WL. Transcatheter closure of patent foramen ovale using the Amplatzer septal occluder to prevent recurrence of neurological decompression illness in divers. *Heart* 1999;81:257–261.

89. Windecker S, Meier B. Patent foramen ovale and atrial septal aneurysm: when and how should it be treated. *Am Coll Cardiol Curr J Rev* 2002;11:97–101.

90. Del Sette M, Angeli S, Leandri M, et al. Migraine with aura and right-to-left shunt on transcranial Doppler: a case control study. *Cerebrovasc Dis* 1998;8:327–330.

91. Wilmshurst P, Nightingale S. Relationship between migraine and cardiac and pulmonary right to left shunts. *Clin Sci (Lond)* 2001;100:215–220.

92. Wilmhurst PT, Nightingale S, Walsh KP, et al. Effect on migraine of closure of cardiac right-to-left shunts to prevent recurrence of decompression illness or stroke or for haemodynamic reasons. *Lancet* 2000;356:1648–1651.

93. Sharafuddin MJA, Gu X, Titus JL, et al. Transvenous closure of secundum atrial septal defects: preliminary results with a new self-expanding Nitinol prosthesis in a swine model. *Circulation* 1997;95:2162–2168.

94. Han Y, Gu X, Titus JL, et al. New self-expanding patent foramen ovale occlusion device. *Catheter Cardiovasc Interv* 1999;47: 370–376.

95. Hijazi ZM, Hakim F, Abu Haweleh A, et al. Catheter closure of perimembraneous ventricular septal defects using new Amplatzer membranous VDS occluder: initial clinical experience. *Catheter Cadiovasc Intervent* 2002;56:508–515.

96. Tasousis GS, Eleftherakis NG, Karanasios ES, et al. Transcatheter closure of perimembraneous ventricular septal defects with the Amplatzer asymmetric ventricular septal defect occluder: preliminary experience in children. *Catheter Cardivasc Interv* 2002;57:100(abst).

97. Duke C, Chan KC. Aortic obstruction caused by device occlusion of patent arterial duct. *Heart* 1999;82:109–111.

98. Fischer G, Stieh J, Ueging A, et al. Transcatheter closure of persistent ductus arteriosus in infants using the Amplatzer duct occluder. *Heart* 2000;86:444–447.

99. Kong H, Gu X, Bass JL, et al. Experimental evaluation of a modified Amplatzer duct occluder. *Catheter Cadiovasc Interv* 2001;53:571–576.

100. Ewert P, Kretschmar O, Nuernberg JH, et al. First closure of a large patent ductus arteriosus in an infant with angulated Nitinol plug. *Catheter Cadiovasc Interv* 2002;57:88–91.

101. Thanopoulos BD, Tsaousis GS, Papadopoulos GS, et al. Tran-

scatheter closure of patent ductus arteriosus using the swivel disk and plug occluders. *Catheter Cadiovasc Intervent* 2002; 57:99(abst).

102. Gavora P, Masura J, Podnar T. Percutaneous closure of patent ductus arteriosus using a new angled Amplatzer duct occluder: initial human experience. *Catheter Cardiovasc Interv* 2002;57:99(abst).

103. Ewert P, Kretschmar O, Nuerenberg JH, et al. Closure of large patent ductus arteriosi in small children with an angulated Nitinol plug. *Catheter Cadiovasc Interv* 2002;57:100(abst).

104. Eltchaninoff H. First-ever percutaneous aortic valve replacement. In: Accardio "Hot Topics" edited by Block PC. August 9, 2002.

52

ROLE OF TRANSESOPHAGEAL ECHOCARDIOGRAPHY IN TRANSCATHETER DEVICE IMPLANTATION FOR THE TREATMENT OF NONCORONARY CARDIAC DEFECTS

GAUTAM K. SINGH

Pioneering works in transcatheter treatment of many congenital and acquired heart diseases began in the 1960s and 1970s (1–4). Since then a remarkable number of catheter-based devices have been developed for the treatment of both coronary and noncoronary cardiac diseases. The expanding therapeutic role of catheter-based devices in the management of noncoronary cardiac defects has created the need for monitoring modalities to aid in the device deployment and assess its effectiveness. These devices are used to close intra- and extracardiac communications, as well as to open and maintain patency of vessels. Conventionally, the monitoring of such interventions has been performed by a combination of radiographic screening and angiography. However, radiologic landmarks are often inadequate in demonstrating the preciseness of device placement in relation to the cardiac defects and the surrounding cardiac structures. Repeated angiography for the monitoring purpose is often impractical during the procedure and reveals the improper device placement only after it has been deployed. Transesophageal echocardiography (TEE) has opened a new acoustic window for assessing cardiac structures not well visualized by transthoracic imaging and fluoroscopy. TEE has proven ideal for continuous monitoring for a wide range of interventional procedures, as the transesophageal probe can be left in position during the entire procedure without interfering with its execution. Visualization of guide wire, catheter, and device positions in relation to the cardiac site of interven-

tion and surrounding structures can be defined precisely in real time. Immediate assessment of the result of the intervention and hemodynamic changes can also be obtained with TEE. Based on published literature, our experience, and that of others, there are some specific indications for the use of TEE in device-based interventions, which are listed in Table 52.1.

Abiding with the scope of this book, discussion about the role of TEE in the device deployment for the management of noncoronary cardiac defects will be limited to indications 1 and 4 in Table 52.1. The role of three-dimensional reconstruction in device deployment is discussed elsewhere in this book.

Gautam K. Singh: Associate Professor, Department of Pediatrics, Saint Louis University; Echo-Laboratory Director, Division of Pediatric Cardiology, Cardinal Glennon Children's Hospital, Saint Louis, Missouri

TABLE 52.1. INDICATIONS FOR THE USE OF TRANSESOPHAGEAL ECHOCARDIOGRAPHY IN DEVICE-BASED INTERVENTION IN NONCORONARY CARDIAC DISEASE

1. Transcatheter device closure of shunt lesions: atrial septal defect, ventricular septal defect, and patent ductus arteriosus
2. Transcatheter creation of intracardiac communication: interatrial communication by Brockenbrough transseptal puncture and blade catheter atrial septectomy
3. Balloon dilation: valvuloplasty and angioplasty
4. Transcatheter device intervention in postoperative congenital heart disease: relief of obstruction in systemic and pulmonary arterial and venous pathways
5. Miscellaneous:
   Reduction of radiation exposure during multiple interventional procedure during the same catheterization
   Patients with renal failure and allergy to contrast material
   Complex and large septal defects closure

TRANSCATHETER DEVICE CLOSURE OF INTRACARDIAC SHUNT

Atrial Septal Defect and Patent Foramen Ovale

The atrial septal defects (ASDs) and persistent patent foramen ovales (PFOs) are considered suitable for transcatheter device closure to prevent later morbidity and mortality, including presumed paradoxical embolism. A number of devices, which are under clinical trials, are being used for the closure of secundum ASD and PFO. The metal component of these devices can be seen by fluoroscopy, but neither the ASD/PFO nor the atrial septum itself can be seen on fluoroscopy. TEE is important for assessment and monitoring of the transcatheter device closure.[1]

1. *Morphology and size of the defect.* The accurate determination of suitability of an ASD for device closure is crucial. The suitability depends on the morphology and size of the defect and the septum. The position of the defect in oval fossa (displacement of the defect to the mouth of vena cava), adequacy of a muscular rim around the defect (lack of it causes embolization of the device), flap valve position (inserted away from the rim), and proximity of the septal insertion of the Eustachian valve (its proximity to the defect may cause it to be caught by the device) may all dictate the suitability of a defect for device closure (5–8). The importance of ASD size was shown in one study in which an effective device closure with a Bard Clamshell device was predicted for those ASDs that, on echocardiographic screening, measured <13 mm in diameter (9). Although rim size and atrial size were not predictive of effective closure with the Clamshell device in the study, an adequate length of the septum and upper and lower rims of the defect are important to accommodate the total diameter of most other devices. For this reason a sinus venosus ASD without a superior rim or primum ASD without an inferior rim or a small septum (due to small left atrium) is not suitable for device closure. TEE provides the acoustic window that discerns the morphology of the ASD and delineates the length of the septum and rims more accurately than any other current on-line monitoring modalities (10–12). For this purpose basal four-chamber, short-axis, and longitudinal views with lateral sweep are extremely helpful (Figure 52.1) to visualize the morphology and size of the ASD/PFO.

Many of the current devices for ASD closure should be two times larger than the stretched size of the ASD/PFO (13,14). The stretched diameter of the ASD is measured by

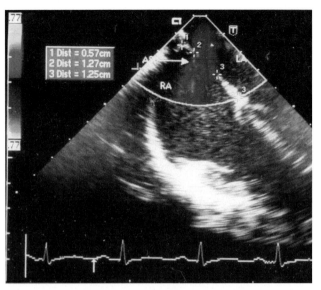

FIGURE 52.1. Transesophageal echocardiographic four-chamber view of the heart in transverse plane, showing the lengths of superior (1) and inferior (3) rims and the size of the atrial septal defect (2). The color flow through the defect (*arrow*) from the left atrium (LA) to the right atrium (RA) helps to delineate the size of the defect. ASD, a trial septal defect. (See Color Figure 52.1.)

the balloon-sizing technique during cardiac catheterization. TEE visualizes the passage of the balloon across the defect in real time (Figure 52.2A) and with the help of color flow mapping discerns the exact size of an inflated balloon that has no residual leaks around it. This is a prerequisite for the selection of an appropriate device size not accurately obtainable from fluoroscopy. A clockwise-rotated four-chamber view and longitudinal view accompanied with color flow mapping of the septum provide the information (Figure 52.2B).

In fenestrated ASD, where multiple defects exist in the septum, the balloon-stretching technique does not accurately measure the ASD size, as the balloon is often trapped between the fenestration strands. TEE, with the sensitive imaging window for posterior cardiac structures, can diagnose the fenestrated ASD (Figure 52.3) and help choose a device that will cover the whole ASD, including the fenestrated area (15,16).

2. *Device position.* TEE clearly visualizes all the steps of device deployment. Modified four-chamber and longitudinal views of the septal defect and atria demonstrate the passage of sheath/catheter across the defect into the left atrium. Appearance of echo-contrast, injected through the sheath, into the left atrium also confirms the position of the tip. TEE ascertains the placement of left atrial disk along the left atrial side of the septum before applying right atrial disk on the right side of the septum during button device deployment or before releasing right atrial components during deployment of other devices (Figure 52.4) (17). TEE can also help adjust the device position away from inlet valves, pulmonary veins, and septum primum.

3. *Residual leakage.* Residual leakage across the device can be detected immediately after its deployment by color flow

---

[1] Since commissioning this chapter, intracardiac echocardiography (ICE) became available. ICE can be used to define the defect and septal rims, and to monitor device implantation and may replace the transesophageal echocardiography since the ICE can be performed without general anesthesia. However, the disposable ICE catheters (e.g., Acunav Diagnostic Ultrasound Catheter, Acuson, Mountain View, CA) are expensive and require 10 to 12 F sheaths for introduction. Miniaturization of ICE catheters and decreased cost may eventually result in selecting ICE as the preferred modality for monitoring device closure of cardiac septal defects.

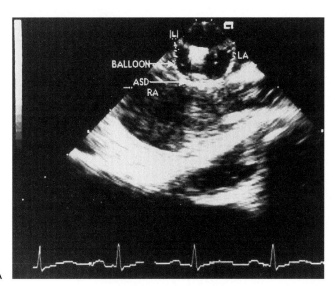
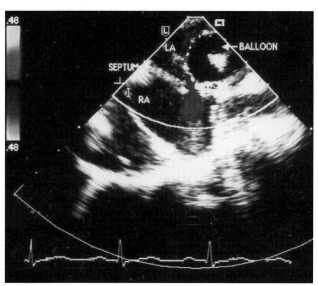

A   B

FIGURE 52.2. A: Transesophageal echocardiographic view in longitudinal plane showing the passage of balloon during the measurement of stretched diameter of the atrial septal defect (ASD) by balloon-sizing technique. **B:** Residual leakage around the balloon, not apparent in two-dimensional echocardiography, became evident on color flow mapping indicated by *arrowheads*. LA, left atrium; RA, right atrium. (See Color Figure 52.2B.)

mapping. Small leakage, often seen immediately after implantation, completely seals within a short period of time. The presence of a large leakage indicates the need for further device intervention, which may be undertaken during the same sitting.

Fluoroscopy cannot demonstrate the spatial relationship of the defect and device and provide immediate information about adequacy of the device deployment as TEE does

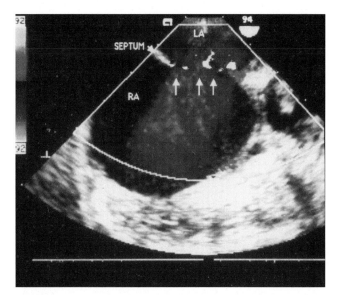

FIGURE 52.3. Basal four-chamber view in transverse plane showing fenestrated atrial septal defects with multiple holes indicated by *arrows*. The color flow through the three defects delineated the fenestrated defect. LA, left atrium; RA, right atrium. (See Color Figure 52.3.)

(Figure 52.5). Real-time feedback by TEE regarding device position facilitates the adjustment of the delivery system until the device position is optimum, which is defined as the achievement of complete placement of right and left atrial components of the device on the respective sides of the septum without impingement of any structures beyond the atrial septum. In a study involving a buttoned device, achievement of optimum position was associated with less occurrence of residual shunts, device unbuttoning, or atrioventricular valve regurgitation (18). The use of TEE guidance was strongly associated with achievement of optimum device position (18). This was also true for the Clamshell device in another study (9). Recent studies have also shown that in most patients in whom transcatheter closure of interatrial communication with the Amplatzer Septal Occluder is possible, the use of TEE to guide device deployment is of paramount importance (19) and the procedure can be safely performed even under TEE guidance without fluoroscopy (20,21).

Ventricular Septal Defect

Similar to the function in ASD/PFO closure, TEE facilitates the device closure of ventricular septal defects (VSDs) in the following areas:

1. *Morphology and size of the VSD.* The morphology of the VSD has a bearing on the feasibility of its closure by a transcatheter device (22,23). A mid-septal muscular VSD may be technically more appropriate for a device closure than an inlet VSD or outlet (supracrystal) VSD near atrioventricular and semilunar valves, respectively.

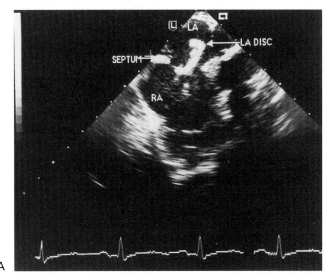

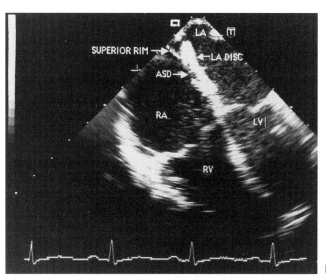

A   B

FIGURE 52.4. A: Transesophageal echocardiographic view in longitudinal plane showing improper positioning of the left atrial (LA) disk across the atrial septal defect during a button device deployment. **B:** Four-chamber view in transverse plane showing proper positioning of left atrial disk in the left atrium away from the mitral valve and hugging the septum. ASD, atrial septal defect; LA, left atrium; LV, left ventricle; RA, right atrium; RV, right ventricle.

Although a transthoracic echocardiogram or angiography may easily define the VSD anatomy, malalignment of the muscular septum apical to VSD and rim size of the defect may be missed (24). A four-chamber view obtained with anteroposterior sweep of the probe stationed at the gastroesophageal junction can define the anatomy of most of the muscular VSDs and inlet VSDs. Longitudinal view between 120 and 135 degrees can profile most of the outlet VSDs. However, apical muscular VSD may be difficult to delineate with TEE.

Balloon sizing may be necessary for the perimembranous VSD, which, like ASD-sizing, can be facilitated by TEE. On the other hand, TEE-measured cross-sectional size alone of a muscular VSD may be adequate for the selection of device.

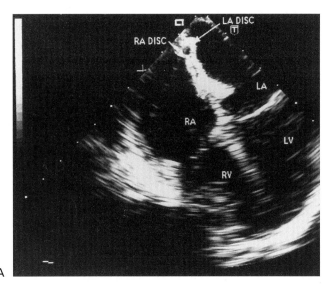

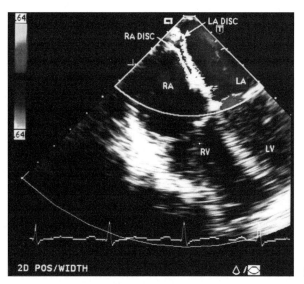

A   B

FIGURE 52.5. A: Four-chamber view in transverse plane showing proper deployment of the button device for the closure of atrial septal defect. The left and right atrial disks are on the respective sides of the septum and away from the inlet valves. **B:** Color flow mapping in the same view shows no residual leakage across the defect and device, indicating the complete closure of the defect. LA, left atrium; LV, left ventricle; RA, right atrium; RV, right ventricle. (See Color Figure 52.5B.)

2. *Multiple VSDs.* If present, their spatial relationships can be better defined by TEE (25). This will dictate the selection of a device size needed to occlude all of them.
3. *Guidance of different stages of the procedure,* including catheter and wire manipulation through VSD.
4. *Monitoring of the positioning of left and right ventricular components of the device* during device delivery and after release.
5. *Assessment of the proximity of the device to the valve structures.*
6. *Assessment of the closure of the defect by detecting residual leakage by color Doppler.*

The usefulness of TEE in the transcatheter closure of the VSD was verified in a study that demonstrated that TEE, in comparison with angiography and fluoroscopy, was more efficient in assessing device position (failure rate, 11% versus 22%), its proximity to valve structure (failure rate, 2% versus 9%), and the residual leakage (failure rate, 20% versus 70%) (24). The study also revealed that the TEE discovered unrecognized cardiac abnormalities in approximately 40% of cases, 16% of which required additional intervention at the time of VSD closure (24). The combination of both TEE and fluoroscopy resulted in improved ability to assess device position, proximity to valves, and residual flow.

Patent Ductus Arteriosus

There is no real advantage offered by TEE monitoring in the device closure of patent ductus arteriosus. It cannot visualize the aorta, pulmonary artery, and arterial duct simultaneously to ascertain the position of the device (26). Moreover, the probe often obstructs the fluoroscopic view during the placement of the device across the duct. An aortogram can ascertain both the position of the limbs of the device prior to its detachment from the delivery system and the effectiveness of the ductus arteriosus occlusion (26).

Transcatheter Device Intervention in Postoperative Congenital Heart Diseases: Relief of Obstruction in Systemic and Pulmonary Venous Pathways

A growing number of patients are surviving after surgical intervention for congenital heart defects (CHDs) and joining the ever-increasing pool of adults with corrected or palliated CHD. This pool is approaching 1 million in the United States alone (27). Many of the postoperative residua and sequelae in this patient population have required device-based intervention. Notable among them is obstruction of venous pathways after atrial (venous) switch operations (Senning and Mustard procedures), which channel systemic venous return to subpulmonary left ventricle and pulmonary venous return to subaortic right ventricle for transposition of the great arteries. Also seen is the obstruction of cavopulmonary circuit, which channels systemic venous blood directly to the pulmonary artery from the right atrium or venae cavae after Fontan procedure for single-ventricle physiology.

TEE studies in both transverse and longitudinal views provide superior definition of the site, extent, and morphology of systemic venous pathway obstruction after Mustard procedure than prior transthoracic echocardiographic and concomitant angiographic studies (28–30). We and others (31) have utilized TEE guidance in stent placement in the stenosed systemic venous baffle after Mustard procedure and found TEE visualization of positioning of the stent particularly helpful, as angiography foreshortens the length and diameter of the narrowing. The basal short-axis view obtained after withdrawing the probe from high transgastric view is consistently useful for this purpose.

In Fontan patients, the systemic venous pathway is well visualized by TEE in longitudinal and angulated long-axis views. TEE can define the extent and site of narrowing of the systemic venous pathway. Compared with transthoracic imaging, TEE with views in multiple planes can better visualize cavopulmonary shunt or atrial shunt, which are other encountered complications from the Fontan procedure (32). However, we have found that, relative to angiography, no additional information, including the choice of stent size, may be gained by TEE monitoring in transcatheter device intervention for distal cavopulmonary vessel obstruction.

LIMITATIONS OF TEE MONITORING

Although safe and well tolerated (33,34), TEE is semiinvasive and requires, unlike in adults, deep sedation, mechanical ventilation, and often general anesthesia in younger patients. Transient hemodynamic changes can be induced by TEE, such as increase in heart rate, systolic left ventricular pressure, and pulmonary artery pressure as well as decrease in pulmonary artery oxygen saturation (35). The latter changes are noted to be more marked in patients with pulmonary hypertension (35), where extra vigilance should be used with TEE.

The nature of intervention requires extended duration of esophageal intubation and commitment of physician and equipment time. Also, since imagery of vessels is less satisfactory compared with angiography, it is of limited value in ductal occlusion and stent placement in distal cavopulmonary circuit.

REFERENCES

1. Dotter CT, Judkins MP. Transluminal treatment of atherosclerotic obstructions: description of a new technique and preliminary report of its application. *Circulation* 1954;30:654–670.

2. Rashkind WJ, Miller WW. Creation of an atrial septal defect without thoracotomy. *JAMA* 1966;196:991–992.

3. Portsmann W, Wierny L, Warnke H, et al. Catheter closure of patent ductus arteriosus: 62 cases treated without thoracotomy. *Radiol Clin North Am* 1971;9:203–218.

4. King TD, Thompson SL, Steiner C, et al. Secundum atrial septal defect: non-operative closure during cardiac catheterization. *JAMA* 1976;235:2506–2509.

5. Ferreira SMAG, Ho SY, Anderson RH. Morphological study of defects of the atrial septum within the oval fossa: implications for transcatheter closure of left-to-right shunt. *Br Heart J* 1992;67:316–320.

6. Chan KC, Godman MJ. Morphological variations of fossa ovalis atrial septal defects (secundum): feasibility for transcatheter closure with the clamshell device. *Br Heart J* 1993;69:52–55.

7. Rome JJ, Keane JF, Stanton BP, et al. Double-umbrella closure of atrial septal defects: initial applications. *Circulation* 1990;82:751–758.

8. Rocchini AP. Transcatheter closure of atrial septal defects: past, present and future. *Circulation* 1990;82:1044–1045.

9. Rosenfeld HM, vander Velde ME, Sanders SP, et al. Echocardiographic predictors of candidacy of successful transcatheter atrial septal defect closure. *Catheter Cardiovasc Diagn* 1995;34:29–34.

10. Kronzon I, Tunick PA, Freeberg RS, et al. Transesophageal echocardiography is superior to transthoracic echocardiography in the diagnosis of sinus venous atrial septal defect. *J Am Coll Cardiol* 1991;17:537–540.

11. Morimoto K. Matsuzaki M, Tohma Y, et al. Diagnosis and quantitative evaluation of secundum-type atrial septal defect by transesophageal Doppler echocardiography. *Am J Cardiol* 1990;66:88–90.

12. Muhiundeen IA, Roberson DA, Silverman NH, et al. Intraoperative echocardiography in infants and children with congenital cardiac shunt lesions: transesophageal versus epicardial echocardiography. *J Am Coll Cardiol* 1990;16:1687–1691.

13. Rao PS, Langhough R, Beekman RH, et al. Echocardiographic estimation of balloon-stretched diameter of secundum atrial septal defect for transcatheter occlusion. *Am Heart J* 1992;124:172–175.

14. Rao PS, Wilson AD, Levy JM, et al. Role of buttoned double disc device in the management of atrial septal defect. *Am Heart J* 1992;123:191–200.

15. Vick GW, Titus J. Defects of atrial septum including the atrioventricular canal. In: Garson A, Bricker JT, McNamara DG, eds. *The science of practice of pediatric cardiology.* Philadelphia: Lea and Febiger, 1990:1023–1054.

16. Ludomirsky A. The use of echocardiography in pediatric interventional cardiac catheterization procedures. *J Interv Cardiol* 1995;8:569–578.

17. Boutin C, Musewe NN, Smallhorn JF, et al. Echocardiographic follow-up of atrial septal defect after catheter closure by double-umbrella device. *Circulation* 1993;88:621–627.

18. Loyd TR, Vermilion RP, Zamora R, et al. Influence of echocardiographic guidance on positioning of the button occluder for transcatheter closure of atrial septal defects. *Echocardiography* 1996;13:117–121.

19. Hizazi ZM, Cao Q, Patel HT, et al. Transesophageal echocardiographic results of catheter closure of atrial septal defects in children and adults using the Amplatzer device. *Am J Cardiol* 2000;85:1387–1390.

20. Ewert P, Daehnert I, Berger F, et al. Transcatheter closure of atrial septal defects under echocardiographic guidance without x-ray: initial experience. *Cardiol Young* 1999;9:136–140.

21. Ewert P. Berger F, Daehnet I, et al. Transcatheter closure of atrial septal defects without fluoroscopy: feasibility of a new method. *Circulation* 2000;101:847–849.

22. Lock JE, Block PC, McKay RG, et al. Transcatheter closure of ventricular septal defects. *Circulation* 1988;78:361–368.

23. Bridges ND, Perry SB, Keane JF, et al. Preoperative transcatheter closure of congenital muscular ventricular septal defects. *N Engl J Med* 1991;324:1312–1317.

24. Van der Velde ME, Perry SB, Sanders SP. Transesophageal echocardiographic with color Doppler during interventional catheterization. *Echocardiography* 1991;8:721–730.

25. Van der Velde ME, Keane JF, Stanton BP, et al. Transesophageal echocardiographic guidance of transcatheter ventricular septal defect closure. *J Am Coll Cardiol* 1994;23:1660–1665.

26. Cheung Y-F, Leung MP, Lee J, et al. An evolving role of transesophageal echocardiography for the monitoring of interventional catheterization in children. *Clin Cardiol* 1999;22:804–810.

27. Perloff JK, Child JS, eds. *Congenital heart disease in adults.* Philadelphia: WB Saunders, 1991.

28. Kaulitz R, Stumper OF, Geuskens R, et al. Comparative values of the precordial and transesophageal approaches in the echocardiographic evaluation of atrial baffle function after an atrial correlation procedure. *J Am Coll Cardiol* 1990;16:686–691.

29. Stumper O, Witsenburg M, Sutherland GR, et al. Transesophageal echocardiographic monitoring of interventional cardiac catheterization in children. *J Am Coll Cardiol* 1991;18:1506–1514.

30. Hosking MCK, Aliheri M, Murdison KA, et al. Transcatheter management of pulmonary venous pathway obstruction with atrial baffle leak following Mustard and Senning operation. *Catheter Cardiovasc Diagn* 1993;30:76–82.

31. Tong AD, Rothman A, Shiota T, et al. Interventional cardiac catheterization under transesophageal echocardiographic guidance. *Am Heart J* 1995;129:827–831.

32. Stumper O, Sutherland GR, Geuskens R, et al. Transesophageal echocardiography in evaluation and management after Fontan procedure. *J Am Coll Cardiol* 1991;17:1152–1158.

33. Seward JB, Khandheria BK, Oh JK, et al. Transesophageal echocardiography: technique, anatomic correlations, implementations and clinical applications. *Mayo Clin Proc* 1988;63:649–680.

34. Hellenbrand WE, Fahey JT, McGowant FX, et al. Transesophageal echocardiographic guidance of transcatheter closure of atrial septal defect. *Am J Cardiol* 1990;66:207–213.

35. Vilacosta I, Iturralde E, San Roman JA, et al. Transesophageal echocardiographic monitoring of percutaneous mitral balloon valvuloplasty. *Am J Cardiol* 1992;70:1040–1044.

Catheter Based Devices: For the Treatment of Non-coronary Cardiovascular Diseases in Adults and Children. Edited by P. Syamasundar Rao and Morton J. Kern, Lippincott Williams & Wilkins, Philadelphia © 2003.

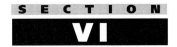

FUTURE DIRECTIONS

53

SUMMARY AND FUTURE DIRECTIONS

MORTON J. KERN
P. SYAMASUNDAR RAO

The conventional treatment of choice for acquired and congenital cardiac defects is surgical correction. Since the early 1950s, concurrent with the development of open-heart surgical techniques, several investigators attempted to develop transcatheter methodologies to replace invasive surgical procedures. A number of transcatheter methods—including pulmonary and tricuspid valvotomy by Rubio-Alverez and his colleagues, gradational dilatation of atherosclerotic lesions of peripheral arteries by Dotter and Judkins, balloon atrial septostomy by Rashkind, occlusion of patent ductus arteriosus (PDA) by Portsmann, device occlusion of atrial septal defects (ASDs) by King, and coil occlusion of blood vessels by Gianturco—have been described. However, it was not until Gruntzig's clinical use of a double-lumen catheter with nonelastic balloon (percutaneous transluminal angioplasty) that interventional technology was applied widely to treat cardiac disease in both adult and pediatric patients. The decade of 1980s witnessed development, proliferation, and refinements of balloon angioplasty techniques, and the 1990s saw the mushrooming of transcatheter device implantation technology. In this book we attempted to bring together the descriptions of all the available transcatheter-implantable devices. This book has not included coronary artery device applications because many other monographs and books deal with that subject.

Following pioneering efforts of King, Rashkind, and their colleagues in the mid-1970s, a number of transcatheter ASD occluding devices have been described. These include the Clamshell septal occluder, buttoned device, monodisk device, modified Rashkind PDA device, ASDOS (ASD occluding system), Angel Wing Das device, Amplatzer Septal Occluder, CardioSEAL device, Starflex device, Helex device, and PFO-Star. Most of the devices have undergone experimentation in animal models to test their feasibility, safety, and efficacy. This experience was followed by clinical trials in human subjects with approval of local Institutional Review Boards (IRBs) and the Food and Drug Administration (FDA) with investigational device exemption (IDE) in the United States. Some of the devices have been discontinued either because of investigators' assessment of lack of safety or efficacy or because of instructions from regulatory authorities. Other devices are modified or redesigned.

Following the description of historical developments of ASD occluding devices by one of us (PSR), Dr. Rome describes the Clamshell device and its utility in occluding the ASDs. Dr. Rao then discusses the buttoned device, its modification and results. The role of ASDOS in closing ASDs was reviewed by Dr. Babic and his colleagues. Drs. Das, Harrison, and O'Laughlin provide insight into the design, application, and modifications of the Angel Wing Das device, now the Guardian Angel device. The method of implantation and results of the Amplatzer Septal Occluder are reviewed by Drs. Hamdan, Cao, and Hijazi. Drs. Bennhagen, McLaughlin, and Benson describe the CardioSEAL and Starflex devices and their role in closure of the ASDs. This is followed by the description of the Helex device by Drs. Latson, Wilson, and Zahn. Dr. Sideris brought wireless devices to our attention. Drs. Ewert and Berger review their experience in closing ASDs without fluoroscopy. Dr. Rao provides a summary of ASD closure devices.

At the time of this writing, the FDA approves none of the devices for general clinical use. At the present time, several devices are under FDA-approved clinical trials with IDE. These include the Amplatzer Septal Occluder, centering-on-demand buttoned device, CardioSEAL, STARflex, and Helex devices.[1]

There are a few studies comparing a limited number of devices, used consecutively as the new devices become available. There are no prospective, randomized clinical trials

Morton J. Kern: Professor of Medicine, Division of Cardiology, Saint Louis University; Director, JG Mudd Cardiac Catheterization Laboratory, Saint Louis University Hospital, Saint Louis, Missouri

P. Syamasundar Rao: Professor of Pediatrics, Medicine, and Cardiology, Department of Pediatrics, University of Texas–Houston Medical School; Director, Division of Pediatric Cardiology, Memorial Hermann Children's Hospital, Houston, Texas

---

[1]Since writing this chapter, the FDA has approved the Amplatzer Septal Occluder to close ostium secundum ASDs.

using all the available devices to provide a comparison of their feasibility, safety, and effectiveness. It also appears unlikely that such a clinical trial is feasible at this juncture.

There are claims of superiority of one device over the others. But a careful comparison of the previously conducted studies in Chapter 11 suggests that the feasibility, safety, and effectiveness of most of the devices are similar. There are minor differences in the size of the delivery sheath, ease of implantation, cost, and availability.

At the present time, the FDA approves none of the devices for general clinical use, with the exception of Amplatzer. Approval of other devices is anticipated in the near future. The availability of several devices may help facilitate randomized clinical studies that may provide data to evaluate which is the better (best) device. However, it is more likely that such trials may not be feasible. Also, it is possible that a particular device may be useful for a given type of defect, whereas another device may be suitable for another type of defect.

In addition to occluding ostium secundum ASD, the devices have been utilized to occlude patent foramen ovale (PFO)/ASD presumed to be the site of paradoxical embolism, PFOs/ASDs causing right-to-left shunt following surgical or transcatheter intervention, Fontan fenestrations, PFOs/ASDs responsible for platypnea-orthodeoxia syndrome, and PFOs causing neurologic decompression illness in divers.

Drs. Schräder, Fossbender, and Strasser describe the role of PFO-Starr in closing the PFOs presumed to be the site of paradoxical embolism causing cerebrovascular accidents (CVAs) and transient ischemic attacks (TIAs) in young people. Dr. Windecker and Meier discuss the issues related to prevention of recurrence of CVAs and TIAs presumably secondary to paradoxical embolism through the atrial septum with particular attention to device closure. Dr. Rao presents a discussion on closure of ASDs/PFOs with right-to-left shunt. Drs. Bitar and Rao describe transcatheter treatment of platypnea-orthodeoxia syndrome. In the final chapter of this section, Dr. Banarjee and his associates discuss the role of three-dimensional echocardiographic reconstruction in transcatheter closure of atrial defects.

Thus device closure of not only ostium secundum ASD, but also atrial defects responsible for actual and presumed right-to-left shunt is feasible, safe, and effective. However, with the current technology it is not feasible to address sinus venosus and ostium primum ASDs.

Since the initial description of transcatheter closure of PDAs by Porstmann and associates, a number of devices have been described to achieve transcatheter occlusion. A number of devices have been designed and tested in animal models but did not reach the stage of human application, and these have been reviewed in Chapter 25. In addition, a number of devices have undergone clinical trials, including Porstmann's Ivalon foam plug, Rashkind's hooked single umbrella, the Rashkind PDA occluding system, Botallo-

occluder, buttoned device, clamshell ASD occluder, Gianturco coils, detachable coils, Duct-Occlud pfm, polyvinyl alcohol foam plug mounted on titanium pin, infant PDA buttoned device, Gianturco vascular occlusion device, Amplatzer Duct Occluder, folding plug buttoned device, and wireless PDA devices. Of these, Porstmann's Ivalon foam plug, both Rashkind's hooked single-umbrella and double-umbrella devices, Botallo-occluder, Clamshell ASD device, regular buttoned device, infant buttoned device, and polyvinyl foam plug were discontinued or modified after initial clinical trials.

Dr. Rao details historical developments in transcatheter PDA occlusion. Dr. Qureshi describes the Rashkind device and its role in closure of PDA prior to the discontinuation. Dr. Rao reviews the various modifications of the buttoned device and the result of closure of PDAs. Drs. Schneider and Moore reviewed Gianturco coil occlusion of PDA. Drs. Sreeram and Yap provide insight into the usage of detachable coils in occluding PDAs. Drs. Lê, Neuss, and Freudenthal describe the Duct-Occlud device and its modification and their utility in ductal closure. The role of the Gianturco-Grifka vascular occlusion device in occluding tubular PDA is discussed by Dr. Grifka. Drs. Sandhu and King describe the Amplatzer Duct Occluder and its role in PDA closure. Finally, Dr. Rao provides a summary of PDA closure devices and presents an approach to the choice of closure methods in occluding PDAs based on its size and shape.

Gianturco coils were initially used on an off-label application and they subsequently became available for general clinical use. Detachable coils and the Gianturco-Grifka vascular occlusion device are currently available for general clinical use. Several PDA-occluding devices are undergoing FDA-approved clinical trials with IDE and include Duct-Occlud, the folding-plug buttoned device, and the Amplatzer Duct Occluder.

Very small and small PDAs can be occluded safely and effectively with either free or detachable Gianturco coils. Some investigators prefer detachable coils because of greater control during delivery and to "prevent" embolization. Careful review of the data, however, suggests that the prevalence of coil dislodgment/embolization is not significantly different from that of free coils, and therefore the advantage cited does not seem to exist. We personally prefer free 0.038-inch Gianturco coils for very small to small PDAs, 0.052-inch coils (delivered with a biopsy forceps via 4F long sheath) for small to moderate PDAs, and devices for moderate-to-large PDAs. As and when data become available on the devices in clinical trials, an appropriate selection of devices for closure of moderate-to-large PDAs will be feasible.

Continued use of and gaining experience with the use of coils for closure of small PDAs and approval of some of the devices for moderate to large PDAs in the near future are anticipated.

Since the report of Rashkind and Cuoso in the mid-1970s of transcatheter closure of experimentally created ventricular septal defects (VSDs) with single- and double-umbrella devices, a number of devices have been used by other workers. The Rashkind PDA occluder, Clamshell Septal Occluder, buttoned device, Amplatzer muscular VSD occluder, CardioSEAL, and STARflex devices and Nit-occlud have been utilized to close the VSD.

Dr. Goh discusses the role that the Rashkind and Clamshell devices played in occluding VSDs before their discontinuation. Dr. Sideris describes the use of the buttoned device in closure of muscular and perimembranous VSDs. Drs. Waight, Cao, and Hijazi review the utility of the Amplatzer muscular VSD occluder in transcatheter occlusion of muscular VSD. Drs. Marshall and Perry provide data on the usefulness of the CardioSEAL and STARflex devices in closing VSDs. Dr. Lê and his colleagues describe a new VSD occluding device, Nit-occlud, and present data on its experimental use and preliminary clinical trials. Dr. Landzberg presents an approach to occlude postmyocardial infarction VSDs. He also provides information on device closure of paravalvular leaks.

None of the devices are available for general clinical use. CardioSEAL is available for use under humanitarian device exemption (HDE). Nit-occlud is in clinical trials in Europe. Other devices—namely, buttoned device, Amplatzer muscular VSD occluder, and STARflex—are in FDA-approved clinical trial with IDE in the United States.

Isolated defects and defects associated with other complex heart disease have been addressed. In the latter situation, catheter closure served as an adjunct to surgery. Congenital and postmyocardial infarction VSDs have been tackled. The experience with VSD closure is not as extensive as that with ASD and PDA closures, presumably related to complexity of the procedure and lack of anatomic suitability of most VSDs for device closure.

Since the advent of the balloon dilatation catheter in 1977 to mechanically alter the shape of coronary artery conduits, the field of interventional cardiology has consistently and steadfastly moved forward, developing new means to address both acquired and congenital heart disease and eliminate the morbidity and mortality of surgery. Approximately 7 years following introduction of the balloon catheter, Palmaz produced a tubular steel-etched stent system that, when expanded with a balloon catheter, formed a metallic scaffold to be permanently implanted, opening the diseased arterial system.

Continued efforts from this landmark achievement have made the stent a mainstay of everyday interventional adult and pediatric cardiology. As the technology of coronary stents evolved, so did the clinical applications. A wide variety of peripheral and central arterial deformities and diseases involving the pulmonary artery, aortic coarctation, patent ductus arteriosus, pulmonary and systemic venous obstruction, as well as bidirectional cavopulmonary shunts, and stenosed synthetic conduits are now treated by stenting. Moreover, the success of placing large-diameter stents,

either covered or uncovered, facilitated nonsurgical treatment of many congenital cardiac conditions, requiring either reconstruction of narrowed conduits or closure of abnormal connections. In both adults and children this technologic advance has become commonplace.

In addition to management of arterial disease, a number of miscellaneous techniques of catheter-based noncoronary interventions are applied to arrhythmia management, pulmonary embolism control with vena caval filters, vascular closure for arterial punctures, and implantation of prosthetic valves through percutaneous approaches. Coupled to device placement is the increased use of refined and enhanced imaging of these clinical dilemmas with transesophageal echocardiography. Both the device and imaging advances propelled the field toward more minimally invasive methods to manage complex heart disease.

As the data on stents have been acquired, it is appropriate to concentrate on the outcomes of stents for the various manifestations of extracardiac and peripheral vascular abnormalities. Late Dr. Hausdorf describes important mechanical and biophysical aspects of stenting as they may be applied to pulmonary arteries, coarctations, ductal connections, and venous obstructions. Drs. Coulson, Everett, and Owada present information on the recent technical developments, including all the available stents and balloons, particularly for use in congenital and postsurgical cardiovascular anomalies.

For clinical management, Drs. McMahon and Nihill describe management of pulmonary artery stenosis and its subbranches using stenting. Drs. Jayakumar and Hellenbrand provide further insight into the management of coarctation using large stents in children. Dr. Ruiz elucidates new stenting techniques to assess and treat patent ductus arteriosus in most of the complex congenital heart defects encountered in the pediatric cardiac catheterization laboratory. Unique to this field is the information regarding the treatment of systemic and pulmonary venous obstruction using self-expanding and balloon-expandable stents, presented by Dr. Ing. Further insight is provided with a specific device, the NuMed CP stent, for congenital heart defects, as described by Dr. Cheatham. Dr. Rao discusses the role of new stents in the treatment of vascular obstructive lesions in children.

Of great interest to the adult interventional cardiologist will be the information on the management of peripheral arterial stenosis. Drs. Vale, Bashir, and Rosenfield describe the wide use of stents in these patients. The application of stents to the carotid artery, now an everyday practice, is reviewed by Dr. Iyer and his associates. Infrarenal aortic aneurysms, once the exclusive province of the vascular surgeon, may now be managed by interventional cardiologists and radiologists using covered stents, as described by Drs. White, Lennox, and May.

In years to come, these methods will be highly influenced by new materials and coatings applied to stents. Drs.

Tsuji and Tamai describe prospects for the future using biodegradable stents.

In the miscellaneous section contributing to our understanding of catheter-based devices for treatment of noncoronary cardiovascular disease, several premier interventionalists place in perspective the current status of devices for arrhythmia management, embolization of unwanted blood vessels, and application of vena caval filters for the prevention of pulmonary embolus. Dr. Sandborn reports his wide experience with vascular closure devices, reviewing the different mechanisms of femoral arterial closure with the immediate and long-term outcomes for these tools. Needless to say, most adult vascular closure devices would not suffice for children but have potential for use. These closure devices have been a great boon to the adult cardiologist concerned with complications of vascular access, especially retroperitoneal hematoma after intense anticoagulation during percutaneous coronary intervention (PCI).

Probably the most important new area in the next decade will be that of prosthetic valve implantation through a transcatheter approach. Drs. Pavčnik, Boudjemline, and Bonnhoeffer describe the percutaneous methods of implanting prosthetic valves in both the aortic and pulmonary positions. Dr. Rao briefly reviews several unique applications of device technology not included in the prior chapters—namely, percutaneous completion of Fontan, use of covered stents to treat aortic coarctation, device closure of aortopulmonary windows, devices to keep that atrial septal defect open, transcatheter management of pulmonary oligemia, and percutaneous closure of left atrial appendage to prevent strokes in patients with atrial fibrillation.

While it is clear that stents have risen as the mainstay of treatment of narrowed conduits in any location within the body, new devices continue to emerge. These devices well described herein are designed to solve problems that formerly could be addressed only by surgery. These devices will be the future of the field. It is important for all interventionalists in this area to observe, follow, and critique the changes in materials, methods, and results for implantation of new occluding devices and stents and valvular substitutes, in a fashion similar to that of surgery, the quality of procedures.

This volume on catheter-based noncoronary device interventions may lead to new ideas and the next developments in noncoronary catheter-based devices. Understanding the current data provides the basis from which improved care can be delivered to both adults and children needing these approaches.

Catheter Based Devices: For the Treatment of Non-coronary Cardiovascular Diseases in Adults and Children. Edited by P. Syamasundar Rao and Morton J. Kern, Lippincott Williams & Wilkins, Philadelphia © 2003.

SUBJECT INDEX

Note: Page numbers followed by f *indicate figures; those followed by* t *indicate tables.*

A

Accent catheters, 292
Accessory pulmonary vein draining to
    inferior vena cava, 211
Accunet filter, 423f
ACS-Multi Link Tetra stent, 317
Adult patients
    Amplatzer Duct Occluder for use in, 217
    Amplatzer muscular ventricular septal
        defect occluder for use in, 249
    Amplatzer Septal Occluder for use in, 58,
        89
    buttoned PDA occluder for use in,
        170–171
    CardioSEAL device for use in, 67–68
    CardioSEAL/STARFlex VSD occlusion
        in, 257
    coil embolotherapy with, 449–456
    Gianturco coils for use in, 182
    HELEX Septal Occluder for use in, 77
    postmyocardial infarction ventricular
        septal rupture in, 265–267, 268
    Rashkind's double-umbrella device for
        use in, 160
    right-to-left shunt ASD closure in, 126
    stent implantation in
        for branch pulmonary stenosis, 301
        for venous stenosis, 321, 322
Alagille syndrome, 297
Allergic reaction, 108
Ampicillin, 106
Amplatz Super Stiff guide wire, 292–293
Amplatzer Duct Occluder, 150–151, 223
    adult patients, 217
    advantages, 217–218
    complications, 217, 224
    current status, 218
    delivery and implantation, 214–216, 215f
    design, 213, 213t, 214f
    outcomes, 216–218, 216t
    patient selection, 213–214, 224
    for pulmonary arteriovenous fistula
        embolization, 459
Amplatzer muscular ventricular septal defect
        occluder
    adult patients, 249
    advantages, 245
    current status, 251
    delivery and implantation, 246–248,
        247f, 249f, 250f
    design, 245–246, 246f
    outcomes, 248–250

patient selection, 246
sizes, 246t
Amplatzer PFO Occluder, 115f, 131
Amplatzer Septal Occluder, 51–59, 87–88,
        87f, 119, 137f
    adult patients, 58
    applications, 51
    ASD closure under echocardiography,
        87–89, 87f, 88f, 89t
    complications, 55, 57–59, 93, 98
    current status, 59
    delivery and implantation, 51, 52–55,
        53f, 54f, 87–88, 87f, 88f
    design, 51, 52f
    distinguishing features, 51
    to maintain atrial fenestration, 517
    modifications, 521
    multiple, 137–140, 140f
    outcomes, 55–58, 56t, 57t, 89, 92t,
        125–126
    for patent foramen ovale closure, 51, 55,
        58, 521
    patient selection, 51, 58
    for right-to-left shunt ASD closure,
        125–126
Amputations, peripheral artery disease-related,
        380
Ancef, 22, 300
Ancure graft, 436
Anesthesia
    in Amplatzer Septal Occluder
        implantation, 52
    in ASDOS, 36
    in buttoned device implantation, 22
    in PFO-Star implantation, 106
    in ventricular septal defect occlusion, 241
AneuRx graft, 275, 436
Aneurysm formation
    aortic coarctation therapy outcomes, 306,
        311
    coil embolization therapy, 454
Aneurysm repair. *See* Aortic aneurysm
    repair, infrarenal
Angel Wings device, 45–49, 136f
    centering mechanism, 45
    complications, 47–48, 98
    delivery and implantation, 45, 46
    design, 45, 48f
    Guardian Angel version, 45, 48–49, 48f
    outcomes, 46–48, 49, 92t
    patient selection, 45–46, 47t
    prolapsed, 138f

for right-to-left shunt ASD closure, 126
Angiogenesis, 381
Angiography
    Amplatzer Septal Occluder implantation,
        53f
    Angel Wings device implantation, 46
    aortic coarctation, 306, 307
    aortoiliac angioplasty/stenting, 386f,
        387f, 388f, 389f
    aortopulmonary collateral vessel
        embolization, 462ff
    ASD closure, 133
    brachiocephalic, 412–413
    buttoned device implantation, 22
    buttoned PDA occluder implantation,
        166
    CardioSEAL/STARFlex implantation, 63,
        65, 254
    carotid artery stenting, 411, 412–413,
        418–419, 419f
    clamshell occluder implantation, 13
    coil embolization of blood vessels, 458
    Gianturco coils, 182f
    HELEX Septal Occluder placement, 73,
        74
    infrarenal aortic aneurysm stent
        implantation, 431, 432f
    mesenteric artery, 404–405
    Nit-Occlud coil system, 260
    over-the-wire, 293–294
    patent ductus arteriosus, 167f
    pulmonary arteriovenous fistula, 459,
        460f
    pulmonary stenosis assessment, 298
    Rashkind's double-umbrella device
        implantation, 157
    stent implantation for pulmonary
        stenosis, 300
    stenting of ductus arteriosus, 317, 318f
    superior vena cava stenting, 323,
        326–327ff
Angioguard filter, 423f
Angioplasty balloon
    catheters, 290–292
    laceration by stent, 285, 287
    See also Balloon angioplasty
AngioSeal, 493
Angiostent, 275
Anticoagulation therapy
    complications, 486
    contraindications, 486
    in stent implantation, 300